AF324842

The Pathogenesis and Treatment of
COVID-19 and Long COVID
with Traditional Chinese Medicine

The Pathogenesis and Treatment of COVID-19 and Long COVID with Traditional Chinese Medicine

PEILIN SUN

Belgium

Contributors:
Hongyan Zhu (UK)
Shulan Tang (UK)
Guanhu Yang (USA)
Liuzhong Ye (UK)
Tianjun Wang (UK)
Mark Kim Loong Tan (UK)

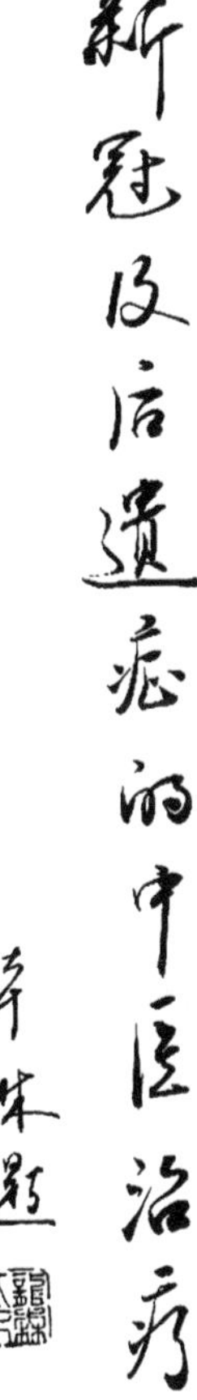

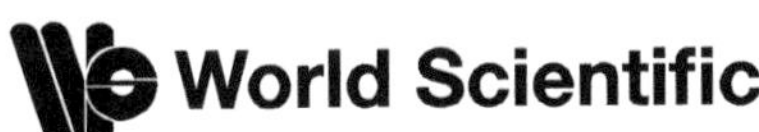

World Scientific

NEW JERSEY · LONDON · SINGAPORE · BEIJING · SHANGHAI · HONG KONG · TAIPEI · CHENNAI · TOKYO

Published by

World Scientific Publishing Europe Ltd.

57 Shelton Street, Covent Garden, London WC2H 9HE

Head office: 5 Toh Tuck Link, Singapore 596224

USA office: 27 Warren Street, Suite 401-402, Hackensack, NJ 07601

Library of Congress Cataloging-in-Publication Data
Names: Sun, Peilin, author.
Title: 880-01 The pathogenesis and treatment of COVID-19 and long COVID with
    traditional Chinese medicine = Xin guan ji hou yi zheng de Zhong yi zhi liao /
    Peilin Sun ; contributors, Hongyan Zhu [and 5 others].
Other titles: 880-02 Xin guan ji hou yi zheng de Zhong yi zhi liao
Description: Hackensack, New Jersey : World Scientific, [2023] |
    Includes bibliographical references.
Identifiers: LCCN 2022010504 | ISBN 9781800612532 (hardcover) |
    ISBN 9781800612549 (ebook for institutions) | ISBN 9781800612556 (ebook for individuals)
Subjects: MESH: COVID-19--therapy | Medicine, Chinese Traditional--methods |
    COVID-19--etiology | COVID-19--complications
Classification: LCC RA644.C67 | NLM WC 506.2 | DDC 616.2/414--dc23/eng/20220314
LC record available at https://lccn.loc.gov/2022010504

British Library Cataloguing-in-Publication Data
A catalogue record for this book is available from the British Library.

For any available supplementary material, please visit
https://www.worldscientific.com/worldscibooks/10.1142/Q0370#t=suppl

Desk Editors: Soundararajan Raghuraman/Shi Ying Koe

Typeset by Stallion Press
Email: enquiries@stallionpress.com

Foreword

It gives me great pleasure to introduce *The Pathogenesis and Treatment of COVID-19 and Long COVID with Traditional Chinese Medicine* by Peilin Sun. As a comprehensive text on this subject it is, to my knowledge, the first of its kind in the English language; given the extent of the suffering caused by the pandemic around the world, it is greatly welcome.

The author, Peilin Sun, has been a prolific contributor to the Chinese medicine profession for many years. He has shared his knowledge generously via the *Journal of Chinese Medicine* since the 1990s, and as editor I have been fortunate to work with him to bring his articles to publication. More recently, Professor Sun responded to the coronavirus pandemic with urgency and an admirable commitment to be of assistance to his colleagues around the world. He swiftly set about researching to understand the nature of the disease the world was faced with and how it might best be treated with traditional Chinese medicine, and has since shared his findings generously. Initially, this material was based on clinical reports from the frontline of care in China, and as the pandemic has progressed and he has built up a significant body of clinical experience in treating this disease, he has shared his valuable insights into the treatment of side-effects of the vaccines and how to intervene in the crucial convalescent phase of COVID-19 to prevent patients' lives being blighted by Long COVID.

Professor Sun's work is characterized by great clarity in clinical thinking and a broadness of perspective that encompasses both the extreme complexity of detail characteristic of Western biomedicine and the holistic, inter-relational approach of Chinese medicine. While he justifiably proudly points out that traditional Chinese medicine is currently one of the best options for the treatment of COVID-19, his astute integrative approach allows biomedicine and traditional Chinese medicine to shine on their own terms to provide the best possible care for patients.

The clinics of Chinese medicine practitioners around the world are filled with patients affected by COVID-19—whether survivors discharged from hospital, those with ongoing health problems due to Long COVID, those with unpleasant lingering side-effects following vaccination, or even those left with mental distress by the isolation of lockdown restrictions. Whether practitioners wish to get a general understanding of the nature of COVID-19 from the perspective of Chinese medicine, or want to successfully treat patients with active COVID-19 infection or specific COVID-related symptoms such as ongoing loss of smell and taste, this book will be invaluable. In fact, the Chinese medicine theory and treatment strategies presented here go far beyond just COVID-19 and could be used to understand and treat most types of infectious disease and their sequelae.

At the time of writing, two years into this pandemic, many of us are now looking toward living alongside COVID-19. Despite the awful cost of this disease around the world, it has reminded us of the huge value of traditional Chinese medicine for the treatment of infectious disease. I sincerely hope that this book helps to relieve human suffering caused by the coronavirus pandemic, and wholeheartedly recommend it to readers.

Daniel Maxwell
Editor, *The Journal of Chinese Medicine*
March 2022

Preface

For the continued reproduction and survival of mankind, infectious diseases are the demons human beings have fought ever since the beginning of human history. Numerous epidemics have occurred in the history of China. Fortunately, none of them have caused large scale mortality rate due to the efficacy of Traditional Chinese Medicine (TCM) in their treatment. TCM have always considered the etiologies of highly infectious and easily prevalent disease as "Yiqi (疫气)-pestilent qi", and named these diseases "Yi disease-plague". Until now, TCM has battled against a multitude of epidemic/pandemic events and has accumulated a valuable store of effective experiences and therapeutic methods. More recently, TCM also played a vital role in the fight against severe acute respiratory syndrome (SARS).

Coronavirus Disease 2019 (COVID-19) is a virulent infectious disease. It is considered a fast emerging, rapidly developing epidemic and is also a Public Health Emergency of International Concern (PHEIC), the highest level of alarm under international law. This sudden pandemic destroyed the peaceful and harmonic life of people around the world. Furthermore, it involved us in a war without the battlefield of military weapons, the smoke fire and the smell of armies in conflict-a war that is a greater threat to human lives and national security, a race against time, and a battle fighting a highly deadly enemy to save lives. Due to the strong contagion rate, varied incubation period, rapid spread, multiple routes of transmission, widespread susceptibility, and great destructiveness of the COVID-19 virus, there is no clear boundary and definite location for this epidemic prevention battle, highlighting and intensifying the severity of this war. Complexity and danger have also made the fighting of the epidemic a comprehensive, multi-level and multi-domain systematic project. At the beginning of the epidemic last year, governments of various countries adopted measures, such as curfews, lockdowns, and home quarantine, hoping to completely smash and control the virus, ultimately reaching zero COVID cases. One and a half years later, the current situation in Western countries proved that the COVID-19 vaccines are not 100% effective, and natural immunity of human beings can be only a firewall to fight the COVID virus. Moreover, the facts have confirmed that the Zero COVID policy cannot be maintained and followed all the time. Once countries start to reopen, this head-on confrontation with the virus will be faced once more. We believe that the stronger the immunity, the more ammunition for the battle, which means more power to resist the attack of the virus and protect human health.

Globally, there is a lot of knowledge about the virus but the knowledge of how to eradicate it or make it harmless is still in its infancy. There is no effective treatment plan for it at this stage. At the start of the outbreak last March, vaccine options were being tested, the human population had not received any vaccine, and there was little or no immunity against COVID-19. At the point of writing this book, vaccination rates in most developed countries has achieved a relative high level, although people still feel frustrated because of the phenomena, i.e., while observing the high efficacy of COVID-19 vaccines in the prevention of severe and critical cases, and new confirmed COVID-19 numbers increasing sharply over the past few weeks up to November 2021 even among those who have been fully vaccinated. This is because the natural immunity is still low to COVID-19. Even when fully vaccinated, people are still at risk of getting infected. Some new variants are emerging and among them, the Delta variant is highly infectious, and has spread all over the world. Many have found it difficult to keep up with new policies and changes to measures. "Zero COVID" by means of isolation, guarantee, and lockdown measures does not seem to be a realistic option anymore, because not every country can stay locked down and closed off indefinitely. Thus, almost all the countries over the world have accepted the strategy of "Living with COVID-19", encouraging people to take personal and social responsibilities properly.

To achieve the goal of "Living with COVID-19" successfully during the battle against this epidemic/pandemic event including Long COVID, TCM stresses the great importance of zheng-qi instead of passive home isolation or a symptomatic treatment. TCM health support and care is to offer a holistic approach and treat each case differently to speed up the recovery, prevent aggravation of illness, and diminish Long COVID complaints as much as possible. At the start of compiling this book, our aim was to introduce the valuable knowledge of TCM in managing Long COVID, but we quickly realized that the treatment of COVID-19 is unique. It shines a spotlight on the whole process of TCM treatment since TCM holds that the presence of Long COVID is the consequent result of COVID-19 when these patients are not properly managed in the acute phases. While we are proud to point out that TCM is currently one of the best options for COVID-19 treatment, cognizance must be made that vaccines are also a good option for the prevention and treatment to reduce mortality rate from the virus infection. TCM will play a more important role with COVID-19 and Long COVID, and TCM will be promoted more in countries around the world. Although not every TCM practitioner is able to treat a patient with acute COVID-19 infection face to face, they could take this book as a reference to review how TCM could manage all the different syndromes and to improve the use of TCM as a means to help.

During clinical practice and when saving patients with severe cases of COVID-19, I worked very closely with a few of my TCM colleagues, and Dr. Hongyan Zhu is among them. She has assisted me a lot during this important time to save the lives of our patients. I must say that without her consistency and persistence, it would be impossible for me to fulfill tasks in my clinic.

I am very grateful to the publisher who offered the opportunity to accept this book and publish it. I owe my deep thanks to all our team members who have spent so much time co-operating with me. Furthermore, Dr. Hongyan Zhu and her husband, Dr. Jinjun Xu, have provided a lot of assistance in editing my text and inserting the Latin names and acupuncture names in the book. Without their effort, this book will definitely be different.

I would like to extend my thanks to Mr. John Bergin (UK) and Dr. Huating Li (Germany), who spent much time reading our text and correcting grammatical errors. They have also given many good suggestions in English expressions. Meanwhile, I highly appreciate Mr. Benlin You (Australia) for his wonderful calligraphy of book title, and Mr. Shunchang Wang (France) for his wise suggestion for the book cover.

My special thanks also go to Mr. Soundararajan Raghuraman, Ms. Shi Ying Koe and Dr. Natalie K. Watson from the publishing house, for their patience, kindness and great assistance. Without their efforts and guidance, it could be impossible for this team to reach the point of publication.

I am also thankful for all the public websites. Through them I could surf, search, study and improve my knowledge. All English names of herbal formulas in this book are obtained from https://www.americandragon.com/.

COVID-19 will eventually become a minor virus, but the information included in this book should not cease to apply at that stage, as it is a guide to the treatment of all viruses and can become part of the future treatments in TCM as a whole.

Peilin Sun
December 2021, Belgium

About the Author

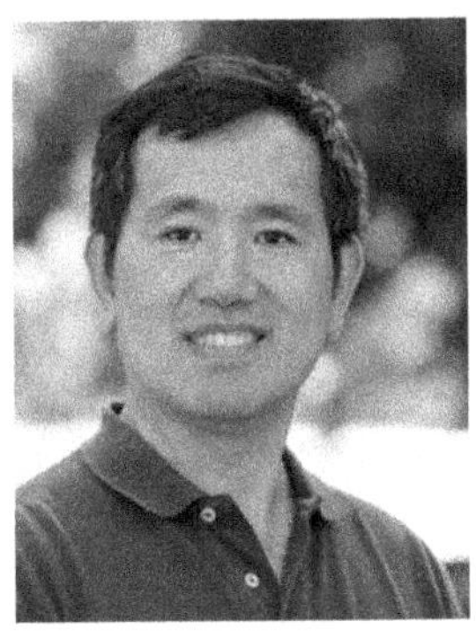

Peilin Sun has been in the field of TCM clinical practice and teaching for more than 40 years. He used to teach at the International Acupuncture Training Centre, Nanjing University of Traditional Chinese Medicine after receiving his master's degree in 1988. He moved to Belgium in 1990 and have been living there till now.

Currently, Professor Sun teaches at the Belgian School of Medicine (www.ICZO.be). He also has teaching responsibilities in other European countries, such as the Netherlands, Germany, France, Austria, Switzerland, Norway, Turkey, and Poland, as well as Canada, USA, and other countries. Meanwhile, he is a visiting professor at a few Traditional Chinese Medicine universities in China. Apart from that, he is also a tutor for the master's and PhD degree program at Nanjing University of TCM and Shulan College of Chinese Medicine, UK.

While working in China, Professor Sun published more than twenty articles. After moving to Belgium, he published more than 50 articles in different international medical journals. He also serves as editor for several international medical journals, and made a keynote lecture at the International Congress of Traditional Chinese Medicine.

Some of his published books include *Bi Syndrome or Rheumatic Diseases Treated by TCM, The Treatment of Pain with Chinese Herbs and Acupuncture, The Management of Postoperative Pain with Acupuncture, Sport Medicine in TCM, Traditionele Chinese Fytotherapie-Courrante Remedies* and *Der Altere Patient in der Chinesischen Medizin—Gesund alt Werden, Alterserkrankungen Vorbeugen und Behandeln.*

List of Contributors

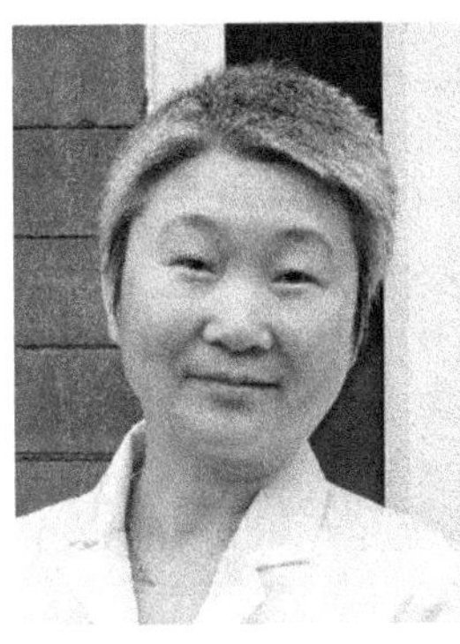

Hongyan Zhu started studying TCM since 1991 and received a bachelor's degree in clinical Traditional Chinese Medicine in 1996 from Anhui College of Traditional Chinese Medicine (now Anhui University of Traditional Chinese Medicine). She then became a resident doctor in Taihe County Hospital of Traditional Chinese Medicine, Anhui Province, Department of Cardiovascular and Cerebrovascular, and carried out clinical work in Chinese medicine. Eager to further her knowledge in the TCM field, she persevered in her studies and subsequently entered Nanjing university of TCM in 1997 and obtained a master's degree in Clinical Chinese Materia Medica in 2000. After that, she successfully published several articles in China.

After attaining her master's degree, she became a clinical adviser in both Chinese and Western medicine in Nanjing Chengong Pharmaceutical Co. Ltd. Then, she moved to the United Kingdom in 2007 and is now the owner and operator of an established TCM clinic. She also published several articles in the UK.

Her main clinical specializations include:

- Clinical acupuncture and Chinese medicine.
- Gynecological issues, respiratory diseases, pain management, and other areas, etc.

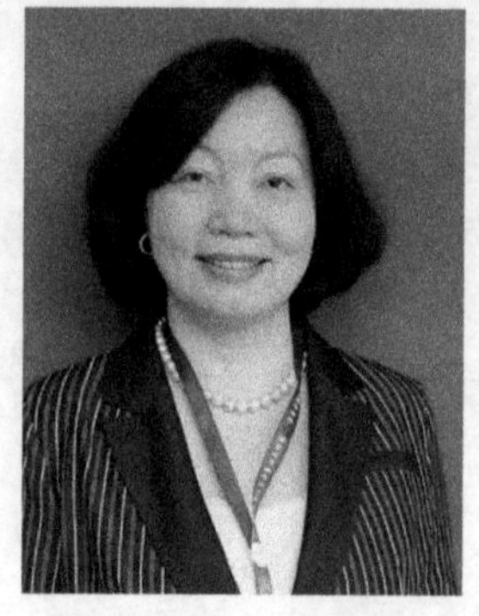

Shulan Tang studied at Nanjing University of Chinese Medicine from 1979 to 1984, where she obtained a bachelor's degree in Medicine. She then went on to further her studies at Beijing University of Chinese Medicine from 1984 to 1987 and gained a master's degree in Medicine. She then worked at South-East University Hospital from 1988 to 1991 as Physician in Charge.

Professor Tang came to Manchester UK in 1991. Since then, she has been practicing and teaching Chinese Medicine in Manchester, UK and across Europe. She is highly successful in treating gynecological and dermatological problems, including difficult and complicated internal diseases. Furthermore, she has a rich experience in teaching Science of Chinese Materia Medica, Science of Chinese Medicine Prescriptions, TCM gynecology, dermatology, Internal Medicine, and other fields. Professor Tang treats her patients from the heart and teaches students with passion. She is a well-respected doctor and professor.

Since the pandemic, she has written more than ten articles including "How to Prevent COVID-19 Using Chinese Medicine", "Treatment Methods of COVID-19 Using Chinese Medicine", and "Treating Long-COVID with Chinese Medicine". She has also conducted over 30 lectures and talks to both TCM professionals and the public about COVID-19 and TCM. Professor Tang has been continuously treating COVID-19 via video call consultation and has had great success using Chinese herbal medicine for Long COVID treatments.

Currently, Professor Tang is the principal of Shulan College of Chinese Medicine, PhD supervisor for Nanjing University of Chinese Medicine, a senior practitioner of the British Acupuncture Council, and the Register of Chinese herbal medicine. She has published over 60 academic articles and is the chief editor of *Chinese Herbal Patent Book*, vice chief editor of the core, international textbook of TCM Gynecology and one of the chief editors of *Understanding, Managing and Treating Female Infertility with Chinese Medicine*.

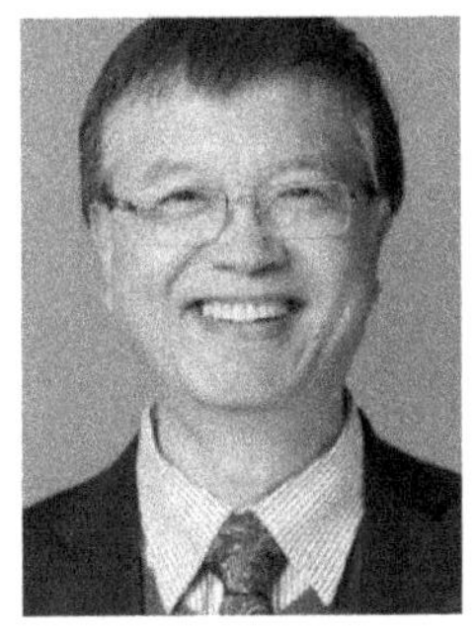

Guanhu Yang graduated from Zhejiang College of Traditional Chinese Medicine (MD) and Nanjing College of Traditional Chinese Medicine (MS), and served as Assistant Professor at Wenzhou Medical University. In 1993, Guanhu joined the staff of Toyama Medical and Pharmaceutical University in Japan, and from there he went to Kanazawa Medical University for his PhD study in lung repair. After completion of his PhD, Dr. Yang continued his research in pulmonary biology at Cincinnati Children's Hospital as a postdoc and then research scientist.

Dr. Yang has been running two acupuncture clinics in Ohio, USA. He is currently a Clinical Assistant Professor (honored/endowed) at Ohio University, and Chair Professor of the US-China Joint Institute for Acupuncture & Rehabilitation Medicine at Wenzhou Medical University. Dr. Yang also have served as director for the SHI acupuncture school, vice president at American TCM Association few years ago, and supervised the doctoral program at American Academy of Acupuncture & Oriental Medicine and other 10 medical university in the World. He is president of Chinese Medicine Luobing Society of American. During his career, Dr. Yang published 10 books and over 70 research articles on basic biology and traditional Chinese medicine, and work as editor and reviewer for numerous renowned *SCI journals*. Dr. Yang also is associate editor for *International Journal of Clinical Acupuncture*. He also is vice president of the World Federation of Chinese Medicine Digestion Committee and Endocrine Committee.

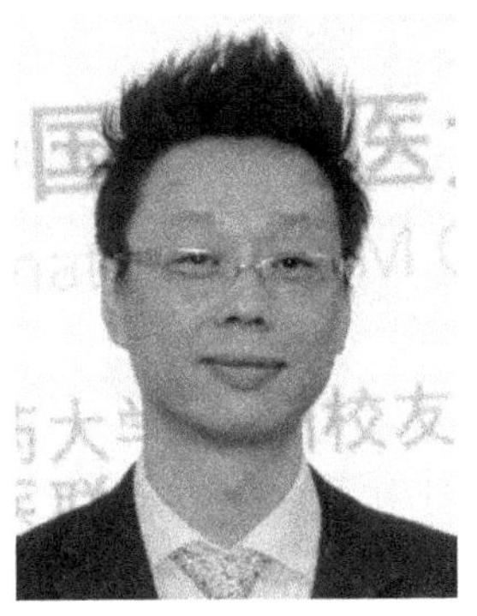

Liuzhong Ye, PhD and Master of TCM from Guangzhou University of TCM in 2003, started his TCM practice as senior consultant in the UK after graduating from Guangzhou. After establishing his own TCM practice in Norwich, Hado in 2008, he started his career as a senior lecturer and module leader of several TCM colleges across Europe, including CNM London, LACA London, Wroclaw

Academy of Acupuncture Poland, and Swiss TCM Academy. He is also appointed as supervisor professor of the Master and PhD scheme of TCM at Shulan College Manchester UK, in association with Nanjing University of TCM China. In addition, he serves as the director of Chinese Acupuncture and Herbal Medicine Alliance (CAHMA) and the General Secretary of British Institute of Scalp Acupuncture.

Professor Ye's specialty in meridian palpation differentiation enabled him to achieve great success in clinical practice and won him high reputation in acupuncture and TCM teaching across the world. He has organized numerous workshops and seminars in many countries on meridian palpation treatment.

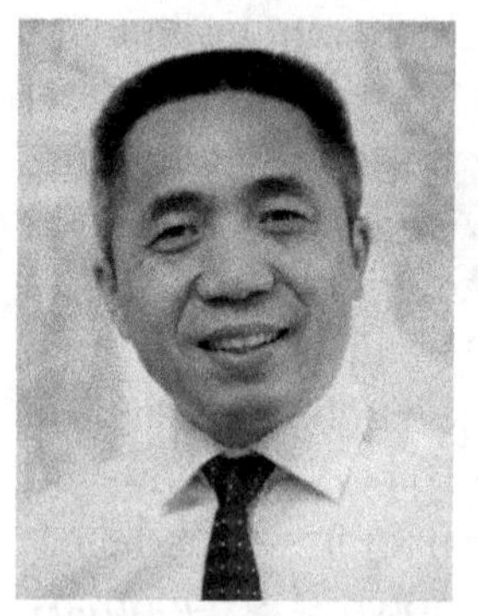

Tianjun Wang graduated from Nanjing University of Chinese Medicine (NJUCM) in 1989. He completed his PhD at NJUCM. Professor Wang moved to the UK and joined the University of East London UK as a Senior Lecturer and was the Director of Acupuncture Clinic from 2007 to 2014. He is a Guest Professor of NJUCM and the Master and PhD course supervisor at the UK Centre of NJUCM. Currently, Professor Wang is the principal of the London Academy of Chinese Acupuncture. He is also the vice president of the Scalp Acupuncture Committee of World Federation of Chinese Medicine Societies (WFCMS) and the President of the Institute of Scalp Acupuncture UK. He owns TJ Acupuncture Clinic and Brain Care Centre in London.

Professor Wang authored and co-authored more than 50 academic papers. He also peer reviewed articles in many international journals. His book *Acupuncture for Brain: Treatment for Neurological and Psychologic Disorders* was published by Springer in 2020.

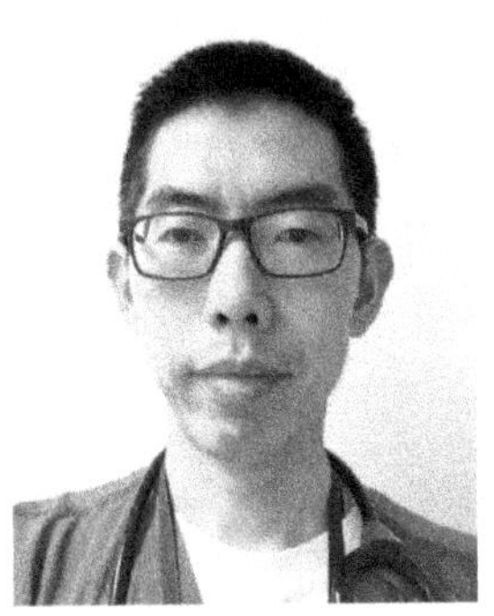

Mark Kim Loong Tan, BSc (Hons), PgD, MD, Dip Nutrition, ND, IVNT, LiAC, ISOM, has been engaged in Western medicine for the last 13 years. At the same time, he is also involved in Nutrition, Naturopathic Medicine, Acupuncture, Orthomolecular Medicine, Qigong, and ancient Tao wisdom from Master Dr. Sha to create Soul Mind Body Medicine and Tao Calligraphy to help humanity.

Currently, Dr. Tan works in the Accident and Emergency Department and his private clinic, applying the above techniques seven days a week to serve more patients. He is a survivor of COVID-19 and had symptoms that lasted for four days without Long COVID symptoms or complications.

On top of that, he is a member of the International Society of Orthomolecular Medicine, Longevitology Academy, Tao Academy, Tao Hands practitioner, Kuan Yin Lineage holder and Love Peace Harmony Foundation.

Contents

Foreword   v
Preface   vii
About the Author   xi
List of Contributors   xiii

1 General Procedures of Treatment of COVID-19   **1**

    1.1 Diagnosis of COVID-19   5
    1.2 Therapeutic Principles   16
    1.3 Selection and Analysis of Formulas and Herbs   23
    1.4 Selection and Combination of Acupuncture Points   35
    1.5 Precautions   43

2 TCM Treatment of Asymptomatic Infections of COVID-19   **47**

    2.1 TCM Analysis Asymptomatic Infections
         of COVID-19   48
    2.2 TCM Treatment   55

3 TCM Treatment of Early Symptoms of COVID-19   **89**

    3.1 TCM Analysis of Early Symptoms of COVID-19   89
    3.2 TCM Treatment   104

4 TCM Treatment of Ordinary Syndromes of COVID-19   **117**

    4.1 TCM Analysis of Ordinary Syndromes
         of COVID-19   117
    4.2 TCM Treatment   121

5 TCM Treatment of Severe Syndromes of COVID-19 **141**

   5.1 TCM Analysis of Severe Syndromes
      of COVID-19 141
   5.2 TCM Treatment 158

6 TCM Treatment of COVID-19 at Convalescent Stage **191**

   6.1 TCM Analysis of COVID-19 at Convalescent Stage 192
   6.2 TCM Treatment 209

7 TCM Treatment of Side Effects of COVID-19 Vaccines **227**

   7.1 TCM Analysis of Side Effects of COVID-19 Vaccines 230
   7.2 TCM Treatment 234

8 COVID-19 Case Study **243**

   8.1 Case 1 243
   8.2 Case 2 250
   8.3 Case 3 258
   8.4 Case 4 265
   8.5 Case 5 272

9 Generalization of Long COVID **279**

   9.1 Definition 283
   9.2 Timeline of Post-acute COVID-19 285
   9.3 Percentage of Post-acute COVID-19 Syndromes 287
   9.4 Symptoms 288
   9.5 Treatment in Modern Medicine 296
   9.6 General TCM Aspects of Post COVID-19
      Syndromes 298

**10 Meridian Palpation Treatment for COVID-19 and
Long COVID Conditions** **301**

   10.1 Method of the Meridian Palpation Differentiation 301
   10.2 Application of Meridian Palpation in
       COVID-19 Setting 302

10.3 Strategy of Meridian Selection and Point Decision   306
10.4 Understanding COVID-19 by Meridian Palpation   312
10.5 Case Study   324

11 TCM Treatment of Long COVID   **327**

11.1 Fatigue   327
11.2 Breathlessness   341
11.3 Joint Pain   354
11.4 Chest Pain   369
11.5 Headache   382
11.6 Myalgia   400
11.7 Cough   415
11.8 Loss of Smell and Taste   431
11.9 Sicca Syndrome   450
11.10 Rhinitis   460
11.11 Red Eyes   471
11.12 Sputum Production   482
11.13 Loss of Appetite   495
11.14 Sore Throat   506
11.15 Dizziness   519
11.16 Diarrhea   532
11.17 Psychological and Neuropsychiatric Disorders   549
11.18 Excessive Sweating   577
11.19 Sleep Disorders   592
11.20 Hearing Loss or Tinnitus   615
11.21 Brain Fog   632
11.22 Hair Loss   645

12 Long COVID Case Study   **659**

12.1 Case 1   659
12.2 Case 2   662
12.3 Case 3   665
12.4 Case 4   670
12.5 Case 5   673
12.6 Case 6   676

1

General Procedures of Treatment of COVID-19

At the end of 2019, a novel coronavirus was identified as the cause of a cluster of pneumonia cases. In February 2020, the World Health Organization (WHO) identified the disease COVID-19, which stands for coronavirus disease 2019. The virus that causes COVID-19 is severe acute respiratory syndrome coronavirus 2 (SARS-CoV-2), previously referred to as 2019-nCoV.

According to the Director-General's opening remarks at the COVID-19 media briefing on 19 April 2021, prior to this statement, new cases of COVID-19 increased for the eighth week in a row, with more than 5.2 million cases reported—the most in a single week so far. Deaths surged for the fifth week, with more than three million deaths reported to WHO.

Furthermore, it took nine months to reach a million deaths; four months to reach two million, and three months to reach three million. These numbers were traumatizing. Each case was a tragedy for families, communities and nations. Infections and hospitalizations among people aged 25 to 59 were increasing at an alarming rate, possibly as a result of highly transmissible variants and increased social mixing among younger adults.[1]

Infectious diseases are the demons that human beings have been fighting since the beginning of human history. Traditional Chinese

---

[1] World Health Organization (WHO). Director-General's opening remarks at the media briefing on COVID-19–19 April 2021. (Press Release) 19 April 2021. https://www.who.int/director-general/speeches/detail/director-generals-opening-remarks-at-the-media-briefing-on-covid-19-19-april-2021.

Medicine (TCM) practitioners have accumulated abundant experiences in the treatment of infectious diseases for thousands of years. Several epidemics occurred in the history of China, but fortunately, the number of casualties have always been kept greatly under control due to the prevalence of TCM during the epidemic period of severe acute respiratory syndrome (SARS), first identified at the end of February 2003. TCM played a vital role in fighting the epidemic and gained valuable experience. Nevertheless, it must be pointed out that in fighting against COVID-19, modern medicine has played an important role in the entire treatment process. For severe and critical patients, targeted oxygen therapy, symptomatic and anti-infective treatments were implemented.

The treatment from TCM is based on the patient's symptoms, signs, time of onset, geographic locations, individual conditions and differentiated by syndrome differentiation. Its aim is quite clear—to slow down and prevent the transformation from severe to critical cases, and promote the transition from severe to common, in order to control the mortality rate. In terms of geographic locations and personalized syndrome differentiation, here is a very good example. At the end of 2019, the epidemic in Wuhan was dominated by damp and toxins. Most of the patients at the early stage were mainly caused by cold-damp. However, for the patients from the same region in February and March 2020, the climate in Wuhan turned hot and humid, forming damp-heat. Thus, the treatment must change its direction and principles. When the Delta variant arrived in China, it occurred in the summer season in Guangdong and Jiangsu provinces. According to TCM, summer is characterized by heat and humidity with a tendency of damaging the qi and yin. In fact, all the clinical symptoms and signs are in line with the evolution of the pathogenesis of damp, heat and toxins. Thus, the treatment is changed to clear heat, reduce fever, resolve damp and eliminate toxins.

COVID-19 is associated with pestilential disease in TCM. Since the outbreak of coronavirus disease-2019 (COVID-19) in December 2019 and based on the climate changes, the features of diagnosis and treatment also changed with TCM. Seven versions of the Diagnosis and Treatment Program for Coronavirus Disease-2019 was issued by the Chinese government with TCM designated as a necessary medical strategy. This Diagnosis and Treatment Program has analyzed the understanding of the etiology, pathogenesis, syndrome differentiation, treatment methods and prescriptions of COVID-19 by TCM.

Clinically, there is no Western medication that has been proven effective in treating COVID-19 to date. Usually, symptomatic treatment or hospitalization is the only option available for severe or critical cases of COVID-19. However, TCM could be considered as a treatment option for patients with COVID-19, at least as a supplementary treatment and support next to the symptomatic management. TCM could also be applied to prevent deterioration of lung functions and some related complaints, such as myalgia, fatigue, loss of smell and taste, emotional disturbance, digestive disorders, physical weakness and neurological dysfunctions.

To examine the literature on TCM used in the treatment, prevention and supportive care in patients with COVID-19, some authors have launched a systematic and comprehensive search on articles published between 1 December 2019 and 1 April 2020. This search included both Chinese and English electronic databases, which includes China National Knowledge Infrastructure, Wanfang Data, CINAHL, Embase, Cochrane, PubMed, PsycINFO. etc. They qualitatively described and synthesized the published research and current clinical practice on the use of TCM for COVID-19 and focused on the following areas: TCM treatment used in SARS, MERS, H1N1; TCM treatment plan for COVID-19; TCM in prevention and treatment at the early stage of COVID-19; TCM emotional therapy; personalized TCM treatment plan. It was confirmed that the combination of Western medicine and TCM in treatment, and treatment based on the local condition, isolation, and personal protective measures are of great significance for the prevention and treatment of COVID-19. Relevant laboratory research and clinical evaluation should be continued to collect scientific evidence on the efficacy of TCM.[2]

---

[2]Xi Vivien Wu, *et al*. Traditional Chinese Medicine as a complementary therapy in combat with COVID-19—A review of evidence-based research and clinical practice. *Journal of Advanced Nursing*. 2021, 77: 1635–1644. https://doi.org/10.1111/jan.14673.

Since the sudden epidemic of coronavirus disease 2019 (COVID-19), the State Administration of Traditional Chinese Medicine in China immediately organized experts to formulate and screen the effective prescriptions of TCM according to the characteristics of the novel coronavirus infection. Qing Fei Pai Du Tang (QFPDT) has been proven to be effective in multi-provincial clinical trials and has been selected as a general prescription for the treatment of COVID-19 in different stages that was later promoted to be used nationwide.

Some authors published their research on Frontiers in Pharmacology on 27 January 2021, in which it highlights the latest advances of QFPDT, focusing on the TCM theory, mechanism analysis, clinical application of QFPDT, and its future perspectives. Moreover, an in-depth discussion of some valuable issues and possible development for future research on QFPDT was also discussed, aiming to provide a novel guide to combat the global epidemic COVID-19. The authors concluded that TCM strategies represented by QFPDT have shown apparent advantages in improving symptoms, promoting virus clearance and shortening hospitalization, as well as surprising efficacy of zero patients progressing from mild to severe cases in a TCM cabin hospital. Clinical data illustrated the effectiveness of TCM strategies proposed by the Chinese government. This major epidemic may bring new opportunities for TCM development. Some other clinical and scientific reports and reviews have also been published in top medical journals. All these reports and reviews could provide practical recommendations for the policy makers in the selection process of the treatment and preventive measures for the global pandemic COVID-19. Further relevant laboratory research and clinical evaluation should be continued to collect scientific evidence on the efficacy of TCM.[3]

---

[3]Wei Ren, *et al.* Research advance on Qingfei Paidu Decoction in prescription principle, mechanism analysis and clinical application. *Frontiers in Pharmacology.* 2021, 11: 589714. https://doi.org/10.3389/fphar.2020.589714.

Another review performed a classified analysis of the efficacy and advantages of TCM for the prevention and treatment of COVID-19 and summarized the mechanisms of TCM in treating COVID-19. The review shows that TCM is effective in preventing COVID-19 and medical staff can prevent an iatrogenic infection by taking a decoction made based on the principles of TCM. As of 13 March 2020, new cases of COVID-19 in China have decreased in number to single digits. TCM's curative effect was outstanding, with a national participation rate of over 90%. More than 70,000 people were cured of COVID-19 and discharged from the hospital. Only approximately 10,000 patients are currently being treated and the total treatment time is about two months. The conclusion is made that TCM is currently the best choice for the treatment and prevention of COVID-19 and it is expected that it will be promoted by countries around the world.[4]

1.1 Diagnosis of COVID-19

1.1.1 In modern medicine

Diagnosis of COVID-19 in modern medicine could be obtained or confirmed by the following procedures.

1.1.1.1 *According to the contact and traveling history*

People who reside in or has traveled within 14 days to a location where there is community transmission of severe acute respiratory syndrome coronavirus 2 (SARS-CoV-2), i.e., large numbers of cases that cannot be linked to specific transmission chains, should be extra careful. This includes people who residence in congregate settings or have association with events where clusters of cases have been reported, as it is a particularly high risk for exposure. Anyone who

---

[4]Zhenyu Zhao, *et al.* Prevention and treatment of COVID-19 using Traditional Chinese Medicine: A review. *Phytomedicine.* 2021, 85: 153308. doi: 10.1016/j. phymed.2020.153308.

had close contact with a confirmed or suspected case of COVID-19 in the prior 14 days, including through work in health care settings should take preventive measures.

1.1.1.2 *According to the clinical symptoms and signs*

Clinical suspicion, including symptomatic patients, lead to a new coronavirus (SARS-CoV-2) outbreak in more than 200 countries, causing viral pneumonia that was extremely infectious and pathogenic. A current meta-analysis also showed that the main clinical symptoms of COVID-19 patients are fever (88.5%), cough (68.6%), myalgia or fatigue (35.8%), expectoration (28.2%) and dyspnea (21.9%). Minor symptoms include headache or dizziness (12.1%), diarrhea (4.8%) and nausea and vomiting (3.9%).[5] The possibility of COVID-19 should be considered primarily in those with new-onset fever or respiratory tract symptoms (e.g., cough and dyspnea). It should also be considered in patients with severe lower respiratory tract illness without any clear cause. Other consistent symptoms include smell or taste disturbances, myalgias, diarrhea, etc.

1.1.1.3 *According to some laboratory tests*

The most accurate way of establishing a diagnosis in modern medicine is to obtain laboratory tests.

When assessing the above symptoms of COVID-19, fever, cough, myalgia, fatigue, or dyspnea (albeit can resemble many other diseases, e.g., influenza, common cold, upper respiratory infection, etc.), diagnostic tests are essential to identify people who have COVID-19. In addition to this, these tests can also help determine who has recovered from COVID-19, as well as track how the virus spreads and monitor the effectiveness of control measures.

Some tests for the virus itself, looking for the RNA (the genetic blueprint) of the SARS-CoV-2 virus that causes COVID-19, should be implemented. As the coronavirus that causes the COVID-19 disease

---

[5] *Ibid.*

spreads across the world, real-time reverse transcription-polymerase chain reaction (real-time RT–PCR), one of the fastest and most accurate laboratory methods for detecting, tracking and studying the COVID-19 virus, has been introduced. Real-time RT–PCR is one of the most widely used laboratory methods for detecting the COVID-19 virus as the detection result is extremely reliable. However, these tests cannot determine whether someone has recovered from the virus, and can potentially miss the virus if it is present in extremely low levels in a patient's body.

Other tests such as looking for antibodies to the virus, i.e., the evidence that the body has produced an immune response to it, are very important as a follow-up measure. It takes time for such antibodies to be created, so antibody tests are not much use in confirming if someone has COVID-19 in the first few days of infection. However, in contrast to the RNA tests, they can be extremely useful in determining whether someone has previously been infected with the new coronavirus, but no longer has the virus present. One factor to note is that different people can have different antibody responses to COVID-19. For instance, an individual with severe disease could develop higher antibody levels than an individual with mild or asymptomatic disease. As a result, a test for antibodies developed using blood samples from individuals with severe COVID-19 may not work as well in detecting antibodies in patients with a mild or asymptomatic version of the disease, where there are far fewer antibodies to detect.

1.1.1.4 *According to some imagine technology*

Some authors carried out one retrospective study, in which data were collected from 131 patients with confirmed coronavirus disease 2019 (COVID-19) from three Chinese hospitals. Their common clinical manifestations, as well as characteristics and evolvement features of chest CT images, were analyzed.[6] A total of 100 (76%) patients

---

[6]Xiaoming Li, *et al.* CT imaging changes of corona virus disease 2019 (COVID-19): A multi-center study in Southwest China. *Journal of Translational Medicine.* 2020, 18: 154. https://doi.org/10.1186/s12967-020-02324-w.

had a history of close contact with people living in an infectious city. The clinical manifestations of COVID-19 included cough and fever. Most of the lesions identified in chest CT images were multiple lesions of bilateral lungs, which were more localized in the peripheral lung. 109 (83%) patients had more than two lobes involved, 20 (15%) patients presented with patchy ground-glass opacities and consolidation of lesions co-existed in 61 (47%) cases. Complications such as pleural thickening, hydrothorax, pericardial effusion, and enlarged mediastinal lymph nodes were detected but only in rare cases. For the follow-up chest CT examinations (91 cases), they found that 66(73%) cases changed very quickly, with an average of 3.5 days. 25(27%) cases presented absorbed lesions, progression was observed in 41(46%) cases, 25(27%) cases showed no significant changes. The conclusion is that chest CT play an important role in diagnosing COVID-19. The imaging pattern of multifocal peripheral ground-glass or mixed consolidation is highly suspicious of COVID-19, which can quickly change over a short period of time.

1.1.2 In TCM

Diagnosis of COVID-19 in TCM could be obtained or confirmed by the following procedures.

Since there is no term for "virus" in TCM, the diagnosis of COVID-19 in TCM is completely different from those in modern medicine. Common symptoms and signs of COVID-19 include:

- fever
- dry cough
- fatigue
- shortness of breath or breathing difficulties
- loss of smell or taste
- muscle pain or headache
- joint pain
- chest pain
- depression or anxiety
- memory, concentration, or sleep problems

- dizziness
- worsened symptoms after physical or mental activities

The data showed that although patients with COVID-19 had a fever, mainly in the early stage of disease, the fever was not high and had the characteristic of "heat not rising". In addition, patients have symptoms such as cough, fatigue, loss of smell and taste, diarrhea and a thickly coated tongue, which are consistent with the characteristics of invasion of external pathogenic factors, such as wind-damp, cold-damp, or damp-heat to the body in TCM. However, it could be impossible to establish a concrete diagnosis by judging upon the above symptoms and signs.

TCM recognizes the human body by system discrimination and cybernetic ways. TCM is characterized as holistic with emphasis on the integrity of the human body, the close relationship between humans and their social and natural environment. TCM focuses on dynamic health balance and maintenance among all zang-fu organs, different tissues and important energetic substances. Besides, TCM applies multiple natural therapeutic methods in the treatment, enhancing the body's resistance to the disease. To achieve a good and efficient therapeutic result, an accurate diagnosis is of extreme importance. In fact, TCM diagnosis of COVID-19 is usually done based upon the following procedures.

1.1.2.1 *Diagnosis according to the etiology*

TCM etiology diagnosis is a branch of procedure concerned with causes that specifically alter the state of relative balance in the body that lead to disease.

In modern medicine, it attempts to isolate purely physical factors as the cause of diseases, such as bacteria and viruses, chemical compounds and other external factors that are responsible for most illnesses. In terms of COVID-19, the SARS-CoV-2 virus is found to be the main cause. Since it is a virus, its treatment is limited, especially when mutation occurs. In the absence of specific drugs, supportive treatment remains the primary treatment for COVID-19.

TCM, however, attributes the cause of most diseases to external cosmological invasion, based upon dysfunction of the internal body, including dietary disorder, emotional factors, personal constitutions, chronic sickness and even various applied treatments. These factors confirm and act according to the principles of yin and yang and the five elements, which stress balance and interconnectedness. TCM gathers all the clinical symptoms and signs, history and all related situations before a conclusion is made to find out what the main etiology is. Treatment is given not to eliminate the symptoms and signs, but the root causes.

1.1.2.2 *Diagnosis according to the pathology*

The purpose of diagnosis according to the pathology is to search diligently for the disease mechanism and treat it accordingly. TCM treatment is fulfilled based on the pathologic diagnosis.

Diagnostic pathology identifies the cause of disease based on morphological, clinical pathology findings, history, and clinical signs, as well as some ancillary test results. It is important in all areas of pathology, including spontaneous and experimentally induced disease.

The struggle disrupts the normal balance between the yin and yang, the qi and blood, and this disturbance in turn affects the physiological activities of all the organ and tissue systems of the body. Moreover, in some cases, the ascent and descent of organ qi become irregular. In other cases, the actions of visceral qi and blood become ineffective, stagnant, or accumulate some excess, etc. In all cases, a variety of abnormal changes ensue, whether in the entire body or in a localized region.

1.1.2.3 *Diagnosis according to the eight principles*

The process of diagnosis is to evaluate and determine the eight patterns of disease with their basic nature, locations, qualities and the tendency of development. The eight principles consist of four pairs of mutual opposites, including yin and yang, interior and exterior, heat and cold, deficiency and excess.

- The pair of yin and yang is the most general classification for pattern diagnosis and description of the relationship between the other three pairs of the principles.
- The pair of interior and exterior differentiation is not made based on etiology of disease but location, which could give an indication of the direction the illness is becoming—more external or migrating deeper into the body.
- The pair of cold and heat describes the nature of a pattern and clinical manifestations.
- The pair of deficiency and excess is made according to the presence or absence of a pathogenic factor and the strength of the body's energetic substances.

1.1.2.4 *Diagnosis according to the organ system*

The body consists of 12 main organs, and they must work together harmoniously to ensure the physical, energetic, emotional and mental balance. Furthermore, each organ is associated with one of the five elements and has its own channel, which contains the points used in acupuncture treatment.

When there is an invasion of external pathogenic factors, different zang-fu organs could be affected, leading to dysfunction or injury. Among these organs, the lung is mainly impaired, resulting in either disorder of the lung in dispersing or descending the qi. Moreover, the spleen and stomach could also be affected, bringing about nausea, vomiting, diarrhea, tiredness, etc. Without the differentiation of the zang-fu organ, it would be impossible to start the treatment properly without distinguishing the organ mainly involved.

1.1.2.5 *Diagnosis according to the six channels, four stages, and San Jiao systems*

Since COVID-19 is mainly caused by invasion of external pathogenic factors, these three methods of differentiation and diagnosis are extremely essential. They are not contradictory but rather supplement each other and can be used jointly to differentiate febrile diseases.

Nevertheless, the theories of the six channels, four stages of wei, qi, ying and xue, and San Jiao systems are methods of differentiating syndromes of febrile diseases caused by external pathogenic factors.

Differentiation of syndromes according to the six channels originally appeared in the Traditional Chinese Medicine classic called the *Shang Han Lun*, written by Zhang Zhongjing in the late Han Dynasty, circa 20–200 A.D. According to the differentiation based upon six channels, various clinical manifestations of febrile disease caused by external pathogenic factors could be classified into Taiyang syndromes, Yangming syndromes, Shaoyang syndromes, Taiyin syndromes, Shaoyin syndromes, and Jueyin syndromes. Thus, to explain the location, the nature of pathological changes, strength and weakness of anti-pathogenic and pathogenic qi and the tendency of disease development, acts as a guide for clinical treatment. This method of differentiation is often used for febrile diseases caused by pathogenic cold.

Differentiation of four stages (wei, qi, ying and xue stages) is applied to classify the clinical manifestations of febrile diseases caused by pathogenic heat—to explain the location and severity of pathological changes, which form the basis of clinical treatment. The system of San Jiao differentiation is mainly formed during the Ming and Qing Dynasties, summarizing clinical manifestations of epidemic febrile diseases caused by damp-heat involving three areas: the upper, middle, and lower portions of the body, to guide clinical treatment.

1.1.2.6 *Diagnosis according to the constitution, climate, and geographic locations*

Young and healthy people can feel unwell for weeks to months after infection, although most people who have coronavirus disease 2019 (COVID-19) recover completely within a few weeks. But COVID-19 symptoms in some people with mild cases of the disease may sometimes persist for months and may cause damage to the lungs, heart, kidney or brain, leading to the risk of long-term health complications.

These patients could often suffer from some constitutional weakness and sickness. Older individuals and those with complex comorbidities are susceptible to COVID-19. All the above situations imply that the personal constitutions of the patients play important roles for COVID-19.

Nonetheless, TCM always pays attention to the correlation between the disease and constitution, climate and geographic locations, considering that their conditions could greatly influence the occurrence and deterioration of the sickness. COVID-19, which is a contagious disease and belongs to the "plague" in the field of TCM, should be no exception in this context. SARS-CoV-2 can be transmitted through various bio-aerosols, large droplets, or direct contact with secretions similar to the influenza virus.[7,8] Virus transmission can be influenced by several geographical factors such as climatic conditions (temperature and humidity) and population density (PD).[9] It was observed that the outbreak is more severe in the countries located in the mid-latitudes where the temperature is considerably low in contrast to the tropical countries. Many researchers from different parts of the world tried to establish a relationship between COVID-19 transmission and various meteorological factors.[10–12]

---

[7]Yuguo Li, *et al*. Role of air distribution in SARS transmission during the largest nosocomial outbreak in Hong Kong. Wiley online library. *Indoor Air*. 2004, 15(2): 83–95. https://doi.org/10.1111/j.1600-0668.2004.00317.x.

[8]Hongchao Qi, *et al*. COVID-19 transmission in Mainland China is associated with temperature and humidity: A time-series analysis. *Science of the Total Environment*. 2020, 728: 138778. https://doi.org/10.1016/j.scitotenv.2020.138778.

[9]Benjamin D. Dalziel, *et al*. Urbanization and humidity shape the intensity of influenza epidemics in U.S. cities. *Science*. 2018, 362(6410): 75–79. doi: 10.1126/science.aat6030.

[10]Muhammad Farhan Bashir, *et al*. Correlation between climate indicators and COVID-19 pandemic in New York, USA. *Science of the Total Environment*. 2020, 728: 138835. https://doi.org/10.1016/j.scitotenv.2020.138835.

[11]David N. Prata, *et al*. Temperature significantly changes COVID-19 transmission in (sub)tropical cities of Brazil. *Science of the Total Environment*. 2020, 729: 138862. https://doi.org/10.1016/j.scitotenv.2020.138862.

[12]Peng Shi, *et al*. Impact of temperature on the dynamics of the COVID-19 outbreak in China. *Science of the Total Environment*. 2020, 728: 138890. https://doi.org/10.1016/j.scitotenv.2020.138890.

In a study conducted in New York, USA, using Kendall and Spearman rank correlation test, it was found that mean temperature, minimum temperature and air quality had a significant association with the COVID-19 pandemic.[13] Moreover, Shi *et al.* reported[14] a significant correlation between daily temperature and daily count of COVID-19 cases in China, and suggested that a temperature above 8–10°C would lead to the reduction of infected cases. Prata *et al.* concluded that a rise in 1°C temperature would result in a decrease in the number of daily confirmed COVID-19 cases in Brazil.[15]

One study, aimed to understand the geographical influence on the spatial distribution of COVID-19 transmission at the regional level in the context of India, was carried out. It is observed in several statistical analyzes that climatic factors have an unavoidable influence on this viral disease in India. The heterogeneity in the spatial occurrence of infections might be attributed to local meteorology with its geographical location and population. However, no single attribute can explain the nature of transmission well. Positive association with solar radiation and temperature, as well as negative association with humidity and rainfall suggests that hot and arid areas in low altitude regions are required to strictly follow-up preventive measures on an emergency basis.[16]

1.1.2.7 *Diagnosis according to the tongue conditions*

Diagnosis based on pulse and tongue conditions is a unique technique in TCM, which is combined during the whole procedure of syndrome differentiation and treatment. However, since COVID-19 is an infectious disease, it is impossible for most of the practitioners of TCM to consult the patients face to face. Thanks to modern

---

[13] Muhammad Farhan Bashir, *et al. op. cit.*

[14] Peng Shi, *et al. op. cit.*

[15] David N. Prata, *et al. op. cit.*

[16] Amitesh Gupta, *et al.* Significance of geographical factors to the COVID-19 outbreak in India. *Modeling Earth Systems and Environment.* 2020, 6: 2645–2653. https://doi.org/10.1007/s40808-020-00838.

technology development, advanced telemedicine is now well-designed and possible in this case, including WeChat, Zoom meetings, Google meetings, and WhatsApp, etc. Besides inquiring about all-important information about the patients, observation of the tongue is at present extremely essential.

The tongue, a component of the inspection method within the four methods of diagnosis in TCM, is a method of diagnosing disease and disease patterns by visual inspection of the tongue and its various features. Tongue diagnosis in COVID-19 is crucial to clinical diagnosis, treatment and prognosis. The tongue provides important clues not only reflecting the conditions of the internal organs, but also predict the conditions of external invasion, indicating the progression or alleviation of the sickness. Tongue diagnosis is based on the "outer reflects the inner" principle, which means external structures reflect the conditions of the internal structures. Besides, by observing the various regions of the tongue, we can identify the organs or tissues affected by COVID-19.

The aspects of the tongue considered in diagnosis in COVID-19 include:

- tongue characteristics
- body color
- body shape
- tongue coating
- tongue moisture

The tongue characteristics include its movement, bristles, cracks and teeth marks.

The tongue is connected to the viscera through meridians, connecting with the zang-fu organ, qi, blood, yin, and yang, as well as the disease degree and disease progression. Tongue diagnosis reveals the conditions of organs, nature of diseases and changes in pathogens. For instance, thick or thin coating during COVID-19 is usually linked to the damp-phlegm. When the thick coating turns into a thin coating after treatment, it implies the disease is improving, otherwise, it is deteriorating and indicates that the treatment is not sufficient. Further, the color of the tongue is also extremely important. A combination of tongue coating and color could reveal the real conditions of the sickness. For instance, when there is a red tongue with a yellow and greasy coating, it indicates invasion of damp-heat, while a thick, white and greasy coating with a pale tongue, usually implies invasion of cold-damp.

Moreover, when the patient's tongue turns dark and purplish, it indicates the reduction of blood circulation and the blood flow rate. Thus, it may result in hypoxia, leading to the occurrence of dyspnea and pressure over the chest, etc. Since tongue diagnosis is mainly conducted by the practitioners with visual observation and description language, personal experience and knowledge play an essential role during tongue diagnosis. Besides, environmental factors also significantly affect the results of tongue diagnosis. A close and careful tongue observation should be performed. Nevertheless, as COVID-19 is a challenging case, diagnosis and treatment is also extremely difficult and important. Thus, tongue diagnosis should be done at least once or twice a day. In crucial situations, it should be done once every four to five hours, to analyze various tongue images to ensure that herbal treatment is adequate and sufficient. Meanwhile, PCR tests need to be conducted several times to obtain a precise diagnosis and follow up their reaction to the treatment.

1.2 Therapeutic Principles

As the world's most comprehensive and deeply researched system of alternative and complementary medicine, TCM provides various kinds of holistic therapies. The body is not only considered as a physical entity but also as a concept with different energetic substances and emotional changes. All these components could be the heuristic models facilitating diagnosis and principles of treatment.

Coronavirus disease 2019 (COVID-19) is a novel, human-infecting β-coronavirus enveloped, positive-sense single-stranded RNA virus, like the severe acute respiratory syndrome (SARS) infection that emerged in November 2002.[17] Once TCM diagnosis of COVID-19 is established based on etiology, pathology, constitutions, geographic and cultural aspects, etc., therapeutic principles should be formed accordingly. Although therapeutic principles vary at different stages of COVID-19 infection, such as asymptomatic, early, ordinary, severe, critical and convalescence, etc., we should focus on one important issue—eliminating the pathogenic factors, restoring normal lung function, ameliorating pulmonary, vascular injury and improving the functioning of the zang-fu organ.

Depending on the etiology, pathology, clinical symptoms and some other important situations, different therapeutic principles should be applied to offer the most appropriate treatment. They could be applied individually or in combination. Here are some main principles.

1.2.1 To dispel wind and eliminate cold

This principle is used to treat general external symptoms in the early stage of COVID-19 due to an invasion of wind-cold. Manifestations are: aversion to cold, slight fever, chills, cough, sore throat or dryness, anosmia, ageusia, myalgia, arthralgia, headache, abdominal pain, thin and white tongue coating, and a superficial and tight pulse.

1.2.2 To disperse wind and clear heat

This principle is used to treat general external symptoms in the early stage of COVID-19 due to invasion of wind-heat. Symptoms are: slight fever, aversion to cold, anosmia, ageusia, non-productive cough, sore throat with redness and burning sensation, body pain or joint pain, headache, slight thirst, thin and yellow tongue coating, red tongue, and a superficial and rapid pulse.

---

[17] Sheng-Teng Huang, *et al.* Principles and treatment strategies for the use of Chinese herbal medicine in patients at different stages of coronavirus infection. *American Journal of Cancer Research.* 2020, 10(7): 2010–2031. eCollection 2020.

1.2.3 To dispel wind and eliminate cold-damp

This principle is used to treat general external symptoms or digestive complaints as their chief symptoms in the early stage of COVID-19 due to an invasion of wind and cold-damp. The manifestations are: aversion to cold, slight fever, cough, anosmia, ageusia, nausea, diarrhea, poor appetite, myalgia, arthralgia, headache with a heavy feeling, a thin, white, greasy tongue coating, and a tight, superficial and slippery pulse.

1.2.4 To dispel wind and clear damp-heat

This principle is applied to treat general external symptoms or digestive complaints as their chief symptoms in the early stage of COVID-19 due to invasion of wind and damp-heat. Expressed as fever, cough, loss of taste and smell, nausea, diarrhea, poor appetite, slight thirst with no desire to drink, painful joints and muscles with heaviness, red tip of the tongue, thin, yellow, and greasy tongue coating, and a superficial, rapid and slippery pulse.

1.2.5 To disperse the lung-qi and relieve cough

This principle is one of the chief therapeutic principles used to treat cough, anosmia and ageusia as their main clinical symptoms in the early stage of COVID-19 due to dysfunction of the lung in dispersing the qi, resulting from invasion of external pathogenic factors, such as wind-heat, wind-cold, cold-damp or damp-heat. Manifested with non-productive cough, anosmia, ageusia, sore throat, aversion to cold, slight fever, headache, poor appetite, myalgia, arthralgia, thin tongue coating and a superficial pulse.

1.2.6 To descend the lung-qi and relieve shortness of breath

This main therapeutic principle during the entire procedure of treatment for COVID-19, is used to treat cough, dyspnea and chest tightness as their main clinical symptoms in clinical, severe, or even in the critical stage of COVID-19. This is due to the failure of the lung in descending the qi, resulting from deterioration of the situations from various kinds of causative factors. The main clinical manifestations are severe cough, dyspnea or even asthma, chest tightness, excitation of profuse foamy or diluted phlegm, edema, scanty urination, greasy tongue coating and a slippery pulse.

1.2.7 To eliminate phlegm and resolve damp

There could be an invasion of wind in combination with damp, cold or heat, either creating cold-damp or damp-heat. Moreover, since the lung is the upper source of water, there could be the formation of damp or water in various parts of the body, mainly in the lung, when there is dysfunction of the lung in dispersing or descending the lung-qi. Nevertheless, any excessive fluid in the lung is again a pathogenic factor, leading to aggravation of the lung's situation.

In the very early stage of COVID-19, there is usually a non-productive cough, which is an indication that there is not much damp in the lung, or the damp is somewhere else outside the lung. In this case, there is no need to use certain herbs to eliminate phlegm in the lung. However, attention should be paid to search if there is damp in the spleen or stomach or at the superficial layer of the body, because one of the chief pathogenic factors of COVID-19 is damp.

Furthermore, when there is a damp invasion at the superficial layer of the body, some herbs should be applied to expel sweat and external pathogenic factors. When the damp impairs the physiological functions of the spleen and stomach in transportation and transformation, there could be nausea, vomiting and diarrhea. This principle of treatment should focus on harmonizing the middle Jiao and resolving the damp. Of course, invasion of damp could also occur in different zang-fu organs, such as the gallbladder, five sense organs (ear and nose, etc.) and brain, resulting in various kinds of clinical manifestations. The same principle of treatment should be combined to deal with complaints.

1.2.8 To clear heat and reduce fever

This principle is applied to treat COVID-19 at the ordinary stage or severe stage with high fever, productive cough with yellow phlegm, chest pain, shortness of breath, insomnia, restlessness, profuse sweat, myalgia, slight constipation, headache, thirst, red tongue, yellow coating on the tongue, and a forceful and rapid pulse. These manifestations are the indication of penetration of heat into the Yangming system with the formation of channel syndrome.

1.2.9 To clear heat and purge the defecation

This principle is applied to treat COVID-19 at the severe or critical stage due to accumulation of excessive heat in the Yangming fu organs, leading to high fever, cough with yellow phlegm, chest pain, dyspnea, insomnia, restlessness, thirst, severe constipation for a few days, abdominal pain with distension, headache, red tongue, yellow and dry tongue coating, and a deep, wiry and rapid pulse.

1.2.10 To clear heat and remove toxins

This principle is applied to treat COVID-19 at an early or ordinary stage due to invasion of toxic heat. It happens often in combination with the accumulation of excessive heat in the body. The manifestations are high fever, sore throat with inflammation, or redness, hotness, swelling, and pain of the eyes or face, burning sensation on skin, restlessness, insomnia, headache, thirst, constipation, red tongue with yellow coating, and a superficial, forceful, and rapid pulse.

1.2.11 To cool the blood and remove toxins

This principle is applied to treat COVID-19 at the ordinary stage or severe stage due to invasion of toxic heat into the blood, causing various kinds of bleeding, such as on the skin, teeth, nose, urine or stool. One instance is Kawasaki disease, also called mucocutaneous lymph node syndrome. The clinical manifestations vary according to different phases; the symptoms and signs of the first phase may include: high fever, irritability, extreme red eyes without a thick discharge, body or genital rash, dry, red cracked lips, and extremely red, swollen, and red skin on the palms of the hands and the soles of the feet, swollen lymph nodes in the neck and perhaps elsewhere, red and swollen tongue, and a wiry and rapid pulse. In the second phase of the disease, the situation could be much worse. TCM care in combination with modern medicine should be applied immediately.

1.2.12 To clear heat in the liver and regulate the gallbladder

This principle is used to deal with COVID-19 at the ordinary stage or severe stage due to invasion of damp-heat to the liver and gallbladder, manifesting as fever, headache, jaundice, hypochondriac pain and distention, nausea, epigastric pain, poor appetite, heaviness of the body, tiredness, red tongue, yellow with greasy coating, slippery and wiry pulse.

1.2.13 To eliminate blood stasis and resolve phlegm

This principle is used to treat COVID-19 at the severe or critical stage, sometimes in the convalescent stage due to stagnation of blood with an accumulation of phlegm. Thrombotic events that frequently occur in COVID-19 are predominantly venous thromboemboli (VTE) and are associated with increasing disease severity and worse clinical outcomes. Distinctive microvascular abnormalities in COVID-19 include endothelial inflammation, disruption of intercellular junctions and microthrombi formation. A distinct COVID-19-associated coagulopathy along with increased cytokines and activation of platelets, endothelium, and complement occurs in COVID-19, which is more frequent with worsening disease severity.[18]

---

[18]Joan Loo, *et al.* COVID-19, immunothrombosis and venous thromboembolism: Biological mechanisms. *Thorax.* 2021, 76(4): 412–420. http://dx.doi.org/10.1136/thoraxjnl-2020-216243.

When there is a stubborn pain in the chest or somewhere else in the body, palpitations, pressure over the chest, difficult breathing, restlessness, purplish color of the tongue, greasy tongue coating, etc., it is necessary to consider applying this principle of treatment.

1.2.14 To warm the body and tonify yang

This principle is applied to treat COVID-19 at the severe or critical stage due to declining of the yang of the heart and kidney, manifesting as shallow and shortness of breathing, very low oxygen saturation in the blood with difficulty in rising, cold hands and feet, weakness, semiconsciousness, restlessness, low voice, pale tongue, thin and wet tongue coating, and a deep, thready, and weak pulse.

1.2.15 To tonify qi and blood

This principle of treatment is applied to treat COVID-19 at the convalescent stage due to deficiency of qi and blood, showing extreme tiredness, weakness, pale complexion, hair loss, poor appetite, poor memory, aversion to cold, thin and white tongue coating, and a thready and weak pulse. Attention should be paid to see if there is still some existence of pathogenic factors, such as damp, phlegm, blood stagnation, heat, etc. If these pathogenic factors are still present, methods should be used to eliminate them first before applying the treatment to tonify the qi and blood.

1.2.16 To warm the interior and eliminate cold

This principle is used to treat COVID-19 at the convalescent stage due to deficiency of qi and yang with the formation of interior cold, manifesting as an aversion to cold, tiredness, cold hands and feet, pale complexion, diarrhea, nocturia, lower back pain, pale tongue, thin and white tongue coating, and a deep, thready, and slow pulse.

1.2.17 Nourish yin and clear deficient heat

This principle of treatment is applied to COVID-19 at the convalescent stage due to deficiency of yin in the lung, heart, liver, and kidney.

Since the liver stores blood and the kidney stores essence, the blood and essence can be mutually nourished, which means that the liver and kidney are derived from the same source (Gan Shen Tong Yuan). Deficiency of yin of the liver and kidney shows the following manifestations: dry cough, tiredness, hair loss, weakness, lower back pain, headache, poor memory, hot flush, night sweat, slight thirst, dry eyes, throat, and stools, red tongue, thin or peeled tongue coating, and a thready and weak pulse. Depending on the specific involvement of the organs, some other symptoms and signs could be observed at the same time. For instance, if there is mainly deficiency of lung-yin, there could be dry nose and throat, dry cough, slight chest pain. For deficiency of heart-yin, there could be more obvious palpitations, insomnia, extrasystole, slight chest pain or discomfort, etc. For deficiency of yin of the liver and kidney, there could be a more obvious headache, dizziness, poor concentration, tinnitus, poor vision, nervousness, easily frightened, frustration, etc.

1.3 Selection and Analysis of Formulas and Herbs

According to reports,[19] as of 1 March 2021, there have been more than 2,700 clinical trials for COVID-19 in the world, evaluating the efficacy of various drugs such as antiviral, immunosuppressant and hormones. However, only the Oxford University study confirmed that the use of corticosteroids could reduce the mortality of oxygen patients. In addition, no treatment has been found to improve the prognosis.

---

[19]Lihua Zhang, *et al.* Association between use of Qingfei Paidu Tang and mortality in hospitalized patients with COVID-19: A national retrospective registry study. *Phytomedicine.* 2021, 85: 153531. doi: 10.1016/j.phymed.2021.153531.

Traditional Chinese medicine and other forms of herbal medicine have been suggested as treatments for COVID-19 patients. The findings of several systematic reviews are summarized and some of them have been published in top-rank journals, including *The Lancet* and *Phytomedicine*, etc. Different researchers have found that herbal and traditional Chinese medicine (alone or in combination with Western medicine) may improve patient outcomes for COVID-19 patients and the effects on mortality for COVID-19 patients. For instance, *Qing Fei Pai Du Tang* (QFPDD), a formula of traditional Chinese medicine, which was suggested to be able to ease symptoms in patients with Coronavirus Disease 2019 (COVID-19), has been recommended by clinical guidelines and is widely used to treat COVID-19 in China. Moreover, the Fuwai Hospital, CAMS & PUMC, China, analyzed the medical records of nearly 10,000 cases in Hubei Province and pointed out in a study published recently that this herbal formula reduced in-hospital mortality rate by 50% for patients with COVID.

The results of the 8,939 patients are below (with 28.7% receiving QFPDD). The crude mortality was 1.2% (95% confidence interval [CI] 0.8% to 1.7%) among the patients receiving QFPDD and 4.8% (95% CI 4.3% to 5.3%) among those not receiving QFPDD. After adjustment for patient characteristics and concomitant treatments, QFPDD use was associated with a relative reduction of 50% in in-hospital mortality (hazard ratio, 0.50; 95% CI, 0.37 to 0.66 $p < 0.001$). This association was consistent across subgroups by sex and age. Meanwhile, the incidence of acute liver injury (8.9% [95% CI, 7.8% to 10.1%] vs. 9.9% [95% CI, 9.2% to 10.7%]; odds ratio, 0.96 [95% CI, 0.81% to 1.14%], $p = 0.658$) and acute kidney injury (1.6% [95% CI, 1.2% to 2.2%] vs. 3.0% [95% CI, 2.6% to 3.5%]; odds ratio, 0.85 [95% CI, 0.62 to 1.17], $p = 0.318$) was comparable between patients receiving QFPDD and those not receiving QFPDD. The major study limitations included that the study was an observational study based on real-world data rather than a randomized control trial, and that the quality of data could be affected by the accuracy and completeness of medical records. In conclusion, QFPDD was associated with a substantially lower risk of in-hospital mortality, without extra risk of acute liver injury or acute kidney injury among patients hospitalized with COVID-19.[20] The research results were published on the internationally renowned medRxiv platform on 27 December 2020 and published in *Phytomedicine* on 31 March 2021.

The rule of selection of formulas and herbs for treatment of COVID-19 at different stages is that selection of the herbal formulas and individual herbs should be done according to differentiation. The following formulas and herbs should be selected.

1.3.1 The formula to cause sweating and relieve the external symptoms

When COVID-19 is in its asymptomatic or initiative stage due to invasion of external pathogenic factors such as wind, cold, heat, damp or toxins, the chief principles of treatment are to promote sweating, in order to dispel the pathogenic factors and relieve the external symptoms.

Herbal Treatment for the Invasion of
Wind-cold:
Jing Fang Bai Du San—*Schizonepeta and Saposhnikovia Powder to Overcome Pathogenic Influences.*

Jing Jie *Herba seu Flos Schizonepetae Tenuifoliae* 10 g
Fang Feng *Radix Ledebouriellae Divaricatae* 10 g
Zi Su Ye *Folium Perillae Frutescentis* 10 g
Cong Bai *Bulbus Allii Fistulosi* 10 g

Herbal Treatment for the Invasion of
Wind-heat:
Sang Ju Yin—*Mulberry Leaf and Chrysanthemum Decoction.*

Sang Ye *Folium Mori Albae* 10 g
Ju Hua *Flos Chrysanthemi Morifolii* 10 g

---

[20] *Ibid.*

Bo He *Herba Menthae Haplocalycis* 5 g
Niu Bang Zi *Fructus Arctii Lappae* 10 g

1.3.2 The formula to promote sweating and eliminate cold-damp

When there is an invasion of cold-damp, the patients with COVID-19 could mainly suffer from muscle pain or joint pain, headache with heaviness, etc. The method should be applied to dispel external cold-damp and relieve the external symptoms.

Herbal Treatment:
Qiang Huo Sheng Shi Tang—*Notopterygium Decoction to Overcome Dampness.*

Qiang Huo *Rhizoma et Radix Notopterygii* 10 g
Du Huo *Radix Angelicae Pubescentis* 10 g
Gao Ben *Rhizoma et Radix Ligustici* 10 g
Cang Zhu *Rhizoma Atractylodis* 10 g
Chuan Xiong *Radix Ligustici Wallichii* 10 g

1.3.3 The formula to eliminate cold-damp and harmonize spleen and stomach

Some patients with COVID-19 could suffer mainly from invasion of cold-damp to the spleen and stomach, manifesting as nausea, vomiting, abdominal pain and distention, loose stools or diarrhea, poor appetite, myalgia and heaviness, headache, and a thin, white, and greasy tongue coating, etc.

Herbal Treatment:
Huo Xiang Zheng Qi San—*Agastache Powder to Rectify the Qi.*

Huo Xiang *Herba Agastaches seu Pogostemi* 10 g
Pei Lan *Herba Eupatorii Fortunei* 10 g
Guan Zhong *Radix Potentillae* 10 g

Hou Po *Cortex Magnoliae Officinalis* 10 g
Cang Zhu *Rhizoma Atractylodis* 10 g
Sha Ren *Fructus Amomi* 3 g

1.3.4 The formula to disperse the lung-qi and relieve cough

One symptom of patients with COVID-19 is dysfunction of the lung and not being able to disperse the lung-qi due to invasion of the lung by external pathogenic factors, either by wind-cold or wind-heat, manifesting as cough, stuffy nose, anosmia, ageusia, sore throat or itching and thin tongue coating.

Herbal Treatment for the Invasion of Wind-heat:
Sang Ju Yin—*Mulberry Leaf and Chrysanthemum Decoction.*

Xing Ren *Semen Pruni Armeniacae* 10 g
Huang Qin *Radix Scutellariae Baicalensis* 10 g
Jie Geng *Radix Platycodi Grandiflori* 10 g
Pi Pa Ye *Folium Eriobotryae Japonicae* 5 g

Herbal Treatment for the Invasion of Wind-cold:
Zhi Sou San—*Stop Coughing Powder.*

Zi Wan *Radix Asteris Tatarici* 10 g
Bai Bu *Radix Stemonae* 10 g
Chen Pi *Pericarpium Citri Reticulatae* 5 g
Zi Su Zi *Fructus Perillae Frutescentis* 10 g

1.3.5 The formula to clear heat and descend the lung-qi

When there is an accumulation of excess heat in the lung, resulting in failure of the lung in descending its qi, there would be fever, severe cough, dyspnea, pressure over the chest, even asthma, expectoration of some yellow phlegm, red tongue, yellow and dry tongue coating, etc.

Herbal Treatment:

Ma Xing Gan Shi Tang—*Ephedra, Apricot Kernel, Gypsum and Licorice Decoction.*

Ma Huang *Herba Ephedrae* 10 g
Xing Ren *Semen Pruni Armeniacae* 10 g
Shi Gao *Gypsum Fibrosum* 20 g
Zhi Mu *Radix Anemarrhenae Asphodeloidis* 10 g
Zhi Zi *Fructus Gardeniae Jasminoidis* 10 g
Huang Qin *Radix Scutellariae Baicalensis* 10 g

1.3.6 The formula to descend the lung-qi and eliminate cold-phlegm

If the lung is impaired by the invasion of external pathogenic factors with an accumulation of cold-phlegm in the lung, leading to dysfunction of the lung in descending the qi, there could be a severe cough, shortness of breath, pressure over the chest, even asthma, expectoration of profuse white, thin, and mucous phlegm, pale tongue, white and greasy tongue coating, etc.

Herbal Treatment:
Xiao Qing Long Tang—*Minor Blue Green Dragon Decoction.*

Ma Huang *Herba Ephedrae* 10 g
Xing Ren *Semen Pruni Armeniacae* 10 g
Xi Xin *Herba cum Radice Asari* 3 g
Gan Jiang *Rhizoma Zingiberis Officinalis* 6 g
Zhi Ban Xia *Rhizoma Pinelliae Ternatae Preparata* 10 g

1.3.7 The formula to clear heat and eliminate damp

When the invasion of damp-heat to the body occurs, it may attack different zang-fu organs and tissues, causing disturbance and blockage of these affected areas. Accordingly, different herbal formulas should be applied in compliance with syndrome differentiation. For instance:

- When it attacks the wei system in the body, it may bring about aversion to cold, slight sweating with difficulty in lowering down the fever, fever, slight cough, headache and body pain with heavy sensation, red tip of the tongue, and a superficial and rapid pulse.
- While the invasion of damp-heat to the middle Jiao could cause fever, aversion to cold, slight cough, nausea, poor appetite, vomiting, stomach pain or abdominal pain, loose stool, heaviness of the body, red tongue, yellow and greasy tongue coating, and a superficial and slippery pulse.
- If there is an invasion of damp-heat to the lower burner, it could cause frequent and painful urination, fever, aversion to cold, lower back pain, red tongue, yellow and greasy coating on the tongue, and a slippery and rapid pulse.
- When there is an invasion of damp-heat to the liver and gallbladder, it could cause aversion to cold, fever, jaundice, tiredness, nausea, epigastric pain and distention, poor appetite, hypochondriac pain and distention, red tongue, yellow and greasy coating on the tongue, and a wiry, slippery, and rapid pulse.

Herbal Treatment:
Lian Po Yin—*Coptis and Magnolia Bark Drink*
or
San Ren Tang—*Three Seed (Nut) Decoction.*

Huang Lian *Rhizoma Coptidis* 5 g
Huang Qin *Radix Scutellariae Baicalensis* 10 g
Zhi Zi *Fructus Gardeniae Jasminoidis* 10 g
Yin Chen Hao *Herba Artemisiae Capillaris* 10 g
Bai Dou Kou *Fructus Amomi Cardamomi* 3 g
Yi Yi Ren *Semen Coicis Lachryma-Jobi* 15 g
Tong Cao *Medulla Tetrapanacis Papyriferi* 5 g
Hua Shi *Talcum* 20 g

Also, certain herbs to resolve damp-heat in different organs should be used in combination.

1.3.8 The formula to clear heat and eliminate phlegm

When COVID-19 is caused by an impaired lung via the accumulation of phlegm-heat, leading to dysfunction of the lung in dispersing and descending the qi, there could be fever, severe cough, shortness of breath, pressure over the chest, even asthma, expectoration of profuse yellow and sticky phlegm, red tongue, yellow and greasy coating on the tongue, etc.

Herbal Treatment:
Qing Qi Hua Tan Tang—*Clear the Qi and Transform Phlegm Decoction.*

Zhe Bei Mu *Bulbus Fritillariae Thunbergii* 10 g
Xing Ren *Semen Pruni Armeniacae* 10 g
Huang Qin *Radix Scutellariae Baicalensis* 10 g
Zhi Zi *Fructus Gardeniae Jasminoidis* 10 g
Kun Bu *Thallus Laminariae seu Eckloniae* 10 g
Hou Po *Cortex Magnoliae Officinalis* 10 g

1.3.9 The formula to clear heat and remove toxins

If there is an invasion of toxic heat, it could manifest as fever, swelling of the face or throat, formation of blisters on the lips or in the mouth, restlessness, insomnia, red tongue, yellow coating on the tongue, etc.

Herbal Treatment:
Yin Qiao San—*Honeysuckle and Forsythia Powder.*

Jin Yin Hua *Flos Lonicerae Japonicae* 12 g
Lian Qiao *Fructus Forsythiae Suspensae* 10 g
Pu Gong Ying *Herba Taraxaci Mongolici cum Radice* 15 g
Da Qing Ye *Folium Isatidis* 10 g
Zhi Zi *Fructus Gardeniae Jasminoidis* 10 g

1.3.10 The formula to cool the blood and remove toxins

If there is invasion of toxic heat to the blood, it may manifest as fever, formation of skin rashes with itching, redness of the skin, restlessness, insomnia, red tongue, thin and yellow tongue coating, etc.

Herbal Treatment:
Qing Ying Tang—*Clear the Nutritive Level Decoction.*

Sheng Di Huang *Radix Rehmanniae Glutinosae Recens* 15 g
Mu Dan Pi *Cortex Moutan Radicis* 10 g
Xuan Shen *Radix Scrophulariae Ningpoensis* 10 g
Chi Shao Yao *Radix Paeoniae Rubrae* 10 g

1.3.11 The formula to clear heat and promote the defecation

When there is accumulation of excessive heat in the Yangming fu organs, the usual clearing method is not sufficient to reduce heat and fever. This is because the heat is already mixed with feces in the body, which obstructed the large intestines with blockage of the qi circulation. The only correct way of managing this situation is to promote defecation and reduce fever as soon as possible. High fever, constipation for a couple of days, abdominal pain and distention, etc. should be presented to confirm this diagnosis.

Herbal Treatment:
Tiao Wei Cheng Qi Tang—*Regulate the Stomach and Order the Qi Decoction*
or
Da Cheng Qi Tang—*Major Order the Qi Decoction.*

Da Huang *Radix et Rhizoma Rhei* 10 g
Mang Xiao *Mirabilitum* 10 g
Hou Po *Cortex Magnoliae Officinalis* 10 g
Zhi Shi *Fructus Immaturus Citri Aurantii* 10 g
Zhi Mu *Radix Anemarrhenae Asphodeloidis* 10 g

1.3.12 The formula to eliminate blood stasis and resolve phlegm

When there is formation of blood stagnation with an accumulation of phlegm, it could cause some serious, life-threatening illness. One of these situations is an aggravation of the cardiovascular disease, or cancer during COVID-19. In most cases, it could cause sudden oxygen desaturation, stabbing chest pain, dyspnea, palpitations, purplish tongue, white or yellow and greasy tongue coating, etc.

The current experience that can be used for reference is that patients with severe acute respiratory syndrome (SARS) still have a certain degree of post-inflammatory pulmonary fibrosis and loss of lung function a year after discharge. Thus, it is necessary to take precautions and interventions as soon as possible for post-inflammatory pulmonary fibrosis in patients who have recovered from new coronary pneumonia. One report pointed out that as of the submission date (6:00 pm on 15 March 2020), 67,023 patients across the country in China have been cured. *Fang Cang* hospitals have wind up operations. These patients who have been discharged from the hospital are currently under follow-up. Pulmonary fibrosis after inflammation in varying degrees and pulmonary fibrosis after inflammation is particularly significant in severely ill patients. Therefore, the rehabilitation of discharged patients require extra attention by medical workers.[21] One of the managements in TCM is to apply some blood circulation herbs and phlegm resolving herbs to open the blood collaterals.

Herbal Treatment:
Dan Shen Yin—*Salvia Drink*
or
Tao Hong Si Wu Tang—*Four Substance (Things) Decoction with Safflower and Peach Pit.*

---

[21]Xi Zhan, *et al.* Postinflammatory pulmonary fibrosis of COVID-19: The current status and perspective.*Chinese Journal of Tuberculosis and Respiratory Diseases* (中华结核和呼吸杂志). 2020, 43(9): 728–732. doi: 10.3760/cma.j.cn112147-20200317-00359.

Hong Hua *Flos Carthami Tinctorii* 10 g
Tao Ren *Semen Pruni Persicae* 10 g
Dan Shen *Radix Salviae Miltiorrhizae* 10 g
Yu Jin *Tuber Curcumae* 10 g
Pu Huang *Pollen Typhae* 10 g

1.3.13 The formula to warm the body and tonify yang

When COVID-19 hits old and weak patients with comorbidities, it could cause severe consequences or even death. One of the signs is the decline of the yang of the heart and kidney. Urgent TCM measures should be taken in combination with modern medicine to rescue the patients.

Herbal Treatment:
Si Ni Tang—*Frigid Extremities Decoction.*

Zhi Fu Zi *Radix Lateralis Aconiti Carmichaeli Praeparata* 10 g
Gan Jiang *Rhizoma Zingiberis Officinalis* 10 g
Gui Zhi *Ramulus Cinnamomi Cassiae* 10 g
Zhi Gan Cao *Radix Glycyrrhizae Preparata* 5 g

1.3.14 The formula to tonify qi and blood

When COVID-19 is at the convalescent stage, it is possible that there is still the existence of some pathogenic factors or some deficiency of vital substances, such as qi and blood, yin, and yang. If these pathogenic factors are eliminated, then methods could be applied to tonify the deficiency.

Deficiency of qi and blood could be dealt with by some tonics. However, the selection of these herbs should be determined by identifying the affection of different zang-fu organs. For instance, in terms of qi deficiency, the lung, heart, spleen, and kidney could be involved, while in terms of blood deficiency, the heart, liver, and kidney, etc. could be affected.

Herbal Treatment:
Si Jun Zi Tang—*Four Gentlemen Decoction.*

Ren Shen *Radix Ginseng* 10 g
Zhi Huang Qi *Radix Astragali Membranacei Praeparata* 10 g
Shan Yao *Radix Dioscoreae Oppositae* 10 g
Dang Gui *Radix Angelicae Sinensis* 10 g
Shu Di Huang *Radix Rhemanniae Glutinosae Praeparata* 15 g
Zhi Gan Cao *Radix Glycyrrhizae Preparata* 5 g

1.3.15 To warm the interior and eliminate cold

When deficiency of qi reaches a certain degree, it could cause deficiency of yang, affecting different zang-fu organs, and leading to the formation of deficient colds. In that case, only tonification of qi is not able to solve yang deficiency and relieve the interior cold. Thus, some herbs to tonify the qi and yang should be applied simultaneously.

Herbal Treatment:
Shi Quan Da Bu Tang—*All-Inclusive Great Tonifying Decoction*
or
Li Zhong Tang—*Decoction (Pill) to Regulate the Middle.*

Ren Shen *Radix Ginseng* 10 g
Zhi Huang Qi *Radix Astragali Membranacei Praeparata* 10 g
Shan Yao *Radix Dioscoreae Oppositae* 10 g
Gan Jiang *Rhizoma Zingiberis Officinalis* 5 g
Rou Gui *Cortex Cinnamomi Cassiae* 3 g
Zhi Fu Zi *Radix Lateralis Aconiti Carmichaeli Praeparata* 6 g

1.3.16 Nourish yin and clear deficient heat

One of the characteristics of COVID-19 is fever, which could exist through the whole process of disease. When it enters the convalescent stage, it could cause a deficiency of qi and yin. Either tonification of qi or tonification of yin should not sufficiently solve this problem. Treatment of a combination of tonifying qi and yin at the same time could be a proper solution. Again, different zang-fu organs could be involved, which needs clear clinical differentiation and management. Too early application of yin tonic could cause obstruction of damp or phlegm in the body.

Herbal Treatment:
Sha Shen Mai Men Dong Tang—*Glehnia and Ophiopogonis Decoction.*

Wu Wei Zi *Fructus Schisandrae Chinensis* 10 g
Tai Zi Shen *Pseudostellariae Radix* 10 g
Xi Yang Shen *Radix Panacis Quinque Folii* 10 g
Bei Sha Shen *Radix Glehniae Littoralis* 10 g
Nan Sha Shen *Radix Adenophorae* 10 g
Yu Zhu *Rhizoma Polygonati Odorati* 10 g
Tian Hua Fen *Radix Trichosanthis Kirilowii* 12 g

1.4 Selection and Combination of Acupuncture Points

Currently, there are many studies on the application of TCM in COVID-19, such as the clinical outcome, pathogenesis and underlying mechanism of TCM application on COVID-19. The general conclusion is: Besides the effective treatment with Chinese herbs for COVID-19 that is of great significance, acupuncture could help make up for the deficiency of the current treatment of COVID-19, which is worth studying. Summarization of the available evidence of the treatment of COVID-19 with acupuncture and evaluation of the efficacy of these treatments have been done. These findings may help clinicians, health professionals, policy-making authorities and organizations make relevant decisions about the treatment of patients with COVID-19 for further study in the future.

Person-to-person transmission directly through respiratory droplets during sneezing or coughing or indirectly through contaminated surfaces[22] causes severe acute respiratory syndrome coronavirus 2 (SARS-CoV-2) to be highly contagious.

The clinical manifestations of COVID-19 vary greatly—from asymptomatic or mild symptoms to the common symptoms at the ordinary stage or even to severe acute respiratory distress syndrome—which may eventually lead to significant respiratory impairment among many other multi-organ dysfunctions.

Acupuncture is one of the main and important components of TCM and has been widely used in the practice for a few thousand years. One of its indications is inflammatory and infectious diseases. As an important method of treatment now, acupuncture plays an indispensable role in the treatment of respiratory diseases in China. Therefore, during the coronavirus disease 2019 (COVID-19) pandemic, acupuncture has been used as a complementary treatment for COVID-19 in China as well as abroad.

Since the outbreak of COVID-19, many publications have proven that acupuncture could be effective in the treatment of this infectious disease. There is one case involving a previously healthy anesthesiologist and medical acupuncturist working in the COVID intensive care unit in New York City, who contracted and was diagnosed with the COVID-19 virus. She subsequently developed self-diagnosed acute symptomatic COVID pneumonia, including symptoms of pleuritic chest pain, hypoxia with shortness of breath, increased respiratory rate, dry cough, orthostatic hypotension and headache. She self-treated with cupping therapy at the onset of symptoms and medical acupuncture at the onset of pulmonary symptoms, leading to her full recovery. The author concludes that acupuncture should be considered as a viable adjunct in supportive care for patients with symptomatic COVID-19 pneumonia.[23]

---

[22]Carlos del Rio, *et al.* COVID-19–New insights on a rapidly changing epidemic. *JAMA.* 2020, 323(14): 1339–1340. doi: 10.1001/jama.2020.3072.

[23]Stephanie I. Cheng. Medical acupuncture as a treatment for novel COVID-19-related respiratory distress: Personal experience from a frontline anesthesiologist. *Medical Acupuncture.* 2021, 33(1): 83–85. http://doi.org/10.1089/acu.2020.1467.

Some scientists have also exerted their efforts to explore the underlying mechanism of acupuncture treatment of COVID-19. Based on bioinformatics/topology, one research paper systematically revealed the multi-target mechanisms of acupuncture therapy for COVID-19 through text mining, bioinformatics, network topology, etc. Two active compounds produced after acupuncture and 180 protein targets were identified. A total of 522 Gene Ontology terms related to acupuncture for COVID-19 were identified, and 61 pathways were screened based on the Kyoto Encyclopedia of Genes and Genomes. The findings suggested that acupuncture treatment of COVID-19 helped to suppress inflammatory stress, improved immunity, and regulated nervous system function, including activation of neuroactive ligand–receptor interaction, calcium signaling pathway, cancer pathway, viral carcinogenesis, *Staphylococcus aureus* infection, etc. The study also found that acupuncture may have additional benefits for COVID-19 patients with cancer, cardiovascular disease and obesity. The study revealed for the first time the multiple synergistic mechanisms of acupuncture on COVID-19. Acupuncture may play an active role in the treatment of COVID-19 and deserve further promotion and application. These results may help to solve this pressing problem currently faced by the world.[24]

In order to determine the efficacy and safety of acupuncture in COVID-19 and provide a high-quality synthesis of current evidence for researchers in this subject area to evaluate whether acupuncture is an effective treatment for patients suffering from COVID-19, one study was carried out to search the following sources for the Randomized Controlled Trials (RCT): The Cochrane Library, PubMed, EMBASE, Web of Science, Chinese Biomedical Literature Database (CBM), Chinese National Knowledge Infrastructure Database (CNKI), Chinese Science and the Wanfang Database. All the above databases have been searched from the available date of inception until the latest issue. No language or publication restriction will be used. Primary

---

[24]Zhenzhen Han, *et al.* Is acupuncture effective in the treatment of COVID-19 related symptoms? Based on bioinformatics/network topology strategy. *Brief Bioinform.* 2021, 22(5). https://doi.org/10.1093/bib/bbab110.

outcomes include chest CT and nucleic acid detection of respiratory samples.[25]

The findings are as follows:

Acupuncture, the main component of TCM, has been widely adopted to treat respiratory diseases in clinical practice and its efficacy has been assessed by a number of randomized controlled trials (RTCs). Acupuncture may play a role in the prevention, treatment, and rehabilitation of the COVID-19, and relieve the symptoms caused by COVID-19. Acupuncture has been demonstrated to effectively relieve common symptoms in the supportive and palliative care, including anxiety disorders, nausea, insomnia, leukopenia, fatigue as well as vomiting, which might also effectively treat abdominal pain and abdominal distension. Coyle *et al.* proposed that acupuncture is an effective therapeutic approach for chronic obstructive pulmonary disease (COPD) associated breathlessness.[26] Possible related symptoms of COVID-19 treated with acupuncture include anxiety disorder, insomnia, leucopenia, fatigue, nausea and vomiting, abdominal pain and abdominal distension, and breathlessness. The recent systematic review and meta-analysis show that acupuncture can relieve breathlessness in subjects with advanced diseases. Therefore, in this meta-analysis review protocol, our goal is to systematically review the efficacy of acupuncture in relieving the symptoms of discomfort, subsequently improving the physiological function and quality of life of patients with COVID-19 combined with dyspnea.

The aims of acupuncture treatment of COVID-19 include eliminating pathologic factors, restoring the physiologic functions and maintaining a dynamic balance of qi, blood, yin, and yang.

---

[25]Chen Yong, *et al.* Acupuncture for corona virus disease 2019 A protocol for systematic review and meta analysis. *Medicine.* 2020, 99(40): p. e22231. doi: 10.1097/MD.0000000000022231.

[26]Meaghan Elizabeth Coyle, *et al.* Acupuncture therapies for chronic obstructive pulmonary disease: A systematic review of randomized, controlled trials. *Alternative Therapies in Health Medicine.* 2014, 20(6): 10–23. https://pubmed.ncbi.nlm.nih.gov/25478799/.

Depending upon the functions, differences and characteristics of the points, selection and combination of acupuncture points should follow the principles listed below.

1.4.1 Point selection of some points to open the extraordinary meridians

Extraordinary meridians (Qi Jing Ba Mai) do not directly communicate with the organs, as they run and distribute differently than these regular meridians without being subjected to the restraint of the 12 regular meridians.

They play significant roles in the practice to treat the dysfunctions of different organs at the same time, emotional problems, and some complicated cases. Nevertheless, COVID-19 is an infectious disease with impairment and involvement of multiple zang-fu organs at the same time. Of course, it is also a complicated and difficult illness. As a matter of fact, extraordinary meridians, next to the application of regular meridians, could be applied in the treatment of COVID-19. The purpose of using this technique is to open these extraordinary meridians and restore massive physiological functions of the zang-fu organs.

During the application of extraordinary meridians, the following pairs of points could be used in the following conditions in COVID-19, such as

- Waiguan SJ-5 + Zulinqi GB-41

This combination is indicated in the situations when there is a disorder of Shaoyang in the shoulders and neck, especially at the lateral aspects of the body. This includes COVID-19 at Shaoyang level, or conditions with stiffness, pain at the neck and shoulder, etc.

- Neiguan P-6 + Gongsun SP-4

This combination is indicated in the situations when there is a disorder of lung, heart, liver, stomach, spleen, and kidney. In fact, the lung is always mainly involved from the beginning to the end of the illness.

• Lieque LU-7 + Zhaohai KID-6

This combination is indicated in the situations when there is a disorder of Ren Mai, manifested as tiredness, weakness, dizziness, palpitations, epigastric discomfort feeling, abdominal distention and diarrhea.

• Houxi SI-3 + Shenmai BL-62

This combination is indicated in the situations when there is the decline of yang of the heart and kidney, both in acute and chronic situations.

Since Du Mai is connected to the brain, this combination could be applied to deal with the foggy feeling in the head and dizziness.

1.4.2 Point selection based upon syndrome differentiation

• The points to cause sweating and relieve the external symptoms

Wind-cold
Hegu L.I.-4, Waiguan SJ-5, Lieque LU-7, Fengchi GB-20, and Fengmen BL-12, etc. A reducing method is applied on these points. Moxibustion is suggested to be applied on the first three points.

Wind-heat
Erjian L.I.-2, Hegu L.I.-4, Waiguan SJ-5, Yuji LU-10, Fengchi GB-20, and Fengmen BL-12, etc. A reducing method is applied on these points.

• The points to promote sweating and eliminate cold-damp
Hegu L.I.-4, Yangchi SJ-4, Waiguan SJ-5, Zhigou SJ-6, Lieque LU-7, Fenglong ST-40, Yinlingquan SP-9, etc. A reducing method is applied on these points.

• The points to eliminate cold-damp and harmonize spleen and stomach
Neiguan P-6, Zhongwan REN-12, Sanyinjiao SP-6, Yinlingquan SP-9, and Fenglong ST-40, etc. A reducing method is applied on these points.

• The points to disperse the lung-qi and relieve cough
Zhongfu LU-1, Lieque LU-7, and Feishu BL-13, etc. A reducing method is applied on these points.

• The points to clear heat and descend the lung-qi
Zhongfu LU-1, Chize LU-5, Lieque LU-7, Feishu BL-13, and Tanzhong REN-17, etc. A reducing method is applied on these points.

• The points to descend the lung-qi and eliminate cold-phlegm
Zhongfu LU-1, Chize LU-5, Lieque LU-7, Feishu BL-13, and Tanzhong REN-17, Fenglong ST-40, and Yinlingquan SP-9, etc. A reducing method is applied on these points.

• The points to clear heat and eliminate damp
Hegu L.I.-4, Yemen SJ-2, Yangchi SJ-4, Zhongwan REN-12, Fenglong ST-40, Sanyinjiao SP-6, Yinlingquan SP-9, and Yanglingquan GB-34, etc. A reducing method is applied on these points.

• The points to clear heat and eliminate phlegm
Hegu L.I.-4, Quchi L.I.-11, Chize LU-5, Zhongwan REN-12, Fenglong ST-40, Sanyinjiao SP-6, and Yinlingquan SP-9, etc. A reducing method is applied on these points.

• The points to clear heat and remove toxins
Erjian L.I.-2, Hegu L.I.-4, Chize LU-5, Yuji LU-10, Sanyinjiao SP-6, and Shaofu HE-8, etc. A reducing method is applied on these points.

• The points to cool the blood and remove toxins
Hegu L.I.-4, Sanyinjiao SP-6, Xuehai SP-10, Taiyuan LU-9, and Shaofu HE-8, etc. A reducing method is applied on these points.

• The points to clear heat and promote the defecation
Hegu L.I.-4, Quchi L.I.-11, Tianshu ST-25, Fenglong ST-40, Jiexi ST-41, and Neiting ST-44, etc. A reducing method is applied on these points.

• The points to eliminate blood stasis and resolve phlegm
Hegu L.I.-4, Taiyuan LU-9, Shaohai HE-3, Tongli HE-5, Yinxi HE-6, Fenglong ST-40, and Sanyinjiao SP-6, etc. A reducing method is applied on these points.

• The points to warm the body and tonify yang
Guanyuan REN-4, Qihai REN-6, Zusanli ST-36, Shaohai HE-3, Shenmen HE-7, Baihui DU-20, and Xinshu BL-15, etc. Moxa should be applied to the first three points. A tonifying method is applied on these points.

• The points to tonify qi and blood
Zusanli ST-36, Qihai REN-6, Taixi KID-3, Sanyinjiao SP-6, Pishu BL-20, Shenshu BL-23, and Xuanzhong GB-39, etc. Moxa should be applied to the first three points. A tonifying method is applied on these points.

• The points to warm the interior and eliminate cold
Zusanli ST-36, Guanyuan REN-4, Qihai REN-6, Shaohai HE-3, Taixi KID-3, Pishu BL-20, Shenshu BL-23, and Xuanzhong GB-39, etc. Moxa should be applied to the first three points. A tonifying method is applied on these points.

• The points to nourish yin and clear deficient heat
Zusanli ST-36, Qihai REN-6, Taixi KID-3, Zhaohai KID-6, Yingu KID-10, and Sanyinjiao SP-6, etc. Moxa should be applied on the first three points. A tonifying method is applied on these points.

1.4.3 Point selection based upon symptomatic treatment

There could be various symptoms during the development of COVID-19, and sometimes previous basic diseases such as hypertension, diabetes, cardiovascular diseases, cancers, or renal diseases, etc. could deteriorate. Besides treatment based upon syndrome differentiation as the chief management, symptomatic treatment could be considered as well to relieve some complaints. For instance,

Neiguan P-6 should be used to treat blood pressure problems or digestive problems. If someone has an irregular heartbeat or palpitations, Shaohai HE-3 could be used. If there is a headache, Fengchi GB-20 could be applied. If blood sugar rises, then Sanyinjiao SP-6 or Zhangmen LIV-13 could be applied.

1.4.4 Point selection to calm the shen and regulate the emotions

TCM also pays high attention to emotional influence in the occurrence and development of any sickness. Although traditionally seven emotions are classified in accordance with the five zang organs, there are many other emotions, which could also induce and aggravate the sickness. During many situations that occurred during COVID-19, such as lack of sufficient PCR tests, fast spreading of the virus, missing an accurate and effective treatment, long periods of lockdown, uncertainty of the future and staying indoors, etc., many patients, both confirmed cases and non-confirmed cases, are suffering from emotional disturbance, including stress, frustration, depression, fear, panic, anxiety and worry. Acupuncture to calm the shen and regulate the emotions should be used. These points include:

- Classic points, such as Shaohai HE-3, Shenmen HE-7, Neiguan P-6, Extra Anmian.
- The points from Benshen, such as Shentang BL-44, that are responsible for shen to treat restlessness, nervousness, too much negative concern, hysteria, agitation, etc.
- Some ghost points to sedate the pathogenic factors and quickly and strongly calm down the emotions.

1.5 Precautions

COVID-19 is a highly contagious disease that could transmit from person-to-person directly. During the TCM treatment, especially acupuncture treatment, preventive measures should be taken to prevent being infected. The infectious period is 10 days from the onset of the first symptom. It is suggested to consult the patients via telemedicine, while herbs could be picked up by family members and delivered to the patient's doorstep.

Besides, the following precautions could be taken into considerations:

- If the practitioner cannot be fully protected from getting infected, the acupuncture treatment can be postponed until the patient is in the convalescent stage.
- During treatment, if possible, provide personalized herbal prescriptions based on the differentiation of symptoms and signs as much as possible.
- When personalized prescriptions cannot be provided or obtained due to various reasons, a patent remedy or some standard herbal prescriptions can be considered.
- Even if a personalized herbal prescription is given to the patient before the convalescent stage, the patient's response, actual situations and prognosis should be closely observed. No delay or improper treatment is permitted.
- Since COVID-19 is an acute infectious disease, the pathogen changes rapidly, and sometimes there may be some differences in clinical manifestations within a few hours. Therefore, herbal prescriptions should not be given for too many days, usually not more than a week. If necessary, the prescription should be modified after one or two days of taking the herb.
- Regardless the stage of COVID-19, caring for the lung is one of the key features of the treatment. Restoring the physiological function is always the most important treatment principle and method. For light or ordinary syndromes, dispersing the lung-qi is most important, often using the herbs listed below.

Ma Huang *Herba Ephedrae* 10 g
Jie Geng *Radix Platycodi Grandiflori* 10 g
Sang Ye *Folium Mori Albae* 10 g

Zi Su Ye *Folium Perillae Frutescentis* 10 g
Xing Ren *Semen Pruni Armeniacae* 10 g

Meanwhile, herbs to eliminate phlegm and stop cough should be combined, such as:

Zhi Ban Xia *Rhizoma Pinelliae Ternatae Preparata* 10 g
Chen Pi *Pericarpium Citri Reticulatae* 5 g
Zi Su Zi *Fructus Perillae Frutescentis* 10 g

But when it enters the severe or critical stage, herbs to descend the lung-qi should be applied, including:

Ma Huang *Herba Ephedrae* 10 g
Xing Ren *Semen Pruni Armeniacae* 10 g
Sang Bai Pi *Cortex Mori Albae Radicis* 10 g
Ting Li Zi *Semen Descurainiae seu Lepidii* 10 g

The fullness of the chest with tightness is the most urgent problem to be solved. Extra herbs should be added, such as:

Hou Po *Cortex Magnoliae Officinalis* 10 g
Zhi Shi *Fructus Immaturus Citri Aurantii* 10 g

Expectoration of profuse phlegm is another complaint from the patients that should be cared for by adding:

Bai Jie Zi *Semen Sinapis Albae* 10 g and Zi Su Zi *Fructus Perillae Frutescentis* 10 g for cold-phlegm.
Zhe Bei Mu *Bulbus Fritillariae Thunbergii* 10 g and Quan Gua Lou *Fructus Trichosanthis* 10 g for heat-phlegm.

2

TCM Treatment of Asymptomatic Infections of COVID-19

In view of the numbers related to COVID-19 globally as of 15 April 2021, 1:40 pm CEST, there were 137,541,598 confirmed cases, 2,960,777 confirmed deaths, and 223 countries, areas, or territories with COVID-19 cases.[1] The World Health Organization (WHO) officially named this disease coronavirus disease 2019 (COVID-19) on 11 February 2020. At the same time, the International Committee on Taxonomy of Viruses (ICTV) announced that the new coronavirus was named severe acute respiratory syndrome coronavirus 2 (SARS-CoV-2). Since the outbreak, COVID-19 has brought major harm and challenges to more than 200 countries and regions around the world.[2,3]

All infectious diseases share one characteristic: the coexistence of asymptomatic infections and symptomatic patients, and this characteristic is also proven and reflected by COVID-19. Asymptomatic infections due to COVID-19 must be accompanied by more symptomatic patients and some asymptomatic infections at the same time.

---

[1]World Health Organization (WHO). Coronavirus disease (COVID-19). 15 April 2021. https://www.who.int/emergencies/diseases/novel-coronavirus-2019.

[2]World Health Organization (WHO). Clinical management of severe acute respiratory infection (SARI) when COVID-19 disease is suspected. 2020. https://www.who.int/publications-detail/clinical-management-of-severe-acute-respiratory-infection-when-novel-coronavirus-(ncov)-infection-is-suspected.

[3]World Health Organization (WHO). Coronavirus disease (COVID-19). Weekly epidemiological update and weekly operational update. 2020. https://www.who.int/emergencies/diseases/novel-coronavirus-2019/situation-reports.

COVID-19 was initially divided into four types: mild, moderate, severe, and critical cases.[4] However, with the global outbreak of coronavirus, there is increasing evidence that many infections of COVID-19 are asymptomatic, but they can transmit the virus to others.

Early recognition of an infected person and cutting off the route of transmission are key points to control COVID-19. However, most asymptomatic infections do not seek medical assistance due to no obvious clinical signs and poor prevention awareness, which contribute to the rapid spread of COVID-19. Therefore, it is a great challenge to prevent and control this specific type of patients globally, which requires more attention around the world.[5]

2.1 TCM Analysis Asymptomatic Infections of COVID-19

2.1.1 Definition of asymptomatic infections

Asymptomatic infections refer to patients who have no fever, cough, fatigue, nasal congestion, runny nose, sore throat, chest pain, diarrhea, and other related clinical symptoms, but their PCR test is positive.[6,7]

---

[4] National Health Commission of People's Republic of China. Diagnostic and treatment plan of coronavirus disease 2019. 7th edn. 2020. http://www.nhc.gov.cn/yzygj/s7653p/202003/46c9294%20a7dfe4cef80dc7f5912eb1989.shtml.

[5] Zhiru Gao, *et al*. A systematic review of asymptomatic infections with COVID-19. *Journal of Microbiology, Immunology and Infection.* 2021, 54(1): 12–16. doi: 10.1016/j.jmii.2020.05.001.

[6] Jasper Fuk-Woo Chan, *et al*. A familial cluster of pneumonia associated with the 2019 novel coronavirus indicating person-to-person transmission: A study of a family cluster. *The Lancet.* 2020, 15, 395(10223): 514–523. doi: 10.1016/S0140-6736(20)30154-9.

[7] Zhiliang Hu, *et al*. Clinical characteristics of 24 asymptomatic infections with COVID-19 screened among close contacts in Nanjing, China. *Science China Life Sciences.* 2020, 63(5): 706–711. https://doi.org/10.1007/s11427-020-1661-4.

These infected patients are mainly detected after close contact with confirmed cases, or those who may consciously be infected with the new coronavirus and are actively tested.

Since asymptomatic infections are contagious, the asymptomatic infections in the incubation period may also become confirmed cases. The incubation period is the approximate time from the first exposure to the virus until clinical symptoms or signs onset, and patients can also transmit the virus in this period.[8] However, recent research found that the viral load detected in asymptomatic populations were similar to that in symptomatic patients, indicating that asymptomatic infections have the potential for transmission, which may occur early in the course of infection.[9]

2.1.2 Significance of asymptomatic infections

Asymptomatic infections have the same infectivity as symptomatic infections.[10] It has been reported that a 53-year-old UK patient with an asymptomatic COVID-19 infection may cause 11 infections.[11] Another report pointed out that one asymptomatic person who experienced 19 days from contact with the source of infection to PCR confirmation may have infected five people.[12]

---

[8] Gao Wenjing, *et al.* Advances on presymptomatic or asymptomatic carrier transmission of COVID-19. *Chinese Journal of Epidemiology.* 2020, 41(0): 485–488. doi: 10.3760/cma.j.cn112338-20200228-00207.e.

[9] Lirong Zou, *et al.* SARS-CoV-2 viral load in upper respiratory specimens of infected patients. *The New England Journal of Medicine.* 2020, 382: 1177–1179. doi: 10.1056/NEJMc2001737.

[10] Yi Chen, *et al.* Epidemiological characteristics of infection in COVID-19 close contacts in Ningbo city. *Chinese Journal of Epidemiology.* 2020, 10, 41(5): 667–671. doi: 10.3760/cma.j.cn112338-20200304-00251.

[11] Anne Gulland. (2020, 2011). Could you be a coronavirus super spreader? The Telegraph: [1] https://www.telegraph.co.uk/health-fitness/body/could-coronavirus-super-spreader/.

[12] Yan Bai, *et al.* Presumed asymptomatic carrier transmission of COVID-19. *JAMA.* 2020, 323(14): 1406–1407. doi:10.1001/jama.2020.2565.

At the press conference on the prevention and control of the new coronavirus pneumonia epidemic in Beijing on the 9 July 2020, Jiang Li (an expert on the national new crown pneumonia medical treatment expert group and director of the Department of Critical Care Medicine, Xuanwu Hospital, Capital Medical University), introduced the newly-occurring outbreak in Beijing. 21 out of the 52 cases of asymptomatic infections were converted to confirmed patients, and a considerable part of them developed the disease after intensive medical observation.[13] Therefore, asymptomatic infections should also be subjected to intensive medical observation to control the spread of the epidemic, in order to detect and treat possible confirmed cases in time. In China, those who have been under intensive medical observation for 14 days,[14] and have a negative PCR test can be released from intensive medical observation. However, if the PCR test remains positive with no clinical symptoms, then it is vital to continue intensive medical observation.

Moreover, Wilder-Smith *et al.* (2005) reported that the asymptomatic ratio of COVID-19 patients may be lower than the asymptomatic ratio of SARS (13.0%),[15] albeit the asymptomatic ratio of MERS (9.8%).[16] At present, there is no evaluation of the role of asymptomatic infection in the spread of the epidemic. The China CDC's analysis of 72,314 cases in mainland China showed that

---

[13] Manzi Zhang, *et al.* The initial 52 cases of asymptomatic infections in the new outbreak cluster 21 cases were referred to confirmed. *Xinhua Net* (新华网). 9 July 2020. http://www.xinhuanet.com/politics/2020-07/09/c_1126217493.htm.

[14] Yunshuang Yang, *et al.* Discussion on TCM treatment strategies for asymptomatic patients with new coronary pneumonia. *Basic Medical Theory Research* (基础医学理论研究). 2020, 2(2): 5–6.

[15] Annelies Wilder-Smith, *et al.* Asymptomatic SARS coronavirus infection among healthcare workers, Singapore. *Emerging Infectious Diseases.* 2005, 11(7): 1142–1145. doi: 10.3201/eid1107.041165.

[16] Jaffar A. Al-Tawfiq. Asymptomatic coronavirus infection: MERS-CoV and SARS-CoV-2 (COVID-19). *Travel medicine and infectious disease.* 2020, 35: 101608. doi: 10.1016/j.tmaid.2020.101608.

asymptomatic infections reached 1.2%,[17] Tian *et al.* reported 5.0%[18] and South Korea reported 10.7%.[19]

COVID-19 is highly contagious and may have either a short or long incubation period. As the COVID-19 epidemic spreads around the world, how we detect and isolate infected persons in a timely manner is very important to effectively control the epidemic. In the early stages of the epidemic in China, the population is initially screened based on whether there are clinical symptoms. The medical staff used fever as the main screening method, and then gradually extended to clinical symptoms such as fever, dry cough, and fatigue. This screening standard ignores the existence of asymptomatic infections, resulting in loopholes in the prevention and control of the epidemic, causing an increase in the number of initial infections.

It is difficult to detect asymptomatic infected persons and keep them quarantined in time. The asymptomatic infection could easily cause an accumulation of infection sources, posing a major challenge to the prevention and control of the epidemic. The study has shown that the presence or absence of clinical symptoms is not significantly related to the severity of COVID-19 patients. There is no difference between the pathophysiological changes caused by 2019-nCoV infection to asymptomatic patients and symptomatic patients. For instance, in a study, 21 patients in the asymptomatic group underwent chest CT examination, of which 12 cases showed bilateral pneumonia, two cases showed unilateral pneumonia, and the remaining seven cases underwent CT examination in a third-party

---

[17] Zhonghua Liu, *et al.* The epidemiological characteristics of an outbreak of 2019 novel coronavirus diseases (COVID-19) in China. *Chinese Journal of Epidemiology.* 2020, 41(2): 145–151. doi: 10.3760/cma.j.issn.0254-6450.2020.02.003.

[18] Sijia Tian, *et al.* Characteristics of COVID-19 infection in Beijing. *Journal of Infection.* 2020, 80(4): 401–406. doi: 10.1016/j.jinf.2020.02.018.

[19] COVID-19 National Emergency Response Center, Epidemiology and Case Management Team, Korea Centers for Disease Control and Prevention. Early epidemiological and clinical characteristics of 28 cases of coronavirus disease in South Korea. *Osong Public Health and Research Perspectives.* 2020, 11(1): 8–14. doi: 10.24171/j.phrp.2020.11.1.03.

hospital, and complete examination records could not be obtained. 580 patients in the symptomatic group underwent chest CT examination, of which 538 cases (92.8%) had bilateral pneumonia, 39 cases (6.7%) had unilateral pneumonia, and three cases (0.5%) had no signs of pneumonia. There was no statistically significant difference in imaging examination results between the two groups (Fisher Exact Probability Method, $p > 0.05$).[20] It therefore could be concluded that besides expanding the criteria for contact tracing and testing to capture potential transmission before symptom onsets, the same vigilance and attention should be maintained in the clinical diagnosis and treatment of asymptomatic infections.

With the development of the epidemic and the deepening of research, it has been found that a small number of patients may be asymptomatic after infection and continue to spread the virus. Therefore, early detection and diagnosis of asymptomatic infections due to COVID-19 is of great significance for disease prevention and control. Hu *et al.*[21] analyzed 24 cases of asymptomatic infections and found that asymptomatic infections can also cause severe pneumonia, suggesting that asymptomatic infections have the effect of increasing transmission and strong concealment. It can be observed from the following case from China in February 2020, which discovered that asymptomatic infection could be very difficult and trained investigators could spend quite a lot of effort trying to collect information from the medical record system.[22]

[20]Wenhao Su, *et al.* Analysis of clinical characteristics of asymptomatic infections of novel coronavirus. *Chinese Journal of Infectious Diseases* (中华传染病杂志). 2020, 38(12): 772–776. doi: 10.3760/ca.j.cn311365-20200319-00356.

[21]Zhibin Hu, *et al.* Discovery and management of latent infections of the new coronavirus. *Chinese Journal of Preventive Medicine* (中华预防医学杂志). 2020, 54(5): 484–485. doi: 10.3760/cma.j.cn112150-20200229-00220.

[22]Si-hui Luo, *et al.* A confirmed asymptomatic carrier of 2019 novel coronavirus. *Chinese Medical Journal* (Engl). 2020, 133(9): 1123–1125. doi: 10.1097/CM9.0000000000000798.

2.1.3 Age-related asymptomatic infections

Studies have found that the mortality rate of patients with COVID-19, severe acute respiratory syndrome (SARS) and the Middle East respiratory syndrome (MERS) are all age-related.[23-25] One case in Wuhan tracked the prevalence of 1,391 children under 15 years old who had been in close contact with infected or suspected cases.[26] The incidence of asymptomatic infections in the children is lower than that of the whole population, proposing that it is related to the special immune response and ACE2 level in children's bodies.[27] Another study have realized that the age group of asymptomatic infections is relatively low, and those less than 30 years old are more likely to be asymptomatic. It shows that the age of the asymptomatic group was 35.0(31.5, 58.0) years, which was lower than the 58.5(45.0, 69.0) years of the symptomatic group, and the difference was statistically significant (U = 4 234.500, p = 0.002).[28] This may be related to the weak innate immune response produced by young people and the differential expression of inflammation-related genes. Young patients' T lymphocytes and B lymphocytes have strong functions, which can better control virus replication and reduce the body's inflammatory

---

[23] Fei Zhou, *et al.* Clinical course and risk factors for mortality of adult inpatients with COVID-19 in Wuhan, China: A retrospective cohort study. *The Lancet.* 2020, 395(10229): 1054–1062. doi: 10.1016/S0140-6736(20)30566-3.

[24] Kin Wing Choi, *et al.* Outcomes and prognostic factors in 267 patients with severe acute respiratory syndrome in Hong Kong. *Annals of Internal Medicine.* 2003, 139(9): 715–723. doi: 10.7326/0003-4819-139-9-200311040-00005.

[25] Ki-Ho Hong, *et al.* Predictors of mortality in Middle East respiratory syndrome (MERS). *Thorax.* 2018, 73(3): 286–289. doi: 10.1136/thoraxjnl-2016-209313.

[26] Xiaoxia Lu, *et al.* SARS-CoV-2 infection in children. *The New England Journal of Medicine.* 2020, 382(17): 1663–1665. doi: 10.1056/NEJMc2005073.

[27] Jieliang Chen. Pathogenicity and transmissibility of 2019-nCoV-A quick overview and comparison with other emerging viruses. *Microbes and Infection.* 2020, 22(2): 69–71. doi: 10.1016/j.micinf.2020.01.004.

[28] Wenhao Su, *et al.* Analysis of clinical characteristics of asymptomatic infection of novel coronavirus. *Chinese Journal of Infectious Diseases* (中华传染病杂志). 2020, 38(12): 772–776. doi: 10.3760/cma.j.cn311365-20200319-00356.

response so that patients fail to develop clinical symptoms.[29,30] When compared with symptomatic patients, there is no statistically significant difference in imaging examination results and laboratory test indicators of asymptomatic infections, suggesting that after asymptomatic infections are infected with 2019-nCoV, the virus only causes a specific immune response without significant tissue damage, so there are no obvious clinical symptoms and signs.[31] Methods such as CT and laboratory examinations can effectively detect asymptomatic infections during the screening of close contacts.

2.1.4 Five situations of asymptomatic infections

Asymptomatic infections include the following five situations:

- The disease is in the incubation period (usually three to seven days, or longer, up to three weeks). In the beginning, there were no clinical symptoms, and the infection had already occurred. After three to seven days, symptoms such as fever, cough, and fatigue start to appear.
- The so-called asymptomatic-infected people experience some discomfort, such as slight muscle pain and the desire to sleep but have no nose and throat problems despite feeling tired, or have a headache. They think that they have a cold or are simply too nervous. These complaints went away after taking painkillers. Actually, their symptoms are the manifestations of this infectious disease, but they were unaware. This situation accounts for a considerable number of patients. If the PCR is tested at this time, it could show a positive result. It means the patient is infected with very mild symptoms.

---

[29] Saskia L. Smits, *et al.* Exacerbated innate host response to SARS-CoV in aged non-human primates. *PLOS Pathogens.* 2010, 6(2): e1000756. doi: 10.1371/journal.ppat.1000756.
[30] Steven M. Opal, *et al.* The immunopathogenesis of sepsis in elderly patients. *Clinical Infectious Diseases.* 2005, 41(Suppl 7): S504–512. doi: 10.1086/432007.
[31] Zhibin Hu, *et al. op. cit.*

- When the PCR test result is positive, patients have to be quarantined for 14 days and follow-up visits to designated hospitals are required. After this period, such patients could still be asymptomatic. The quarantine will be terminated when the PCR test is negative. But in some circumstances in some countries, these patients will be free of quarantine even after 10 days.
- A small number of patients are confirmed with positive PCR tests, but they don't show any symptoms. After a month, their PCR remains positive. They have not produced antibodies and are called virus carriers.
- Confirmed cases discharged from the hospital show positive PCR tests through follow-up examinations despite having no clinical symptoms and signs, and their imaging shows no signs of pneumonia. Either their pneumonia absorption improved or there are residual unabsorbed lesions.

2.2 TCM Treatment

2.2.1 TCM views of management

As there are no obvious clinical symptoms and signs, asymptomatic patients bring not only difficulties to the prevention and control of the epidemic, but also great challenges to traditional Chinese medicine based on syndrome differentiation. Although asymptomatic patients are "asymptomatic and discernible" on a macro level, their classification, pathogenesis, TCM syndrome differentiation methods, and treatment principles through microscopic syndrome differentiation can still be analyzed so as to conduct syndrome differentiation and treatment. In addition, it is worth pointing out that the so-called "asymptomatic" is only a self-perceived feeling. TCM's understanding of symptoms also includes other aspects of the "four diagnoses", especially tongue and pulse manifestations. Applying the diagnostic methods of traditional Chinese medicine, experienced practitioners may obtain an objective and comprehensive understanding of "asymptomatic" to provide a basis for clinical diagnosis and treatment.

2.2.1.1 *Importance of zheng-qi*

COVID-19 with an asymptomatic situation is a kind of epidemic febrile disease caused by incubating pathogens. *Huang Di Nei Jing* 《黄帝内经》—Yellow Emperor's Inner Canon points out that if there is impairment to the body by cold in winter, there would be febrile diseases in spring. This statement laid the foundation for the onset of latent xie-qi. Youke Wu (1582–1652), an outstanding physician in the Ming Dynasty, forwarded the theory of li qi (epidemic qi) as the cause of infectious diseases, bringing forth new ideas in the etiology, transmission, and treatment of these diseases. He proposed in his book *Wen Yi Lun* 《瘟疫论》—Treaties on pestilence in 1642 that "there is a mysterious epidemic qi between Heaven and Earth, which accumulates in the mo yuan (interpleural-diaphragmatic space), resulting in the occurrence of pandemics".

COVID-19, a disease caused by an epidemic infection in modern medicine, is considered as a sickness in TCM, due to the invasion of external pathogenic factors through the mouth and nose, the corridor of the lung and stomach, to the body. When it attacks the body and mainly stays at the superficial layer of the body, in which the zheng-qi is still relatively strong, it could lead to an immediate and drastic imbalance of the qi and blood, yin and yang, leading to impairment of the zang-fu organs, qi, blood, body fluid, and channels. At this moment, there could be the appearance of clinical symptoms and signs. However, when the pathogenic factors are not yet too strong, and zheng-qi is still relatively very strong—or the pathogenic qi is relative too strong while zheng-qi is not so strong—they could directly invade the deep layer of the body, bringing about accumulation of these pathogenic factors in the body with not so violent and drastic conflict between the zheng-qi and xie-qi. Even so, the zheng-qi is constantly attempting to overwhelm the xie-qi, showing no clinical symptoms and signs.

It could be seen from the above statements that occurrence, its severity, development, aggravation, or alleviation of asymptomatic infection is mainly determined by the conditions of zheng-qi and xie-qi, but also influenced by various conditions such as diet and emotion, physical constitutions, and therapeutic intervention.

There are four possible patterns of continuous conflict between zheng-qi and xie-qi, illustrating the mechanism of asymptomatic infections in TCM:

- Although the PCR test is positive, its pathogenic qi is still mild and the zheng-qi of the patient is sufficient. The patient is considered asymptomatic when he is able to fight against, control, and dispel the pathogenic qi.
- Zheng qi is insufficient, and the pathogens are relatively strong, in which xie-qi is able to enter deeply into the body and hide in the *Mo Yuan*. In this situation, the battle between zheng-qi and xie-qi is not violent and obvious. Although the disease will not occur temporarily, it could start at any time when xie-qi grows and becomes strong, or when the zheng-qi is also improving. This condition often happens to confirmed cases which are still in the incubation period, resulting in an asymptomatic reaction.
- The xie-qi is mild, and the zheng-qi is also insufficient, resulting in weak conflict between these two factors without showing some obvious symptoms. Even so, the diseases are developing quietly and deeply. In such cases, the PCR test could be positive, and chest imaging could show multiple ground glass shadows in the lungs. The cases could be worsening and become severe or critical. Early attention and intervention are needed. One study demonstrated that chest CT have confirmed there are lung lesions among the 159 asymptomatic patients. 7 of the 38 patients, who were rechecked on chest CT, had lesion progression within a short period of time with a poor prognosis.[32]
- In the recovery period, the zheng-qi is insufficient, and xie-qi is also weak, resulting in a nostalgic reaction of xie-qi. This situation is common in the confirmed patients who are discharged after recovery. However, their PCR tests soon become positive again or even constantly remain positive, with or without imaging lesions of the lungs.

---

[32]Wang YF, *et al.* (2020). CT image features of asymptomatic patients with novel coronavirus pneumonia. *Medical Edition, Journal of Wuhan University* (武汉大学学报(医学版)). 2020, 41(3): 353–356.

2.2.1.2 *Physical constitutions*

Besides zheng-qi playing a key role in the occurrence and development of COVID-19 and its asymptomatic infection, physical constitutions of the patients are also extremely important.

Prof. Qi Wang, one of the most famous TCM specialists in China put forward nine types in physical constitution, including peace, qi deficiency, yang deficiency, yin deficiency, phlegm-damp, damp-heat, qi-stagnation, blood stasis, and special hereditary quality, and gave TCM prevention care and treatment according to the different constitution of all the patients.[33]

The physical constitutions, except the first peaceful type, are mostly a result of disorder in qi, blood, yin, and yang with certain dysfunction of zang-fu organs. They could be identified and regulated by TCM. Based on the concepts of syndrome differentiation and sickness management, methods should be applied to adjust the imbalance in qi, blood, yin and yang, and disharmony of the zang-fu organs so as to maintain a dynamic healthy condition. This is also the principle of treatment for asymptomatic infections.

2.2.1.3 *The aims of the treatment*

It can be concluded that all methods and attempts should be used to maintain a healthy condition for zheng-qi. Meanwhile, procedures should also be applied to eliminate xie-qi as much as possible.

2.2.1.3.1 *To eliminate the xie-qi completely*

When the asymptomatic infection starts, it implies that there was an invasion of pathogenic factors, which directly entered the interior organs or tissues of the body and became a latent issue. COVID virus is an external pathogenic factor, and it usually causes the occurrence

---

[33]Qi Wang. The classification of 9 basic TCM constitution types and the basis for their diagnosis. *Journal of Beijing University of Traditional Chinese Medicine* (北京中医药大学学报). 2005, 28(4): 1–8.

of Taiyang syndrome, showing some external symptoms and signs. These symptoms include an aversion to cold, slight fever, running nose, cough, muscle pain, superficial pulse, etc. However, it could hide inside the body and induce some sickness without any obvious notice. Therefore, the TCM system of four methods of diagnosis and syndrome differentiation should be applied with a careful examination to detect any trace abnormality. After a thorough study on the etiologies and pathologies with successful treatment of COVID-19 by using Chinese herbs and acupuncture, sufficient knowledge has been gained to formulate some strategies in dealing with various syndromes. Wind, cold, heat, damp, and toxins are the main pathogenic factors that need to be eliminated completely and urgently.

2.2.1.3.2 *To support zheng-qi ultimately*

The condition of zheng-qi is always the key factor, which determines the battle with the pathogenic factor. When these pathogenic factors invades the body, it implies that zheng-qi is somewhat insufficient, disturbed, or in disharmony. Zheng-qi is a collective term for all kinds of factors to fight against the invasion. Therefore, it is necessary to identify which zheng-qi is in trouble and why it is in imbalance.

Actually, zheng-qi is constantly fighting against and eliminating these pathogenic factors. It doesn't mean that zheng-qi is always deficient, which implies that there is no need to tonify the zheng-qi by using different tonics here. Even if there is a deficiency of zheng-qi, it is also not a good moment to tonify the zheng-qi, since COVID-19 is a rather excessive case, which needs to be dealt with by applying the method of elimination as its main approach in the treatment. The conclusion is clear that supporting the zheng-qi is not the same as its tonification.

2.2.1.3.3 *To prevent further aggravation efficiently*

As proven by the above scientific studies, the asymptomatic infection could develop into some severe or critical cases. Any methods and procedures should be taken seriously to cease its development.

To prevent infections from worsening, care and attention should be paid specially to protect the lung and avoid any aggravation of this organ in dispersing and descending the qi and water. Meanwhile, the relations between the lung and its related organs also need to be regulated properly. It means that the consequence of the development of COVID-19 should be taken into consideration when forming the treatment strategies.

2.2.1.3.4 *To balance the physical and mental conditions sufficiently*

COVID-19 disturbs and damages not only the physiological functions of the lung, but also many other zang-fu organs, different channels, and collaterals, as well as the mental state of patients. A mixture of these complaints often shows complications of the situation. Sometimes, mental disturbance such as anxiety, panic, restlessness, palpitation, and insomnia, etc could be a major problem besides lung difficulty. Sophisticated treatment could bring about a good benefit to the patient.

As pointed out already on the "macro" level, asymptomatic patients with COVID-19 don't have obvious self-perceived clinical symptoms or signs. However, on the "microscopic" level, the body is already in a pathological state with possible dysfunction of qi, blood, yin and yang, etc. According to the general pathological changes in patients who suffer from COVID-19, which could show some manifestations of phlegm, heat, and fire with involvement of different zang-fu organs, the asymptomatic patients could develop into the same pathological state when they are left untreated in time.

2.2.1.4 **Treatment strategies**

Although asymptomatic infection of COVID-19 could be confirmed by PCR test and the disease has not been fully presented for the time being, it does not mean that there will be no outbreak. It is just in a budding state and surface at any time. TCM could be applied together with care in daily life, diet, and exercise, to intervene in time to get rid of hidden potential dangers and restore health. The intention of all these kinds of management is to put prevention first, i.e., treating the diseases before they occur, which is an important concept in TCM. The strategies of this preventive management include the following contents.

2.2.1.4.1 *To eliminate pathogenic factors*

COVID-19 could be caused by many pathogens, although the invasion of damp and toxins, in combination with wind, cold or heat, are the basic factors. Treatment should focus on the elimination of pathogenic factors. Of course, there is a difference between the treatment for patients with clinical symptoms and those who are asymptomatic. During the treatment for patients with clinical symptoms, management for COVID-19 at different stages should be differentiated and taken. However, for asymptomatic patients, their treatment mainly aims to eliminate hidden pathogenic factors, but not using the dispelling method as that often happens in the treatment for symptomatic patients.

The following herbs are used to eliminate damp:

Cang Zhu *Rhizoma Atractylodis* 10 g
Bai Zhu *Rhizoma Atractylodis Macrocephalae* 10 g
Chen Pi *Pericarpium Citri Reticulatae* 5 g
Hou Po *Cortex Magnoliae Officinalis* 10 g
Fu Ling *Sclerotium Poriae Cocos* 10 g

Depending upon the location and mixture of this damp with some other pathogenic factors, some herbs should be combined, including the following.

If there is an invasion of external cold-damp, then add:
Fang Feng *Radix Ledebouriellae Divaricatae* 10 g
Gui Zhi *Ramulus Cinnamomi Cassiae* 10 g
Qiang Huo *Rhizoma et Radix Notopterygii* 10 g
Du Huo *Radix Angelicae Pubescentis* 10 g

If there is an invasion of external damp-heat, then add:
Sang Ye *Folium Mori Albae* 10 g
Huang Qin *Radix Scutellariea Baicalensis* 10 g
Zhi Zi *Fructus Gardeniae Jasminoidis* 10 g

If there is an invasion of external damp to the middle Jiao, then add:
Huo Xiang *Herba Agastaches seu Pogostemi* 10 g
Pei Lan *Herba Eupatorii Fortunei* 10 g
Zi Su Ye *Folium Perillae Frutescentis* 10 g
Yi Yi Ren *Semen Coicis Lachryma-Jobi* 12 g
Bai Dou Kou *Fructus Amomi Cardamomi* 3 g

If there is an invasion of external damp to the lower Jiao, then add:
Hua Shi *Talcum* 10 g
Tong Cao *Medulla Tetrapanacis Papyriferi* 10 g
Che Qian Zi *Semen Plantaginis* 10 g

Following herbs are used to remove toxins:
Lian Qiao *Fructus Forsythiae Suspensae* 10 g
Jin Yin Hua *Flos Lonicerae Japonicae* 10 g
Pu Gong Ying *Herba Taraxaci Mongolici cum Radice* 10 g

2.2.1.4.2 *Protect and restore the physiological functions of the lung*

The pathogenesis of COVID-19 is rather complicated, but its main pathogenic consequence is dysfunction of the lung in dispersing and descending the qi, leading to cough, shortness of breath, and expectoration of sputum. In the beginning, there could be only disturbance to the lung in dispersing the qi, sore throat, dry cough or cough with slight sputum, while anosmia and ageusia etc. may occur. When it is not properly treated, the lung could fail to descend the qi, bringing about pressure in the chest, shortness of breath, extreme tiredness, water retention in the lung or other organs, as well as bring forward many serious conditions. These pathogenic results could be predicted when this disease is developing, especially on some elderly patients or those who have existing basic diseases. Therefore, some methods should be applied to prevent the aggravation of these lung conditions by using some herbs in advance. Usually, two or three such herbs could be applied in the preventive herbal prescription.

Following herbs are used to protect and restore the lung in dispersing the qi:
Ma Huang *Herba Ephedrae* 10 g
Gui Zhi *Ramulus Cinnamomi Cassiae* 10 g
Jie Geng *Radix Platycodi Grandiflori* 10 g
Xing Ren *Semen Pruni Armeniacae* 10 g
Zi Su Ye *Folium Perillae Frutescentis* 10 g

Following herbs are used to protect and restore the lung in descending the qi:
Ma Huang *Herba Ephedrae* 10 g
Gui Zhi *Ramulus Cinnamomi Cassiae* 10 g
Xing Ren *Semen Pruni Armeniacae* 10 g
Zi Su Zi *Fructus Perillae Frutescentis* 10 g

2.2.1.4.3 *Unblock the San Jiao*

With disharmony and blockage of the San Jiao in qi, transformation and transmission is generally recognized and accepted as its pathogenesis. Thus, to protect the lungs, harmonizing and unblocking the San Jiao are the most important treatment options.

Damp may easily transform into fire or cold, which could be influenced by the constitutions, diets, climate, and geographic locations. As the temperature rises or falls, damp may become damp-heat or cold-damp, showing fatigue, sleepiness, chest tightness, stomach discomfort, nausea, loose stools, white, greasy coating, and slippery pulse, etc. Nevertheless, those patients who suffer from obesity, weak spleen, stomach and San Jiao system, could possibly have blockage in the San Jiao.

Following herbs are used to unblock the San Jiao:
Xing Ren *Semen Pruni Armeniacae* 10 g
Bai Dou Kou *Fructus Amomi Cardamomi* 5 g
Yi Yi Ren *Semen Coicis Lachryma-Jobi* 12 g

2.2.1.4.4 *Support the zheng-qi*

Whether the asymptomatic infection develops into symptomatic infection mostly depends upon the condition of zheng-qi. The diseases caused by COVID-19, invasion of pathogenic factors, onset and occurrence of diseases, deterioration of physiological situations, and even possible death, are all related to the condition of zheng-qi. Zheng-qi is always in its position to protect the body and fight against any pathogenic invasion and aggravation. It doesn't mean that asymptomatic infection could leave zheng-qi alone without proper care. Supporting the zheng-qi could maintain a dynamic position to eliminate this pathogenic invasion and aggravation.

Following herbs are used to support the qi:
Zhi Huang Qi *Radix Astragali Membranacei Praeparata* 10 g
Dang Shen *Radix Codonopsis Pilosulae* 10 g
Shan Yao *Radix Dioscoreae Oppositae* 10 g
Jiao Bai Zhu *Rhizoma Atractylodis Macrocephalae (grill)* 10 g
Fu Ling *Sclerotium Poriae Cocos* 10 g
Bai Bian Dou *Semen Dolichoris Lablab* 10 g

Following herbs are used to tonify the blood:
Dang Gui *Radix Angelicae Sinensis* 10 g
Huang Jing *Rhizoma Polygonati* 10 g
Da Zao *Fructus Zizyphi Jujubae* 10 g

Following herbs are used to nourish the yin:
Shan Yao *Radix Dioscoreae Oppositae* 12 g
Gou Qi Zi *Fructus Lycii* 10 g
Bei Sha Shen *Radix Glehniae Littoralis* 10 g
Nan Sha Shen *Radix Adenophorae* 10 g

Following herbs are used to benefit the body fluid:
Tian Hua Fen *Radix Trichosanthis Kirilowii* 10 g
Ge Gen *Radix Puerariae* 10 g

Following herbs are used to reinforce the yang:
Rou Gui *Cortex Cinnamomi Cassiae* 5 g
Zhi Fu Zi *Radix Lateralis Aconiti Carmichaeli Praeparata* 10 g
Gan Jiang *Rhizoma Zingiberis Officinalis* 5 g
Du Zhong *Cortex Eucommiae Ulmoidis* 10 g

Besides, some relevant herbs should be combined to regulate the internal zang-fu organs to strengthen them so as to avoid deterioration of physiological functions. For instance, if someone suffers from hypertension with liver yang hyperactivity and is confirmed as an asymptomatic case, herbs should be added to the above prescription to calm down the liver yang, such as Gou Teng *Ramulus cum Uncis Uncariae*, Tian Ma *Rhizoma Gastrodiae Elatae*, Xia Ku Cao *Spica Prunellae Vulgaris*, etc. If someone suffers from diabetes and has a PCR positive test, herbs should be added to lower blood sugar level, such as Tian Hua Fen *Radix Trichosanthis Kirilowii*, Ge Gen *Radix Puerariae*, etc. In this way, zang-fu organs are well protected and regulated to maintain a good condition of zheng-qi.

2.2.1.4.5 *Regulate the emotion*

The physical body consists of jing, qi and shen, and their conditions could influence each other. Besides methods taken to treat the physical diseases, management to take care of the emotions and the shen should also be seriously considered.

Shen presides over activities that take place in the mental, spiritual, and creative planes. Shen in TCM includes broad and narrow senses. The former refers to all kinds of mental activities, reactions, and attitudes to the world and environments, embodying consciousness, emotions, and thought. The latter refers to the aspect of our being that is spiritual, including different emotions.

When COVID-19 is diagnosed, even if it is an asymptomatic infection, fear, anxiety, nervousness, restlessness, insomnia, panic, etc. could occur, especially in elderly patients. Regulation and attention should be taken to care and manage these emotions and calm the shen in order to support the patient.

Following herbs are used to regulate the shen:
Yuan Zhi *Radix Polygalae Tenuifoliae* 10 g
Fu Shen *Sclerotium Poriae Cocos Paradicis* 10 g
Hou Po *Cortex Magnoliae Officinalis* 10 g
Bai He *Bulbus Lilii* 10 g
Shi Chang Pu *Rhizoma Acori Graminei* 10 g

2.2.2 Treatment according to syndrome differentiation

During the clinical consultation in February 2020, experts found that many asymptomatic patients tested positive for nucleic acid. However, some confirmed patients were asymptomatic after treatment, but still had a positive PCR test result. In order to shorten the course of the disease and discharge patients from the hospital as soon as possible, Professor Wang Xixing and members of the expert team from Shan Xi province believe that those who are asymptomatic with the new coronavirus and those whose PCR tests did not turn negative after the symptoms of new coronary pneumonia improve, belong to the group with qi deficiency and persistence of toxins. The treatment should be based on tonifying qi, nourishing the lungs, clearing away heat and removing toxins. Yi Qi Qu Du Ke Li—Granules 益气祛毒颗粒 (The prescription consists of Huang Qi *Radix Astragali Membranacei*, Dang Shen *Radix Codonopsis Pilosulae*, Cang Zhu *Rhizoma Atractylodis*, Sheng Ma *Rhizoma Cimicifugae*, Jin Yin Hua *Flos Lonicerae Japonicae*, Chai Hu *Radix Bupleuri* and Mai Men Dong *Tuber Ophiopogonis Japonici* etc.) to tonify the qi and remove toxins were firstly tested on a patient who was unable to turn PCR negative for a long time. After taking three doses (for three days) of this formula, the throat swab of the nucleic acid test was negative for two consecutive times, and he was discharged smoothly. On 17 February 2020, after taking three to six doses of this herbal medicine, another six patients had their throat swabs, blood, and sputum tested by nucleic acid, and they all turned negative. After a series of clinical use, the effect was confirmed. By 28 February, Yi Qi Qu Du Ke Li started to be widely used in clinical trials in Hubei.[34]

Due to possible viral transmission, it is generally recommended that the herbs should be taken for at least three to four weeks to cover the possible incubation period and restore the zheng-qi completely. If necessary and possible, PCR control could be carried out to determine whether it turns negative.

Following treatments are given to most asymptomatic patients with no obvious clinical signs or are not consciously aware about their symptoms. However, in TCM, some trace symptoms and signs could be discovered at the micro level.

2.2.2.1 *Invasion of wind-heat*

Slight aversion to wind, feeling warm, slight thirst, restlessness, or very slight muscle pain or headache, red tip of the tongue, with or without a superficial and rapid pulse.

Principles of Treatment:
Dispel wind-heat and disperse the lung-qi.

Herbal Treatment:
Sang Ju Yin-*Mulberry Leaf and Chrysanthemum Decoction.*

Sang Ye *Folium Mori Albae* 10 g
Ju Hua *Flos Chrysanthemi Morifolii* 10 g

---

[34]Bo Zhang. Our province launched a traditional Chinese medicine for promoting nucleic acid to turn negative, which is the first in the country. *Taiyuan Evening News* (太原晚报). 1 March 2020. http://www.tynews.com.cn/system/2020/03/01/030187933.shtml.

Huang Qin *Radix Scutellariae Baicalensis* 10 g
Jie Geng *Radix Platycodi Grandiflori* 10 g
Lian Qiao *Fructus Forsythiae Suspensae* 10 g
Zhe Bei Mu *Bulbus Fritillariae Thunbergii* 10 g
Xing Ren *Semen Pruni Armeniacae* 10 g

Explanation:
- Sang Ye and Ju Hua promote sweating to dispel wind-heat and relieve external symptoms. They could prevent further invasion of wind-heat into the deep layer of the body.
- Huang Qin and Lian Qiao clear the heat in the upper Jiao and remove the toxins.
- Jie Geng disperses and protects the lung-qi. Meanwhile, it resolves the phlegm in the lung and relieves possible coughing. Xing Ren disperses and descends the lung-qi at the same time, and could prevent the failure of lung-qi in descending. In this way, the lung is well protected.
- Zhe Bei Mu is applied here to resolve the heat-phlegm because it works in combination with Jie Geng to eliminate potential cough due to heat-phlegm.

Modifications:
- In the case of an obvious sore throat, add Niu Bang Zi *Fructus Arctii Lappae* 10 g and Bo He *Herba Menthae Haplocalycis* 5 g to improve throat condition and relieve the sore throat.
- In the case of too much cough, add Zhi Ban Xia *Rhizoma Pinelliae Ternatae Preparata* 10 g and Gua Lou Pi *Pericarpium Trichosanthis* 10 g to eliminate phlegm and relieve the cough.
- In the case of strong loss of smell, add Cang Er Zi *Fructus Xanthii Sibirici* 10 g and Xin Yi Hua *Flos Magnoliae* 10 g to open the nasal orifice and relieve the loss of smell.
- In the case of obvious loss of taste, add Sha Ren *Fructus Amomi* 5 g and Shi Chang Pu *Rhizoma Acori Graminei* 10 g to benefit the orifice and improve the tastebuds.

2.2.2.2 *Invasion of wind-cold*

Slight aversion to cold, very slight running nose, muscle pain, or headache, thin and white tongue, with or without a superficial and tight pulse.

Principles of Treatment:
Dispel wind-cold and disperse the lung-qi.

Herbal Treatment:
Jing Fang Bai Du San-*Schizonepeta and Saposhnikoviae Powder to Overcome Pathogenic Influences.*

Jing Jie *Herba seu Flos Schizonepetae Tenuifoliae* 10 g
Fang Feng *Radix Ledebouriellae Divaricatae* 10 g
Zi Su Ye *Folium Perillae Frutescentis* 10 g
Du Huo *Radix Angelicae Pubescentis* 10 g
Qiang Huo *Rhizoma et Radix Notopterygii* 10 g
Jie Geng *Radix Platycodi Gran* 10 g
Xing Ren *Semen Pruni Armeniacae* 10 g
Zi Su Zi *Fructus Perillae Frutescentis* 10 g
Fu Ling *Sclerotium Poriae Cocos* 10 g

Explanation:
- Jing Jie, Fang Feng and Zi Su Ye are used to dispel wind-cold and relieve external symptoms.
- Du Huo and Qiang Huo promote sweating to dispel wind-cold and relieve muscle pain.
- Jie Geng, Xing Ren and Zi Su Zi disperse the qi of the lung and protect the lung in its descending qi.
- Fu Ling tonifies the zheng-qi and resolves phlegm.

Modifications:
- In the case of an obvious sore throat, add Niu Bang Zi *Fructus Arctii Lappae* 10 g and She Gan *Rhizoma Belamcandae Chinensis* 10 g to improve throat condition and relieve the sore throat.

- In the case of too much cough, add Zhi Ban Xia *Rhizoma Pinelliae Ternatae Preparata* 10 g to eliminate phlegm and relieve the cough.
- In the case of strong loss of smell, add Cang Er Zi *Fructus Xanthii Sibirici* 10 g and Xin Yi Hua *Flos Magnoliae* 10 g to open the nasal orifice and relieve the loss of smell.
- In the case of an obvious loss of taste, add Sha Ren *Fructus Amomi* 5 g and Shi Chang Pu *Rhizoma Acori Graminei* 10 g to benefit the orifice and improve the tastebuds.

2.2.2.3 *Invasion of cold-damp to the middle Jiao*

Slightly poor appetite, loose stool, sometimes possible nausea, slight muscle pain or heaviness, thin, white, and greasy tongue coating, with or without a slippery and slow pulse.

Principles of Treatment:
Resolve cold-damp and harmonize the middle Jiao.

Herbal Treatment:
Huo Xiang Zheng Qi San-*Agastache Powder to Rectify the Qi.*

Huo Xiang *Herba Agastaches seu Pogostemi* 10 g
Pei Lan *Herba Eupatorii Fortunei* 10 g
Cang Zhu *Rhizoma Atractylodis* 10 g
Chen Pi *Pericarpium Citri Reticulatae* 5 g
Zhi Ban Xia *Rhizoma Pinelliae Ternatae Preparata* 10 g
Jie Geng *Radix Platycodi Grandiflori* 10 g
Fu Ling *Sclerotium Poriae Cocos* 12 g
Hou Po *Cortex Magnoliae Officinalis* 10 g
Sha Ren *Fructus Amomi* 3 g
Bai Dou Kou *Fructus Amomi Cardamomi* 3 g

Explanation:
- Huo Xiang and Pei Lan dispel cold-damp and resolve damp in the middle Jiao.

- Cang Zhu, Zhi Ban Xia and Chen Pi resolve damp in the middle Jiao and harmonize the spleen and stomach.
- Jie Geng and Zhi Ban Xia could eliminate phlegm in the lung and prevent coughing.
- Hou Po eliminates damp in the middle Jiao and resolves fullness in the abdomen and stomach.
- Fu Ling promotes urination to eliminate damp in the body and strengthens the zheng-qi.
- Sha Ren and Bai Dou Kou regulate the qi and eliminate the damp in the middle Jiao.

Modifications:
- In the case of an obvious heaviness of the body or body pain, add Qiang Huo *Rhizoma et Radix Notopterygii* 10 g and Du Huo *Radix Angelicae Pubescentis* 10 g to eliminate external damp and relieve the body pain.
- In the case of too much cough, add Zhi Ban Xia *Rhizoma Pinelliae Ternatae Preparata* 10 g and Zi Su Zi *Fructus Perillae Frutescentis* 10 g to eliminate phlegm and relieve the cough.
- In the case of obvious nausea and poor appetite, add Zi Su Ye *Folium Perillae Frutescentis* 10 g and Sheng Jiang *Rhizoma Zingiberis Officinalis Recens* 5 g to descend the stomach-qi and relieve nausea.
- In the case of excessive diarrhea, add Ge Gen *Radix Puerariae* 10 g to ascend the clear-yang and relieve diarrhea.

2.2.2.4 *Invasion of damp-heat to the middle Jiao*

Slightly poor appetite, loose stool, sometimes possible nausea, slight muscle pain or heaviness, slight red tongue, thin, yellow, and greasy tongue coating, with or without a slippery and rapid pulse.

Principles of Treatment:
Clear heat, dispel damp, and harmonize the middle Jiao.

Herbal Treatment:
Lian Po Yin-*Coptis and Magnolia Bark Drink.*

Huang Lian *Rhizoma Coptidis* 5 g
Dan Dou Chi *Semen Sojae Praeparatum* 10 g
Zhi Zi *Fructus Gardeniae Jasminoidis* 10 g
Hou Po *Cortex Magnoliae Officinalis* 10 g
Chang Pu *Rhizoma Acori Graminei* 10 g
Xing Ren *Semen Pruni Armeniacae* 10 g
Zhe Bei Mu *Bulbus Fritillariae Thunbergii* 10 g
Zhi Ban Xia *Rhizoma Pinelliae Ternatae Preparata* 10 g
Chen Pi *Pericarpium Citri Reticulatae* 5 g
Fu Ling *Sclerotium Poriae Cocos* 12 g

Explanation:
- Huang Lian, Dan Dou Chi, and Zhi Zi clear heat and resolve damp.
- Xing Ren, Zhe Bei Mu and Zhi Ban Xia protect the lung, eliminate phlegm in the lung and relieve the disturbance to the lung.
- Hou Po, Chen Pi and Chang Pu resolve the damp in the middle Jiao and relieve the fullness of the abdomen and stomach.
- Fu Ling promotes urination to eliminate damp in the damp and strengthens the zheng-qi.

Modifications:
- In the case of constant high fever, add Zhi Mu *Radix Anemarrhenae Asphodeloidis* 10 g to clear the heat and reduce the fever.
- In the case of excessive cough with yellow phlegm, add Huang Qin *Radix Scutellariae Baicalensis* 10 g to clear the heat, eliminate phlegm and relieve the cough.
- In the case of excessive white phlegm, add Zi Su Zi *Fructus Perillae Frutescentis* 10 g and Ting Li Zi *Semen Descurainiae seu Lepidii* 10 g to eliminate phlegm and stop the cough.

- In the case of too much diarrhea, add Che Qian Zi *Semen Plantaginis* 10 g and Ge Gen *Radix Puerariae* 10 g to eliminate damp-heat in the lower Jiao and relieve diarrhea.

2.2.2.5 *Deficiency of qi*

Slight tiredness, sweating easily, slightly poor appetite and sleepiness, possible lightness in the head or weakness of muscle, slight loose stool, thin and white tongue coating, with or without weak pulse.

Principles of Treatment:
Tonify the qi and strengthen the body.

Herbal Treatment:
Yu Ping Feng San-*Jade Windscreen Powder* and Si Jun Zi Tang-*Four Gentlemen Decoction.*

Zhi Huang Qi *Radix Astragali Membranacei Praeparata* 10 g
Dang Shen *Radix Codonopsis Pilosulae* 10 g
Fang Feng *Radix Ledebouriellae Divaricatae* 10 g
Jiao Bai Zhu *Rhizoma Atractylodis Macrocephalae (grill)* 10 g
Fu Ling *Sclerotium Poriae Cocos* 15 g
Zi Su Ye *Folium Perillae Frutescentis* 10 g
Jing Jie *Herba seu Flos Schizonepetae Tenuifoliae* 10 g
Jie Geng *Radix Platycodi Grandiflori* 10 g
Xing Ren *Semen Pruni Armeniacae* 10 g
Zhi Ban Xia *Rhizoma Pinelliae Ternatae Preparata* 10 g
Zhi Gan Cao *Radix Glycyrrhizae Preparata* 3 g

Explanation:
- Zhi Huang Qi, Fang Feng and Jiao Bai Zhu, the complete compositions of Yu Ping Feng San, are used to tonify the wei qi and strengthen the skin pores.

- Dang Shen, Fu Ling, and Zhi Gan Cao, together with Jiao Bai Zhu, the complete composition of Si Jun Zi Tang, tonify the qi of the spleen and stomach in general to improve the resistance to the pathogenic factors.
- Jing Jie, Zi Su Ye, together with Fang Feng are used to dispel wind and relieve any external symptoms.
- Jie Geng, Xing Ren and Zhi Ban Xia are used to dispel the lung-qi and eliminate phlegm in the lung, consequently protecting the physiological function of the lung.

Modifications:
- In the case of excessive white phlegm, add Zi Su Zi *Fructus Perillae Frutescentis* 10 g and Ting Li Zi *Semen Descurainiae seu Lepidii* 10 g to eliminate phlegm and stop cough.
- In the case of profuse cough with yellow phlegm, add Huang Qin *Radix Scutellariae Baicalensis* 10 g to clear the heat, eliminate phlegm and relieve the cough.
- In the case of poor appetite, add Shen Qu *Massa Medica Fermentata* 15 g and Ji Nei Jin *Endothelium Corneum Gigeriae Galli* 10 g to improve the appetite.
- In the case of excessive diarrhea, add Ge Gen *Radix Puerariae* 10 g to eliminate damp and relieve diarrhea.

2.2.3 Treatment according to constitutions

The following treatments are given to asymptomatic patients with no clinical signs at all. Since their infections have been confirmed by PCR and they are under a quarantine period, they should be supported according to their constitutions.

2.2.3.1 *Peace type*

This constitution has the following characteristics:

- a strong physique
- a moderate body posture

- good complexion
- energetic state
- well-proportioned body
- moisturized complexion, skin and lips
- shiny hair
- bright eyes
- able to smell and taste normally
- low fatigue levels
- good tolerance to cold and heat
- sleep well
- good appetite
- easy-going and cheerful personality
- strong ability to adapt to the natural and social environment
- normal tongue, tongue coating, and pulse

Principles of Treatment:
Strengthen the body and tonify the wei qi.

Herbal Treatment:
Yu Ping Feng San-*Jade Windscreen Powder.*

Zhi Huang Qi *Radix Astragali Membranacei Praeparata* 10 g
Fang Feng *Radix Ledebouriellae Divaricatae* 10 g
Jiao Bai Zhu *Rhizoma Atractylodis Macrocephalae (grill)* 10 g
Zi Su Ye *Folium Perillae Frutescentis* 10 g
Jing Jie *Herba seu Flos Schizonepetae Tenuifoliae* 10 g
Jie Geng *Radix Platycodi Grandiflori* 10 g
Xing Ren *Semen Pruni Armeniacae* 10 g
Zhi Gan Cao *Radix Glycyrrhizae Preparata* 3 g

Explanation:
- Zhi Huang Qi, Fang Feng and Jiao Bai Zhu, the complete compositions of Yu Ping Feng San, are used to tonify the wei qi and strengthen the skin pores.
- Zi Su Ye and Jing Jie, together with Fang Feng are used to dispel wind and relieve external invasion.

- Jie Geng and Xing Ren are used to dispel the lung-qi and eliminate phlegm in the lung so as to protect the physiological functions of the lung.

2.2.3.2 *Qi deficiency type*

This constitution has the following characteristics:

- general weakness
- thin or softness of the muscles
- myalgia
- weakness of limbs
- fatigue
- dyspnea
- no desire to talk or have a low voice
- spontaneous sweating or easy sweating
- catches the common cold frequently
- pale complexion
- poor vision
- pale lips
- thin or brittle hair
- dizziness
- forgetfulness
- normal or loose stool, or prolapse of rectum and internal organs
- normal or frequent urination
- introverted personality
- emotional instability or emotional exhaustion
- mental fog, timid and not adventurous
- intolerance of cold
- cold hands and feet
- pale and swollen tongue with teeth marks on the sides
- weak pulse

Principles of Treatment:
Activate the spleen and kidney and tonify qi.

Herbal Treatment:
Si Jun Zi Tang-*Four Gentlemen Decoction.*

Ren Shen *Radix Ginseng* 10 g
Bai Zhu *Rhizoma Atractylodis Macrocephalae* 10 g
Shan Yao *Radix Dioscoreae Oppositae* 10 g
Fu Ling *Sclerotium Poriae Cocos* 12 g
Zhi Huang Qi *Radix Astragali Membranacei Praeparata* 10 g
Dang Gui *Radix Angelicae Sinensis* 10 g
Jing Jie *Herba seu Flos Schizonepetae Tenuifoliae* 10 g
Fang Feng *Radix Ledebouriellae Divaricatae* 10 g
Zi Su Ye *Folium Perillae Frutescentis* 10 g
Jie Geng *Radix Platycodi Grandiflori* 10 g
Xing Ren *Semen Pruni Armeniacae* 10 g
Zhi Gan Cao *Radix Glycyrrhizae Preparata* 3 g

Explanation:
- Ren Shen, Bai Zhu, Fu Ling and Zhi Gan Cao, the complete composition of Si Jun Zi Tang, are used to activate the spleen and stomach and to promote the production of qi.
- Huang Qi raises the qi and tonify the qi of the middle Jiao and relieves the tiredness. When Huang Qi, Bai Zhu and Fang Feng are used together, they can also strengthen the skin and improve the wei qi, which is very important to improve the resistance to fight against a common cold.
- Shan Yao tonifies the qi, benefits the kidney and reinforces the jing.
- Since qi and blood share a good relationship between each other and when there is a deficiency of qi, there would be a deficiency of blood to a certain degree. Thus, Dang Gui is used to benefit the jing and tonify the blood.
- Zi Su Ye, Jing Jie and Fang Feng, are used to dispel wind and relieve external invasion.

- Jie Geng and Xing Ren are used to dispel the lung-qi and eliminate phlegm in the lung, in order to protect the physiological function of the lung.

2.2.3.3 *Yang deficiency type*

This constitution has the following characteristics:

- aversion to cold
- sensitivity to cold weather
- cold hands and feet
- preference for warm food and drinks
- lack of energy
- excessive sleep
- pale complexion and lips
- darkness of lower eyelid
- hair loss
- easy sweating
- loose stool
- clear and profuse urine
- nycturia
- impotence
- frigidity
- water retention
- edema
- pale tongue, thin and white coating
- thready, deep, and slow pulse

Principles of Treatment:
Tonify the yang and dispel the cold.

Herbal Treatment:
Da Bu Yuan Jian-*Great Tonify the Primal Decoction.*

Shu Di Huang *Radix Rhemanniae Glutinosae Praeparata* 12 g
Ren Shen *Radix Ginseng* 6 g

Gou Qi Zi *Fructus Lycii* 10 g
Shan Zhu Yu *Fructus Corni Officinalis* 10 g
Shan Yao *Radix Dioscoreae Oppositae* 10 g
Dang Gui *Radix Angelicae Sinensis* 10 g
Du Zhong *Cortex Eucommiae Ulmoidis* 10 g
Jing Jie *Herba seu Flos Schizonepetae Tenuifoliae* 10 g
Fang Feng *Radix Ledebouriellae Divaricatae* 10 g
Zi Su Ye *Folium Perillae Frutescentis* 10 g
Jie Geng *Radix Platycodi Grandiflori* 10 g
Xing Ren *Semen Pruni Armeniacae* 10 g
Zhi Gan Cao *Radix Glycyrrhizae Preparata* 3 g

Explanation:
- Shu Di Huang, Shan Yao, Shan Zhu Yu and Gou Qi Zi are used to tonify the kidney-qi and benefit the jing.
- Du Zhong reinforces the yang of the kidney and dispels the cold. It can also strengthen the lower back to relieve lower back pain and weakness.
- Ren Shen and Dang Gui tonify the qi and blood, so as to improve the zheng-qi in general.
- Zi Su Ye, Jing Jie and Fang Feng are used to dispel wind and relieve external invasion.
- Jie Geng and Xing Ren are used to dispel the lung-qi and eliminate phlegm in the lung, so as to protect the physiological function of the lung.
- Zhi Gan Cao regulates the formula and tonifies the qi of the body.

2.2.3.4 *Yin deficiency type*

This constitution has the following characteristics:

- thin body
- warm or hot hands and feet
- restlessness
- dry mouth, throat and lips

- occasionally dry eyes
- thirsty
- dry stool
- dizziness
- tinnitus
- insomnia
- night sweating
- small and red tongue, with scanty coating or peeled coating
- thready, deep, and rapid pulse

Principles of Treatment:
Nourish the yin, clear the deficient heat, and benefit the kidney.

Herbal Treatment:
Liu Wei Di Huang Wan-*Six-Ingredient Pill with Rehmannia.*

Shu Di Huang *Radix Rhemanniae Glutinosae Praeparata* 12 g
Shan Zhu Yu *Fructus Corni Officinalis* 10 g
Shan Yao *Radix Dioscoreae Oppositae* 10 g
Gou Qi Zi *Fructus Lycii* 10 g
Wu Wei Zi *Fructus Schisandrae Chinensis* 10 g
Mai Men Dong *Tuber Ophiopogonis Japonici* 10 g
Jing Jie *Herba seu Flos Schizonepetae Tenuifoliae* 10 g
Fang Feng *Radix Ledebouriellae Divaricatae* 10 g
Zi Su Ye *Folium Perillae Frutescentis* 10 g
Jie Geng *Radix Platycodi Grandiflori* 10 g
Xing Ren *Semen Pruni Armeniacae* 10 g

Explanation:
- Shu Di Huang, Shan Yao, and Shan Zhu Yu are used to tonify the kidney and benefit the jing.
- Gou Qi Zi, Mai Men Dong and Wu Wei Zi tonify the Yin and benefit the body fluid.
- Zi Su Ye, Jing Jie and Fang Feng are used to dispel wind and relieve external invasion.

- Jie Geng and Xing Ren are used to dispel the lung-qi and eliminate phlegm in the lung so as to protect the physiological function of the lung.

2.2.3.5 *Phlegm-damp type*

This constitution has the following characteristics:

- obesity
- swollen abdomen
- fullness in the stomach
- greasy skin
- often cough with expectoration of phlegm
- loose stool, sticky stool on the toilet
- indulgence in sweet or fatty food
- sticky or sweet feeling in the mouth, or poor appetite
- sleepiness
- lassitude
- uncomfortable body weight
- swollen tongue, white and greasy tongue coating
- slippery pulse

Principles of Treatment:
Activate the spleen and stomach and resolve the damp.

Herbal Treatment:
Ping Wei San-*Calm the Stomach Powder, plus*
Er Chen Tang-*Decoction of Two Old (Cured) Drugs.*

Cang Zhu *Rhizoma Atractylodis* 10 g
Hou Po *Cortex Magnoliae Officinalis* 10 g
Chen Pi *Pericarpium Citri Reticulatae* 5 g
Qing Pi *Pericarpium Citri Reticulatae Viride* 10 g
Zhi Ke *Fructus Citri Aurantii* 10 g
Zhi Ban Xia *Rhizoma Pinelliae Ternatae Preparata* 10 g

Fu Ling *Sclerotium Poriae Cocos* 10 g
Jing Jie *Herba seu Flos Schizonepetae Tenuifoliae* 10 g
Fang Feng *Radix Ledebouriellae Divaricatae* 10 g
Zi Su Zi *Fructus Perillae Frutescentis* 10 g
Jie Geng *Radix Platycodi Grandiflori* 10 g
Xing Ren *Semen Pruni Armeniacae* 10 g

Explanation:
- Cang Zhu, Hou Po and Zhi Ban Xia eliminate damp and resolve phlegm.
- Qing Pi, Chen Pi and Zhi Ke eliminate damp and promote the qi circulation and relieve the fullness of the abdomen caused by damp accumulation.
- Fu Ling activates the spleen and stomach and eliminates damp.
- Jing Jie and Fang Feng are used to dispel wind and relieve external invasion.
- Jie Geng and Xing Ren are used to dispel the lung-qi and eliminate phlegm in the lung so as to protect the physiological function of the lung.

2.2.3.6 *Damp-heat type*

This constitution has the following characteristics:

- greasy and warm skin, prone to acne or skin infection
- heaviness of the body
- bitter taste in the mouth
- poor appetite, nausea
- halitosis
- diarrhea with burning sensation
- restlessness
- deep yellow urine
- leukorrhea
- red tongue, yellow and greasy coating
- slippery and rapid pulse

Principles of Treatment:
Clear the heat, eliminate damp, and remove the toxins.

Herbal Treatment:
Lian Po Yin-*Coptis and Magnolia Bark Drink.*

Huang Lian *Rhizoma Coptidis* 5 g
Hou Po *Cortex Magnoliae Officinalis* 10 g
Zhi Ban Xia *Rhizoma Pinelliae Ternatae Preparata* 10 g
Zhi Zi *Fructus Gardeniae Jasminoidis* 10 g
Shi Chang Pu *Rhizoma Acori Graminei* 10 g
Dou Chi *Semen Sojae Praeparatum* 10 g
Lu Gen *Rhizoma Phragmitis Communis* 10 g
Huang Qin *Radix Scutellariae Baicalensis* 10 g
Lian Qiao *Fructus Forsythiae Suspensae* 10 g
Jie Geng *Radix Platycodi Grandiflori* 10 g
Xing Ren *Semen Pruni Armeniacae* 10 g

Explanation:
- Lian Po Yin is applied to clear the heat, eliminate damp, resolve disharmony in the middle Jiao and benefit the stomach. This formula is good to eliminate damp-heat in the middle Jiao and of course, it has a weak function to dispel external invasion.
- Huang Qin and Lian Qiao are added into the prescription to dispel wind-heat and relieve toxins.
- Jie Geng and Xing Ren are used to disperse the lung-qi and descend the lung-qi so as to protect the physiological function of the lung.

2.2.3.7 *Qi stagnation type*

This constitution has the following characteristics:

- long-term unsatisfactory emotions
- introverted personality
- sensitivity and suspicious

- depression
- headache
- fullness of the chest and abdomen
- belching
- poor appetite
- hypochondriac pain and distention
- insomnia
- cyst in the breast
- painful and irregular menstruation
- a thin and white coating
- a wiry pulse

Principles of Treatment:
Emotional balance, promote the qi circulation, and relieve qi stagnation.

Herbal Treatment:
Xiao Yao San-*Rambling Powder.*

Chai Hu *Radix Bupleuri* 10 g
Bai Shao Yao *Radix Paeoniae Lactiflorae* 10 g
Dang Gui *Radix Angelicae Sinensis* 10 g
Zhi Ke *Fructus Citri Aurantii* 10 g
Xiang Fu *Rhizoma Cyperi Rotundi* 10 g
Chen Pi *Pericarpium Citri Reticulatae* 5 g
Qing Pi *Pericarpium Citri Reticulatae Viride* 5 g
Jing Jie *Herba seu Flos Schizonepetae Tenuifoliae* 10 g
Fang Feng *Radix Ledebouriellae Divaricatae* 10 g
Zi Su Zi *Fructus Perillae Frutescentis* 10 g
Jie Geng *Radix Platycodi Grandiflori* 10 g
Xing Ren *Semen Pruni Armeniacae* 10 g

Explanation:
- Chai Hu and Bao Shao Yao smooth the liver and regulate the qi in the liver.

- The liver is the organ, which is called a yin organ with a yang activity. Dang Gui benefits the liver blood and promotes blood circulation so as to relieve the spasm in the liver due to liver-qi stagnation.
- Zhi Ke and Xiang Fu promote the qi circulation and relieve the fullness in the abdomen.
- Chen Pi and Qing Pi are used to promote the qi circulation and eliminate damp due to the stagnation of qi.
- Jing Jie and Fang Feng are used to dispel wind and relieve external invasion.
- Jie Geng and Xing Ren are used to dispel the lung-qi and eliminate phlegm in the lung so as to protect the physiological function of the lung.

2.2.3.8 *Blood stasis type*

This constitution has the following characteristics:

- dull or purplish complexion
- dark skin, or hyperpigmentation
- prone to ecchymosis
- prone to pain
- dull or purple lips
- dull tongue
- dysmenorrhea
- amenorrhea, multiple clots in the menstrual blood, or the menstrual color is purple and black
- uterine bleeding, or bleeding tendency
- vomiting blood
- stabbing pain somewhere in the body
- thin and white coating, purplish tongue or purplish vein under the tongue
- thready and unsmooth pulse

Principles of Treatment:
Promote the qi and blood circulation, eliminate blood stasis, and relieve the pain.

Herbal Treatment:
Tao Hong Si Wu Tang-*Four Substance (Things) Decoction with Safflower and Peach Pit.*

Tao Ren *Semen Pruni Persicae* 10 g
Hong Hua *Flos Carthami Tinctorii* 10 g
Dang Gui *Radix Angelicae Sinensis* 10 g
Chuan Xiong *Radix Ligustici Wallichii* 10 g
Chi Shao Yao *Radix Paeoniae Rubrae* 10 g
Shu Di Huang *Radix Rhemanniae Glutinosae Praeparata* 10 g
Yu Jin *Tuber Curcumae* 10 g
Pu Huang *Pollen Typhae* 10 g
Jing Jie *Herba seu Flos Schizonepetae Tenuifoliae* 10 g
Fang Feng *Radix Ledebouriellae Divaricatae* 10 g
Jie Geng *Radix Platycodi Grandiflori* 10 g
Xing Ren *Semen Pruni Armeniacae* 10 g

Explanation:
- Tao Hong Si Wu Tang is a typical herbal formula to promote blood circulation and eliminate blood stasis without harming the blood.
- However, this formula is not so strong to eliminate blood stasis. Pu Huang and Yu Jin are added to promote blood circulation, eliminate blood stasis, and relieve the pain.
- Jing Jie and Fang Feng are used to dispel wind and relieve external invasion.
- Jie Geng and Xing Ren are used to dispel the lung-qi and eliminate phlegm in the lung, in order to protect the physiological function of the lung.

2.2.3.9 *Special hereditary quality type*

This constitution has the following characteristics:

- no special features, deformities, or congenital physical defects
- hereditary diseases with possible mental disturbance
- prone to drug allergies and hay fever

- poor adaptability to the external environment
- intolerance of wind and cold
- comorbidities
- irritable, impatient, forgetfulness
- prone from bleeding
- epilepsy, stroke, chest pain, and other disease

Principles of Treatment:
Strengthen the constitution, eliminate pathological changes, and restore physiological functions.

Since there are various kind of patterns related to this type, treatment and herbal formulas should be given accordingly by adding certain herbs to relieve the external invasion and protect the physiological functions of the lung. These herbs can be the same as the herbs used above, including Jing Jie *Herba seu Flos Schizonepetae Tenuifoliae*, Fang Feng *Radix Ledebouriellae Divaricatae*, Jie Geng *Radix Platycodi Grandiflori*, and Xing Ren *Semen Pruni Armeniacae*, etc.

3

TCM Treatment of Early Symptoms of COVID-19

3.1 TCM Analysis of Early Symptoms of COVID-19

The SARS-CoV-2 virus is the virus strain that causes the severe acute respiratory syndrome. It is contagious in humans, and the World Health Organization (WHO) has designated the ongoing pandemic of COVID-19 a Public Health Emergency of International Concern, and new outbreaks can emerge rapidly.[1-3]

In terms of the contagious capacity of SARS-CoV-2, Wölfel *et al.* have done some scientific research and pointed out that SARS took 7–10 days after onset until peak RNA concentrations (of up to 5×10^5 copies per swab) were reached. In the present study, peak concentrations were reached before day five, and were more than 1,000 times higher. Extended tissue tropism of SARS-CoV-2 with replication in the throat is strongly supported by the studies of sgRNA-transcribing cells in throat swab samples, particularly during the first five days of developing symptoms. Critically, the majority of patients in the present study seemed to be already beyond their shedding peak in upper respiratory tract samples when first tested, while shedding of

---

[1] World Health Organization (WHO). WHO Director-General's opening remarks at the media briefing on COVID-19—11 March 2020. (Press Release) 11 March 2020. Archived from the original on 11 March 2020. Retrieved 12 March 2020.
[2] Sui-Lee Wee, *et al.* WHO declares global emergency as Wuhan coronavirus spreads. *The New York Times.* 30 January 2020. https://www.nytimes.com/2020/01/30/health/coronavirus-world-health-organization.html.
[3] Jasper Fuk-Woo Chan, *et al. op. cit.*

infectious virus in sputum continued through the first week of symptoms. Based on the present findings, early discharge with ensuing home isolation could be chosen for patients who are beyond day ten of symptoms with less than 100,000 viral RNA copies per ml of sputum. These research results were published online on "Nature" on 1 April 2020.[4]

Although comprehensive testing is key to confirm COVID-19, which plays an extreme role in the decision on quarantine procedures and treatment as soon as possible, it is, on the other hand, almost impossible for most of the countries to currently carry out this technique thoroughly due to various reasons. Iceland is the only exception as the government allows everyone in the country to be tested for the virus. The government says it spent years perfecting its approach.[5]

It therefore appears that it is more important to have full awareness of the early symptoms of COVID-19 infection, so that we avoid the risk of spreading it to a wider scale in a more proactive and health monitoring sense, apart from the common methods introduced by most countries like social distancing and self-isolating. Most of the countries in the world remain conservative on whether to receive a proper medical treatment with the infection in the early stage. Apparently, identification and understanding of the early symptoms could determine how well the whole world copes with the outbreak and could help provide accurate information for healthcare and prevention strategies.

3.1.1 Manifestations of early symptoms of COVID-19 infection

While the COVID-19 pandemic is still spreading fast across the world, it has only been a time span of four months since it was first

---

[4]Roman Wölfel. Virological assessment of hospitalized patients with COVID-2019. *Nature.* 2020, 581: 465–469.

[5]Kelly McLaughlin. Iceland is allowing everyone in the country to be tested for the coronavirus. The government says it spent years perfecting its approach. *Insider.* 2 April 2020. https://www.businessinsider.com/iceland-coronavirus-pandemic-approach-could-help-other-countries-2020-4?r=US&IR=T.

identified and announced to the public in December 2019 by China. We, as humans, still have very little knowledge about the virus. Now it becomes essential that once we can identify the early symptoms of the infection, we target it with immediate tailored treatment, inhibiting further progression of the infection and reducing the activity of the virus replication. By doing so, it can be expected that the impact of the infection could be greatly reduced. Since the list of most commonly reported symptoms on COVID-19 patients across the world during this pandemic is still incomplete and ongoing, we searched through the published literature globally and attempted to give the TCM's in-depth insight on it.

It is still a long time before people are fully aware of Long COVID being associated with early symptoms. Our study indicates that the relevant symptoms include not only the commonly recognized ones, like fever and respiratory manifestations or the major flu-related symptoms, but also some digestive, urological, physical, mental and musculoskeletal issues. On top of that, other less identifiable symptoms like anosmia, ageusia, skin rash, chilblain-like wound, eye irritations and different levels of nervous system impairments may be involved too. Although there is a lack of inner logic connection between each individual symptom in the western context, these clinical manifestations have various underlying mechanisms in TCM.

Regarding the early symptoms, different countries take a different approach towards it. In the UK, the NHS still insists on its website that only fever, cough and difficulty breathing are the key symptoms of COVID-19 infection. Only if a patient presents the above symptoms will NHS medical professionals consider admitting the patient for COVID-19 test and hospital treatments. This method has completely excluded all other mild symptoms on the early stage of the infection, which in our opinion, may greatly contribute to the consequence that the UK is among those holding the highest COVID-19 casualty alongside the US as of 24 April 2020, with 18,738 deaths, reaching the fifth highest in the world.[6]

---

[6]Worldometer COVID-19 data. https://www.worldometers.info/coronavirus/about.

In comparison, the US National Centre for Disease Control and Prevention (CDC), pays higher attention to patients whose symptoms appear 2 to 14 days after exposure to the virus, including fever, cough, shortness of breath or difficulty breathing, chills, repeated shaking with chills, muscle pain, headache, sore throat, the new loss of taste or smell.[7]

Medical researchers are taking a more systematic view of the complexity of the virus. Hussin A. Rothan summarized that the symptoms of COVID-19 infection appear after an incubation period of approximately 5.2 days. The period from the onset of COVID-19 symptoms to death ranged from 6 to 41 days with a median of 14 days.

It lists two groups of symptoms:

1. Systematic disorders: Fever, cough, fatigue, sputum production, headache; haemoptysis, acute cardiac injury, hypoxemia, dyspnea, lymphopenia, diarrhea.
2. Respiratory disorders: Rhinorrhea, sneezing, sore throat; pneumonia, ground-glass opacities; RNA anemia, acute respiratory distress syndrome.

The chapter particularly pointed out that COVID-19 infection presented more symptoms of gastrointestinal symptoms like diarrhea than other coronavirus like SARS-CoV and MERS-CoV. This shows that digestive and urinary symptoms with COVID-19 infection need more attention.[8]

However, these are not sufficient to cover all the symptoms especially in the very early stage of the infection, as we are fighting against an intense battle against the progress of the virus. As the pandemic develops, there are increasingly more discoveries on potential symptoms and signs of the infection being reported across the world

---

[7]Centers for Disease Control and Prevention (CDC). Symptoms of COVID-19. Updated 22 February 2021. https://www.cdc.gov/coronavirus/2019-ncov/symptoms-testing/symptoms.html.

[8]Hussin A. Rothan, *et al.* The epidemiology and pathogenesis of coronavirus disease (COVID-19) outbreak. *Journal of Autoimmunity.* May 2020, 109: 102433. Published online 26 February 2020. doi: 10.1016/j.jaut.2020.102433.

since its global outbreak. It is worth mentioning that some of these newly-reported COVID-19 symptoms are not widely identified and reported in China. The reason for the difference between China and the other countries is worth discussing in the future.

The New York Times reported doctors from different countries with a surge in COVID-19 cases, including South Korea, Italy, Germany, UK, and US. The report urged for doctors to screen patients with symptoms such as loss of sense of smell and taste, even those with no noticeable nasal congestion. The percentage of the presence of anosmia among the COVID-19 positive patients is between 30–59% according to different research.[9,10] Loss of taste or smell appeared around 24–72 hours before more typical symptoms, such as fever.[11]

Some patients also reported rash like frostbite or toes turning blue/purple in Italy, Spain and the Middle East.[12,13] But the percentage of skin rash occurrence on COVID-19 positive patients shows a big difference between the studies of China and the other countries, with western countries being much higher.[14]

---

[9]Roni Caryn Rabin. Lost sense of smell may be peculiar clue to coronavirus infection. *The New York Times*. 22 March 2020. https://www.nytimes.com/2020/03/22/health/coronavirus-symptoms-smell-taste.html?_ga=2.188496424.1813510712.1587638610-1648265835.1587638610.

[10]Cristina Menni, *et al.* Loss of smell and taste in combination with other symptoms is a strong predictor of COVID-19 infection. *MedRxiv*. 2020. https://doi.org/10.1101/2020.04.05.20048421.

[11]Luigi A. Vaira, *et al.* Anosmia and ageusia: Common findings in COVID-19 patients. *Laryngoscope*. 2020, 130(7): 1787. doi: 10.1002/lary.28692.

[12]Enrique D Fernandez-Nieto, *et al.* Comment on: Cutaneous manifestations in COVID-19: A first perspective. Safety concerns of clinical images and skin biopsies. *Journal of the European Academy of Dermatology and Venereology*. 2020, 34(6): e252–e254. doi: 10.1111/jdv.16470.

[13]Anwaar Alramthan, *et al.* A case of COVID-19 presenting in clinical picture resembling chilblains disease. First report from the Middle East. *Clinical and Experimental Dermatology*. 2020, 45(6). doi: 10.1111/ced.14243.

[14]Antoine Mahe, *et al.* A distinctive skin rash associated with coronavirus disease 2019. *Journal of the European Academy of Dermatology and Venereology*. 2020, 34, e241–290. doi: 10.1111/jdv.16471.

Skin changes can be found throughout the whole process of COVID-19 infections. Furthermore, Magro *et al.* (2020) studied five cases of severe COVID-19 associated respiratory failure, of which three had a purpuric skin rash, and pointed out the potential key role of microvascular injury and thrombosis in the pathogenesis of COVID-19.[15]

There were also reports of red and irritated eyes in some cases. Cheema *et al.* (2020) reported the first case of COVID-associated keratoconjunctivitis in North America, presenting red eyes and watery eye discharge without any fever and respiratory symptoms.[16]

The damages and impact of COVID-19 on the nervous system and particularly the brain is also raising people's concerns. There have been very little and scattered published articles on the relevant CNS (Central Nerve System) symptoms on COVID-19 cases, although signs like nausea, headache and vomiting are commonly recorded on patients. In a review, Asadi-Pooya *et al.* (2020) quoted that about 25% of the COVID-19 infected patients present CNS manifestations.[17] Nonetheless, a study on 214 COVID-19 infected patients in China showed that 36.4% of them displayed neurological symptoms, including CNS manifestations like dizziness, headaches, impaired consciousness, acute cerebro-vascular disease, ataxia, seizures, and peripheral manifestations like taste and smell impairment, vision impairment, neuralgia as well as musculoskeletal injury.[18] To add some more evidence between COVID-19 and CNS impairment, a team led

---

[15] Cynthia Magro, *et al.* Complement associated microvascular injury and thrombosis in the pathogenesis of severe COVID-19 infection: A report of five cases. *Translational Research: The Journal of Laboratory and Clinical Medicine.* 2020, 220: 1–13. doi: 10.1016/j.trsl.2020.04.007.

[16] Marvi Cheema, *et al.* Keratoconjunctivitis as the initial medical presentation of the novel coronavirus disease 2019 (COVID-19). *Canadian Journal of Ophthalmology.* 2020, 55(4): E125–E129. doi: 10.1016/j.jcjo.2020.03.003.

[17] Ali A. Asadi-Pooya, *et al.* Central nervous system manifestations of COVID-19: A systematic review. *Journal of the Neurological Sciences.* 2020, 413: 116832. doi: 10.1016/j.jns.2020.116832.

[18] Kevin Roe. Explanation for COVID-19 infection neurological damage and reactivations. *Transboundary and Emerging Diseases.* 2020, 67: 1414–1415. doi: 10.1111/tbed.13594.

by Dr. Oxley in the Department of Neurosurgery, Mount Sinai Health System, New York, investigated five cases of large vessel stroke over a two-week period in COVID-19 patients under 50 with either no or mild COVID-19 symptoms. This represents a seven-fold increase in what would normally be expected, and the relevant article will be published online at the end of April in *The New England Journal of Medicine*, says the *Medscape Medical News*.[19] This study provides a clue implying that COVID-19 may attack large vessels in the younger population to cause thrombosis and clotting at an early stage of the infection. However, it is still early to conclude that COVID-19 leads to a higher risk of stroke in the early stage of the infection.[20]

These reports from all over the world, from the view of Western medicine, reflect a broad variety of different clinical symptoms on different anatomic systems. However due to the limitation on the scale and quantity of observations by individual clinicians in different countries and regions, these symptoms represent some level of similarity and coincidence. Each symptom identified is still lacking strong supporting evidence in connection with certain pathogenesis, in terms of when and why they show on one patient but not on the others. Therefore, it will be very helpful if we can find a new viewing point to understand this disease.

3.1.2 TCM's mechanisms on early symptoms of COVID-19 infection

In fact, TCM has a much more logical line of insight on these seemingly random and scattered manifestations, that all these clinical manifestations have various intersecting and underlying mechanisms. TCM treatment is thus totally established based upon these understandings.

---

[19]Damian McNamara. COVID-19 linked to large vessel stroke in young adults. *Medscape*. 24 April 2020. https://www.medscape.com/viewarticle/929345.

[20]Libin. We have a deeper understanding of response strategies—Academician Tong Xiaolin "interprets" the TCM treatment plan in the "New Coronavirus Pneumonia Diagnosis and Treatment Plan" (Trial Fourth Edition). *Xinhua Net* (新华网). 28 January 2020. http://www.xinhuanet.com/2020-01/28/c_1125508711.htm.

In general, when the EPF (external pathogenic factors) enter the body, they develop and progress following certain patterns, rarely involving multiple internal organs and channels at the same time. As a result, well-trained TCM practitioners could easily and promptly identify these external symptoms and signs associated with the relevant patterns. However, when it comes to a pandemic EPF, even though it appears as an external invasion pattern at the start, the pathogenic factors can rapidly fall into multiple internal organ and system disorders, creating a mixture of complications involving multiple malfunctions. COVID-19 is a live example.

Coronavirus pneumonia, for starters, presents a typical pattern of cold-damp with evil toxins. Since it is a mixture of external pathogenic factors, coronavirus inevitably shares some features of external symptoms and signs, laying a solid foundation for a treatment principle to dispel and eliminate the external evils.

When studying this disease, it will be interesting to start by looking into the climate of Wuhan, when COVID-19 first broke out in December 2019. The local weather was very rainy and wet, with an average temperature higher than previous records of winters, with not much sunlight. Reviews on tongue images of patients with COVID-19 also show the similarity of a white and greasy coating—and some of them, not many—have a yellow thick and greasy coating. This confirms the presence of cold and damp, especially at the beginning of its infection.[21]

Taking all the early symptoms listed above into consideration, TCM's understanding of the development of EFP invasion shows a perfect insight. 《Simple Question-Chapter 63》: "when an evil settles in the physical appearance, it will first lodge in the skin and its hair. It stays there and does not leave. Then it enters more deeply and lodges in the tertiary vessels (*sun mai*). It stays there and does not leave. Then it enters further and lodges in the network vessels (*luo mai*). It stays there and does not leave. Then it enters further and lodges in the conduit vessels (*jing mai,* channels). It then links up with the five depots (*wu zang,* internal yin organs) internally and

---

[21] Cristina Menni, *et al. op. cit.*

spreads into the Intestines and the stomach. With both the yin and the yang (regions/channels) being affected, the five depots (*wu zang, internal yin organs*) will be harmed".

This chapter provides a clear clue of the mechanisms of evil EPF's invasion into the body:

- EPF first enters the body on stage one via skin and the cutaneous section to disturb the wei-qi level.
- EPF then lodges into the channel and collateral vessel level in stage two. Because the cutaneous section belongs to the jing-luo complex system, it is clear that stage one and two are both the disorders on the channel system—a superficial level of disorder. Regarding invasion on these two early stages, if a tailored treatment to dispel and eliminate the EPF from the channel system can be applied promptly, it will cease or at least slow down the further development of the invasion, and this is the importance of our emphasis on the early intervention on COVID-19 infections.
- The invasion ends in stage three, after affecting the stomach and Intestines. The invasion settles finally in the five *yin* organs (*wu zang*) and damage of five *yin* organs, leading to more severe systematic illness.

However, when considering its epidemic character, it is important to emphasize that COVID-19, although bearing the nature of external cold-damp factors, is not the same type of "cold" or "flu" that we encounter in everyday clinical practice. It occurs and progresses extremely fast, in an unusual, unpredictable, and hard to control pattern, involving much higher mortality than usual. Many patients with severe cases could face death within 20 days from the beginning when early symptoms appear. Therefore TCM calls it *"han shi yi* (寒湿疫)", the term y*i* (疫) means "plague" and "epidemic". "Evil toxins" is the name we give to describe another aspect of its pathogenesis. Due to the nature of the evil toxins mixed with cold-damp, y*i*, the plague enters the body quickly, develops, and changes rapidly. Sometimes it can even skip the first two stages and collapse into stage three within a very short period, affecting organs that present symptoms of a mixture of cold-damp and toxic heat.

Consequently, it becomes even more crucial that identifying and acknowledging the first two earliest stages and properly applying relevant tailored preventive intervention is the key to win the battle in fighting this infective viral illness.

Based on the three yang and three yin channel system, *Shang Han Lun's* six channel differentiation provides a great approach in analyzing COVID-19 pathogenesis. Especially when we look at the early symptoms of it, differentiation of the three-*yang*-channel enables us to have a broader view to link together all those scattered symptoms in the early stage of the infection. Three *yang*-channel-system represents the individual channels of six *yang* organs (*liu fu*), laying on the outer side of the body, which serve as the defending front line against the external invasion. Illnesses of the three-yang channel system manifest two aspects of the disorders:

- The symptoms on body parts and areas along with the distribution of the relevant channels.
- The malfunction symptoms of the relevant *yang* organs.
- The three-*yang*-channel system clearly draws a line on the process of external invasion between stages one, two and three in which the internal yin organs are affected and harmed. In other words, stage three represents the three-*yin*-channel system that is stated in *Shang Han Lun*.

In addition, invasion can attack one or a cluster of several channels, and the *yin yang* internal-external paired channels tend to have patterns with more direct interlapping influence on each other in the process of the epidemic infection, which happens very frequently with the COVID-19 pandemic. This all adds more complexity to the disease.

3.1.3 Six channel differentiations

Following are the six channel differentiations related to the COVID-19 early-stage symptoms.

3.1.3.1 *Taiyang channel syndrome*

Aversion to cold, slight fever, headache, runny nose, loss of smell, neck pain, muscle pain or stiffness of the muscles, dry cough, tickling throat, a thin, white and greasy coating, a superficial and slippery pulse, etc.

In COVID-19 cases, we saw a lot of patients with pain at the forehead (close to Ex-Yintang) and the top of head, and often with upper or middle back pain as the very early symptoms. Watery eyes and urinary dysfunction can be related to Taiyang syndrome too.

3.1.3.2 *Taiyang and Yangming channel syndrome*

Next to Taiyang's symptoms (slight aversion to cold, high fever, headache, neck pain, muscle pain, cough), carrying a mixed nature of damp, cold, and toxic heat can present two types of symptoms:

- Damp is related to vomiting, diarrhea with pungent smell, and fatigue.
- Toxic heat is related to fever, red face, restlessness, insomnia, constipation, yellow and dry coating on the tongue, and a rapid and forceful pulse.

In COVID-19 cases, we saw patients with the sudden loss of smell or taste, purple toes or chilblain patches appearing on regions where the stomach and large intestine meridians distribute. Because of Yangming-Taiyin lung inter-connection, it is common to see patients presenting skin rashes in the early stage, as well as blisters under the damp category. It is worth mentioning that the further development of Yangming heat from skin can invade into the blood. Furthermore, it may end in Kawasaki disease, where inflammation on blood vessels and the heart are widely involved (this is classified as Shaoyin or Jueyin *yin* depleted complication, as a later stage pattern).

3.1.3.3 *Taiyang and Shaoyang channel syndrome*

Patients present an aversion to cold and fever, headache, neck pain, muscle pain or stiffness of the muscles, cough with the fullness of chest, bitter taste in the mouth, poor appetite, depressive, sore and dryness in the throat, vomiting, ataxia, a thin, yellow, and greasy coating on the tongue, and a wiry and slippery pulse.

In COVID-19 cases, we often see patients with neck and shoulder pains, temporal headaches with repetitive patterns of fever, red eyes or eye irritations, and disturbance. Blockage energy in Shaoyang can cause chest tightness and palpitation too.

3.1.3.4 *Taiyang, Yangming and Shaoyang channel syndrome*

Patients present an aversion to cold, slight fever, headache, neck pain, muscle pain or stiffness of the muscles, cough, redness of the face, sore throat, bitter taste in the mouth, a white and greasy/yellow and greasy coating on the tongue, and a rapid and slippery pulse.

Obviously, this is a combination of all the three yang-channel syndromes, usually an extensive development of the previous three patterns. We should take some measures to prevent the aggravation of above conditions.

As mentioned above, we frequently see yin yang complex patterns in COVID-19 patients in the early stage of contacting the virus, as the evil EPF develops much faster. The most common combined yin yang patterns are listed below.

3.1.3.5 *Taiyang and Taiyin channel syndrome*

Patients present a slight aversion to cold, little fever, headache, muscle pain, cough, sore throat, tiredness, the fullness of the abdomen with slight pain, lack of taste, poor appetite, loose stools or less pungent diarrhea, weakness of the muscle, pale tongue with a white and greasy coating, and a thin, weak, and slippery pulse.

With the involvement of damp and a weakened Taiyin spleen, patients present much more noticeable fatigue with the heaviness of the body, cold limbs, and stronger, longer-lasting loss of appetite, or even anosmia.

3.1.3.6 *Taiyang and Shaoyin channel syndrome*

Patients present an aversion to cold, no fever, headache, cough, throat pain, cold and purple hands and feet, extreme tiredness, somnolence, weak heartbeat, semi-consciousness, a pale and wet coating on the tongue, and a thin, slow, and weak pulse.

With the involvement of cold and a weakened Shaoyin kidney and heart, patients present much more noticeable low spirit, lethargy, purple lips, and palpitation with mild exertion. Besides, the involvement of toxic heat can damage the Shaoyin channel and cause yin depletion, featuring deep red skin rash or bleeding complications, although this is usually a later stage condition not covered completely in this article. At this complex state, it could manifest into a critical condition soon. Therefore, urgent attention is needed once this complex pattern is identified.

In addition to the six-channel differentiation by *Shang Han Lun*, *zang-fu* differentiation may give a more detailed analysis of stage three development. It mainly involves the three organs: lung, spleen and San Jiao, at the beginning of COVID-19 infection.

The functions of the lung are to maintain respiration, disperse and descend the lung-qi, provide an opening into the nose, dominate the skin, and regulate the water passage. On the other hand, the spleen has physiological functions in producing qi and blood, transporting and transforming food and fluid, dominating the muscles and four limbs, providing an opening to the mouth, harmonizing with the stomach, and controlling the blood circulation within the vessels. San Jiao functions in harmonizing the San Jiao, regulating the corridor of yuan-qi and water, distributing the qi to all parts of the body. If the qi distribution and water metabolism of the San Jiao become disturbed or blocked, water retention could happen, which leads to various dysfunctions throughout the whole body across the different Jiao(s). The nature of pathogenesis of COVID-19—damp, cold and toxic heat—are closely connected to the disorders of body fluid and water metabolism. Nonetheless, we find that the lung, spleen, and San Jiao are the most essential organs often involved at the beginning of the infection. The cold-damp pathogens may dominate the beginning stage of the illness, leading to disturbance and blockage of water metabolism. Toxic heat then dominates a later stage that burns out the body fluid, leading to severe yin depletion. However, in many fast-progressing cases, the two factors often mingle together.

When the lung becomes impaired or blocked, the following happens:

- Disruption of its dispersing function

  - Aversion to cold, or chillness, slight fever, cough, and itching in the throat.

- Failure of the lung to open into the nose

  - Loss of smell, stuffy nose, runny nose, and nasal bleeding.

- Dysfunction of the lung in descending the qi

  - The fast development of chest congestion, increasing pressure in the chest, and hypoxemia.

- Blockage of wei qi

  - Muscle pain, joint pain, sweating, and sensitivity to wind.

- Disruption of its role as the upper source of water

  - Rapid build-ups of fluid in the lung, scanty urination, and mild edema.

When the spleen is affected, the following happens:

- Dysfunction of transportation and transformation

  - Poor appetite, loss of taste, nausea, vomiting, formation of thin and white phlegm (mucus) in the mouth, bloating of the abdomen, soft or loose stool, or diarrhea, signs of buildup of damp in the body, including blisters on the feet or somewhere on the body.

- Poor function of qi and blood production

  - Lassitude, fatigue, difficulty walking for a short distance, pale complexion, and cold hands and feet.

- Lack of domination of the muscles and four limbs

  - Muscle weakness and lack of force in the four limbs.

- Failure of the spleen in controlling the blood

  - Bruises and haemoptysis.

  When the San Jiao is affected, the following happens:

- Disturbance of yuan-qi distribution

  - Tiredness, weakness, mental fatigue, lacking the power to do things. In some cases, even activities as simple as reading, writing, or moving for a very short distance (e.g., 20 meters), could become a challenging effort.

- Blockage of the water metabolism

  - Rapid water retention in the lung, formation of phlegm and mucus in the lung, fast buildup of general water retention, edema on the lower limbs, scanty urination, heart palpitation, shortness of breath, the fullness of abdomen, or constipation.

The prognosis of the infection depends on the patient's constitution, age, and underlying sickness. The invasion of cold-damp, toxins, and heat may enter through either cold-dominant or heat-dominant directions. The cold-dominant direction takes the system to excessive accumulation of mucus in the lung and/or kidney system, resulting in ARDS or heart and kidney failure. The heat-dominant direction takes the system to the over-burning of multiple organs, resulting in general cytokine storm and multiple organ failure. By foreseeing the possible consequence of the development of relevant pathology, a proper intervention of herbal or acupuncture treatment—as early as possible—will be able to shorten the process of the illness and avoid further progress into critical conditions. Unlike the ordinary flu, COVID-19 has a much faster and higher chance to drive the whole system into an extensive crisis. From this point of view, it is no doubt that promptly identifying the early-stage symptoms and managing the original pathogen with proper intervention can prevent drastic system deterioration and reduce mortality rate.

3.2 TCM Treatment

The main key focus of TCM treatment for early stage symptoms of COVID-19 is to dispel the pathogenic factors, namely cold-damp, toxins and heat, and restore the functions of lung, spleen, San Jiao, and other relevant organs. We want to particularly emphasize on the application of Ghost points in acupuncture treatment. The idea of a combination of Ghost points, Shaoshang LU-11 with Yinbai SP-1 comes from the ancient analogy that the evil epidemic EPF are acting as "ghosts" finding their way into the human body. We are also keen on eight extraordinary confluence points that have multi-dimension actions on both the 12 primary channels and extraordinary vessels.

3.2.1 Taiyang channel syndrome

Principle of Treatment:
Dispel cold-damp, remove toxins, disperse the lung-qi and relieve external symptoms.

Herbal Treatment:
Qiang Huo Sheng Shi Tang-*Notopterygium Decoction to Overcome Dampness.*

Fang Feng *Radix Ledebouriellae Divaricatae* 10 g
Jing Jie *Herba seu Flos Schizonepetae Tenuifoliae* 10 g
Qiang Huo *Rhizoma et Radix Notopterygii* 10 g
Du Huo *Radix Angelicae Pubescentis* 10 g
Gao Ben *Rhizoma et Radix Ligustici* 10 g
Bai Zhi *Radix Angelicae Dahuricae* 10 g
Chuan Xiong *Radix Ligustici Wallichii* 10 g
Chai Hu *Radix Bupleuri* 5 g
Zhi Ke *Fructus Citri Aurantii* 10 g
Zi Su Ye *Folium Perillae Frutescentis* 10 g
Xing Ren *Semen Pruni Armeniacae* 10 g
Zhi Gan Cao *Radix Glycyrrhizae Preparata* 3 g

Herbal Modifications:
- Cang Zhu *Rhizoma Atractylodis* 10 g, Huo Xiang *Herba Agastaches seu Pogostemi* 10 g, Qing Hao *Herba Artemisiae Annuae* 10 g and Jin Yin Hua *Flos Lonicerae Japonicae* 10 g could be added into the formula to strengthen the effect of eliminating cold-damp and toxins.
- In the case of obvious dry cough, add Tian Hua Fen *Radix Trichosanthis Kirilowii* 5 g and Mai Men Dong *Tuber Ophiopogonis Japonici* 10 g to moisten the lung and reduce the dry cough.
- In the case of severe anhidrosis, add Ma Huang *Herba Ephedrae* 10 g and Gui Zhi *Ramulus Cinnamomi Cassiae* 10 g to promote sweating and relieve the external symptoms.

- In the case of severe throat pain, add She Gan *Rhizoma Belamcandae Chinensis* 10 g to relieve the throat pain.
- In the case of loss of smell, add Cang Er Zi *Fructus Xanthii Sibirici* 10 g and Xin Yi Hua *Flos Magnoliae* 10 g to open the nasal orifice and improve the nose function.
- In the case of loss of taste, add Sha Ren *Fructus Amomi* 5 g to eliminate cold-damp and improve the tastebuds.

Acupuncture Points:
- Ghost points: Shaoshang LU-11 and Yinbai SP-1, puncturing superficially.
- Lieque LU-7 + Zhaohai KID-6, Waiguan SJ-5 + Zulinqi GB-41 with even methods.
- Hegu L.I.-4, Fengchi GB-20, Zhigou SJ-6, Feishu BL-13, Zhongwan Ren-12, Fenglong ST-40 and Zusanli ST-36 with reducing methods.

Points Modifications:
- In the case of an obvious dry cough, add Jingqu LU-8 to moisten the lung and reduce the dry cough.
- In the case of severe anhidrosis, add moxa on Hegu L.I.-4, Feishu BL-13, and Zusanli ST-36 to promote sweating and relieve the external symptoms.
- In the case of muscle pain, add Feiyang BL-58 and Kunlun BL-60 to harmonize the collaterals and relieve the muscle pain.
- In the case of severe sore throat, add Lianquan REN-23 to relieve the throat pain.
- In the case of loss of smell, add Yingxiang L.I.-20 and Juliao ST-3 to open the nasal orifice and improve the nose function.

3.2.2 Taiyang and Yangming channel syndrome

Principle of Treatment:
Clear heat, remove toxins, disperse the lung-qi, and clear the heat.

Herbal Treatment:
Da Qing Long Tang-*Major Green Dragon Decoction.*

Ma Huang *Herba Ephedrae* 10 g
Gui Zhi *Ramulus Cinnamomi Cassiae* 10 g
Qiang Huo *Rhizoma et Radix Notopterygii* 10 g
Xing Ren *Semen Pruni Armeniacae* 10 g
Zi Su Zi *Fructus Perillae Frutescentis* 10 g
Ting Li Zi *Semen Descurainiae seu Lepidii* 10 g
Bai Jie Zi *Semen Sinapis Albae* 10 g
Lai Fu Zi *Semen Raphani Sativi* 10 g
Shi Gao *Gypsum Fibrosum* 20 g
Hou Po *Cortex Magnoliae Officinalis* 10 g
Zhi Shi *Fructus Immaturus Citri Aurantii* 10 g

Herbal Modifications:
- Cang Zhu *Rhizoma Atractylodis* 10 g, Huo Xiang *Herba Agastaches seu Pogostemi* 10 g, Qing Hao *Herba Artemisiae Annuae* 10 g and Jin Yin Hua *Flos Lonicerae Japonicae* 10 g could be added into the formulas to strengthen the effect of eliminating cold-damp and toxins.
- In the case of high fever, add Zhi Mu *Radix Anemarrhenae Asphodeloidis* 10 g and Huang Qin *Radix Scutellariae Baicalensis* 10 g to clear the heat in Yangming and reduce the fever.
- In the case of severe thirst, add Tian Hua Fen *Radix Trichosanthis Kirilowii* 10 g to benefit the body fluid and relieve the thirst.
- In the case of yellow phlegm, add Zhe Bei Mu *Bulbus Fritillariae Thunbergii* 10 g and Niu Bang Zi *Fructus Arctii Lappae* 10 g to resolve heat-phlegm and reduce cough.
- In case of haemoptysis, add Bai Ji *Rhizoma Bletillae Striatae* 10 g and Xian He Cao *Herba Agrimoniae Pilosae* 10 g to cool blood and stop bleeding.
- In the case of constipation, add Da Huang *Radix et Rhizoma Rhei* 10 g to clear the heat and promote defecation to relieve constipation.

Acupuncture Points:
- Ghost points: Shaoshang LU-11 and Yinbai SP-1, puncturing superficially.

- Lieque LU-7 + Zhaohai KID-6, Neiguan P-6 + Gongsun SP-4 with even method.
- Chize LU-5, Feishu BL-13, Tanzhong Ren-17, Yuji LU-10, Hegu L.I.-4, Quchi L.I.-11, Tianshu ST-25 and Neiting ST-44 with reducing methods.

Points Modifications:
- In the case of high fever, add Dazhui Du-14 to clear the heat and reduce fever.
- In the case of a blocked nose and nasal bleeding, add Yingxiang L.I.-20 to open the nasal orifice and stop the bleeding.
- In the case of loss of taste, add Dicang ST-4 to regulate the channel and harmonize the collateral to improve the tastebuds.
- In the case of skin red rashes or irritations (heat oriented), add Xuehai SP-10 and Geshu BL-17 to clear the heat and eliminate heat in the blood.
- In the case of excessive yellow phlegm, add Yuji LU-10 to eliminate heat-phlegm and stop coughing.
- In the case of haemoptysis, add Kongzui LU-6 to cool the blood and stop bleeding.

3.2.3 Taiyang and Shaoyang channel syndrome

Principle of Treatment:
Dispel cold-damp, remove toxins, disperse the lung-qi, and harmonize Shaoyang.

Herbal Treatment:
Chai Hu Gui Zhi Tang-*Bupleuri and Ramuli Cinnamomi Decoction.*

Gui Zhi *Ramulus Cinnamomi Cassiae* 10 g
Bai Shao Yao *Radix Paeoniae Lactiflorae* 10 g
Qiang Huo *Rhizoma et Radix Notopterygii* 10 g
Gao Ben *Rhizoma et Radix Ligustici* 10 g
Fang Feng *Radix Ledebouriellae Divaricatae* 10 g

Chai Hu *Radix Bupleuri* 10 g
Huang Qin *Radix Scutellariae Baicalensis* 10 g
Lian Qiao *Fructus Forsythiae Suspensae* 10 g
Xing Ren *Semen Pruni Armeniacae* 10 g
Zhi Ban Xia *Rhizoma Pinelliae Ternatae Preparata* 10 g
Dang Shen *Radix Codonopsis Pilosulae* 10 g
Bai Zhi *Radix Angelicae Dahuricae* 10 g
Zhi Gan Cao *Radix Glycyrrhizae Preparata* 3 g

Herbal Modifications:

- Cang Zhu *Rhizoma Atractylodis* 10 g, Huo Xiang *Herba Agastaches seu Pogostemi* 10 g, Qing Hao *Herba Artemisiae Annuae* 10 and Jin Yin Hua *Flos Lonicerae Japonicae* 10 g could be added into the formula to strengthen the effect of eliminating cold-damp and toxins.
- In the case of redness in the eyes or eye irritation, add Xia Ku Cao *Spica Prunellae Vulgaris* 10 g to clear the heat in the liver and relieve the eye complaints.
- In the case of severe vomiting and a bitter taste in the mouth, add Xuan Fu Hua *Flos Inulae* 10 g (packed with gauze) to descend the stomach-qi and relieve the vomiting.
- In the case of emotional depression, add He Huan Pi *Cortex Albizziae Julibrissin* 10 g to smooth the qi circulation and tranquilize the shen.
- In the case of ataxia, add Tian Ma *Rhizoma Gastrodiae Elatae* 10 g to subdue the wind and improve the balance of the body.

Acupuncture Points:

- Ghost points: Shaoshang LU-11 and Yinbai SP-1, puncturing superficially.
- Lieque LU-7 + Zhaohai KID-6, Waiguan SJ-5 + Zulinqi GB-41, Neiguan P-6 + Gongsun SP-4 with an even method.
- Chize LU-5, Feishu BL-13, Yuji LU-10, Yanglingquan GB-34, Xiaxi GB-43, and Sanyinjiao SP-6 with reducing methods.

Points Modifications:

- In the case of much dry cough, add Jingqu LU-8 to moisten the lung, disperse the lung-qi and relieve the dry cough.
- In the case of redness in the eyes or eye irritation, add Guanchong SJ-1 and Xingjian LIV-2 to clear the heat in the liver and relieve the eye complaints.
- In the case of severe vomiting and a bitter taste in the mouth, add Qiuxu GB-40 and Zhongwan REN-12 to descend the stomach-qi and relieve the vomiting.
- In the case of emotional depression, add Qimen LIV-14 and Shaohai HE-3 to smooth the qi circulation, and tranquillize the shen.
- In the case of chest tightness or pressure over the chest, add Tanzhong REN-17 and Ximen P-4 to descend the qi, regulate the chest and relieve the chest tightness and pressure.

3.2.4 Taiyang, Yangming and Shaoyang channel syndrome

Principle of Treatment:
Dispel cold-damp, remove toxins, clear heat, disperse the lung-qi and harmonize Shaoyang.

Herbal Treatment:
Chai Ge Jie Ji Tang-*Bupleurum and Kudzu Decoction to Release the Muscle Layer.*

This pattern is mostly seen in the clinic or practice. After launching the "Screening Study of Effective Prescriptions of Traditional Chinese Medicine for the Prevention and Treatment of New Coronavirus Pneumonia" in Shanxi, Hebei, Heilongjiang and Shaanxi with a very effective therapeutic result, the State Administration of Traditional Chinese Medicine in China has encouraged TCM doctors to apply an herbal formula named Qing Fei Pai Du Tang (QFPDD — *Lung Cleansing & Detoxifying Decoction*) to treat patients with COVID-19 pneumonia.

Qing Fei Pai Du Tang (QFPDD) is a new compound formula composed of four classic prescriptions, containing warm, pungent, cold, light and fragrant herbs to disperse the lung, stop cough, clear heat, resolve damp and remove toxins. It contains:

Ma Huang *Herba Ephedrae* 10 g
Xing Ren *Semen Pruni Armeniacae* 10 g
Shi Gao *Gypsum Fibrosum* 30 g
Zhi Gan Cao *Radix Glycyrrhizae Preparata* 5 g
Gui Zhi *Ramulus Cinnamomi Cassiae* 10 g
Ze Xie *Alismatis Rhizoma* 10 g
Zhu Ling *Polyporus* 10 g
Bai Zhu *Rhizoma Atractylodis Macrocephalae* 10 g
Fu Ling *Sclerotium Poriae Cocos* 15 g
Chai Hu *Radix Bupleuri* 10 g
Huang Qin *Radix Scutellariae Baicalensis* 10 g
Zhi Ban Xia *Rhizoma Pinelliae Ternatae Preparata* 10 g
Sheng Jiang *Rhizoma Zingiberis Officinalis Recens* 10 g
Zi Wan *Radix Asteris Tatarici* 10 g
Kuan Dong Hua *Flos Tussilaginis Farfarae* 10 g
She Gan *Rhizoma Belamcandae Chinensis* 10 g
Xi Xin *Herba cum Radice Asari* 3 g
Huo Xiang *Herba Agastaches seu Pogostemi* 10 g
Shan Yao *Radix Dioscoreae Oppositae* 10 g
Zhi Shi *Fructus Immaturus Citri Aurantii* 10 g
Chen Pi *Citri reticulatae Pericarpium* 5 g

Directions:
- Decoct one package of crude herbs each day and take the decoction once in the morning and once in the evening (40 minutes after a meal). If conditions permit, take half a bowl of rice soup after drinking the decoction.
- Three days of treatment constitutes one course. Usually, only one or two courses of treatment are required.

- If the patient does not have a high fever, the amount of Shi Gao Gypsum Fibrosum can be reduced. Conversely, if the fever is high, the amount of Shi Gao Gypsum Fibrosum should be increased.

Acupuncture Points:
- Ghost points: Shaoshang LU-11 and Yinbai SP-1, puncturing superficially.
- Lieque LU-7 + Zhaohai KID-6, Neiguan P-6 + Gongsun SP-4 with even method.
- Chize LU-5, Feishu BL-13, Yuji LU-10, Hegu L.I.-4, Quchi L.I.-11, Fengchi GB-20, Yanglingquan GB-34, and Neiting ST-44 with reducing methods.

Points Modifications:
Selections are as above patterns.

3.2.5 Taiyang and Taiyin channel syndrome

Principle of Treatment:
Dispel cold-damp, remove toxins, disperse the lung-qi, and strengthen the Taiyin system.

Herbal Treatment:
Huo Xiang Zheng Qi Tang-*Agastache Decoction to Rectify the Qi.*

Huo Xiang *Herba Agastaches seu Pogostemi* 10 g
Pei Lan *Herba Eupatorii Fortunei* 10 g
Zi Su Ye *Folium Perillae Frutescentis* 10 g
Hou Po *Cortex Magnoliae Officinalis* 10 g
Bai Zhu *Rhizoma Atractylodis Macrocephalae* 10 g
Gan Jiang *Rhizoma Zingiberis Officinalis* 5 g
Cang Zhu *Rhizoma Atractylodis* 10 g
Fu Ling *Sclerotium Poriae Cocos* 12 g
Chen Pi *Pericarpium Citri Reticulatae* 5 g
Bai Zhi *Radix Angelicae Dahuricae* 10 g

Bai Zhu *Rhizoma Atractylodis Macrocephalae* 10 g
Sheng Jiang *Rhizoma Zingiberis Officinalis Recens* 5 g
Zhi Gan Cao *Radix Glycyrrhizae Preparata* 3 g

Herbal Modifications:
- Qing Hao *Herba Artemisiae Annuae* 10 g and Jin Yin Hua *Flos Lonicerae Japonicae* 10 g could be added into the formula to strengthen the effect of eliminating cold-damp and toxins.
- In the case of loss of taste, add Sha Ren *Fructus Amomi* 5 g to eliminate cold-damp and improve the tastebuds.
- In the case of severe diarrhea, add Ge Gen *Radix Puerariae* 10 g to ascend the clear-qi and descend the turbid-qi.
- In the case of severe tiredness, add Shan Yao *Radix Dioscoreae Oppositae* 10 g to activate the spleen and tonify spleen-qi to improve the energy.
- In the case of bruises and haemoptysis, add Xian He Cao *Herba Agrimoniae Pilosae* 10 g and Bai Ji *Rhizoma Bletillae Striatae* 10 g to stop bleeding.
- In the case of frostbite/chilblain (cold-oriented), add Bai Jie Zi *Semen Sinapis Albae* 10 g and Rou Gui *Cortex Cinnamomi Cassiae* 3 g to warm the channels and eliminate blockage in the collaterals.

Acupuncture Points:
- Ghost points: Shaoshang LU-11, Yinbai SP-1, puncturing superficially.
- Waiguan SJ-5 + Zulinqi GB-41, Neiguan P-6 + Gongsun SP-4 with even method.
- Zhigou SJ-6, Feishu BL-13, Yanglingquan GB-34, Zhongwan Ren-12, Fenglong ST-40, Tianshu ST-25, Yinlingquan SP-9, Zusanli ST-36 with even method. Moxa on ST-36.

Points Modifications:
- In the case of severe fatigue, add Pishu BL-20 and Qihai Ren-6 with moxa to activate the spleen and tonify spleen-qi to improve the energy.

- In the case of loss of taste, add Dicang ST-4 and Chongyang ST-42 to regulate the channel and harmonize the collateral to improve the tastebuds.
- In the case of severe diarrhea, add Shangjuxu ST-37 to stop diarrhea.
- In the case of loss of appetite, add Taibai SP-3 to activate the spleen and improve appetite.
- In the case of excessive mucus in the mouth, add Tiantu REN-22 to descend the qi and relieve the mucus.
- In the case of frostbite/chilblain (cold-oriented), moxa on jing Well points of nearest relevant meridians or on the tip of the nearest toe.
- In the case of skin blisters, add Taiyuan LU-9 and Taibai SP-3 to eliminate cold-damp in the skin and muscle and relieve the skin blisters.

3.2.6 Taiyang and Shaoyin channel syndrome

Principle of Treatment:
Dispel cold-damp, remove toxins, disperse the lung-qi and tonify the Shaoyin.

Herbal Treatment:
Ma Huang Fu Zi Xi Xin Tang-*Ephedra, Prepared Aconite and Asarum Decoction,* or
Ma Huang Fu Zi Gan Jiang Tang-*Ephedra, Prepared Aconite and Dry Ginger Decoction.*

Ma Huang *Herba Ephedrae* 10 g
Zhi Fu Zi *Radix Lateralis Aconiti Carmichaeli Praeparata* 10 g
Xi Xin *Herba cum Radice Asari* 3 g
Gao Ben *Rhizoma et Radix Ligustici* 10 g
Xin Yi Hua *Flos Magnoliae* 10 g
Chuan Xiong *Radix Ligustici Wallichii* 10 g
Xing Ren *Semen Pruni Armeniacae* 10 g
Zhi Ban Xia *Rhizoma Pinelliae Ternatae Preparata* 10 g
Sheng Jiang *Rhizoma Zingiberis Officinalis Recens* 5 g

If Ma Huang is missing, Xiang Ru 10 g could act as a replacement. If Zhi Fu Zi is missing, Gan Jiang 10 g could be a replacement. If Xi Xin is missing, Bai Zhi 10 g could be used instead.

Herbal Modifications:
- Cang Zhu *Rhizoma Atractylodis* 10 g, Huo Xiang *Herba Agastaches seu Pogostemi* 10 g and Qing Hao *Herba Artemisiae Annuae* 10 g could be added into the formulas to strengthen the effect of eliminating cold-damp and relieve the external symptoms.
- In the case of a weak heartbeat, add Gui Zhi *Ramulus Cinnamomi Cassiae* 10 g and Zhi Gan Cao *Radix Glycyrrhizae Preparata* 10 g to warm the heart and strengthen the heartbeat.
- In the case of scanty urination or edema on the lower limbs, add Fu Ling *Sclerotium Poriae Cocos* 15 g, Zhu Ling *Sclerotium Polypori Umbellati* 10 g and Ze Xie *Rhizoma Alismatis Orientalis* 10 g to promote urination and relieve edema.
- In the case of semi-consciousness, a combination of Chinese herbs and Western medicine should be applied.

Acupuncture Points:
- Ghost points: Shaoshang LU-11, Yinbai SP-1, puncturing superficially.
- Lieque LU-7 + Zhaohai KID-6, Neiguan P-6 + Gongsun SP-4 with even method.
- Hegu L.I.-4 and Feishu BL-13 with reducing method.
- Xinshu BL-15, Shenshu BL-23, Qihai REN-6, Guanyuan REN-4, Taixi KID-3 and Zusanli ST-36 with a tonifying method with moxa on KID-3, REN-4 and REN-6.

Points Modifications:
- In the case of a weak heartbeat, add Xinshu BL-15 with moxa to warm the heart and strengthen the heartbeat.
- In the case of scanty urination, or edema on the lower limbs, add Shuidao ST-29 and Yinlingquan SP-9 to promote urination and relieve edema.

- In the case of semi-consciousness, adding Shaofu HE-8 and Yongquan KID-1 with a tonic method could be applied.
- In the case of hypoxemia with difficulty inhaling, add Yingu KID-10 and Tanzhong REN-17 to tonify the qi, relax the chest and improve inhalation.

In this chapter, we set foot on the path of understanding the early stage of COVID-19 infections. By analyzing the early symptoms of the infection from a systematic TCM point of view, we are able to obtain a comprehensive reading on the relevant pathogenesis and pathology of it and give our suggestions on the relevant treatments. We are convinced that a proper early intervention of correct differential treatments strictly under TCM principles can play a very important role in controlling the infection and reducing mortality. TCM's early intervention should not be underestimated and neglected in the current pandemic situation.

4

TCM Treatment of Ordinary Syndromes of COVID-19

4.1 TCM Analysis of Ordinary Syndromes of COVID-19

When COVID-19 develops into an ordinary type, it must meet some criteria and make a clear difference between an ordinary type and a severe type. According to the diagnosis and treatment plan for pneumonia of new coronavirus infection (trial version 4),[1] set by the General Office of the National Health Commission, Office of the State Administration of Traditional Chinese Medicine on 27 January 2020, the clinical classifications of ordinary type include fever, symptoms of the respiratory tract, etc. and imaging with the appearance of pneumonia, which is different with that of severe types, such as

- Respiratory distress, RR $\geq$ 30 beats/min.
- In the resting state, the oxygen saturation is $\leq$93%.
- Arterial partial pressure of oxygen (PaO2)/Fraction of inspired oxygen (FiO2) $\leq$300 mmHg (1 mmHg = 0.133 kPa).

Ordinary types of COVID-19 in the clinical stage often occur mainly due to external contraction of severe pathogenic factors, including pestilent toxins, which invade the exterior and the

---

[1] Diagnosis and treatment plan for pneumonia of new coronavirus infection (trial version 4) (新型冠状病毒感染的肺炎诊疗方案(试行第四版)). https://www.gov.cn/zhengce/zhengceku/2020-01/28/5472673/files/0f96c10cc09d4d36a6f9a9f0b42d972b.pdf.

respiratory tracts. It is also related to some other reasons, such as improper or delayed treatment or other underlying diseases.

4.1.1 Symptoms features of ordinary types of COVID-19

4.1.1.1 *The chief cause*

At this stage, the invasion of external pathogenic factors is still the chief cause, leading to disharmony between the ying and wei system, or disorder in the San Jiao system with dysfunction of the lung in dispersing the lung-qi, resulting in fever, a mostly dry or productive cough, myalgia, fatigue, poor appetite, nausea, vomiting or diarrhea.

4.1.1.2 *Deterioration of clinical symptoms*

Most of the clinical symptoms become worse, especially fever and cough, but still not at a very severe stage. There is no high fever, severe cough, expectoration of profuse phlegm, and constipation.

4.1.1.3 *Disturbance of lung in dispersing the qi*

Dysfunction of the lung in dispersing the qi is the main pathogenic result, and is seldom severe although it involves the descending function of the lung. Therefore, there is no asthma, shortness of breath, chest tightness, etc.

4.1.2 Treatment features of ordinary types of COVID-19

4.1.2.1 *The main task*

The main task is to restore the physiological functions of the lung. At this moment, herbs should be used to disperse the lung-qi, such as Jie Geng *Radix Platycodi Grandiflori*, Sang Ye *Folium Mori Albae*, Xing Ren *Semen Pruni Armeniacae*, Niu Bang Zi *Fructus Arctii Lappae*, Cang Er Zi *Fructus Xanthii Sibirici*, Xin Yi Hua *Flos Magnoliae*, etc. Acupuncture points, such as Lieque LU-7, Fengmen BL-12, Feishu BL-13, etc, should be applied. Usually, the method to descend the lung-qi is not necessary. However, attention should be paid to observe the situation just in case it deteriorates.

4.1.2.2 *Necessary to dispel external pathogens*

Meanwhile, the main treatment principles should be included to dispel external pathogenic factors and remove the pestilent toxins.

4.1.2.3 *Damp remains one of the main pathogens*

Damp varies in cold-damp and damp-heat. Besides, damp may exist in different organs and tissues, such as the lung, stomach, spleen, and San Jiao. Corresponding principles of treatment, herbs and acupuncture points should be applied accordingly.

4.1.2.4 *Precautions should be taken in the treatment*

No matter what the cause at this stage is, high doses of herbs bitter in taste and cold in nature are not recommended, because they would intensify the obstruction of yang and retain pathogens. The correct treatment is to apply herbs to dispel the pathogenic factors via sweating, rather than using herbs to clear and purge.

4.1.2.5 *The spleen and stomach should be cared for*

In addition, many COVID-19 patients also suffer from poor appetite, nausea, vomiting, or diarrhea. These herbs with a cold nature could cause aggravation of the above symptoms. On the contrary, herbs that can regulate the San Jiao, harmonize the middle Jiao and eliminate damp or regulate the ascending and descending functions of the spleen and stomach, should be selected.

4.1.2.6 *Damp and heat should be treated simultaneously*

During the treatment of damp-heat, since there is a bond between these two pathogens, it is necessary to apply clearing and eliminating methods simultaneously. Any attempt to only clear heat or eliminate damp is insufficient. Just as Ye Tianshi (1666–1745) said, "damp and heat can be cleared by expelling wind; damp and heat can be eliminated by draining as well. When there is no binding of heat and damp, it is easier to handle".

4.1.2.7 *Tonic is not needed*

In terms of fatigue, it is due to an invasion of pathogenic factors, a disturbance to the lung in dispersing the qi, and disharmony of the spleen and stomach. It is not caused by weakness or deficiency of qi and blood. Thus, the application of any tonics is not recommended. If tonics are applied too early, it could cause retaining of the external pathogenic factors and further obstruction of the damp in the body.

4.1.2.8 *Personalized treatment is essential*

It is emphasized and suggested that a personalized treatment based upon individual should be encouraged in the whole process of the treatment. If that is impossible, standard herbal formulas or patent remedies could be used.

4.1.2.9 *Emotions need to be managed*

With the development of the disease, emotional disturbance could surface gradually. Besides the elimination of these pathogenic factors, herbs and acupuncture points should be used to support the emotion and regulate the shen.

4.1.2.10 *Prevention should not be forgotten*

Prevention should be taken in the treatment to avoid the aggravation of situations, such as close observation of clinical manifestations, reaction during the treatment, general conditions (such as energetic feeling, sleeping, appetite, drinking, urine, defecation, and movement of the limbs, etc.) should also be noticed.

4.1.2.11 *Combination of TCM and modern medicine*

If necessary, a combination of TCM and modern medicine could be applied in time, especially for elderly patients or patients with severe underlying illnesses.

4.2 TCM Treatment

4.2.1 Invasion of wind-cold with damp and toxins

Heavy aversion to cold, slight fever, stuffy nose, severe dry cough, sore throat, hidrosis, headache, myalgia or arthralgia with slight heaviness, absence of thirst or preference of warm drinks, thin, white, and slight greasy coating on the tongue, and a superficial and tight pulse.

Principle of Treatment:
Dispel wind-cold, eliminate damp and toxins, disperse the lung-qi and relieve the cough.

Herbal Treatment:
Qiang Huo Sheng Shi Tang-*Notopterygium Decoction to Overcome Dampness*, plus
Xing Su San-*Apricot Kernel and Perilla Leaf Powder.*

Qiang Huo *Rhizoma et Radix Notopterygii* 10 g
Du Huo *Radix Angelicae Pubescentis* 10 g
Gao Ben *Rhizoma et Radix Ligustici* 10 g
Cang Zhu *Rhizoma Atractylodis* 10 g
Man Jing Zi *Fructus Viticis* 10 g
Jie Geng *Radix Platycodi Grandiflori* 10 g
Xing Ren *Semen Pruni Armeniacae* 10 g
Zi Su Ye *Folium Perillae Frutescentis* 10 g
Bai Jie Zi *Semen Sinapis Albae* 10 g

Zhi Ban Xia *Rhizoma Pinelliae Ternatae Preparata* 10 g
Chen Pi *Pericarpium Citri Reticulatae* 5 g
Fu Ling *Sclerotium Poriae Cocos* 12 g
Zhi Ke *Fructus Citri Aurantii* 5 g

Explanations:
- Qiang Huo, Du Huo and Gao Ben dispel wind-cold, resolve damp, and relieve external symptoms.
- Cang Zhu assists the above herbs to resolve damp and relieve muscle pain and heaviness.
- Zi Su Ye promotes sweating and relieves external symptoms.
- Jie Geng, Xing Ren, Bai Jie Zi, Zhi Ban Xia, Chen Pi and Fu Ling eliminate damp-phlegm and relieve cough.
- Man Jing Zi relieves headache due to external invasion.
- Zhi Ke harmonizes qi circulation in the chest and abdomen and relieves the pain in the chest and abdomen.

Acupuncture treatment:
- Neiguan P-6 + Gongsun SP-4 with even methods.
- Hegu L.I.-4, Waiguan SJ-5, Zhigou SJ-6, Lieque LU-7, Feishu BL-13, Chize LU-5, Fenglong ST-40, Yanglingquan GB-34, and Sanyinjiao SP-6 with a reducing method.

Explanations:
- P-6 + SP-4 are used to regulate the qi circulation in the chest, assist respiration and relieve the cough.
- Hegu L.I.-4, the yuan-source point of the large intestine channel, SJ-5, the luo-connecting point of the San Jiao channel, and LU-7, the luo-connecting point of the lung channel respectively, are used to promote sweating and dispel external pathogenic factors.
- SJ-6, jing-river point of the San Jiao channel, is used to dispel external pathogenic factors, promote the discharge of damp in the body.
- BL-13, the back-shu point of the lung, together with LU-5, the he-sea point of the lung channel, is used to disperse the lung-qi and restore the physiological functions of the lung.

- ST-40, the luo-connecting point of the stomach channel, GB-34, the he-sea point of the gallbladder channel, and SP-6, the crossing point of the three yin channels of the foot, are used to eliminate external damp, regulate the middle Jiao and relieve painful muscle and joints.

4.2.2 Invasion of wind-heat with damp and toxins

Persistent fever, slight aversion to cold, thirst, throat pain and redness, headache, body pain with a warm feeling, much body pain or joint pain with slight heaviness, slight sweating, dry cough, slight expectoration of yellow or white phlegm, red tongue with a yellow and dry coating, and a superficial and rapid pulse.

Principle of Treatment:
Dispel wind, clear heat, eliminate damp and toxins, disperse the lung-qi, and relieve the cough.

Herbal Treatment:
Sang Ju Yin-*Mulberry Leaf and Chrysanthemum Decoction*, plus Zhi Sou San-*Stop Coughing Powder.*

Sang Ye *Folium Mori Albae* 10 g
Ju Hua *Flos Chrysanthemi Morifolii* 10 g
Jie Geng *Radix Platycodi Grandiflori* 10 g
Huang Qin *Radix Scutellariae Baicalensis* 10 g
Xing Ren *Semen Pruni Armeniacae* 10 g
Bo He *Herba Menthae Haplocalycis* 3 g
Cang Zhu *Rhizoma Atractylodis* 10 g
Zhi Zi *Fructus Gardeniae Jasminoidis* 10 g
Fu Ling *Sclerotium Poriae Cocos* 12 g
Bai Bu *Radix Stemonae* 10 g
Zi Wan *Radix Asteris Tatarici* 10 g

Explanations:
- Sang Ye and Ju Hua clear heat, dispel wind, and relieve external symptoms.

- Bo He clears wind-heat, benefits the throat and relieves throat pain.
- Huang Qin and Zhi Zi clear wind-heat and remove toxins.
- Jie Geng, Xing Ren, Zi Wan and Bai Bu dispel lung-qi, eliminate phlegm in the lung and relieve coughing.
- Cang Zhu and Fu Ling eliminate damp and activate the spleen to resolve damp in the body.

Acupuncture Treatment:
- Neiguan P-6 + Gongsun SP-4 with even methods.
- Erjian L.I.-2, Hegu L.I.-4, Waiguan SJ-5, Lieque LU-7, Yuji LU-10, Feishu BL-13, Chize LU-5, Yanglingquan GB-34, and Fenglong ST-40 with a reducing method.

Explanations:
- P-6 + SP-4 are used to regulate the qi circulation in the chest, assist respiration and relieve the cough.
- L.I.-4, the yuan-source point of the large intestine channel, LU-7 and SJ-5, the luo-connecting point of the lung channel and San Jiao channel respectively, are used to promote sweating to dispel external pathogenic factors.
- BL-13 and LU-5, the back-shu point and the he-sea point of the lung channel respectively, are the chief points to descend the lung-qi and relieve difficulty to expectorate the phlegm, shortness of breath, and chest tightness.
- LU-10 and L.I.-2, the ying-stream point of the lung channel and large intestine channel respectively, are used to clear the heat and reduce fever in the lung and relieve the cough.
- GB-34, the he-sea point of the Gallbladder channel, and ST-40, the luo-connecting point of the stomach channel, are used to eliminate external damp, regulate the middle Jiao, and relieve myalgia and arthralgia.

4.2.3 Invasion of cold-damp and toxins

Aversion to cold and fever, absence of sweating and headache, severe dry cough, expectoration of some white phlegm, much pain in the limbs and joints, sore throat and tightness, headache, heaviness of the body, ageusia, lack of thirst, nausea, vomiting, loose stool or diarrhea, abdominal pain and distension, thin, white, and greasy coating on the tongue, and a superficial and slippery pulse.

Principle of Treatment:
Eliminate cold, resolve damp, release the external symptoms, and stop coughing.

Herbal Treatment:
Jiu Wei Qiang Huo Tang-*Nine-Herb Decoction with Notopterygium.*

Qiang Huo *Rhizoma et Radix Notopterygii* 10 g
Fang Feng *Radix Ledebouriellae Divaricatae* 10 g
Cang Zhu Rhizoma Atractylodis 10 g
Zi Su Ye *Folium Perillae Frutescentis* 5 g
Ge Gen *Radix Puerariae* 10 g
Xi Xin *Herba cum Radice Asari* 3 g
Chuan Xiong *Radix Ligustici Wallichii* 10 g
Bai Zhi *Radix Angelicae Dahuricae* 10 g
Bai Shao *Radix Paeoniae Lactiflorae* 5 g
Huang Qin *Radix Scutellariae Baicalensis* 5 g
Gan Cao *Radix Glycyrrhizae Uralensis* 3 g

Explanations:
- Qiang Huo, Fang Feng and Zi Su Ye dispel wind, promote sweating, and eliminate external cold-damp.
- Cang Zhu eliminates cold-damp and relieves diarrhea.
- Bai Zhi, Xi Xin and Chuan Xiong promote sweating, warm the meridians, and relieve pain due to invasion of cold-damp.
- Bai Shao Yao and Huang Qin regulate Shaoyang and eliminate toxins in the body.
- Ge Gen and Sheng Ma harmonize the middle Jiao, descend turbid-qi and relieve vomiting and diarrhea.
- Gan Cao harmonizes the herbs in the prescription.

Acupuncture Treatment:

- Neiguan P-6 + Gongsun SP-4 with even methods.
- Hegu L.I.-4, Yangchi SJ-4, Waiguan SJ-5, Zhigou SJ-6, Lieque LU-7, Feishu BL-13, Chize LU-5, Fenglong ST-40, and Yanglingquan GB-34 with a reducing method.

Explanations:

- P-6 + SP-4 are used to regulate the qi circulation in the chest, assist respiration and relieve the cough.
- L.I.-4, the yuan-source point of the large intestine channel, SJ-5, the luo-connecting point of the San Jiao channel, and LU-7, the luo-connecting point of the lung channel respectively, are used to promote sweating, dispel external pathogenic factors and relieve external symptoms.
- SJ-4 and SJ-6, the yuan-source point and jing-river point of the San Jiao channel respectively, are used to dispel external pathogenic factors and promote the discharge of damp in the body.
- BL-13, the back-shu point of the lung, together with LU-5, the he-sea point of the lung channel, together with LU-7, is used to disperse the lung-qi and restore the physiological functions of the lung.
- ST-40, the luo-connecting point of the stomach channel, GB-34, the he-sea point of the gallbladder channel, are used to dispel external damp and benefit the joints.

4.2.4 Invasion of toxic heat

Persistent fever, mild aversion to cold, dry mouth, thirst, dry cough with scanty sputum occasionally with blood streaks, absence of sweat or little sweat, headache, general body pain, fatigue, restlessness, dry stools, red tongue with a thin, yellow, and dry coating, and a rapid pulse.

Principle of Treatment:

Dispel heat, reduce fever, disperse the lung-qi and relieve cough.

Herbal Treatment:
Yin Qiao San-*Honeysuckle and Forsythia Powder,* plus
Zhi Zi Chi Tang-*Gardenia and Prepared Soybean Decoction.*

Jin Yin Hua *Flos Lonicerae Japonicae* 10 g
Lian Qiao *Fructus Forsythiae Suspensae* 10 g
Jie Geng *Radix Platycodi Grandiflori* 10 g
Sang Ye *Folium Mori Albae* 10 g
Bo He *Herba Menthae Haplocalycis* 3 g
Niu Bang Zi *Fructus Arctii Lappae* 10 g
Huang Qin *Radix Scutellariae Baicalensis* 10 g
Zhi Zi *Fructus Gardeniae Jasminoidis* 10 g
Dan Dou Chi *Semen Sojae Praeparatum* 10 g
Lu Gen *Rhizoma Phragmitis Communis* 12 g
Sheng Di Huang *Radix Rehmanniae Glutinosae Recens* 12 g

Explanations:
- Jin Yin Hua, Lian Qiao and Zhi Zi dispel heat, reduce fever, and remove toxins.
- Jie Geng, Sang Ye, Bo He, Niu Bang Zi and Huang Qin clear heat in the lung, benefit the throat and relieve cough.
- Dan Dou Chi promotes sweating and reduces fever.
- Lu Gen and Sheng Di Huang clear heat and benefit the body fluid to relieve thirst.

Acupuncture Treatment:
- Neiguan P-6 + Gongsun SP-4 with even methods.
- Erjian L.I.-2, Hegu L.I.-4, Quchi L.I.-11, Dazhui DU-14, Chize LU-5, Feishu BL-13, Yuji LU-10, Neiting ST-44, and Sanyinjiao SP-6 with a reducing method.

Explanations:
- P-6 + SP-4 are used to regulate the qi circulation in the chest, assist respiration and relieve the cough.
- L.I.-2, L.I.-4 and L.I.-11, the ying-stream point, the yuan-source point and the he-sea point of the large intestine channel respec-

tively, together with DU-14, the meeting point of all the yang channels in the body, are used to clear heat, remove toxins and reduce fever.

- LU-5 and BL-13, the he-sea point of the lung channel and the back-shu point of the lung respectively, together with LU-10, the ying-stream point of the lung channel, are used to clear heat in the lung and disperse the lung-qi.
- ST-44 and SP-6, the ying-stream point of the stomach channel and the crossing point of three yin channels of the foot, are used to clear heat, remove the toxins, and reduce fever.

4.2.5 Invasion of damp-heat and toxins

Fever aggravated in the afternoon, dry cough, sore throat, impeded or sticky sweating which does not lower down the fever, heaviness of the body and limbs, nausea, vomiting, stomach distention, poor appetite, loose stool or diarrhea, bitter taste or sticky and greasy sensation in the mouth, scanty and difficult urination, red tongue with a yellow and greasy coating or a mixture of white and yellow greasy coating, and a slippery and rapid pulse.

Principle of Treatments:
Clear heat, resolve damp, harmonize the middle Jiao, and relieve cough.

Herbal Treatment:
Gan Lu Xiao Du Yin-*Sweet Dew Special Pill to Eliminate Toxins,* plus Lian Po Yin-*Coptis and Magnolia Bark Drink.*

Hua Shi *Talcum* 20 g
Huang Qin *Radix Scutellariae Baicalensis* 10 g
Yin Chen Hao *Herba Artemisiae Capillaris* 10 g
Hou Po *Cortex Magnoliae Officinalis* 10 g
Lian Qiao *Fructus Forsythiae Suspensae* 12 g
Bo He *Herba Menthae Haplocalycis* 5 g

She Gan *Rhizoma Belamcandae Chinensis* 10 g
Jie Geng *Radix Platycodi Grandiflori* 10 g
Shi Chang Pu *Rhizoma Acori Graminei* 10 g
Huo Xiang *Herba Agastaches seu Pogostemi* 10 g
Bai Dou Kou *Fructus Amomi Cardamomi* 3 g
Bing Lang *Semen Arecae Catechu* 10 g
Zhi Mu *Radix Anemarrhenae Asphodeloidis* 10 g
Gan Cao *Radix Glycyrrhizae Uralensis* 3 g

Explanations:
- Hua Shi, Hou Po, Huag Qin, Lian Qiao, Zhi Mu and Yin Chen Hao clear heat, eliminate damp, reduce fever, and remove toxins.
- Bo He clears heat and benefits the throat.
- She Gan and Jie Geng eliminate phlegm and relieve cough.
- Huo Xiang, Bai Bian Dou, Bing Lang harmonize the middle Jiao and relieve diarrhea.
- Shi Chang Pu relieves damp in the middle Jiao and relieves possible dizziness due to damp invasion.
- Gan Cao eliminates toxins and harmonizes the herbs in the prescription.

Acupuncture Treatment:
- Neiguan P-6 + Gongsun SP-4 with even methods.
- Hegu L.I.-4, Quchi L.I.-11, Waiguan SJ-5, Zhigou SJ-6, Chize LU-5, Feishu BL-13, Zhongwan REN-12, Tianshu ST-25, Fenglong ST-40, Yanglingquan GB-34, and Yinlingquan SP-9 with reducing methods.

Explanations:
- P-6 + SP-4 are used to regulate the qi circulation in the chest, assist respiration and relieve the cough.
- L.I.-4, the yuan-source point of the large intestine channel, SJ-5, the luo-connecting point of the San Jiao channel, and SJ-6, jing-river point of the San Jiao channel, are used to clear heat, eliminate damp, and relieve the external symptoms.

- L.I.-11, the he-sea point of the large intestine, is used to eliminate heat and reduce fever.
- LU-5 and BL-13, the he-sea point of the lung channel, and the back-shu point of the lung respectively, are used to disperse lung-qi, restore the physiological functions of the lung and relieve cough.
- REN-12, ST-25, ST-40, the gathering point of the fu organs and the front-mu point of the stomach, the front-mu point of the large intestine, and the luo-connecting point of the stomach channel respectively, GB-34, the he-sea point of the gallbladder channel, together with SP-9, the he-sea point of the spleen channel, is used to eliminate damp-heat, harmonize the middle Jiao and gallbladder and relieve vomiting and diarrhea.

4.2.6 Accumulation of heat in the lung

High fever, no aversion to cold, dry severe cough or cough with slight yellow phlegm, thirst, possible blood streaks in the phlegm, redness of face, sweating, restlessness, dry stool, red tongue with a yellow coating, and a deep and rapid pulse.

Principle of Treatments:
Clear heat, reduce fever, disperse the lung-qi, and relieve cough.

Herbal Treatment:
Ma Xing Shi Gan Tang-*Ephedra, Apricot Kernel, Gypsum and Licorice Decoction.*

Ma Huang *Herba Ephedrae* 10 g
Xing Ren *Semen Pruni Armeniacae* 10 g
Sheng Shi Gao *Gypsum Fibrosum* 20 g
Zhe Bei Mu *Bulbus Fritillariae Thunbergii* 10 g
Huang Qin *Radix Scutellariae Baicalensis* 10 g
Zhi Mu *Radix Anemarrhenae Asphodeloidis* 10 g
Zhi Ban Xia *Rhizoma Pinelliae Ternatae Preparata* 10 g
Sheng Di Huang *Radix Rehmanniae Glutinosae Recens* 12 g

Explanations:
- Ma Huang and Xing Ren descend the lung-qi and relieve cough.
- Sheng Shi Gao, Huang Qin and Zhi Mu clear heat in the lung, remove toxins and reduce fever.
- Zhe Bei Mu and Zhi Ban Xia eliminate heat-phlegm in the lung and relieve cough.
- Sheng Di Huang clears heat, reduces fever, and removes toxins.

Acupuncture Treatment:
- Neiguan P-6 + Gongsun SP-4 with even methods.
- Hegu L.I.-4, Quchi L.I.-11, Dazhui DU-14, Feishu BL-13, Chize LU-5, Yuji LU-10, Fenglong ST-40, and Sanyinjiao SP-6 with a reducing method.

Explanations:
- P-6 + SP-4 are used to regulate the qi circulation in the chest, assist respiration and relieve cough.
- L.I.-4 and L.I.-11, the yuan-source point and the he-sea point of the large intestine channel respectively, together with Dazhui DU-14, the meeting point of all the yang channels of the body, are used to clear heat and reduce fever.
- BL-13 and LU-5, the back-shu point of the lung and the he-sea point of the lung channel respectively, are used to clear heat in the lung and relieve the cough.
- ST-40 and SP-6, the luo-connecting point of the stomach channel and the crossing point of the three yin channels of the foot respectively, are used to clear heat and eliminate phlegm in the lung.

4.2.7 Accumulation of phlegm-heat in the lung

High fever, no aversion to cold, severe cough with profuse yellow phlegm, thirst, possible blood streaks in the phlegm, slight pressure over the chest, redness of the face, restlessness, nausea, red tongue with a yellow and greasy coating, and a deep, rapid, and slippery pulse.

Principle of Treatments:
Clear heat, eliminate phlegm, disperse the lung-qi, and relieve cough.

Herbal Treatment:
Qing Qi Hua Tan Tang-*Clear the Qi and Transform Phlegm Decoction.*

Dan Nan Xing *Pulvis Arisaematis cum Felle Bovis* 10 g
Quan Gua Lou *Fructus Trichosanthis* 10 g
Huang Qin *Radix Scutellariae Baicalensis* 10 g
Zhe Bei Mu *Bulbus Fritillariae Thunbergii* 10 g
Hou Po *Cortex Magnoliae Officinalis* 5 g
Zhi Zi *Fructus Gardeniae Jasminoidis* 10 g
Zhi Ban Xia *Rhizoma Pinelliae Ternatae Preparata* 10 g
Xing Ren *Semen Pruni Armeniacae* 10 g
Chen Pi *Pericarpium Citri Reticulatae* 5 g
Fu Ling *Sclerotium Poriae Cocos* 10 g

Explanations:
- Dan Nan Xing, Quan Gua Lou and Zhe Bei Mu clear heat, eliminate phlegm and relieve cough.
- Huang Qin and Zhi Zi clear heat in the lung and reduce fever.
- Xing Ren descends the lung-qi and relieve cough.
- Hou Po relaxes the chest and relieves slight pressure over the chest.
- Zhi Ban Xia, Chen Pi and Fu Ling eliminate damp, resolve phlegm, and relieve cough.

Acupuncture Treatment:
- Neiguan P-6 + Gongsun SP-4 with even methods.
- Hegu L.I.-4, Quchi L.I.-11, Dazhui DU-14, Chize LU-5, Yuji LU-10, Feishu BL-13, Tianshu ST-25, Fenglong ST-40, and Sanyinjiao SP-6 with a reducing method.

Explanations:
- P-6 + SP-4 are used to regulate the qi circulation in the chest, assist respiration and relieve cough.
- L.I.-4 and L.I.-11, the yuan-source point and the he-sea point of the large intestine channel respectively, together with DU-14, the meeting point of all the yang channels of the body, are used to clear heat in the body and reduce fever.
- LU-5, BL-13 and LU-10, the he-sea point of the lung channel and the back-shu point, and the ying-stream point of the lung channel respectively, are used to clear heat in the lung, disperse the lung-qi and relieve cough.
- ST-25, the front-mu point of the large intestine, ST-40 and SP-6, the luo-connecting point of the stomach channel, and the crossing point of the three yin channels of the foot respectively, are used to clear heat, reduce fever, and eliminate phlegm in the lung.

4.2.8 Accumulation of cold-phlegm in the lung

Fever, aversion to cold, severe cough with profuse white and foamy phlegm, no thirst, cold limbs, heaviness in the chest, tiredness, nausea, pale tongue with white and greasy coating, and a deep, slow, and slippery pulse.

Principle of Treatments:
Eliminate cold, resolve phlegm, disperse the lung-qi and relieve cough.

Herbal Treatment:
San Zi Yang Qin Tang-*Three Seed Decoction to Nourish One's Parents.*

Bai Jie Zi *Semen Sinapis Albae* 10 g
Zi Su Zi *Fructus Perillae Frutescentis* 10 g
Ting Li Zi *Semen Descurainiae seu Lepidii* 10 g
Xing Ren *Semen Pruni Armeniacae* 10 g
Jie Geng *Radix Platycodi Grandiflori* 10 g

Zhi Shi *Fructus Immaturus Citri Aurantii* 10 g
Hou Po *Cortex Magnoliae Officinalis* 10 g
Zhi Ban Xia *Rhizoma Pinelliae Ternatae Preparata* 10 g
Chen Pi *Pericarpium Citri Reticulatae* 5 g
Fu Ling *Sclerotium Poriae Cocos* 10 g

Explanations:
- Bai Jie Zi, Zi Su Zi and Ting Li Zi eliminate cold-phlegm, descend the lung-qi and relieve cough.
- Jie Geng and Xing Ren eliminate phlegm in the lung, restore the physiological functions of the lung and relieve cough.
- Zhi Shi and Hou Po eliminate phlegm in the lung, promote qi circulation and relieve the heaviness in the chest.
- Zhi Ban Xia, Chen Pi and Fu Ling eliminate damp in the body and resolve phlegm.

Acupuncture Treatment:
- Neiguan P-6 + Gongsun SP-4 with even methods.
- Lieque LU-7, Chize LU-5, Taiyuan LU-9, Feishu BL-13, Zhongwan REN-12, Zusanli ST-36, Fenglong ST-40, Sanyinjiao SP-6, and Yinlingquan SP-9 with a reducing method. Moxibustion could be applied on BL-13, ST-36 and ST-40.

Explanations:
- P-6 + SP-4 are used to regulate the qi circulation in the chest and assist respiration and relieve cough.
- LU-7 and LU-5, the luo-connecting point and he-sea point of the lung channel respectively, and BL-13, the back-shu point of the lung, are used to disperse the lung-qi, eliminate phlegm in the lung and relieve cough.
- REN-12, the gathering point of the fu organs, ST-36 and ST-40, the he-sea point and the luo-connecting point of the stomach channel respectively, together with SP-6, the crossing point of three yin channels of the foot, and SP-9, the he-sea point of the spleen channel, are applied to eliminate damp-phlegm in the body, harmonize the middle Jiao and relieve cough.

- Moxibustion is used to warm the interior, eliminate cold and assist the above points to resolve cold-phlegm in the body.

4.2.9 Symptomatic managements

4.2.9.1 *Fever*

Fever, one of the alarming symptoms of COVID-19, is considered the most common initial symptom of COVID-19. The incubation period of COVID-19 is generally between 5–7 days and could last as long as 10–14 days. From the onset of the illness, fever generally persists 5–7 days because of fierce combat between the zheng-qi and xie-qi, in which zheng-qi is still relatively strong. From the onset of first symptoms till the convalescent stage, it varies from person to person. Sometimes it could last very long. Therefore, we could say that TCM could promote early arrival of the convalescent stage. The purpose of TCM treatment is to support zheng-qi and promote early arrival of the convalescent stage.

In cases of fever, besides using antipyretic in modern medicine, sometimes antibiotics with improper usage (especially the combined use of a broad spectrum of antibiotics), are prescribed. When these medicines are used properly, they could improve the general physical conditions significantly. However, they are considered to have a cold nature, which could directly damage the yang of the spleen and stomach, or even the yang of heart and kidney if improperly used.

TCM controls the body temperature by using different methods and procedures. In the ordinary syndromes in the clinical stages, in most cases, fever is not caused only by exterior pathogenic factors, but it is already in combination with disorders of internal organs. This means that it is inadequate to only apply the dispelling method during this stage. Syndrome differentiations are made to clear heat and reduce fever, including the following methods:

- Disperse the lung-qi and reduce fever.
- Eliminate damp and relieve the blockage of yang.
- Clear heat and eliminate damp.

- Clear heat and remove toxins.
- Clear qi and reduce fever.

Although TCM has some strong herbs that can be used to reduce fever symptomatically, such as Shi Gao *Gypsum Fibrosum* and Zhi Mu *Radix Anemarrhenae Asphodeloidis*, etc., or L.I.-4, L.I.-11 and DU-14, it is never practiced in that way. Clinically, the individual symptom is always treated in combination with a group of symptoms during a syndrome differentiation. It can be seen from above that symptomatic treatment will only reduce fever for a short period, which is not recommended in TCM.

It has also been noticed recently since the appearance of COVID-19 variants that clinical symptoms of COVID-19, especially the initiative symptoms, have begun to change. For instance, originally, fever is always one of the early symptoms of COVID-19, and fever control is also one of the main tasks to deal with in the treatment. Fever control is usually considered as one of the key turning points in the improvement of the disease. However, during the development of the Delta variant, fever is often absent. Meanwhile, there are other new symptoms that are not similar to that of the original strain of the virus, such as skin rashes, nasal bleeding and redness of the eye, etc., which are all caused by invasion of pestilential heat into the ying system. In that case, fever is usually not the key clinical symptom. If the methods introduced above are still applied, they would not be able to help the patient, causing aggravation of the illness. The proper treatment should be to clear heat, remove the toxins, cool the ying system, and prevent heat in the blood. Besides the above symptoms of heat in the ying system, it can also be observed that the patients with Delta variant could suffer from cough, sore throat, anosmia, ageusia, running nose, and myalgia, which are the typical signs of invasion of the external pathogens to the lung with dysfunction of the lung in dispersing the qi. As to their symptoms, such as diarrhea and abdominal pain, etc., they are the signs of invasion of external pathogens to the spleen and stomach. Thus, TCM diagnosis of Delta variant at this stage could be the dysfunction of the lung in dispersing qi with invasion of the pestilential heat to the ying system.

4.2.9.2 *Dry cough*

Cough is the second most common symptom observed in approximately 76% of COVID-19 patients. It is a dry or productive cough with white sputum and with bloodspots in a few patients.

This dry cough is not caused by wind-dryness, because when the TCM diagnosis is the invasion of wind-dryness, there should be some other symptoms to support this pathology, such as dryness of the nose, thirst, and dry coating on the tongue. However, these symptoms are missing here in the initial stage. Therefore, it is not necessary to apply the following herbs to moisten the dryness, such as Mai Men Dong *Tuber Ophiopogonis Japonici*, Bei Sha Shen *Radix Glehniae Littoralis* and Tian Hua Fen *Radix Trichosanthis Kirilowii*, etc. The acupuncture points, such as Jingqu LU-8, Taiyuan LU-9, Sanyinjiao SP-6 and Zhaohai KID-6, etc., are also not necessary.

Bloodspots with cough are caused by damage of the external pathogenic factors, and it could be due to wind-cold, wind-heat or other factors invading the blood vessels. Clinically, blood cooling herbs or bleeding-stopping herbs should not be applied in this case, including Sheng Di Huang *Radix Rehmanniae Glutinosae Recens*, Xuan Shen *Radix Scrophulariae Ningpoensis*, Mu Dan Pi *Cortex Moutan Radicis*, Bai Ji *Rhizoma Bletillae Striatae*, Ce Bai Ye *Cacumen Biotae Orientalis* and Xue Yu Tan *Crinis Carbonisatus*, etc. When these external pathogenic factors are expelled and the lung functions are restored, bloodspots will be under control. Of course, if there is severe bleeding, which is usually not the case, it is something else. TCM never gives an over-treatment.

4.2.9.3 *Muscular pain*

Muscular pain is seen in approximately 44% of patients. It is caused by the stagnation of qi in different meridians with blockage of some vessels by external invasion. It is an extreme sign, indicating there is an invasion of EPF. Clinically, herbs or acupuncture points should be used to dispel the pathogenic factors, and harmonize the meridians and qi circulation. Herbs such as Qiang Huo *Rhizoma et Radix Notopterygii*, Du Huo *Radix Angelicae Pubescentis*, Gao Ben *Rhizoma et Radix Ligustici*, Chuan Xiong *Radix Ligustici Wallichii*, etc. could be applied. Points such as Lieque LU-7, Hegu L.I.-4, Waiguan SJ-5, and Fengchi GB-20, etc. are good points to dispel external pathogenic factors and relieve the muscle pain at some time. It is inappropriate at this moment to only use the method to promote the qi or blood circulation.

4.2.9.4 *Fatigue*

Fatigue could be one of the chief symptoms in the early stage of COVID-19. However, it may remain during ordinary syndromes. similar to the treatment in the early stage, TCM will not offer any qi or blood tonics to the patients for their tiredness because this complaint is not caused by deficiency of qi or blood, but by disturbance to the physiological functions of the lung and spleen, especially the function of the lung in dispersing the qi in the body. When the lung functions recover after treatment, the patient will gradually feel less tired. This explains why in the therapeutic prescription, there is no qi or blood tonic being used. If these tonics are prescribed too early, they could aggravate the situation and slow down the healing process of treatment.

4.2.9.5 *Dysfunction of the throat and nose*

Throat pain is accompanied by a group of symptoms related to external invasion, which is caused by dysfunction of the lung in dispersing the qi to the throat and blockage of the meridian in the throat. When throat pain is not that severe, then treatment should be focused on general conditions. Treatment could be improved when the general pathology is under control. However, if it is severe, then some herbs (such as She Gan *Rhizoma Belamcandae Chinensis*, Yu Hu Die *Oroxylum indicum (L.) Vent*, and Pang Da Hai *Semen Sterculiae Scaphigerae*, etc.) could be used or acupuncture points (Tiantu REN-22, Lianquan REN-23, and Renying ST-9) should be applied.

Sudden loss of smell and taste sometimes could represent an alarming sign of COVID-19. Some patients may only have this sign. A PCR test should be considered to exclude COVID-19. In other patients, there could be nose blockage and dry cough. The main mechanism of these complaints is due to the invasion of the external pathogenic factors with dysfunction of the lung in dispersing the qi. These symptoms will be simultaneously alleviated when methods are used to dispel external factors and disperse the qi. However, when these complaints are too severe, extra attention could be used to relieve them. Herbs such as Xin Yi Hua *Flos Magnoliae*, Cang Er Zi *Fructus Xanthii Sibirici*, and E Bu Shi Cao *Herba Centipeda Minima* can be used. Acupuncture points (Yingxiang L.I.-20, Extra Bitong, and Juliao ST-3, etc.) could be applied. Besides, knowledge about the extra meridian should be considered to identify if these complaints are caused by a disorder of extra meridians. Treatment for important complaints and complications, COVID-19 associated loss of smell and taste from the same chapter should be mentioned.

It has also been noticed that among early symptoms from COVID-19, blocked nose without a running nose is included. However, as far as the Delta variant is concerned, this symptom changes into a running nose. In fact, the whole TCM treatment remains the same, which means that no extra herbs should be added to solve this complaint.

Another new COVID-19 symptom caused by the Delta variant is nasal bleeding. This is important, because it appears together with bleeding from the throat, skin rashes and redness of the eyes, etc. All these symptoms are the indication that there is an invasion of pestilential heat into the ying system. Treatment strategy should be amended to cool blood and stop bleeding, besides dispersing the lung-qi. Herbs such as Sheng Di Huang *Radix Rehmanniae Glutinosae Recens*, Xuan Shen *Radix Scrophulariae Ningpoensis*, Mu Dan Pi *Cortex Moutan Radicis*, Chi Shao Yao *Radix Paeoniae Rubrae*, and Bai Ji *Rhizoma Bletillae Striatae* could be added to the prescription, and acupuncture points Sanyinjiao SP-6, Xuehai SP-10, Geshu BL-17, and Shaofu HE-8, should be applied.

4.2.9.6 *Skin rashes*

Although the mechanism of this symptom is the same as the bleeding from the nose and throat explained above, skin rashes are due to cutaneous bleeding. It is not exactly the same as nasal or throat bleeding, which belongs to the dysfunction of the lung system. When skin rashes happen, it implies something more serious, and great attention should be paid. Herbs and acupuncture points to remove the toxins should be also added. Moreover, the physiological functions of the heart and liver, as well as the spleen should be cared for.

4.2.9.7 *Abdominal pain and diarrhea*

In ordinary syndromes, abdominal pain and diarrhea are often caused by damp, either by cold-damp or damp-heat. These symptoms are not existing independently, but in combination with some symptoms of the lung. It means that besides caring for the lung, (i.e., to restore the physiological function of the lung in dispersing the qi and eliminating the pathogenic factors), methods to activate the spleen, eliminate damp and relieve the pain should be used. Herbs such as Cang Zhu *Rhizoma Atractylodis*, Ge Gen *Radix Puerariae*, Huo Xiang *Herba Agastaches seu Pogostemi*, and Pei Lan *Herba Eupatorii Fortunei* should be used. In addition, the following acupuncture points could be applied:

- Tianshu ST-25, Shuidao ST-28, Yinlingquan SP-9, Zusanli ST-36, and Fenglong ST-40 with reducing method for cold-damp.
- Huang Lian *Rhizoma Coptidis*, Hou Po *Cortex Magnoliae Officinalis*, Hua Shi *Talcum*, Cang Zhu *Rhizoma Atractylodis*, together with Tianshu ST-25, Shuidao ST-28, Yanglingquan GB-34, Dadu SP-2, Yinlingquan SP-9, and Fenglong ST-40 with reducing method for damp-heat could be considered.

5

TCM Treatment of Severe Syndromes of COVID-19

5.1 TCM Analysis of Severe Syndromes of COVID-19

5.1.1 Diagnosis of severe syndromes of COVID-19

5.1.1.1 *Diagnosis criteria*

The "Diagnosis and Treatment Plan" promulgated by the General Office of the National Health Commission and the Office of the State Administration of Traditional Chinese Medicine has clear regulations for the diagnosis of severe cases of COVID-19. This includes the occurrence of "multiple organ failure" which might be possible in addition to septic shock, difficult-to-correct metabolic acidosis, and coagulopathy, etc.

Nonetheless, when suffering from different types of severe syndromes, patients may be too weak to travel to a clinic or get hospitalized. Because of this, it is inconvenient to carry out a face-to-face consultation. Thus, the clinical observation and herbal treatment of TCM could be done through telemedicine using online techniques.

5.1.1.2 *Viral variants related to severe cases*

It is worth noticing that the WHO listed four virus variants worthy of global attention on 31 May 2021. They are the Alpha variant (first discovered in the UK), the Beta variant (first discovered in South Africa), the Gamma variant (first found in Brazil), and the Delta variant (first discovered in India). According to *United Nation News*—Global perspective Human stories, as of 28 July 2021, "of the four COVID-19 mutations that WHO has designated 'variants of concern', the UN agency said that the Alpha variant is present in 182 countries, Beta in 131, Gamma in 81 and after reaching 8 new countries in the past week, the Delta variant is now in 132 countries".[1]

As of July 2021, there are four variants of concerns (VOCs): Alpha, Beta, Gamma and Delta, and four variants of interests (VOIs): Eta, Iota, Kappa, and Lambda. These variants are considered to be potential threats to human society. The Lambda variant was first detected in Argentina on 8 November 2020. The fact that the percentage of the Lambda sequence is increasing in South American countries including Peru, Chile, and Argentina, suggests that the Lambda variant is spreading predominantly in these countries. Lambda is highly infectious and is more susceptible to an infection-enhancing antibody.

The Lambda variant is not only highly infectious but also has high resistance against antiviral immunity. These observations suggest that acquiring at least two virological features—increased viral infectivity, and evasion from antiviral immunity—is pivotal to the efficient spread and transmission in the human population.[2] Lambda accounts for nearly 82% of the coronavirus case samples in Peru reported during May and June, according to the Pan American Health Organization (PAHO),[3] which has the world's highest coronavirus mortality rate. In neighboring Chile, it accounts for almost a third of new cases.[4]

---

[1]COVID-19 infections rise, Delta variant spreads to 132 countries. *United Nation News*. 28 July 2021. https://news.un.org/en/story/2021/07/1096572.

[2]Izumi Kimura, *et al.* SARS-CoV-2 Lambda variant exhibits higher infectivity and immune resistance. *bioRxiv*. 28 July 2021. https://doi.org/10.1101/2021.07.28.454085.

[3]Luke Hurst. Lambda: What do we know about the latest COVID variant flagged by the WHO? Updated: 7 July 2021. https://www.euronews.com/2021/07/06/lambda-what-do-we-know-about-the-latest-covid-variant-flagged-by-the-who.

[4]Clive Cookson. Lambda Covid variant's "unusual" mutations puzzle scientists. *Financial Times*. 2 July 2021. https://www.ft.com/content/b3ea5177-9312-418b-acb7-af16a3bdcd22.

On 31 July 2021, the Scientific Advisory Group for Emergencies (SAGE) and top UK government scientists, said it is a "realistic possibility" that future variants could prove as fatal as MERS, which has a death rate of 35%, and the chance of deadly COVID-19 mutations increases depending on the prevalence of the virus. The advisory body warned that future strains could become resistant to vaccines if they originate from the beta variant and combine with the Alpha or Delta variants, in a process called recombination. Even with vaccines being expected to neutralize serious symptoms among COVID-19 patients, the report said a higher death rate is to be expected in the case of new deadly variants, given that vaccines do not provide total sterilizing immunity.[5]

Among four variants of concerns (VOCs), the Delta variant virus of SARS-CoV-2, first appearing in India in late 2020, is even more aggressive and has quickly swept across the world, becoming the main epidemic strain in more than 80 countries or regions around the world as of 20 July 2021 and is still spreading rapidly.

Yet, many studies have shown that its infectious ability has increased greatly, and the protective effect of vaccines has also reduced significantly. Judging from the recent outbreaks that struck Guangzhou, Shenzhen, and Dongguan in China, when compared with previous viruses, the clinical characteristics of the Delta mutant in infected patients include extremely high viral loads, extremely short incubation periods, and faster conversion to critical illness after infection. It takes a long time for PCR tests to turn negative. Researchers have found that people infected with the Delta variant produce far more viruses than those infected with the original version of SARS-CoV-2, making it very easy to spread. One study reported that the virus was first detectable in people with the Delta variant four days after exposure, compared with an average of six days among people with the original strain, suggesting that Delta replicates much faster. Individuals infected with Delta also had viral loads

---

[5] UK scientists: Future COVID-19 variants could have 35% fatality rates. *Arab News.* 31 July 2021. https://www.arabnews.com/node/1903196/world.

up to 1260 times higher than those in people infected with the original strain.

The combination of a high number of viruses and a short incubation period makes sense as an explanation for Delta's heightened transmissibility, which is more than twice of the original strain of SARS-CoV-2. The short incubation makes contact tracing more difficult in countries such as China, which systematically tracks each infected person's contacts and requires them to go under quarantine. Meanwhile, a number of other questions about the Delta variant remain unanswered. Is it more likely to cause severe disease than the original strain? How good is it at evading the immune system? Some of this information will emerge as researchers look more closely at broader and more diverse populations of people infected with Delta and other variants.[6]

The good news is that one study has confirmed some vaccines could be very effective in preventing this Delta virus, which was published in *The New England Journal of Medicine* on 21 July 2021.

It pointed out that vaccine effectiveness against the Alpha and Delta variants is grouped according to dose and vaccine type, showing that effectiveness was notably lower after the first vaccine dose among persons with the Delta variant 30.7% than among those with the Alpha variant 48.7%. Results for the first dose were similar for both vaccines, with an absolute difference in vaccine effectiveness against the Delta variant as compared with the Alpha variant (11.9% with the BNT162b2 vaccine and 18.7% with the ChAdOx1 nCoV-19 vaccine). The difference in vaccine effectiveness was much smaller among persons who had received the second dose of the vaccine. In the "any vaccine" analysis, the vaccine effectiveness was 87.5% with the Alpha variant and 79.6% with the Delta variant. With the BNT162b2 vaccine, a small difference in effectiveness between variants was seen after the second dose: 93.7% with the Alpha variant and 88.0% with the Delta variant. The effectiveness with

---

[6] Sara Reardon. How the Delta variant achieves its ultrafast spread. *Nature*. 21 July 2021. https://doi.org/10.1038/d41586-021-01986-w.

two doses of the ChAdOx1 nCoV-19 vaccine was lower than with the BNT162b2 vaccine. However, with the ChAdOx1 nCoV-19 vaccine, the difference in effectiveness between the Alpha and Delta variants was small (74.5% and 67.0% respectively).[7] However, according to Israel's Health Ministry, the vaccine protected 64% of inoculated people from infection during an outbreak of the Delta variant, down from 94% before. It was 94% effective at preventing severe illness in the same period, compared with 97% before.[8] Nevertheless, the effectiveness at preventing severe illness is still quite high.

5.1.1.3 *TCM diagnosis systems*

When the disease is caused by invasion of external pathogenic factors, no matter if it is light or severe (including COVID-19 at the severe stage), the following systems are applied to establish a TCM diagnosis. These systems include the six channels, or wei, qi, ying, and xue systems, or San Jiao, etc. Each system is indicated in specific conditions. For instance, for invasion of wind and cold, six-channel system is mainly used. If there is an invasion of wind-heat, then wei, qi, ying, and xue system is applied. If there is an invasion of damp and heat, then the San Jiao system is often considered. However, COVID-19 doesn't follow one of the above systems strictly, which means that this disease could involve all these systems at the same time. The reason for this complicated procedure in diagnosis is because COVID-19 is caused by a mixture of pestilential toxins with different other pathologies, in which invasion of cold-damp or damp-heat remains the main causative factors. Meanwhile, the

---

[7]Jamie Lopez Bernal, *et al.* Effectiveness of Covid-19 vaccines against the B.1.617.2 (Delta) variant. 2021. *N Engl J Med.* 2021, 385: 585–594. doi: 10.1056/NEJMoa2108891.

[8]Dov Lieber. Pfizer vaccine less effective against delta infections but prevents severe illness, Israeli data show. *The Wall Street Journal.* 6 July 2021. https://www.wsj.com/articles/pfizers-covid-19-vaccine-is-less-effective-against-delta-variant-israeli-data-show-11625572796.

constitutional conditions or weaknesses of the patient are the root factors for the deterioration of COVID-19.

5.1.1.4 *Variety of clinical patterns in the severe stage*

When the disease is in its severe stage, it is characterized by complexity, variability, severity, and lung impairment. The most important pathology at this stage is the failure of the lung to descend the lung-qi with dysfunctions of zang-fu organs in qi and blood.

When the disease is in its severe stage, it shows different clinical patterns due to the complexity of the causative factor and different underlying constitutions, including:

- Cold at the exterior with heat at the interior.
- Heat at the exterior with cold at the interior.
- Cold at the exterior with the formation of yin–fluid (饮) at the interior.
- Existence of pathogens at Shaoyang level.
- Accumulation of heat in the lung and stomach.
- Formation and blockage of phlegm-heat in the lung.
- Obstruction of damp in the spleen and stomach.
- Accumulation of damp-heat in the middle Jiao.
- Accumulation and obstruction of excessive heat in Yangming.
- Decline of yang of the heart and kidney.

5.1.1.5 *General TCM management*

Since the outbreak of the new coronavirus pneumonia in December 2019, the General Office of the National Health Commission of China and the Office of the State Administration of Traditional Chinese Medicine have successively promulgated the "New Coronavirus Infection Pneumonia Diagnosis and Treatment Plan" (often referred to as the "Diagnosis and Treatment Plan"). Editions three to eight clarify the TCM treatment plan and propose that the new coronavirus pneumonia belongs to the category of plague in

TCM. The joint participation of Chinese and Western medicine in the treatment has become an important part of the treatment of new coronavirus pneumonia. It is one of the main contents of the "China Plan" for the fight against the pandemic, and it has also become a highlight of the prevention and control of this pandemic.

Yanhong Yu, Secretary of the Party Leadership of the State Administration of Traditional Chinese Medicine, announced at a press conference of the State Council Information Office on 23 March 2020, that observations of clinical efficacy have shown that the total effective rate of traditional Chinese medicine has reached more than 90%. Traditional Chinese medicine can effectively relieve symptoms, reduce the development of mild and common types into severe syndromes, increase the cure rate, reduce the mortality rate, and promote the recovery of patients in the convalescent period.[9] After screening and research, Jin Hua Qing Gan Granules, Lian Hua Qing Wen Capsules/Granules, Xue Bi jing Injection, Qing Fei Pai Du Decoction, Hua Shi Bai Du Decoction, and Xuan Fei Bai Du Decoction, the so-called "three medicines and three prescriptions", proved effective.[10]

Zhongde Zhang, a member of the expert team of the National Health Commission, vice president of Guangzhou University of Traditional Chinese Medicine, and vice president of Guangdong Provincial Hospital of TCM, pointed out that the pathogenic mechanism of the virus is still damp-heat and toxins. Previously, the treatment was mainly to remove damp, and also to clear away heat and toxins. This time, according to the different symptoms, the main purpose is mainly to clear away heat, to remove damp and eliminate toxins. With the mutation of the virus, the passage of time, the

---

[9]Yang Wang. The information office of the state council held a press conference on the important role of traditional Chinese medicine in the prevention and treatment of new coronary pneumonia and effective drugs. 23 March 2020. Central People's Government of the People's Republic of China. http://www.gov.cn/xinwen/2020-03/23/content_5494694.htm.

[10]These Chinese medicine prescriptions are effective in the treatment of new coronary pneumonia. The "three medicines and three prescriptions" write a Chinese medicine anti-epidemic plan. *China Daily* (中国日报). 18 March 2020. http://www.xinhuanet.com/2020-03/18/c_1125729859.htm.

change in seasons, and some other important factors, the pathogenesis analysis and prescription of Chinese medicine need to be adjusted continuously to adapt to the new syndrome differentiation treatment.[11]

From February 2020 to the present, the authors have witnessed the outbreak of new coronary virus pneumonia in Europe, the continuous increase in the number of confirmed cases and deaths, the panic amongst people, and the active anti-epidemic efforts of governments at all levels. They are also very fortunate to be active with colleagues in Europe, participating in the treatment of severe patients with new coronary virus pneumonia using traditional Chinese medicine, and have successfully treated more than 100 severely critical patients through online systems. However, there are still patients with new coronary virus pneumonia at home and abroad, infected with the same virus, with mutated viruses from the United Kingdom, South Africa, and Brazil variants in the second wave of epidemics. In terms of the rate of incidence and changes in the disease, the second wave of epidemics is worse than the first wave. The epidemic situation is relatively serious. In addition, European patients with severe syndromes of new coronary virus pneumonia bear their own characteristics in terms of etiology and pathogenesis, and TCM treatment is also slightly different from that in mainland China. It is always necessary to implement syndrome differentiation and treatment as the center, according to the condition and symptoms of the patients and avoid sticking to prescriptions and patent remedies without modifications. Personalized herbal prescriptions to treat patients should be advocated.

In short, during the TCM management of syndromes in severe stages, in addition to removing the pathogenic factors and restoring the qi and blood function of the zang-fu organs, the main task is to descend lung-qi, resolve phlegm and relax the chest, which

---

[11]Yulong Qin. Traditional Chinese medicine has a good effect on new coronary pneumonia caused by delta mutant strain. *China Traditional Chinese Medicine News Reporter* (中国中医药报), 6 July 2021. http://www.gdhtcm.com/sitecn/mtbd/14297.html.

should be carried out throughout the treatment process for each syndrome. It is important that a combination of TCM with modern medicine in some severe cases be implemented to ensure a good level of oxygen saturation and prevent deterioration of the illness. When TCM treatment is properly practiced, its accurate syndrome differentiation and efficiency could be obtained immediately, reflecting that all theoretical and experience of TCM applied in the diagnosis and treatment of COVID-19 are practical and valuable.

5.1.2 Pathogenesis characteristics of severe and critical syndromes

According to the analysis of authoritative experts that are published in China, COVID-19 belongs to the category of "plague", and its case is characterized as "damp and toxins". The basic pathogenesis is an external invasion of epidemic toxins, dysfunction of the lung, and impairment of zheng-qi with damp, heat, toxins, weakness, and stagnation as their pathologic features. According to the clinical manifestations of their syndromes, COVID-19 could be divided into five stages: light, ordinary, severe, critical, and convalescent stages. From the perspective of the number of infections and mortality, the number of people infected with COVID-19 in China is more than 80,000, and the mortality rate is about 3%.[12] Judging from the treated European patients with severe and critical syndromes, their causative factors are more complicated (including invasion of external six-pathogenic factors with toxins, especially cold-damp, or damp-heat), resulting in dysfunction of the lung in dispersing the qi in the early stage. Due to the lack of proper treatment or delayed treatment, these pathologic conditions quickly deteriorated, leading to failure of the lung in descending the qi, dysfunction of the San Jiao, disharmony of

---

[12]Boli Zhang, *et al.* Experience of Chinese medicine in the treatment of new coronary pneumonia. *State Administration of Traditional Chinese Medicine.* 1 April 2020. http://www.satcm.gov.cn/xinxifabu/meitibaodao/2020-04-01/14418.html.

the spleen and stomach, disorder of the liver and gallbladder, or damage to the yang of the heart and kidney.

Compared with ordinary syndrome, the causative factors and pathogenesis of severe and critical syndromes are much more complicated, in which external pathogenic factors are usually not yet expelled, but the impairment to multiple internal zang-fu organs already happened at the same time. Nonetheless, some of the clinical manifestations of severe and critical syndromes are almost similar to those from the ordinary syndrome, albeit belonging to severe and critical syndromes, because their dyspnea and pressure over the chest could be observed and relatively low oxygen saturation could be tested. Any further delayed or improper treatment could directly cause aggravation of the situation.

It is very important to diagnose and apply precise treatment because the syndrome types are more complex than COVID-19, with severe and critical syndromes making it difficult for TCM treatment. Among them, physical constitutions, age, and underlying diseases, etc., are to a large extent the main factors that determine the trend and prognosis of the disease.

Generally speaking, the pathogenesis of patients with severe to critical COVID-19 in Europe has the following characteristics, which is not similar to that from mainland, China.

5.1.2.1 *Complexity*

Compared with China, Europe is not the same in terms of regional environment, climate change, lifestyle and personal diet, or physical fitness and emotional state. These obvious differences are important for patients in terms of invasion of pathogens and changes in pathogenesis. The causative factors of patients with severe and critical syndromes are complex, and are often caused by the combination of internal and external factors. The combination of new and old illnesses also makes the pathogenesis very complicated. It is rare to see patients with severe and critical syndromes with a single cause, or involvement of only one organ. Failure of the lung in its descending, disorder of metabolism in water, stagnation of qi and blood, and impairment of multiple zang-fu organs, are the usual situations and consequences of the diseases at these stages. In addition, during the course of the disease, the pathogenesis changes are always in constant change. Close attention is paid to the shortness of breath, chest tightness, blood oxygen saturation and fever control. Meanwhile, appetite, physical strength, emotions, and sleep, etc., which could be severely affected at the same time, are also necessarily cared for. TCM treatment with herbal prescription should be modified and regulated accordingly within three to five days.

In view of the complexity of the pathogenesis, its treatment methods are significantly different from the previous general disease due to external invasion or internal disorders.

- Since the pathogens are mainly cold-damp or damp-heat, in combination with toxins, it is rare to encounter the syndromes with a simple transmission according to the theory of the six-channels system. It means if there is an invasion of wind-cold, mixed with the damp, appearance of Taiyang syndrome, Shaoyang syndrome or Yangming syndrome will be more common. In severe or critical situations, there could be direct impairment of the yang of the heart and kidney. During these transmission procedures, there could be some obstruction of qi transformation due to the existence of damp, showing manifestation of the fullness of the chest and abdomen, abdominal distention, loose stool or diarrhea, nausea, or vomiting, etc.
- If it is mainly caused by heat or damp, it is more common that wei, qi, ying, and xue system, or San Jiao system could be mainly damaged, showing hyperactivity of qi and ying or obstruction of the upper and middle Jiao.
- Since the pathogenic factors include wind, cold, heat, damp, and toxins, it is rare to have syndromes that only follow a six-channel system, or wei, qi, ying, and xue system or only the San Jiao system. In most cases, there is a mixture of different systems at the same time.

- No matter whatever system is involved, failure of the lung in descending the qi is the key pathological result, which needs careful management constantly. It can also be seen easily that there is no one patent remedy or one fixed and standard herbal prescription, which has not yet been modified accordingly, that meets the needs of the patients with severe and critical syndromes.

5.1.2.2 *Changeability*

Once highly suspected or positive PCR is confirmed, the patients usually start following procedures in Europe, including quarantine, self-isolation, and self-administration of antipyretic to fight against fever. These procedures are common at the beginning of the pandemic due to limited PCR tests and to avoid patient overload at the hospital. Of course, these measures are often obviously very limited in protecting the immune system, resisting viruses, restoring lung function, and preventing multiple organ damage. On the contrary, they could be the chief reason for aggravating the condition and delaying treatment if no close observation is obtained.

Furthermore, those patients who have not received timely and appropriate treatment or refused to be admitted out of fear of hospital treatment (especially those who are frail, the elderly and those with comorbidities), are very likely to develop a severe or a critical syndrome soon. Dramatic deterioration often happens within a few hours. For example, what manifests in the morning will be different in the evening, in which blood oxygen saturation could drop sharply, pulmonary embolism, myocardial infarction, or cerebral infarction may follow at any moment. Shortness of breath, fever, cough, increased chest tightness, cold hands and feet, sweat and weak pulse, and even fainting may follow as well. Any delayed treatment or lack of proper treatment could lead to aggravation of the disease and even death.

In a common cold or flu, even if there is a high fever for a couple of days or a week, it rarely deteriorates rapidly. However, it is different in COVID-19 cases, in which a persistent high fever that lasts for a few days could immediately cause flaring of heat, hyperactivity of Fire in the qi and ying systems, severe cough with dyspnea, and chest tightness due to failure of the lung in descending the qi. Any inadequate TCM treatment could lead to the occurrence of the critical syndrome, manifesting as dyspnea, pale complexion, extreme cold hands and feet, cold sweat, fading pulse, or even semi-consciousness. During severe or critical syndromes, one of the common phenomena is that some basic diseases start to become aggravated. Examples include the sharp increase in blood sugar level of diabetic patients, the blood pressure of someone with hypertension that cannot be controlled by the routine antihypertensive drugs, the heart function that declines rapidly in patients with heart issues, or the tumor markers deteriorate rapidly. Therefore, how to effectively control the severe syndrome, prevent it from developing into the critical syndrome and actively treat the critical syndrome, are the top priority of TCM practitioners. Patients with COVID-19, who have received TCM treatment overseas, need to be admitted to the hospital for treatment once they enter the critical syndrome. If conditions permit when they are admitted into the hospital, it is best to combine TCM treatment with modern medicine. In the West, some hospitals and doctors are more enlightened and open to TCM. After knowing the background of qualified Chinese medicine, TCM is also involved in the treatment of critical illness.

5.1.2.3 *Severity*

Due to the sudden occurrence of the COVID-19 pandemic, even in economically and technologically advanced Europe, there are still limited medicine available in the treatments, and most of these are based upon symptomatic support. In addition, most patients with self-isolation lack modern tracking methods and technology, which implies that its treatment is somehow left behind social and medical needs.

Home isolation and relying on paracetamol to manage COVID-19 is the chief treatment plan in many countries for most of the confirmed patients or highly suspicious patients. This could be relatively sufficient for the majority of the patients. However, these two methods could put some patients in danger, including those with comorbidities, the elderly, extremely weak patients, patients with cardiac diseases, diabetes, obesity, transplantation, etc. If left untreated, these patients with COVID-19 could rapidly develop into some serious conditions (including uncontrolled high fever, intensified coughing, chest tightness, dyspnea, irritability, extreme fatigue, poor appetite, nausea, vomiting, severe diarrhea, decreased oxygen saturation levels, sudden collapse or confusion, etc.), which are all symptoms from severe or critical syndromes. It could also be observed that both tongue color and coating could change their natures dramatically. It is very possible to observe a red, yellow, and greasy coating tongue a few hours ago suddenly turn into a pale, white and wet coating tongue, accompanied with cold hands, cold body, low body temperature, somnolence, and a deep, thready, fading pulse.

Even when the ambulance finally arrived at the the house, the patients could be so exhausted and too weak to get out of the bed and walk themselves to the ambulance. These patients could pass away in a very short time if no emergency treatment was administered. During the first wave of lockdowns in some severe epidemics, e.g., Italy and Spain, about half of the patients who died of COVID-19 came from nursing homes. The elderly remains as the high-risk group in this epidemic. The morbidity of severe and critical syndromes, as well as their mortality rate, are significantly higher than those of young people without underlying diseases.[13]

Furthermore, for patients who panic because of high morbidity and mortality numbers, this anxiety is also an important factor that

---

[13] Robert Booth. Half of coronavirus deaths happen in care homes, data from EU suggests. *The Guardian.* 13 April 2020. https://www.theguardian.com/world/2020/apr/13/half-of-coronavirus-deaths-happen-in-care-homes-data-from-eu-suggests.

aggravates emotional changes, causing some to experience extreme restlessness, anxiety, insomnia, palpitations, restless and the feeling that "death is coming at any time". These factors could greatly influence the immunity and physical conditions of such patients. A study published in *The Lancet* by Dutch researchers in December 2020 tracked the mental health of 1,517 respondents before and after the COVID-19 pandemic and showed that the pandemic has aggravated depression, anxiety, and loneliness among those with no or mild mental illness.[14] In short, once severe syndrome and critical syndrome occur, their mortality rate will increase significantly.

5.1.2.4 *Lung impairment*

The new coronavirus pneumonia is different from the common cold or infection, as well as other viral infections, such as SARS and MERS. One of the most affected and damaged body part is the lung. TCM believes that the lung is a delicate organ, which is responsible for dispersing the qi and descending the qi, providing an opening into the nose, connecting the skin and vessels, regulating the water passage, etc. When COVID-19 develops into severe or critical syndromes, the above functions of the lung could be damaged simultaneously, manifesting as extreme shortness of breath, severe chest tightness, difficulty in spitting out phlegm, expectoration of a large amount of white foamy sputum or yellow phlegm, scanty urination, peripheral oedema, or even cyanosis and fainting. In some circumstances, even if oxygen is provided in the hospital, the patients could still feel chest tightness and shortness of breath.

The lung is closely connected to other organs, and in correspondence to the five elements in TCM, is considered as the Metal Element. Once the lung fails to descend the qi in severe conditions, it will

---

[14]Kuan-Yu Pan, *et al.* The mental health impact of the COVID-19 pandemic on people with and without depressive, anxiety, or obsessive-compulsive disorders: A longitudinal study of three Dutch case-control cohorts. *The Lancet Psychiatry.* 2021, 8(2), 121–129. https://doi.org/10.1016/S2215-0366(20)30491-0.

naturally affect the other organs, leading to dysfunctions in these affected organs. This is when the entire physiological function of the body will be impaired, and the pathological conditions start to deteriorate.

It is worth mentioning that during severe or critical syndromes, it is very rare to observe that only one physiological function of the lung is affected, but impairment of multiple functions of the lung is often the pathological result. Thus, besides the disturbed descending function of the lung, various physiological functions are also impaired, presenting with complicated symptoms and signs. During the TCM treatment, restoring the lung in descending is the top priority in all treatment options.

5.1.3 Treatment precautions

COVID-19 is a highly contagious disease, which could cause person-to-person transmission directly. During the TCM treatment, especially acupuncture treatment, preventive measures should be taken to prevent being infected. The infectious period is ten days from the onset of the first symptom. It is suggested to consult the patients via telemedicine, and herbs could be collected and delivered to the door by family members or friends directly to the patient. Also, the following precautions could be taken into considerations.

5.1.3.1 *Acupuncture treatment*

If the practitioner's infection safety cannot be fully protected, the acupuncture treatment can be postponed until the patient is in the convalescent stage.

5.1.3.2 *Personalized prescription*

During treatment, if possible, provide personalized herbal prescriptions based on the differentiation of symptoms and signs as much as possible.

5.1.3.3 *Patent remedies*

When personalized prescriptions cannot be provided or obtained due to various reasons, a patent remedy or some standard herbal prescriptions can be considered.

5.1.3.4 *Close observation*

Even if a personalized herbal prescription is given to the patient before the convalescent stage, the patient's response, actual situations, and prognosis should be closely observed. No delay or improper treatment is permitted.

5.1.3.5 *Avoid a fixed prescription*

Since COVID-19 is an acute infectious disease, the pathogen changes rapidly, and sometimes there may be some differences in clinical manifestations within a few hours. Therefore, herbal prescriptions should not be given for too many days, usually less than a week. If necessary, the prescription should be modified after one or two days after taking the herb.

5.1.3.6 *Always consider the lung*

Regardless of the stage of COVID-19, care for the lung during the treatment is one of the key features of the treatment, i.e., to repair the physiological function is always the most important treatment principle and method. For light or ordinary syndromes, dispersing the lung-qi is most important, often using the following herbs:

Ma Huang *Herba Ephedrae*
Jie Geng *Radix Platycodi Grandiflori*
Sang Ye *Folium Mori Albae*
Zi Su Ye *Folium Perillae Frutescentis*
Xing Ren *Semen Pruni Armeniacae*

Meanwhile, some herbs to eliminate phlegm and stop cough should be combined to relieve cough, such as:
Zhi Ban Xia *Rhizoma Pinelliae Ternatae Preparata*
Chen Pi *Pericarpium Citri Reticulatae*
Zi Su Zi *Fructus Perillae Frutescentis*

But when it enters the severe or critical syndromes, these herbs to descend the lung-qi should be applied, including:
Ma Huang Herba *Ephedrae*
Xing Ren *Semen Pruni Armeniacae*
Sang Bai Pi *Cortex Mori Albae Radicis*
Ting Li Zi *Semen Descurainiae seu Lepidii*

The fullness of the chest with tightness is the most urgent problem to be solved, extra herbs should be added, such as:
Hou Po *Cortex Magnoliae Officinalis*
Zhi Shi *Fructus Immaturus Citri Aurantii*

Expectoration of profuse phlegm is another complaint from the patients that should be cared by adding:
Bai Jie Zi *Semen Sinapis Albae* and Zi Su Zi *Fructus Perillae Frutescentis* for cold-phlegm
Zhe Bei Mu *Bulbus Fritillariae Thunbergii* and Quan Gua Lou for heat-phlegm

5.2 TCM Treatment

For the TCM treatment of new coronavirus pneumonia, some experts follow the syndrome differentiation based upon six-channels systems,[15] and some propose the syndrome differentiation based on

---

[15]Xikui Zhang, *et al*. Analysis of the six channels syndrome for differentiation and treatment of novel coronavirus pneumonia. *Fujian Traditional Chinese Medicine* (福建中医药). 2020, 51(2): 1–3. http://subject.med.wanfangdata.com.cn/UpLoad/Files/202002/9bee4dfbc2cd41f29e7a941a419198f4.pdf.

the wei, qi, ying and xue systems,[16] and some follow the syndrome differentiation based upon the perspective of San Jiao system.[17]

However, when COVID-19 develops into severe or critical syndrome, its pathological changes are more complicated and serious. There may be a syndrome with a combination of two different channels simultaneously, or the syndrome with one channel is not yet healed, but another channel starts to be involved. There is the possibility of a mixture of three yang channels with involvement of Shaoyin channel at the same time, or involvement of Taiyang channel with an accumulation of damp-heat in the lower Jiao, or syndrome of Shaoyang channel with an accumulation of damp-heat in the middle Jiao, etc.

In the contents and descriptions of *Shang Han Lun—Treatise on Febrile Diseases*, lung failure and damage to the relation between the lung and other related organs are not the main pathogenesis to be discussed and treated. Therefore, it is necessary to point out that syndrome differentiation and treatment that is based solely upon a six-channel system could not be completely applied in the TCM management of COVID-19. The theory of differentiation based upon the zang-fu organ systems should also be combined. Meanwhile, due to the constant high fever with hyperactivity of qi and ying, and the predominance of damp with blockage of the functions of the qi at various levels, it is also necessary to combine the differentiation based upon wei, qi, ying, and xue system or the San Jiao system. It can be seen clearly that differentiations based upon a single system—no matter what kind of system—in severe and critical syndrome is

---

[16]Juze Lin, *et al.* Based on the combination of Weiqiyingxue syndrome differentiation and visceral syndrome differentiation for the treatment of novel coronavirus pneumonia. *Tianjin Traditional Chinese Medicine* (天津中医药). 2020, 37(3): 251–254. http://www.tjzhongyiyao.com/html/tjzyy/2020/3/20200304.htm.

[17]Yuhao Wang, *et al.* Discussion on the transmission rule of COVID-19 based on damp-heat tri-Jiao syndrome differentiation by XUE Xue. *Journal of Zhejiang University of Traditional Chinese Medicine* (浙江中医药大学学报). 2020, 7: 599–604. https://xuebao.zcmu.edu.cn/ch/reader/view_abstract.aspx?file_no=20200701&flag=1.

never enough and comprehensive to deal with COVID-19 syndromes. However, restoring the lung in descending function remains the core treatment.

5.2.1 Exterior cold with interior heat

This syndrome is caused by invasion of wind-cold or cold-damp to those who have constitutional heat, no matter excessive or deficient heat. This situation could lead to blockage of the interior heat (fire) by exterior cold, resulting in the occurrence of symptoms of an exterior cold with symptoms of interior heat at the same time. Antipyretic from modern medicine will not always work for this syndrome, because the interior heat could be eliminated by which implies that its treatment is somehow left behind social and medical needs.

If this type of syndrome occurs during the non-epidemic period, it could be a simple case. However, when it happens during the pandemic period, it could be a serious condition, showing incomplete disappearance of external symptoms with the formation of the severe syndrome. Its clinical manifestations are constant high fever for more than one week, accompanied by a slight aversion to cold, obvious shortness of breath, severe pressure over the chest, and low blood oxygen saturation often between 90% and 92%. It's key and correct differentiation is done based upon the following clinical symptoms and history of infection.

5.2.1.1 *Exterior cold with interior excessive heat*

Invasion of wind-cold to the lung and wei system with an accumulation of excessive heat in the lung and stomach. Slight aversion to cold, high fever, severe cough with profuse white, foamy or sticky phlegm (that is difficult to be expectorated), chest tightness, redness of the face, restlessness, vomiting, loss of appetite, abdominal distention, constipation, and a red tongue with white coating.

Principle of Treatment:
Dispel cold, clear heat, descend the lung-qi, and relieve cough.

Herbal Treatment:
Da Qing Long Tang-*Major Blue Green Dragon Decoction.*

Xiang Ru *Herba Elsholtziae seu Moslae* 10 g
Gui Zhi *Ramulus Cinnamomi Cassiae* 10 g
Qiang Huo *Rhizoma et Radix Notopterygii* 10 g
Xing Ren *Semen Pruni Armeniacae* 10 g
Zi Su Zi *Fructus Perillae Frutescentis* 10 g
Ting Li Zi *Semen Descurainiae seu Lepidii* 10 g
Bai Jie Zi *Semen Sinapis Albae* 10 g
Lai Fu Zi *Semen Raphani Sativi* 10 g
Shi Gao *Gypsum Fibrosum* 20 g
Huang Qin *Radix Scutellariae Baicalensis* 10 g
Hou Po *Cortex Magnoliae Officinalis* 10 g
Zhi Shi *Fructus Immaturus Citri Aurantii* 10 g

In Europe, some Chinese herbs are banned, such as Ma Huang *Herba Ephedrae* and Xi Xin *Herba cum Radice Asari*, and can only be replaced by Xiang Ru. In addition, even Ban Xia is also prohibited in some countries. So, substitute herbs could be used as alternatives, such as Qing Pi, etc. Most of the above herbs are not so often applied to treat COVID-19 in the early stage with light syndromes. But in severe or critical syndromes, they could not be missed because the treatment must be prompt, adequate and sufficient to deal with the impairment of the lung in descending the qi and eliminating the external pathogenic factors.

Acupuncture Treatment:
- Neiguan P-6 + Gongsun SP-4 with even methods.
- Hegu L.I.-4, Wai guan SJ-5, Lieque LU-7, Feishu BL-13, Zhongfu LU-1, Chize LU-5, Quchi L.I.-11, Fenglong ST-40, Sanyinjiao SP-6, and Neiting ST-44 with a reducing method.

Explanations:
- P-6 + SP-4 are used to descend the lung-qi and relieve chest tightness, while regulating digestion and eliminating excess water in the body.

- L.I.-4, the yuan-source point of the large intestine channel, SJ-5, the luo-connecting point of the San Jiao channel, and LU-7, the luo-connecting point of the lung channel respectively, are used to promote sweating and dispel external pathogenic factors.
- BL-13 and LU-1, the back-shu point and the front-mu point of the lung channel respectively, together with LU-5, the he-sea point of the lung channel, are used to descend the lung-qi and relieve the fullness of the chest.
- L.I.-11, the he-sea point of the large intestine channel, SP-6, the crossing point of the three yin channels of the foot, and ST-44, the ying-spring point of the stomach channel, are used to clear the excessive heat in the body and reduce fever.
- ST-40, the luo-connecting point of the stomach channel, is used to eliminate phlegm in the lung.

5.2.1.2 *Invasion of cold-damp to the lung and wei system with an accumulation of excessive heat in the lung and stomach*

Slight aversion to cold, high fever, heaviness of the body and limbs, arthralgia, severe cough with profuse white and foamy phlegm, the fullness of the chest with chest tightness, redness of the face, thirst, restlessness, constipation, abdominal distention with pain, and a red tongue with white coating.

Principle of Treatment:
Dispel cold, eliminate damp, clear heat, descend the lung-qi, and relieve cough.

Herbal Treatment:
Jiu Wei Qiang Huo Tang-*Nine-Herb Decoction with Notopterygium.*

Qiang Huo *Rhizoma et Radix Notopterygii* 12 g
Fang Feng *Radix Ledebouriellae Divaricatae* 10 g
Cang Zhu *Rhizoma Atractylodis* 10 g

Bai Zhi *Radix Angelicae Dahuricae* 10 g
Huang Qin *Radix Scutellariae Baicalensis* 10 g
Zhi Mu *Radix Anemarrhenae Asphodeloidis* 10 g
Zhe Bei Mu *Bulbus Fritillariae Thunbergii* 10 g
Xing Ren *Semen Pruni Armeniacae* 10 g
Xiang Fu *Rhizoma Cyperi Rotundi* 10 g
Quan Gua Lou *Fructus Trichosanthis* 10 g
Jie Geng *Radix Platycodi Grandiflori* 10 g
Hou Po *Cortex Magnoliae Officinalis* 10 g
Zhi Shi *Fructus Immaturus Citri Aurantii* 10 g
Sheng Di Huang *Radix Rehmanniae Glutinosae Recens* 12 g

Acupuncture Treatment:
Same acupuncture points as above, adding Yangchi SJ-4 and Zhigou SJ-6, the yuan-source point, and the point for water passage respectively (used with a reducing method to dispel external damp), and Yanglingquan GB-34 with a reducing method to eliminate external damp and benefit the joints.

5.2.1.3 *Incomplete elimination of exterior cold, which transferred to heat and entered the interior*

Aversion to cold, high fever, headache with body pain, fullness of the chest, shortness of breath, cough with a lot of white and sticky phlegm (that is difficult to be expectorated), dizziness, thirst, restlessness, and a red tongue with white coating.

Principle of Treatment:
Dispel cold, clear heat, descend the lung-qi, and relieve shortness of breath.

Herbal Treatment:
Chai Ge Jie Ji Tang-*Bupleurum and Kudzu Decoction to Release the Muscle Layer.*

Chai Hu *Radix Bupleuri* 10 g
Ge Gen *Radix Puerariae* 10 g

Bai Zhi *Radix Angelicae Dahuricae* 10 g
Jie Geng *Radix Platycodi Grandiflori* 10 g
Qiang Huo *Rhizoma et Radix Notopterygii* 10 g
Shi Gao *Gypsum Fibrosum* 30 g
Huang Qin *Radix Scutellariae Baicalensis* 10 g
Bai Shao Yao *Radix Paeoniae Lactiflorae* 10 g
Xing Ren *Semen Pruni Armeniacae* 10 g
Bai Jie Zi *Semen Sinapis Albae* 10 g
Lai Fu Zi *Semen Raphani Sativi* 10 g
Zi Su Zi *Fructus Perillae Frutescentis* 10 g
Ting Li Zi *Semen Descurainiae seu Lepidii* 10 g
Hou Po *Cortex Magnoliae Officinalis* 10 g

When there is an invasion of exterior pathogenic factors, and the damages to Taiyang only last a very short time before it quickly changes into the heat to enter the deeper interior, then the Shaoyang or Yangming channels could be affected, leading to severe fighting between the anti-pathogenic qi and pathogenic qi. These pathogenic results could often be seen in severe and critical syndromes.

This formula was originally designed to treat an invasion of wind-heat with the accumulation of heat in the interior, leading to the occurrence of illness of three yang channels (Taiyang, Shaoyang and Yangming). The herbs applied in this formula were equally divided into these three directions to relieve the symptoms of three yang channels. If this syndrome happens during COVID-19, it often is already in severe or critical conditions. Of course, this formula without any modifications could not be directly prescribed to the patients, because the formula did not cover the situation of failure of the lung in descending the qi with the formation of phlegm in the lung. Thus, these herbs should be added.

Acupuncture Treatment:
• Neiguan P-6 + Gongsun SP-4 with even methods.
• Hegu L.I.-4, Lieque LU-7, Feishu BL-13, Zhongfu LU-1, Chize LU-5, Yuji LU-10, Quchi L.I.-11, Fenglong ST-40, Yanglingquan GB-34, and Xiaxi GB-43 with a reducing method.

Explanations:

- P-6 + SP-4 are used to descend the lung-qi, relieve fullness of the chest and shortness of breath. They can also regulate digestion and eliminate excess water in the body.
- L.I.-4 and LU-7, the yuan-source point of the large intestine channel and the luo-connecting point of the lung channel respectively are used to promote sweating to dispel external pathogenic factors.
- BL-13 and LU-1, the back-shu point of the lung and the front-mu point of the lung channel, together with LU-5, the he-sea point of the lung channel, which are all the chief points to descend the lung-qi and relieve the fullness of the chest.
- LU-10, the ying-spring point of the lung channel, L.I.-11, the he-sea point of the large intestine channel, GB-34 and GB-43, the he-sea point and the ying-spring point of the gallbladder channel, are used to clear heat in the three yang channels and reduce fever.
- ST-40, the luo-connecting point of the stomach channel, is used to eliminate phlegm in the lung.

5.2.1.4 *Exterior cold with the formation of deficient heat*

Aversion to cold or wind, fever, slight sweating which could not lower down fever, weak cough, difficulty to expectorate the phlegm, very tired and weak, shortness of breath palpitations, insomnia, anxiety, dry mouth, thirst, constipation, red tongue with scanty coating, and cracks on the tongue.

Principle of Treatment:
Dispel cold, nourish yin, clear heat, and descend the lung-qi.

Herbal Treatment:
Jia Jian Wei Rui Tang-*Modified Solomon's Seal Decoction.*

Fang Feng *Radix Ledebouriellae Divaricatae* 10 g
Bai Zhu *Rhizoma Atractylodis Macrocephalae* 10 g
Xi Yang Shen *Radix Panacis Quinque Folii* 10 g

Mai Men Dong *Tuber Ophiopogonis Japonici* 10 g
Sheng Di Huang *Radix Rehmanniae Glutinosae Recens* 10 g
Qiang Huo *Rhizoma et Radix Notopterygii* 10 g
Bai Zhi *Radix Angelicae Dahuricae* 10 g
Huang Qin *Radix Scutellariae Baicalensis* 10 g
Zhi Mu *Radix Anemarrhenae Asphodeloidis* 10 g
Zhe Bei Mu *Bulbus Fritillariae Thunbergii* 10 g
Xing Ren *Semen Pruni Armeniacae* 10 g
Jie Geng *Radix Platycodi Grandiflori* 10 g
Quan Gua Lou *Fructus Trichosanthis* 10 g
Hou Po *Cortex Magnoliae Officinalis* 10 g
Zhi Shi *Fructus Immaturus Citri Aurantii* 10 g

These patients usually don't have a very high fever, but sometimes it could be very dangerous because most of those patients have some basic diseases, as well as obvious yin deficiency in TCM. Their blood saturation is usually very low, and remains low, often around 90% to 92% or even lower, and does not rise quickly. When the blood saturation drops under 90% suddenly, it is considered a mixture of cold and heat, failure of zheng-qi to prevail over xie-qi, formation of blood stasis in the blood vessels, and restlessness of the heart and shen. The patients should be taken into the hospital to receive a combination of modern medicine and TCM. Any delayed or improper treatment could lead to fatal consequences. In this case, some herbs to promote blood circulation and resolve blood stasis should be applied in the herbal prescription, including:

Hong Hua *Flos Carthami Tinctorii* 10 g
Dan Shen *Radix Salviae Miltiorrhizae* 15 g
Pu Huang *Pollen Typhae* 10 g
Yu Jin *Tuber Curcumae* 10 g

Patients with cancer, diabetes, or cardiovascular diseases should pay extra attention to prevent the occurrence of blood stagnation. It means that two or three of the above blood circulating herbs could be applied in advance for these patients with COVID-19. When blood stasis happens or if there is already an illness of thrombosis somewhere in the body, the treatment becomes more passive instead of preventive.

Acupuncture Treatment:
- Neiguan P-6 + Gongsun SP-4 with even methods.
- Hegu L.I.-4, Lieque LU-7, Feishu BL-13, Zhongfu LU-1, Chize LU-5, and Fenglong ST-40 with a reducing method.
- Jingqu LU-8, Sanyinjiao SP-6, Taixi KID-3, Zhaohai KID-6, KID-7, and REN-6 with tonifying methods.

Explanations:
- P-6 + SP-4 are used to descend the lung-qi and relieve shortness of breath, and meanwhile, regulate digestion and eliminate excess water in the body.
- L.I.-4 and LU-7, the yuan-source point of the large intestine channel and the luo-connecting point of the lung channel respectively are used to promote sweating to dispel external pathogenic factors.
- BL-13, LU-1, and LU-5, the back-shu point of the lung and the front-mu point of the lung channel, together with LU-5, the he-sea point of the lung channel, are the chief points to descend the lung-qi and relieve difficulty to expectorate the phlegm and shortness of breath.
- ST-40, the luo-connecting point of the stomach channel, is used to eliminate phlegm in the lung.
- LU-8, the metal point of the lung channel, SP-6, the crossing point of the three yin channels of the foot, together with KID-3, the yuan-source point of the kidney channel, KID-6, a good point to nourish the yin, and KID-7, the metal point of the kidney channel, together with REN-6 are used to reinforce the yin of the body and clear the deficient heat.

5.2.2 Exterior heat with interior cold

Aversion to cold, cold limbs, weak voice, shortness of breath, sudden occurrence of fever, stuffy nose, throat pain, headache, body pain, chest tightness, cough with expectoration of profuse white foamy phlegm, weak and exhausted feeling, incapable of getting out of bed, the fullness of abdomen, diarrhea, poor appetite, vomiting, and a pale tongue with a thin and slightly yellow coating.

This syndrome is often caused by constitutional deficiency of lung-qi, in combination with deficiency of yang of the heart, spleen and kidney. At the same time, there is a sudden invasion of damp-heat, toxins and, leading to failure of the lung to descend the qi.

Principle of Treatment:
Clear heat, warm the interior, tonify yang of the heart and kidney, and descend the lung-qi.

Herbal Treatment:
Ma Xing Shi Gan Tang-*Ephedra, Apricot Kernel, Gypsum and Licorice Decoction.*

Ma Huang *Herba Ephedrae* 10 g
Xing Ren *Semen Pruni Armeniacae* 10 g
Shi Gao *Gypsum Fibrosum* 30 g
San Bai Pi *Cortex Mori Albae Radicis* 10 g
Zi Su Zi *Fructus Perillae Frutescentis* 10 g
Kuan Dong Hua *Flos Tussilaginis Farfarae* 10 g
Zhi Ban Xia *Rhizoma Pinelliae Ternatae Preparata* 10 g
Hou Po *Cortex Magnoliae Officinalis* 10 g
Rou Gui *Cortex Cinnamomi Cassiae* 5 g
Zhi Fu Zi *Radix Lateralis Aconiti Carmichaeli Praeparata* 10 g
Gan Jiang *Rhizoma Zingiberis Officinalis* 10 g
Zhi Gan Cao *Radix Glycyrrhizae Preparata* 5 g

It is obvious that this prescription is a mixture of cooling herbs and warming herbs at some time. It looks like a contradiction, but is a reflection of serious situations of patients with this syndrome. If Ma Xing Shi Gan Tang is applied without supporting the interior yang, it could damage the internal yang and cause aggravation of yang of the heart and kidney, resulting in a dangerous syndrome, i.e., a decline of yang of the heart and kidney. In that case, critical syndrome follows.

Acupuncture Treatment:
- Neiguan P-6 + Gongsun SP-4 with even methods.
- Erjian L.I.-2, Hegu L.I.-4, Lieque LU-7, Yuji LU-10, Feishu BL-13, Chize LU-5, and Fenglong ST-40 with a reducing method.
- Zusanli ST-36, Shaofu HE-8, KID-3, and REN-6 with a tonifying method.
- Moxibustion should be applied on ST-36, KID-3, and REN-6.

Explanations:
- P-6 + SP-4 are used to descend the lung-qi and relieve chest tightness.
- L.I.-4 and LU-7, the yuan-source point of the large intestine channel and the luo-connecting point of the lung channel respectively, are used to promote sweating to dispel external pathogenic factors.
- BL-13 and LU-5, the back-shu point and the he-sea point of the lung channel respectively, LU-10 and L.I.-2, the spring point of lung channel and large intestine channel repsectively, are the chief points to descend lung-qi, clear heat and relieve difficulty in expectorating the phlegm, shortness of breath and chest tightness.
- ST-40, the luo-connecting point of the stomach channel, is used to eliminate phlegm in the lung.
- ST-36, the he-sea point of the stomach channel, and REN-6 are used in combination with HE-8, the ying-spring point of the heart channel, and KID-3, the yuan-source point of the kidney channel, to tonify the yang of the heart and kidney and eliminate interior cold. Moxibustion strengthens the effect of tonifying points and dispels the interior cold.

5.2.3 Exterior cold with interior cold fluid

Chest pressure with tightness, shortness of breath, asthma, expectoration of white and foamy phlegm, swelling of the face, edema on the low limbs, scanty urine, severe palpitations, unstable emotions, purplish lips, insomnia, physical tiredness, vomiting, diarrhea, and a pale tongue with a white and greasy coating.

Patients with constitutional obesity could suffer from phlegm and damp or accumulation of phlegm or cold fluid in the lung with chronic cough and shortness of breath. Once there is an invasion of wind-cold or invasion of cold-damp with the toxins, it may cause the influence of the exterior and interior, bringing about the failure of the lung to descend the qi, thus various symptoms and signs occur. In normal circumstances, it will not cause life-threatening problems, but during the period of COVID-19, situations become different. The descending function of the lung is mainly impaired, and the other physiological functions of the lung are also mostly impaired, combined with the involvement of damages in the other organs, such as the heart, spleen, and kidney. Once there is a combination of impairment of the lung with disorders of heart and kidney, its severe syndrome or critical syndrome could be complicated.

Principle of Treatment:
Dispel external cold, resolve phlegm, eliminate cold fluid, and descend lung-qi.

Herbal Treatment:
Xiao Qing Long Tang-*Minor Blue Green Dragon Decoction*, plus San Zi Yang Qin Tang-*Three Seed Decoction to Nourish One's Parents.*

Ma Huang *Herba Ephedrae* 10 g
Gui Zhi *Ramulus Cinnamomi Cassiae* 10 g
Xi Xin Herba cum Radice Asari 3 g
Gan Jiang *Rhizoma Zingiberis Officinalis* 10 g
Zhi Ban Xia *Rhizoma Pinelliae Ternatae Preparata* 10 g
Wu Wei Zi *Fructus Schisandrae Chinensis* 10 g
Xing Ren *Semen Pruni Armeniacae* 10 g
Ting Li Zi *Semen Descurainiae seu Lepidii* 10 g
Hou Po *Cortex Magnoliae Officinalis* 10 g
Gua Lou Pi *Pericarpium Trichosanthis* 10 g
Che Qian Zi *Semen Plantaginis* 10 g
Ze Xie *Rhizoma Alismatis Orientalis* 10 g

Qian Niu Zi *Semen Pharbitidis* 10 g
Long Chi *Dens Draconis* 15 g
Zhen Zhu Mu *Concha Margaritiferae Usta* 15 g

No matter if Xiao Qing Long Tang descends the lung-qi and relieves asthma, or San Zi Yang Qin Tang resolves phlegm, both herbal treatments cannot control the complicated situations from this syndrome. Therefore, Xing Ren and Ting Li Zi are added to descend the lung and eliminate phlegm. Hou Po and Gua Lou Pi are used to relax the chest and regulate the qi in the lung. Che Qian Zi, Ze Xie, and Qian Niu Zi are used to promote urination and relieve edema. Long Chi and Zhen Zhu Mu are used to calm the shen and relieve palpitations.

Acupuncture Treatment:
- Neiguan P-6 + Gongsun SP-4, Lieque LU-7 + Zhaohai KID-6 with even methods.
- Hegu L.I.-4, Wai guan SJ-5, Feishu BL-13, Chize LU-5, Fenglong ST-40, Tanzhong REN-17, Sanyinjiao SP-6, and Yinlingquan SP-9 with a reducing method.
- REN-6 and Zusanli ST-36 with a tonifying method.

Explanations:
- P-6 + SP-4, LU-7 + KID-6 are used to descend the lung-qi, reduce fluid in the chest and relieve chest tightness.
- L.I.-4 and SJ-5, the yuan-source point of the large intestine channel and the luo-connecting point of the San Jiao channel respectively are used to promote sweating to dispel external pathogenic cold.
- BL-13, LU-5, and REN-17, the back-shu point and the he-sea point of lung channel respectively, together with REN-17, the gathering point of the qi in the body, are the chief points to descend the lung-qi, eliminate fluid in the chest and relieve difficulty to expectorate the phlegm, shortness of breath and chest tightness.
- ST-40, the luo-connecting point of the stomach channel, is used to eliminate phlegm in the lung.

- SP-6, the crossing point of the three yin channels of the foot, and SP-9, the he-sea point of the spleen channel, are used to eliminate fluid and excessive water in the body.
- REN-6, an essential point for qi in the body, and ST-36, the he-sea point of the stomach channel, are used to tonify the qi and yang in the body and eliminate cold.

5.2.4 Invasion of pathogens to Shaoyang channel

Chest tightness with a heavy feeling, shortness of breath, cough with yellow phlegm (which is sticky and difficult to be expectorated), high fever (especially in the afternoon), low-grade fever, bitter taste in the mouth, dizziness, hypochondriac pain and distension, poor appetite, discomfort feeling at the epigastric region, nausea, vomiting, poor appetite, abdominal distention, diarrhea, burning feeling when urinating or urgent urination, and a red tongue with a yellow and greasy coating.

Relatively speaking, many European patients are full of emotions with strong personal characters. Besides, they prefer highly-flavored food that are sweet and greasy, and love to drink alcohol and coffee. These could all lead to the tendency of damp-heat formation. During COVID-19, these pathogenic factors and results could influence the illness, bringing about a mixture of external invasion and internal pathogens, thus aggravation of the disease occurs.

Principle of Treatment:
Harmonize the Shaoyang and San Jiao, eliminate damp-heat, and descend lung-qi.

Herbal Treatment:
Xiao Chai Hu Tang-*Minor Bupleurum Decoction*, plus
San Ren Tang-*Three Seed (Nut) Decoction.*

Ma Huang *Herba Ephedrae* 10 g
Xing Ren *Semen Pruni Armeniacae* 10 g
Sang Bai Pi *Cortex Mori Albae Radicis* 10 g

Zhe Bei Mu *Bulbus Fritillariae Thunbergii* 10 g
Huang Qin *Radix Scutellariae Baicalensis* 10 g
Gua Lou Pi *Pericarpium Trichosanthis* 10 g
Chai Hu *Radix Bupleuri* 5 g
Bai Shao Yao *Radix Paeoniae Lactiflorae* 5 g
Zhi Ban Xia *Rhizoma Pinelliae Ternatae Preparata* 10 g
Sheng Jiang *Rhizoma Zingiberis Officinalis Recens* 5 g
Bai Dou Kou *Fructus Amomi Cardamomi* 3 g
Yi Yi Ren *Semen Coicis Lachryma-Jobi* 10 g
Tong Cao *Medulla Tetrapanacis Papyriferi* 10 g
Hua Shi *Talcum* 15 g
Zhi Zi *Fructus Gardeniae Jasminoidis* 10 g
Yin Chen Hao *Herba Artemisiae Capillaris* 10 g

Xiao Chai Hu Tang harmonizes the Shaoyang, and San Ren Tang eliminates damp-heat in the San Jiao. They do not regulate and correct the situations of failure of the lung in descending the qi. Therefore Ma Huang, Xing Ren, Sang Bai Pi, Zhe Bei Mu, Huang Qin, and Gua Lou Pi are added into the prescription as the chief herbs to deal with the main pathogenic results. If Yangming excess is also present, manifesting as constipation and abdominal distention, Da Huang and Mang Xiao could be added to promote defecation and relieve constipation.

Acupuncture Treatment:
- Waiguan SJ-5 + Zulinqi GB-41, Neiguan P-6 + Gongsun SP-4 with even methods.
- Hegu L.I.-4, Lieque LU-7, Feishu BL-13, Chize LU-5, Fenglong ST-40, Tanzhong REN-17, Taichong LIV-3, Qimen LIV-14, Yanglingquan GB-34, Qiuxu GB-40, Sanyinjiao SP-6, and Yinlingquan SP-9 with a reducing method.

Explanations:
- SJ-5 + GB-41 is used to harmonize the Shaoyang and relieve the disturbance of external pathogenic factors to the liver and gallbladder.

- P-6 + SP-4 are used to descend the lung-qi and relieve chest tightness.
- L.I.-4 and LU-7, the yuan-source point of the large intestine channel, and the luo-connecting point of the lung channel respectively are used to promote the sweating to dispel external pathogenic factors.
- BL-13, LU-5 and REN-17, the back-shu point and the he-sea point of lung channel respectively, together with REN-17, the gathering point of the qi in the body, are the chief points to descend the lung-qi, eliminate fluid in the chest and relieve difficulty to expectorate the phlegm, shortness of breath and chest tightness.
- ST-40, the luo-connecting point of the stomach channel, is used to eliminate phlegm in the lung.
- LIV-3 and LIV-14, the yuan-source point from the liver channel and the front-mu point the liver respectively, together with GB-34 and GB-40, the he-sea point and yuan-source point of the gallbladder channel respectively are used to promote the qi circulation, harmonize the liver and gallbladder, and restore the physiological functions of the liver and gallbladder.
- SP-6 and SP-9, the crossing point and the he-sea point of the spleen channel respectively, are used to promote digestion and relieve nausea and diarrhea.

5.2.5 Accumulation of heat in the lung and stomach

Constant high fever, severe cough, scanty yellow and sticky phlegm, the fullness of chest with pain, shortness of breath, restlessness, insomnia, thirst, dry stool, and a red tongue with yellow and dry coating or a slightly greasy coating.

Habitual poor diet, such as overindulgence in highly-flavored food, sweet and greasy food, or alcoholic drinking, or even addiction to drugs, etc., could cause the formation of excessive heat in the lung and stomach. When there is an invasion of external pathogenic factors, especially heat, there could be a mixture of external heat and internal heat in the lung and stomach, leading to aggravation of COVID-19 symptoms.

Principle of Treatment:
Clear heat in the lung and stomach, resolve phlegm, and descend the lung-qi.

Herbal Treatment:
Ma Xing Gan Shi Tang-*Ephedra, Apricot Kernel, Gypsum and Licorice Decoction.*

Ma Huang *Herba Ephedrae* 10 g
Xing Ren *Semen Pruni Armeniacae* 10 g
Shi Gao *Gypsum Fibrosum* 30 g
Sang Bai Pi *Cortex Mori Albae Radicis* 10 g
Zhe Bei Mu *Bulbus Fritillariae Thunbergii* 10 g
Huang Qin *Radix Scutellariae Baicalensis* 10 g
Huang Lian *Rhizoma Coptidis* 5 g
Zhi Mu *Radix Anemarrhenae Asphodeloidis* 10 g
Zhi Zi *Fructus Gardeniae Jasminoidis* 10 g
Gua Lou Pi *Pericarpium Trichosanthis* 10 g
Hou Po *Cortex Magnoliae Officinalis* 10 g
Zhi Gan Cao *Radix Glycyrrhizae Preparata* 5 g

Acupuncture Treatment:
- Neiguan P-6 + Gongsun SP-4, Lieque LU-7 + Zhaohai KID-6 with even methods.
- Hegu L.I.-4, Zhongfu LU-1, Feishu BL-13, Chize LU-5, Tanzhong REN-17, Quchi L.I.-11, Zhongwan REN-12, Tianshu ST-25, Fenglong ST-40, ST42, Neiting ST-44, and Sanyinjiao SP-6 with a reducing method.

Explanations:
- P-6 + SP-4 are used to descend the lung-qi and relieve chest tightness.
- LU-7 + KID-6 are used to relax the chest and benefit the lung.
- L.I.-4 and L.I.-11, the yuan-source point and the he-sea point of the large intestine channel respectively, are used to clear heat and reduce fever.

- LU-1, LU-5, and BL-13, the front-mu point and the he-sea point of the lung channel respectively, the back-shu point of the lung, are used to clear heat in the lung and descend the lung-qi.
- REN-12, the gathering point of the fu organs and the front-mu point of the stomach, ST-25, ST42, and ST-44, the front-mu point of the large intestine, the yuan-source point of the stomach channel, and the ying-spring point of the stomach channel, are used to clear heat in the stomach and large intestine.
- ST-40 and SP-6, the luo-connecting point of the stomach channel and the crossing point of the three yin channels of the foot respectively are used to clear heat and eliminate phlegm in the lung.

5.2.6 Accumulation of phlegm-heat in the lung

Constant high fever, severe cough with profuse yellow and sticky phlegm (that is difficult to be expectorated), the fullness of chest with pain and tightness, shortness breath, restlessness, and a red tongue with a yellow and greasy coating.

It frequently occurs on patients who have always been suffering from obesity with retention of damp and phlegm in the body, often have cough with yellow phlegm, bitter taste in the mouth, dryness, and an uncomfortable feeling in the throat. When there is an invasion of wind-heat or damp-heat, it could cause aggravation of the situations with the quick transformation of external heat into the internal heat, leading to failure of the lung in descending the lung-qi and accumulation of phlegm-heat in the lung.

Principle of Treatment:
Clear heat in the lung, resolve phlegm, descend the lung-qi and relieve shortness of breath.

Herbal Treatment:
Ding Chuan Tang-*Arrest Wheezing Decoction.*

Ma Huang *Herba Ephedrae* 10 g
Bai Guo *Semen Ginkgo Bilobae* 10 g

Kuan Dong Hua *Flos Tussilaginis Farfarae* 10 g
Huang Qin *Radix Scutellariae Baicalensis* 10 g
Xing Ren *Semen Pruni Armeniacae* 10 g
Sang Bai Pi *Cortex Mori Albae Radicis* 10 g
Zi Su Zi *Fructus Perillae Frutescentis* 10 g
Zhi Ban Xia *Rhizoma Pinelliae Ternatae Preparata* 10 g
Zhe Bei Mu *Bulbus Fritillariae Thunbergii* 10 g
Zhi Zi *Fructus Gardeniae Jasminoidis* 10 g
Hai Ge Ke *Concha Cyclinae Sinensis* 15 g
Da Qing Ye *Folium Isatidis* 10 g
Jin Yin Hua *Flos Lonicerae Japonicae* 10 g

Basically speaking, Ding Chuan Tang is a very good herbal formula to deal with this syndrome. However, it is still not powerful enough to treat COVID-19. Some extra herbs to clear the heat and eliminate phlegm in the lung should be added to the prescription to strengthen the therapeutic effects.

Acupuncture Treatment:
- Neiguan P-6 + Gongsun SP-4, Lieque LU-7 + Zhaohai KID-6 with even methods.
- Hegu L.I.-4, Quchi L.I.-11, Zhongfu LU-1, Chize LU-5, Yuji LU-10, Feishu BL-13, Tanzhong REN-17, Tianshu ST-25, Fenglong ST-40, and Sanyinjiao SP-6 with a reducing method.

Explanations:
- P-6 + SP-4 are used to descend the lung-qi and relieve chest tightness.
- LU-7 + KID-6 are used to relax the chest and benefit the lung.
- L.I.-4, L.I.-11, and ST-25, the yuan-source point and the he-sea point of the large intestine channel, and front-mu point of the large intestine, are used to clear heat, promote defecation, and reduce fever.
- LU-1, LU-5, and BL-13, the front-mu point, the he-sea point of the lung channel, the back-shu point of the lung respectively, are used to clear heat in the lung and descend the lung-qi.

- LU-10, the ying-stream point of the lung channel, is used to clear heat in the lung and relieve the cough.
- REN-17, the gathering point of the qi, is used to descend the lung-qi and relax the chest to relieve chest tightness.
- ST-40 and SP-6, the luo-connecting point of the stomach channel, and the crossing point of the three yin channels of the foot are used to clear heat and eliminate phlegm in the lung.

5.2.7 Accumulation and blockage of damp in the lung and stomach

Severe cough, expectoration of profuse white and sticky phlegm, fullness and tightness of the chest, heaviness of the body and head, lassitude, poor appetite, abdominal distention, loose stool or diarrhea, and a white and greasy coating on the tongue.

In TCM's view, European diets are made up of highly-flavored, greasy, fatty and sweet food, contain too much dairy products, paired with frequent alcoholic drinking, which could cause the formation of damp-phlegm in the body with the tendency of obesity and overload the spleen and stomach. In addition, there is a lack of sunshine during all the seasons, too much rain and high cold and humidity levels. These pathogenic factors could lead to retardation of transformation and transformation of the spleen and stomach. When COVID-19 occurs, external pathogenic factors could aggravate the above conditions, resulting in deterioration of the functions of the spleen and stomach. Meanwhile, due to improper publicity by the media saying that a profuse protein diet is needed during COVID-19 to stimulate the physiological function of the immune system, many patients start to consume a lot of protein-rich food (such as eating five eggs, one kg of meat, or drinking one liter of milk daily). These kind of diet could become an excessive load to the spleen and stomach if their original digestion system is weak, resulting in aggravation of formation of damp-phlegm.

It is also considered in TCM that the spleen is the production organ for damp phlegm while the lung is the container organ of the damp phlegm. When there is the formation of too much damp-phlegm, it could affect the lung, leading to dysfunction of the lung in descending the qi. During COVID-19, this situation could become worse if external invasion to the lung occurs. Moreover, if the patients are treated with some antibiotics for necessity, it could make the entire situation of damp phlegm worse.

Principle of Treatment:
Resolve damp, eliminate phlegm, descend the lung-qi, and relieve shortness of breath.

Herbal Treatment:
Huo Po Xia Ling Tang-*Agastaches, Magnolia Bark, Pinellia and Poria Decoction,* plus
San Zi Yang Qin Tang-*Three Seed Decoction to Nourish One's Parents.*

Huo Xiang *Herba Agastaches seu Pogostemi* 10 g
Hou Po *Cortex Magnoliae Officinalis* 10 g
Xing Ren *Semen Pruni Armeniacae* 10 g
Zhi Shi *Fructus Immaturus Citri Aurantii* 10 g
Zhi Ban Xia *Rhizoma Pinelliae Ternatae Preparata* 10 g
Zi Su Zi *Fructus Perillae Frutescentis* 10 g
Lai Fu Zi *Semen Raphani Sativi* 10 g
Bai Jie Zi *Semen Sinapis Albae* 10 g
Cang Zhu *Rhizoma Atractylodis* 10 g
Fu Ling *Sclerotium Poriae Cocos* 10 g
Chen Pi *Pericarpium Citri Reticulatae* 5 g
Zhi Gan Cao *Radix Glycyrrhizae Preparata* 3 g

Hou Po Xia Ling Tang is indicated in the invasion of damp to the middle Jiao, and it has almost no effect to descend the lung-qi. Thus, San Zi Yang Qin Tang to eliminate phlegm and descend the lung-qi should be added into the prescription to lead the therapeutic effect to the lung.

Acupuncture Treatment:
- Neiguan P-6 + Gongsun SP-4, Lieque LU-7 + Zhaohai KID-6 with even methods.
- Zhongfu LU-1, Chize LU-5, Taiyuan LU-9, Feishu BL-13, Zhongwan REN-12, Tanzhong REN-17, Tianshu ST-25, Fenglong ST-40, Taichong LIV-3, Sanyinjiao SP-6, and Yinlingquan SP-9 with a reducing method.

Explanations:
- P-6 + SP-4 are used to descend the lung-qi and relieve chest tightness.
- LU-7 + KID-6 are used to relax the chest and benefit the lung.
- LU-1, LU-5, LU-9 and BL-13, the front-mu point, the he-sea point, the yuan-source point of the lung channel, the back-shu point of the lung respectively, are used to descend the lung-qi, resolve damp-phlegm in the lung and relieve cough.
- REN-17, the gathering point of the qi, is used to descend the lung-qi and relax the chest to relieve chest tightness.
- REN-12, ST-25, and ST-40, the gathering point of the fu organs and the front-mu point of the stomach, the front-mu point of the large intestine, the luo-connecting point of the stomach channel respectively, together with SP-6 and SP-9, the crossing point and the he-sea point of the spleen channel respectively, are used to eliminate damp in the spleen and stomach, descend the stomach-qi and relieve diarrhea.
- LIV-3, the yuan-source point of the liver channel, is used to promote and regulate the qi in the body and relieve the qi stagnation due to the accumulation of damp.

5.2.8 Accumulation of damp-heat in the middle Jiao

Fever with a heaviness of the body and limbs (which becomes worse in the afternoon), throat redness and pain, cough with yellow and sticky phlegm (that is difficult to expectorate), shortness of breath, tightness of the chest, restlessness, insomnia, nausea, vomiting, poor appetite, burning sensation in the stomach, loose stool or diarrhea, abdominal distention, lassitude, and a red tongue with yellow and greasy coating.

The spleen and stomach are situated at the middle Jiao, connecting the upper burner and lower burner at the same time, and providing the essential substances of qi and blood. Invasion of damp-heat could take place via the mouth directly, resulting in dysfunctions of the lung, spleen, and stomach.

Principle of Treatment:
Clear heat, resolve damp, harmonize the middle Jiao, descend the lung-qi, and relieve shortness of breath.

Herbal Treatment:
Lian Po Yin-*Coptis and Magnolia Bark Drink.*

Huang Lian *Rhizoma Coptidis* 5 g
Hou Po *Cortex Magnoliae Officinalis* 10 g
Zhi Ban Xia *Rhizoma Pinelliae Ternatae Preparata* 10 g
Shi Chang Pu *Rhizoma Acori Graminei* 10 g
Zhi Zi *Fructus Gardeniae Jasminoidis* 10 g
Lu Gen *Rhizoma Phragmitis Communis* 10 g
Gua Lou Pi *Pericarpium Trichosanthis* 10 g
Huang Qin *Radix Scutellariae Baicalensis* 10 g
Zhe Bei Mu *Bulbus Fritillariae Thunbergii* 10 g
Xing Ren *Semen Pruni Armeniacae* 10 g
Sang Bai Pi *Cortex Mori Albae Radicis* 10 g

Lian Po Yin is only good at clearing the heat and resolving damp in the middle Jiao, it has no effect to descend the lung-qi in COVID-19. Therefore, some extra herbs should be added to the prescription to clear the heat, eliminate phlegm in the lung and descend the lung-qi. Otherwise, shortness of breath, tightness of the chest, and severe cough with yellow phlegm will not improve.

It is possible that sometimes there is some confusion between using Bai Hu Tang or Lian Po Yin. In fact, there is an obvious big difference. Bai Hu Tang is indicated as excessive heat in the lung and stomach, while Lian Po Yin is indicated as an invasion of damp-heat to the middle Jiao. It can be seen from here that Bai Hu Tang should not be applied to treat all kinds of syndrome with fever. Syndrome differentiation is quite essential. On the contrary, if Bai Hu Tang is applied in this syndrome by mistake, it could reduce the fever, but not be able to eliminate damp, causing aggravation of the illness.

Acupuncture Treatment:
- Neiguan P-6 + Gongsun SP-4 with even methods.
- Chize LU-5, Feishu BL-13, Zhongwan REN-12, Tanzhong REN-17, Quchi L.I.-11, Tianshu ST-25, Fenglong ST-40, Yanglingquan GB-34, Qiuxu GB-40, Sanyinjiao SP-6 and Yinlingquan SP-9 with a reducing method.

Explanations:
- P-6 + SP-4 are used to descend the lung-qi and relieve chest tightness.
- LU-5 and BL-13, the he-sea point of the lung channel, and the back-shu point of the lung respectively are used to descend the lung-qi, resolve damp-phlegm in the lung and relieve cough.
- REN-17, the gathering point of the qi, is used to descend the lung-qi and relax the chest to relieve chest tightness.
- L.I.-11, REN-12, ST-25, ST-40, the he-sea point of the large intestine channel, the gathering point of the fu organs and the front-mu point of the stomach, the front-mu point of the large intestine, and the luo-connecting point of the stomach channel respectively, together with SP-6 and SP-9, the crossing point of the three yin channels of the foot and the he-sea point of the spleen channel respectively, are used to eliminate damp-heat in the middle Jiao and relieve the vomiting and diarrhea.
- GB-34 and GB-40, the he-sea point and yuan-source point of the gallbladder channel respectively, are used to eliminate damp-heat in the body and promote digestion.

5.2.9 Accumulation of excessive heat in the Yangming

5.2.9.1 *Formation of heat in the Yangming channel*

Constant high fever for more than one week, redness of the face, painful body and limbs, thirst, dry mouth, severe cough with profuse yellow phlegm, chest pain with tightness, restlessness, profuse sweating, headache, and a red tongue with yellow and dry coating.

This syndrome often occurs in patients who have been suffering from the accumulation of excessive heat in the stomach and large intestine due to improper diet, such as the intake of too little vegetables, overeating of red meat and alcoholic drinking, with a preference for sweet, highly-flavored and deep-fried food. When this is invaded by external pathogenic factors, they could transform into heat quickly, starting to mix with the interior heat in the Yangming. However, it is lucky that there is not yet the formation of excessive heat with the stool in the large intestine. Otherwise, this situation could cause another syndrome discussed below, i.e., formation of Yangming fu excess.

Principle of Treatment:
Clear heat, reduce fever, descend the lung-qi, and relieve shortness of breath.

Herbal Treatment:
Bai Hu Tang-*White Tiger Decoction.*

Sheng Shi Gao *Gypsum Fibrosum* 30 g
Zhi Mu *Radix Anemarrhenae Asphodeloidis* 10 g
Sang Bai Pi *Cortex Mori Albae Radicis* 10 g
Zhi Zi *Fructus Gardeniae Jasminoidis* 10 g
Tian Hua Fen *Radix Trichosanthis Kirilowii* 10 g
Sheng Di Huang *Radix Rehmanniae Glutinosae Recens* 15 g
Hou Po *Cortex Magnoliae Officinalis* 10 g
Xing Ren *Semen Pruni Armeniacae* 10 g
Zhe Bei Mu *Bulbus Fritillariae Thunbergii* 10 g

Zhi Ban Xia *Rhizoma Pinelliae Ternatae Preparata* 10 g
Geng Mi *Oryzae Sativae* 10 g
Zhi Gan Cao *Radix Glycyrrhizae Preparata* 3 g

It is quite clear that the herbal formula Bai Hu Tang is for sure a good prescription to clear the heat and reduce fever. However, it will not be able to descend the lung-qi and relieve severe cough. Besides, it could resolve phlegm in the lung. Therefore, some extra herbs to clear heat and eliminate phlegm in the lung should be added to the prescription. Otherwise, fever is reduced, but the lung situation deteriorates.

Acupuncture Treatment:
- Neiguan P-6 + Gongsun SP-4 with even methods.
- Chize LU-5, Feishu BL-13, Zhongwan REN-12, Tanzhong REN-17, Hegu L.I.-4, Quchi L.I.-11, Fenglong ST-40, Neiting ST-44, Dazhui DU-14, and Sanyinjiao SP-6 with a reducing method.

Explanations:
- P-6 + SP-4 are used to descend the lung-qi and relieve chest tightness.
- LU-5 and BL-13, the he-sea point of the lung channel and the back-shu point of the lung respectively, are used to descend the lung-qi and relieve cough.
- REN-17, the gathering point of the qi, is used to descend the lung-qi and relax the chest to relieve chest tightness.
- L.I.-4, L.I.-11, and REN-12, the yuan-source point and the he-sea point of the large intestine channel, the gathering point of the fu organs, and the front-mu point of the stomach respectively, are used to clear heat in the stomach, reduce fever and promote defecation.
- DU-14, the meeting of all the yang channels in the body, is used to clear heat and reduce fever.
- ST-40, the luo-connecting point of the stomach channel, is used to resolve phlegm in the lung and stop coughing.

- ST-44 and SP-6, the ying-stream point of the stomach channel, and the crossing point of three yin channels of the foot are used to clear heat in the stomach and reduce fever.

5.2.9.2 *Formation of Yangming fu excess*

Constant high fever for more than one week, redness of the face, painful body and limbs, thirst, dry mouth, restlessness, severe constipation for a couple of days, abdominal pain and distention, severe cough with profuse yellow phlegm, chest pain with tightness, restlessness, profuse sweating, headache, and a red tongue with a yellow and dry coating, or even formation of some brown and dry coating on the tongue.

This syndrome is often the result of prolonged persistence of excessive heat in the Yangming channel, which is not properly managed in time, leading to a mixture of stool and excessive heat in the fu organ. This is more severe than the above Yangming channel syndrome.

Principle of Treatment:
Promote defecation, clear heat, descend the lung-qi, and relieve shortness of breath.

Herbal Treatment:
Da Cheng Qi Tang-*Major Order the Qi Decoction.*

Da Huang *Radix et Rhizoma Rhei* 10 g
Mang Xiao *Mirabilitum* 10 g
Hou Po *Cortex Magnoliae Officinalis* 10 g
Zhi Shi *Fructus Immaturus Citri Aurantii* 10 g
Zhi Mu *Radix Anemarrhenae Asphodeloidis* 10 g
Zhi Zi *Fructus Gardeniae Jasminoidis* 10 g
Xing Ren *Semen Pruni Armeniacae* 10 g
Sang Bai Pi *Cortex Mori Albae Radicis* 10 g
Zhe Bei Mu *Bulbus Fritillariae Thunbergii* 10 g

When this formula is used properly, defecation occurs quickly, usually in a couple of hours, and fever reduces also immediately when defecation becomes normal. Improvement of cough, shortness of breath, and chest tightness follows.

The key features of applying this formula include constant high fever and constipation. If missing of these two features, then it is contraindicated in the treatment of COVID-19.

Acupuncture Treatment:
- Neiguan P-6 + Gongsun SP-4 with even methods.
- Chize LU-5, Feishu BL-13, Tanzhong REN-17, Hegu L.I.-4, Quchi L.I.-11, Tianshu ST-25, Shangjuxu ST-37, Fenglong ST-40, Neiting ST-44, Dazhui DU-14, and Sanyinjiao SP-6 with a reducing method.

Explanations:
- P-6 + SP-4 are used to descend the lung-qi and relieve chest tightness.
- LU-5 and BL-13, the he-sea point of the lung channel and the back-shu point of the lung respectively, are used to descend the lung-qi and relieve cough.
- REN-17, the gathering point of the qi, is used to descend the lung-qi and relax the chest to relieve chest tightness.
- L.I.-4, L.I.-11, and REN-12, the yuan-source point and the he-sea point of the large intestine channel, the gathering point of the fu organs, and the front-mu point of the stomach respectively, are used to clear heat in the stomach, reduce fever and promote defecation.
- DU-14, the meeting of all the yang channels in the body, is used to clear heat and reduce fever.
- ST-40, the luo-connecting point of the stomach channel, is used to resolve phlegm in the lung and stop coughing.
- ST-25, the front-mu point of the large intestine, ST-37, the lower sea point of the large intestine, ST-44, the ying-spring point of the stomach, and SP-6, the crossing point of the three yin channels of

the foot, are used to clear heat in the stomach, promote defecation and reduce fever.

5.2.10 Decline of Yang from the heart and kidney

Constant and weak cough, lack of energy, extreme exhausted feeling, unable to expectorate some phlegm and stand up, shortness of breath, white and foamy phlegm, or white and sticky phlegm, fullness of the chest with tightness, low body temperature or slight fever, cold hands and feet, aversion to cold, poor appetite, loose stool, somnolence, profuse cold sweating, low blood oxygen saturation often below 90%, and a pale tongue with wet coating. If it is not urgently treated in the hospital, it could be life-threatening.

This syndrome is often caused by delayed or refused treatment for COVID-19 after onset of clinical symptoms, or for patients who are elderly and weak, or with underlying chronic sickness. When there is an invasion of external pathogenic factors, it could quickly enter the deep interior, forming a situation of failure of zheng-qi to control the xie-qi. In TCM it is called simultaneous sickness of Taiyang and Shaoyin channel.

Principle of Treatment:
Greatly tonify yang of the heart and kidney, descend the lung-qi, and resolve the phlegm.

Herbal Treatment:
Si Ni Tang-*Frigid Extremities Decoction*, plus
Ma Huang Fu Zi Xi Xin Tang-*Ephedra, Prepared Aconite and Asarum Decoction.*

Ma Huang *Herba Ephedrae* 10 g
Zhi Fu Zi *Radix Lateralis Aconiti Carmichaeli Praeparata* 10 g
Xi Xin Herba cum Radice Asari 3 g
Gan Jiang *Rhizoma Zingiberis Officinalis* 10 g
Rou Gui *Cortex Cinnamomi Cassiae* 5 g
Wu Wei Zi *Fructus Schisandrae Chinensis* 10 g

Hou Po *Cortex Magnoliae Officinalis* 10 g
Xing Ren *Semen Pruni Armeniacae* 10 g
Jie Geng *Radix Platycodi Grandiflori* 10 g
Zhi Shi *Fructus Immaturus Citri Aurantii* 10 g
Ting Li Zi *Semen Descurainiae seu Lepidii* 10 g

In a lot of countries, the first three herbs are prohibited, so some other herbs to warm the yang of the heart and kidney can be substituted, such as
Xiang Ru *Herba Elsholtziae seu Moslae* 10 g
Ren Shen *Radix Ginseng* 10 g
Ba Ji Tian *Radix Morindae Officinalis* 10 g
Xian Mao *Rhizoma Curculiginis Orchioidis* 10 g
Yin Yang Huo *Herba Epimedii* 10 g
Long Gu *Os Draconis* 20 g

Acupuncture Treatment:
- Neiguan P-6 + Gongsun SP-4, Lieque LU-7 + Zhaohai KID-6 with even methods.
- Chize LU-5, Feishu BL-13, Tanzhong REN-17, and Fenglong ST-40 with a reducing method.
- Zusanli ST-36, Shaofu HE-8, Laogong P-8, Taixi KID-3, Guanyuan REN-4, and Qihai REN-6 with a tonifying method.
- Moxibustion should be applied on ST-36, Taixi KID-3, REN-4, and REN-6.

Explanations:
- P-6 + SP-4 are used to descend the lung-qi and relieve chest tightness.
- LU-7 + KID-6 are used to benefit the lung and relieve shortness of breath.
- LU-5, BL-13 and REN-17, the he-sea point of the lung channel, the back-shu point of the lung, and the gathering point of the qi respectively, are the chief points to descend the lung-qi and relieve shortness of breath and chest tightness.

- ST-40, the luo-connecting point of the stomach channel, is used to eliminate phlegm in the lung and relieve cough.
- ST-36, the he-sea point of the stomach channel, REN-4 and REN-6, two essential points to strengthen the body, are used in combination with HE-8 and P-8, the ying-spring point of the heart and pericardium channel respectively, and KID-3, the yuan-source point of the kidney channel, are used to tonify the yang of the heart and kidney and eliminate interior cold.
- Moxibustion strengthens the effect of tonifying points and dispels the interior cold.

6

TCM Treatment of COVID-19 at Convalescent Stage

Coronavirus disease 2019 (COVID-19) is a pandemic that has rapidly spread worldwide. Previous reports on COVID-19 primarily focused on epidemiological and clinical characteristics of confirmed cases or hospital discharged patients. Increasingly, confirmed patients are being discharged according to the current diagnosis and treatment protocols, and follow-up of convalescent patients is important to know about the outcome.[1] Thus, it is quite necessary to conduct some retrospective studies to investigate the clinical features, recovery quality, functionalities and their treatment procedures, as well as inflammation and immune biomarkers of COVID-19 convalescent patients with or without re-positive SARS-CoV-2 nucleic acid detection. Convalescence could be considered as one of the most significant periods for the patients. It is important in TCM that any improper management during this period could possibly lead to the remaining of pathogens, further disturbance or damage to the body, and the existence of long-term sequences, such as Long COVID.

---

[1] Hui Zhu, *et al.* Clinical features of COVID-19 convalescent patients with re-positive nucleic acid detection. *J Clin Lab Anal.* 2020, 34: e23392. https://doi.org/10.1002/jcla.23392.

6.1 TCM Analysis of COVID-19 at Convalescent Stage

6.1.1 Definition

Coronavirus disease 2019 (COVID-19), caused by severe acute respiratory syndrome coronavirus 2 (SARS-CoV-2), is a new human disease, which has swept the world since the end of 2019. Although most patients with new coronary pneumonia can recover and be discharged after treatment in the hospital, clinical data show that in addition to causing lung inflammation and tissue damage, the new coronavirus also affects: (i) the digestive system, which causes patients to experience symptoms such as diarrhea, vomiting, and loss of appetite (ii) damage to the nervous system, which leads to insomnia, poor memory, loss of taste and smell (iii) damage to the kidney function, which causes edema and (iv) reduce the number of sperm cells in men, which affects fertility. A number of investigations and research findings in recent days have found that patients who have recovered from new coronary pneumonia still show various symptoms, which might retain for six months or more after convalescence.

Convalescence, synonyms for recovery and recuperation, means the same as the Latin convalēscere, meaning "to regain health", gradual healing after sickness or injury. Convalescence for an illness is often accompanied by various medicines, sufficient rest, proper diet, an emotional coach, and some physical exercise.

The patients during the convalescence period are required to visit the doctor for regular check-ups. A negative COVID-19 test does not mean convalescence or recovery.

6.1.2 Timeline of convalescence of COVID-19

Policymakers, surveillance, and public-health agencies must prioritize agreement on criteria for a definition of convalescence of COVID-19 and the structures in which these criteria could be implemented. In terms of the timeline of convalescence of COVID-19, it is generally accepted that the acute COVID-19 infection phase refers to the period of the first 4–5 weeks immediately after the onset of the symptoms of COVID-19. Acute post-COVID symptoms last from week 5 to week 12, long post-COVID symptoms last from week 12 to week 24, and persistent post-COVID symptoms last more than 24 weeks. From the above, it could be concluded that convalescence of COVID-19 refers to the period from week five to week 12 from the onset of the first symptom. However, it could also be up to 6 months, or even longer. "With other common viral illnesses, such as flu, we would expect recovery to mean going back to pre-infection levels of functionality and quality of life. This means we must follow up on all patients with confirmed (by test) or highly probable (by symptoms) COVID-19 and find out whether they have returned to their previous "normal" within a specified time from the onset of their symptoms. The "recovery" definition must include duration, severity, and fluctuation of symptoms, as well as functionality and quality of life. Everyone who is symptomatic would remain a "case" until they fulfilled the recovery criteria or died.[2]

6.1.3 Convalescence is defined differently for each patient

In many cases, convalescence or recovery is implied by discharge from the hospital or testing negative for the virus. Some researchers consider COVID-19 patients to be fully recovered after the day they get discharged from the hospital. In fact, this way of classification is incomplete because of the following arguments:

- There is still a gap in quantifying and characterizing COVID-related illness in those not hospitalized.
- Non-hospitalized cases, who are under the radar or loosely termed "mild", are not followed up with.

---

[2]Nisreen A. Alwan. A negative COVID-19 test does not mean recovery. *Nature.* 2020, 584: 170. https://doi.org/10.1038/d41586-020-02335-z.

- Some patients who are young or previously healthy might experience only a few days of flu-like symptoms, while some patients with underlying diseases—although they might be very sick—could refuse to be hospitalized for different reasons. They are usually not included for convalescence.
- Millions of patients worldwide who are still alive and got ill without being tested or hospitalized are simply not being counted.

It is therefore to conclude certain that defining and measuring recovery from COVID-19 should be more sophisticated than checking for hospital discharge or testing negative for active infection or positive for antibodies.[3] There are some young patients without any underlying diseases and weak constitutions who suffered only from shortness of breath and fatigue as their main complaints during COVID-19. However, after more than a year, they still have problematic physical and mental weakness, and could not function like before. These young patients should be included in the patients who need some convalescence support and various guidance.

6.1.4 Features of convalescence of COVID-19

6.1.4.1 *Variation of convalescence duration*

The convalescent process of COVID-19 refers not only to recovery from a lung disturbance or damage but also recovery from many aspects. It's duration, fluctuation of symptoms, and restoration in functionality and quality of life, etc., are also the contents to be concerned about. Since convalescence ranges from week 5 to week 12 after the onset of the first symptoms, seven weeks as its interval is a long period of time. The longer its duration, the more complaints the patient could suffer from. Duration of convalescence usually depends on whether COVID-19 is a mild, moderate, or severe case. The patient may need to be admitted into ICU or even be put on a ventilator. It means that the severity of COVID-19 could be one of the chief factors in determining the duration of the convalescence.

---

[3] Yang Wang. *op. cit.*

Besides, its medical treatment, underlying diseases, personal constitutions, emotions, and diets, etc., also play an extremely important role in this process.

- Around 80% of COVID patients (so-called mild cases), only show some slight symptoms or even asymptomatically. They could recover within one week to ten days.
- Some patients with mild COVID cases could be free of symptoms, but others could still suffer from some symptoms for a few more weeks or even months. Symptoms lasting several weeks and impairing a person's usual function should not be called mild.
- Patients with moderate cases of COVID-19 infection (who sometimes need to visit a hospital or emergency department), could experience longer physical fatigue and other symptoms, such as cough and shortness of breath, etc. Their recovery process lasts for several weeks or longer.
- In some patients, the disease may become worse and develop into pneumonia, or the immune system may release a very powerful "cytokine storm" to destroy the virus. This strong inflammatory response can lead to the so-called acute respiratory distress syndrome (ARDS), which damages lung tissue and even causes respiratory failure. They need to be hospitalized to receive comprehensive treatment. Once the disease reaches and causes damage to multiple organs, they also need hospitalization. Recovering from severe COVID-19 may take up to months or years for physical strength and lung function to return to normal.

6.1.4.2 *Necessity of further close observation*

In most cases, when the hospitalized patients with COVID-19 are discharged, they need at least one or two tests, and some hospitals even need three tests to confirm that PCR has turned negative. But there are some hospitals that start discharging the patients two or three days (without carrying out PCR tests) after their fever or chest tightness are under relative control.

According to the European Centre for Disease Prevention and Control, the exact duration of infectivity of COVID-19 patients is not yet known with certainty. Several studies have shown that most transmission happens around the onset of symptoms and that SARS-CoV-2 can initially be detected in upper respiratory samples around two days before the onset of symptoms. In studies of non-severe cases, the virus was successfully isolated for ten days from the onset of symptoms. In an analysis of 72 infector-infected pairs in South Korea, the estimated median transmission onset was 1.31 days (standard deviation (SD) 2.64 days), following the onset of initial symptoms with a peak of 0.72 days. Among hospitalized/severe COVID-19 patients, isolation of SARS-CoV-2 was possible until day 20 after the onset of symptoms, with a median of 8 days (interquartile range (IQR) 5–11 days). The probability of detecting infectious SARS-CoV-2 dropped below 5% after 15.2 days after the onset of symptoms (95% confidence interval (CI) 13.4–17.2). In this study, the risk of having a positive SARS-CoV-2 culture was three times higher in immunocompromised patients than in other patients, which suggests that immunocompromised patients may shed SARS-CoV-2 for prolonged periods. Older age and a more severe infection have been associated with a higher viral load. However, it was also recently demonstrated that children have viral loads similar to that of adults, and asymptomatic patients have viral loads similar to that of symptomatic patients.[4]

In some countries, e.g., China, hospitals must follow very strict rules before they can discharge patients. These discharged patients should remain in quarantine for another 14 days and they can be released from quarantine if their PCR tests are still negative.[5]

In fact, there are many patients with COVID-19 who are young or mild cases, and did not need any hospitalization, in which their

---

[4]European Centre for Disease Prevention and Control. Guidance for discharge and ending of isolation of people with COVID-19. 16 October 2020. Stockholm: ECDC, 2020. https://www.ecdc.europa.eu/sites/default/files/documents/Guidance-for-discharge-and-ending-of-isolation-of-people-with-COVID-19.pdf.

[5]Shaobin He *et al.* Positive RT-PCR test results in 420 patients recovered from COVID-19 in Wuhan: An observational study. *Front. Pharmacol.* 7 October 2020. https://doi.org/10.3389/fphar.2020.549117.

clinical symptoms and PCR tests are left uncontrolled or not followed-up with. For these cases, they also need a close observation because they potentially could also spread the virus if their PCR remains positive with the infectious virus. Although not all the cases with positive PCR could carry the infectious virus, it is tedious to detect in the laboratory if the virus is infectious or noninfectious. Thus, it is not widely carried out in this way. Therefore, as long as PCR is positive, the patients are quarantined in China.

6.1.4.3 *Duration of remained positive PCR tests*

During the convalescence, it is quite possible that the PCR remains positive. Is the patient still contagious? A positive PCR does not always mean that the patient presents any danger to society. It depends on whether the virus is infectious or not.

A PCR test is a technique to find the virus. The PCR alone cannot answer if this virus is active, i.e., infectious, or virulent? In viral culture, viruses are injected into the laboratory cell lines to see if they cause cell damage and death, thus releasing a whole set of new viruses that can go on to infect other cells. That is, if the PCR detects the virus in the human sample, this detection might correspond to a virus that is now incapable of infecting cells and reproducing. Biologists can tell if the virus is infectious by injecting it into culture cells. If these cells are not affected by the virus and the virus does not reproduce in them, then the PCR test found a virus that is no longer active.[6]

Recovered patients can continue to have SARS-CoV-2 RNA detected in their upper respiratory specimens for up to 12 weeks after symptom onset. Available data indicate that adults with mild to moderate COVID-19 remain infectious no longer than ten days after symptom onset. Most adults with more severe to critical illness or severe immunocompromise are likely to remain infectious no longer

---

[6]The Centre for Evidence-Based Medicine. PCR positives: What do they mean? 17 September 2020. https://www.cebm.net/covid-19/pcr-positives-what-do-they-mean/.

than 20 days after symptom onset. However, there have been several reports of people shedding replication-competent virus beyond 20 days due to severe immunocompromise.[7] There could be exceptions. After almost 10 months, 43 positive RT-PCR tests, and several near-death experiences, a man in UK, Bristol has tested negative for COVID-19. With this, he came to hold an unfortunate record of being an active COVID-19 patient for the longest duration.[8]

During the pandemic, some hospitals require their staff to continue to work when their PCR tests are positive. For instance—a hospital in Liege, which is situated in the east near the border with the Netherlands and at the center of a coronavirus hotspot with the highest coronavirus incidence rate in Belgium—was asking its nurses to carry on working as long as they are not displaying symptoms even if they test positive for COVID-19.[9]

Even though it is generally accepted that it is no longer contagious ten days after symptom onset for patients with mild to moderate COVID-19, precautions are still required to prevent COVID-19. Most communities and social environments these days require certificates to prove a negative COVID-19 PCR test result before allowed to enter some public places. Starting July 21, the "health pass" (Pass Sanitaire) will be compulsory in France for access to leisure and cultural venues with more than 50 people, including cinemas and museums. From the beginning of August, it will be necessary to show your health pass to have coffee or eat lunch at a restaurant—even on an outdoor terrace—or to shop at a mall. Customers will have to provide either a QR code proving they are fully vaccinated, a negative PCR or

---

[7] Centers for Disease Control and Prevention (CDC). Ending isolation and precautions for people with COVID-19: Interim guidance. 14 September 2021. https://www.cdc.gov/coronavirus/2019-ncov/hcp/duration-isolation.html.

[8] 10 months. That's how long this UK man tested positive for Covid. *India Today* 24 June 2021. https://www.indiatoday.in/world/story/10-months-that-s-how-long-this-uk-man-tested-positive-for-covid-read-his-story-1818967-2021-06-24.

[9] Shona Murray, Joanna Gill. Nurses with COVID-19 asked to carry on working at under pressure hospital in Belgium. *Euronews.* 28 October 2020. https://www.euronews.com/2020/10/28/coronavirus-nurses-with-covid-19-asked-to-carry-on-working-at-under-pressure-hospital-in-b.

antigen test that is less than 48 hours old or proof that they have recovered from COVID-19 in the last six months. According to the government's draft bill, restaurants could be fined up to €45,000 and proprietors face up to a year in prison if they fail to comply.[10]

6.1.4.4 *Relapse of possible PCR tests*

One study aimed to investigate the clinical characteristics and to analyze the epidemiological features of coronavirus disease 2019 (COVID-19) patients during convalescence. In the study, they enrolled 71 confirmed COVID-19 cases who were discharged from the hospital and transferred to isolation wards from 6 February to 26 March 2020. The patients were all employees of Zhongnan Hospital of Wuhan University or their family members of which three cases were <18 years of age. Clinical data were collected and analyzed statistically. Forty-one cases (41/71, 57.7%) comprised of medical faculty. Young and middle-aged patients (aged <60 years) accounted for 81.7%(58/71). The average isolation period for all adult patients was 13.8 ± 6.1 days. During convalescence, RNA detection results of 35.2% of patients (25/71) turned from negative to positive. The longest RNA reversed-phase time was seven days.[11]

Another retrospective study was performed on 98 convalescent patients with COVID-19 who were treated in a single medical center, HwaMei Hospital, University of Chinese Academy of Sciences, Zhejiang, China. By 2 April 2020, epidemiological and clinical data were collected. The clinical features of patients during their hospitalization and two-week post-discharge quarantine were collected. Among these patients, 17(17.3%) were detected with positive severe acute respiratory syndrome coronavirus 2 (SARS-CoV-2) nucleic acid

---

[10]Grégoire Sauvage. France prepares to introduce COVID-19 "health pass" for access to cultural venues. *France24*. 16 July 2021. https://www.france24.com/en/europe/20210716-as-france-extends-use-of-covid-health-pass-what-are-its-eu-neighbours-doing.

[11]Bingman Liu *et al.* Epidemiological characteristics of COVID-19 patients in convalescence period. *Epidemiol Infect.* 2020, 148: e108. doi: 10.1017/S0950268 820001181.

during two-week post-discharge quarantine. The median time from discharge to SARS-CoV-2 nucleic acid re-positive was four days (IQR, 3–8.5). The median time from symptoms onset to final respiratory SARS-CoV-2 detection of the negative result was significantly longer in the re-positive group (34 days [IQR, 29.5–42.5]) than in the non-re-positive group (19 days [IQR, 16–26]). On the other hand, the levels of CD3-CD56+ NK cells during hospitalization and two-week post-discharge were higher in a re-positive group than in the non-re-positive group (repeated measures ANOVA, $p = 0.018$). However, only one case in the re-positive group showed exudative lesion recurrence in pulmonary computed tomography (CT) with recurred symptoms. The conclusion is that it is still possible for convalescent patients to test positive for SARS-CoV-2 nucleic acid detection, but most of the re-positive patients showed no deterioration in pulmonary CT findings. Continuous quarantine and close follow-up for convalescent patients are necessary to prevent possible relapse and spread of the disease to some extent.[12]

6.1.4.5 *Continuation of medical care*

During the convalescence, some patients could have almost no clinical symptoms, but it doesn't mean that their entire physical or mental conditions are completely restored. They need some time to recover, especially for those who have moderate or severe cases. When they do show some clinical symptoms, no matter only one symptom or a few symptoms, comprehensive treatment could be considered, in which TCM could be one of the choices.

In the same study listed above, 52.9% of adult patients (36/68) had no obvious clinical symptoms, and the remaining ones had mild and non-specific clinical symptoms (e.g., cough, sputum, sore throat, disorders of the gastrointestinal tract, etc.) after discharge from a hospital. Chest CT signs in 89.7% of adult patients (61/68) gradually improved, and in the others, the lesions were eventually absorbed and improved after short-term repeated progression. The main chest

---

[12]Hui Zhu, *et al. op. cit.*

CT manifestations of adult patients were normal (GGO or fiber streak shadow), and six patients (8.8%) had extrapulmonary manifestations, but there was no significant correlation with RNA detection results ($r = -0.008$, $p > 0.05$). The drug treatment was mainly symptomatic support therapy, and antibiotics and antiviral drugs were ineffective. It is necessary to re-evaluate the isolation time and standard to terminate isolation for discharged COVID-19 patients.[13]

6.1.4.6 *Maintenance of personal hygiene*

Even after discharge from hospital and recovering from COVID-19, it is still necessary to take care of personal hygiene, measure body temperature regularly, observe own physical health for any symptoms, follow up on medical controls, wear a mask when in public (especially at a crowded place), disinfect the bathroom surfaces before using the bathroom (including the flusher and faucet handle), wash hands with soap and water, and keep the room with good air ventilation.

6.1.4.7 *Difference in non-severe and severe patients*

Both clinical symptoms and their laboratory test and imagine technology results are different from patient to patient, especially for patients with non-severe COVID-19 and patients with severe COVID-19. Of course, these differences also exist during the convalescent period. Therefore, careful follow-up treatment plans based on the different clinical characteristics of convalescent patients should be established accordingly.

In one retrospective study aimed to evaluate the clinical characteristics of discharged COVID-19 patients, researchers extracted data for 134 convalescent patients with COVID-19 in Guizhou Provincial Staff Hospital from 15 February to 31 March 2020. Cases were analyzed using demographic, clinical, and laboratory data as well as radiological features. Out of 134 convalescent patients with

---

[13] Bingman Liu, *et al. op. cit.*

COVID-19, 19(14.2%) were severe cases, while 115(85.8%) were non-severe cases. The median patient age was 33 years (IQR, 21.8 to 46.3), and the cohort included 69 men and 65 women. Compared with non-severe cases, severe patients were older and had more chronic comorbidities, especially hypertension, diabetes, and thyroid disease ($p < 0.05$). Leukopenia was present in 32.1% of the convalescent patients and lymphocytopenia was present in 6.7%, both of which were more common in severe patients. 48(35.8%) of discharged patients had elevated levels of alanine aminotransferase, which was more common in adults than in children (40.2% vs. 13.6%, $p = 0.018$). A normal chest CT was found in 61 (45.5%) patients during rehabilitation. Severe patients had more ground-glass opacity, bilateral patchy shadowing, and fibrosis. No significant differences were observed in the positive rate of IgM and/or IgG antibodies between severe and non-severe patients. Their conclusions are that leukopenia, lymphopenia, ground-glass opacity, and fibrosis are common in discharged severe COVID-19 patients, and liver injury is common in discharged adult patients.[14]

6.1.5 Importance of convalescence

6.1.5.1 *Combating between zheng-qi and xie-qi*

During the convalescence, the pestilential qi has been primarily eliminated or suppressed, and zheng-qi has been disturbed or damaged at the same time, and has not yet completely restored. However, the fight between zheng-qi and xie-qi is still present, indicating that methods should be used to eliminate the remaining pathogens and to strengthen the qi of the body. During this period, fever subsides, and patients experience slight pressure over the chest, shortness of breath, loss of smelling and taste, spontaneous or night sweating, weak voice or dry cough, fatigue, poor appetite, loose stool or diarrhea, and

---

[14]Siqin Zhang, *et al.* Clinical characteristics of 134 convalescent patients with COVID-19 in Guizhou, China. *Respir Res.* 2020, 21: 314. https://doi.org/10.1186/s12931-020-01580-0.

various kinds of emotional disturbance. In some severe cases, their physiological functions are seriously damaged. The shadow of the lung has not been fully absorbed, and sometimes there are symptoms due to withdrawal of hormones. Nevertheless, treatment priority at this period should be reinforcing zheng-qi.

Reinforcing zheng-qi doesn't mean that only tonics without caring to eliminate remaining pathogenic factors should be used. On the contrary, in the early stage of convalescence, sometimes the main TCM treatment is to eliminate the remaining pathogens, including damp, heat, cold, pestilent toxins and blood stasis. Moreover, fatigue doesn't imply that it is only caused by deficiency of qi or blood, since remaining and accumulation of damp or phlegm could lead to fatigue as well.

6.1.5.2 *Acceleration of recovery procedures*

The advantages of TCM in the treatment of COVID-19 include effective improvement of symptoms, retardation of the development from mild and moderate to severe, raising of cure rate, and reduction of complications and mortality rate. According to the different syndromes and severity levels of individual cases during convalescence, TCM has also showed favorable effects in amelioration of pathological evolution, and acceleration of recovery procedures for patients.

A clinical trial, led by renowned Chinese pulmonologist Zhong Nanshan, has shown that consuming Lian Hua Qing Wen (LH) capsules (the botanical TCM product), and undergoing the standard therapy can speed up recovery in COVID-19 patients. Patients were randomized to receive usual treatment alone or in combination with LH capsules (4 capsules, thrice daily) for 14 days. The primary endpoint was the rate of symptom (fever, fatigue, coughing) recovery. 284 patients were included (142 in each treatment and control group) in the full-analysis set. The recovery rate was significantly higher in the treatment group as compared with the control group (91.5% vs. 82.4%, $p = 0.022$). The median time to symptom recovery was markedly shorter in the treatment group (median: 7 vs. 10 days, $p < 0.001$). Time taken to recover from fever (2 vs. 3 days), fatigue

(3 vs. 6 days) and coughing (7 vs. 10 days) was also significantly shorter in the treatment group (all $p < 0.001$). The rate of improvement in chest computed tomographic manifestations (83.8% vs. 64.1%, $p < 0.001$) and clinical cure (78.9% vs. 66.2%, $p = 0.017$) was also higher in the treatment group. However, both groups did not differ in the rate of conversion to severe cases or viral assay findings (both $p > 0.05$). No serious adverse events were reported.[15] However, it has not proved to be effective in preventing severe infection from happening or reducing median viral assay conversion time.

6.1.5.3 *Prevention of pathological condition deterioration*

When the patients enter convalescence, they usually still suffer from some dysfunctions of some internal zang-fu organs with disturbance of meridians and circulation of qi and blood. It depends on their zheng-qi to fight against all the remaining pathogenic factors and restore dysfunctions of zang-fu organs.

TCM has always been used as a main method in the treatment of epidemic diseases since ancient times in China. Meanwhile, empirical evidence and successful experiences to eliminate toxins, restore healthy qi, harmonize yin and yang and strengthen body resistance in the prevention and treatment of combating fatal epidemic disease have been accumulated by TCM physicians. Today, the treatment for the patients with COVID-19 is mainly based upon a symptomatic management, or a combination of antiviral and antibiotics. However, it is evident that there is no specific medication to treat or prevent the serious complications of patients with COVID-19. To date, specific antiviral treatment for COVID-19 is not yet developed. However, previous experience of using TCM to treat SARS, MERS and H1N1 could provide excellent guidance for healthcare practitioners in the treatment of COVID-19.

---

[15]Ke Hu, *et al.* Efficacy and safety of Lianhua Qingwen capsules, a repurposed Chinese herb, in patients with Coronavirus disease 2019: A multicenter, prospective, randomized controlled trial. *Phytomedicine.* 2021, 85: 153242. https://doi.org/10.1016/j.phymed.2020.153242.

During convalescence, since the interval between symptoms onset and the recovery period is still relatively too short (week four and week five for acute phase), there is a great possibility that pathogenic factors are still partially existing while zheng-qi is already damaged. This is a crucial stage, which could influence or determine future conditions of the patients. When improper treatment is given, or there is a lack of correct cooperation between the patients and medical practitioners, long COVID could happen, which may greatly interfere with the quality of life and functionality of work for the patients.

6.1.5.4 *Possible donation of convalescent plasma*

COVID-19 is currently a big threat to global health with no specific antiviral agents available for its treatment. Convalescent plasma therapy is proposed by some experts. The basic idea behind is that people who have had an illness and recovered from it have antibodies to it and are immune. Convalescent plasma is the blood from recovered patients, and in therapy it is transferred intravenously to people who do not have antibodies to the disease and they in turn, can be immune to the disease. Convalescent plasma is a way of artificially inducing passive immunity by transferring blood plasma from patients who have had a disease to uninfected patients. This can then grant the recipient immunity towards the disease because of antibodies present in the blood plasma. Convalescent plasma therapy is one of the proposed treatments for COVID-19, although recent studies have debated its effectiveness.[16]

One study explored the feasibility of convalescent plasma transfusion to rescue severe patients. The results from ten severe adult cases showed that one dose (200 mL) of CP was well tolerated and could significantly increase or maintain the neutralizing antibodies at a high level, leading to disappearance of viremia in seven days. Meanwhile, clinical symptoms and paraclinical criteria rapidly

---

[16]Sara Ryding. What is convalescent plasma donation? *News-Medical.* 14 April 2021. https://www.news-medical.net/health/What-is-Convalescent-Plasma.aspx.

improved within three days. Radiological examination showed varying degrees of absorption of lung lesions within seven days. These results indicate that CP can serve as a promising rescue option for severe COVID-19, while the randomized trial is warranted.[17]

One study, on the other hand, shows some indication that convalescent plasma can be used successfully before hospitalization to stop the virus, but cannot do much later when the damage has already been done, and the antibodies cannot repair. A randomized (a total of 160 patients), double-blind, placebo-controlled trial of convalescent plasma with high IgG titers against severe acute respiratory syndrome coronavirus 2 (SARS-CoV-2) in older adult patients within 72 hours after the onset of mild COVID-19 symptoms, was conducted. The conclusion was that early administration of high-titer convalescent plasma against SARS-CoV-2 to mildly ill older adults reduced the progression of COVID-19. No solicited adverse events were observed.[18]

One research proposed the same positive evidence as above, pointing out that worldwide matched-control studies have generally found convalescent plasma to improve COVID-19 patient survival. RCTs have demonstrated a survival benefit when transfused early in the disease course but showed limited or no benefit later in the disease course when patients required greater supportive therapies. RCTs have also revealed that convalescent plasma transfusion contributes to improved symptomatology and viral clearance. To further investigate the effect of convalescent plasma on patient mortality, the study performed a meta-analytical approach to pool daily survival data from all controlled studies that reported Kaplan–Meier survival plots. Qualitative inspection of all available Kaplan–Meier survival data and an aggregate Kaplan–Meier survival plot revealed a directionally

---

[17]Kai Duan, *et al.* Effectiveness of convalescent plasma therapy in severe COVID-19 patients. *PNAS.* 2020, 117(17): 9490–9496. https://doi.org/10.1073/pnas.2004168117.

[18]Romina Libster, *et al.* Early high-titer plasma therapy to prevent severe COVID-19 in older adults. *N Engl J Med.* 2021, 384: 6106–6118. doi: 10.1056/NEJMoa2033700.

consistent pattern among studies arising from multiple levels of the epistemic hierarchy, whereby convalescent plasma transfusion was generally associated with greater patient survival. Given that convalescent plasma has a similar safety profile as standard plasma, convalescent plasma should be implemented within weeks of the onset of future infectious disease outbreaks.[19]

6.1.6 Principles of treatment at convalescent stage

At present, huge data have confirmed after return visits and investigations that some patients still suffer from symptoms after being discharged from the hospital, such as fatigue, anorexia, weakness, emotional abnormality, and abnormal biochemical and imaging examinations. There are varying degrees of lung function impairment, interstitial pneumonia changes, and even lung fibers. Since ancient times, TCM has had the idea of "preventing deterioration after sickness, preventing relapse of the disease, and prevention before the disease". Effective control of the disease varies depending on the health and functional recovery of patients. It is very necessary to pay attention to the comprehensive recovery of the health of patients physically and mentally after being discharged from the hospital. TCM comprehensive rehabilitation guidance can promote the recovery of the disease, improve the quality of life, and cut off the source of the recurrence of the disease.

The recovery period is a unique stage in TCM, and the treatment during this period fully reflects the thinking and characteristics of Chinese philosophy. Treatment includes various kinds of intervention strategies with comprehensive content and strong maneuverability, such as Chinese herbal decoction, herbal patent remedies, acupuncture, diet therapy, emotional therapy, breathing and meridian exercises, etc. As far as acupuncture is concerned, it includes the following

---

[19]Stephen A. Klassen, *et al.* Convalescent plasma therapy for COVID-19: A graphical mosaic of the worldwide evidence. *Front. Med.* 2021, 8: 684151. https://doi.org/10.3389/fmed.2021.684151.

common therapies, such as acupuncture, moxibustion, meridian massage, ear-point pressing, Gua Sha, and cupping, etc. On top of that, syndrome of qi deficiency of the lung and spleen and syndrome of qi and yin deficiency are two most important types that need to be cared for besides further elimination of pathogenic factors.

6.1.6.1 *General aims of treatment*

Most pathogenic factors are eliminated for the patients with COVID-19 at convalescent period. However, if we include the first day of symptoms onset till the beginning of convalescent period, convalescent period is in about week 5 to week 12. It is really too short to recover completely, and it is normal that the patients could still suffer from some symptoms. The general aim of treatments are to tonify qi and benefit yin, to resolve phlegm and regulate the lung, to activate the spleen and eliminate damp, to promote blood circulation and eliminate blood stasis, and to calm the shen and harmonize the emotions. All these TCM procedures could relieve cough, promote inflammation absorption, prevent pulmonary fibrosis, restore lung function, improve physical strength, and support emotional weakness.

6.1.6.2 *Elimination of remaining pathogens*

The pathogenic factors of COVID-19 include cold, damp, heat, toxins. Its pathological changes include excess, deficiency, disorder of qi and blood, and dysfunction of water metabolism, etc. When the patients enter the convalescent period, no matter if their previous cases were asymptomatic, mild, ordinary, severe or critical, it could be highly possible that these pathogenic factors are not eliminated entirely, and their pathological changes are not yet thoroughly restored. Nevertheless, their zheng-qi are greatly disturbed or damaged. Balance should be found to identify which treatment is most suitable for the patients. When tonification is given too early in the condition that their remaining pathogenic factors are not completely removed, it could cause prolonged persistence of these pathogens, which could be harmful for the future improvement. On the other hand, when methods to strongly attack the pathogens are still mainly applied instead of using treatment to tonify the zheng-qi for those who has almost no pathogens and are suffering from zheng-qi deficiency, this treatment could cause further damage to the patient.

6.1.6.3 *Consideration of individuality*

It is true that recovery of COVID-19 takes some time, however, measures should be taken to promote this procedure. In addition, not only physical fatigue and pain, loss of smell and taste should be treated. We also need to care about the patient's emotional aspects, dietary correction, and exercise coaching. Each patient is an individual, who is different from someone else suffering from COVID-19. Personal manifestations, feelings and reactions to the treatment are the differences which need personalized treatment or management. In this sense it could be observed that TCM treats personal sickness instead of sickness. Each patient has undergone different stages and severity of the sickness, varying approaches of management and treatment, emotions, dietary habits, constitutions, underlying sickness, and even cultural background. Therefore, their clinical manifestations could be different from each other. If these conditions are neglected, the treatment will not be proper and accurate, which is not in line with the principles of TCM.

Besides treatment based upon syndrome differentiations, seasonal environment and geographic location are also important and should be taken into consideration during TCM treatment.

6.2 TCM Treatment

6.2.1 Incomplete elimination of damp and toxins

Feverish feeling over the body but with no raised temperature, sore throat, dry and weak cough, slight tightness of the chest, fatigue, lassitude, poor appetite, spontaneous sweating, body aches, remaining of positive PCR test or by reexaminations, pale tongue with a white or greasy coating, and a slippery and rapid pulse.

Principle of Treatment:
Clear heat, disperse the lung-qi, resolve damp, and harmonize the middle Jiao.

Herbal Treatment:
Cang Fu Dao Tan Tang-*Atractylodes-Poria Phlegm-Dissipating Decoction.*

Cang Zhu *Rhizoma Atractylodis* 10 g
Xiang Fu *Rhizoma Cyperi Rotundi* 10 g
Zhi Ke *Fructus Citri Aurantii* 10 g
Zhi Ban Xia *Rhizoma Pinelliae Ternatae Preparata* 10 g
Fu Ling *Sclerotium Poriae Cocos* 10 g
Chen Pi *Pericarpium Citri Reticulatae* 5 g
Hou Po *Cortex Magnoliae Officinalis* 5 g
Jie Geng *Radix Platycodi Grandiflori* 10 g
Xing Ren *Semen Pruni Armeniacae* 5 g
Yu Jin *Tuber Curcumae* 10 g
Hong Hua *Flos Carthami Tinctorii* 10 g
Ge Gen R*adix Puerariae* 10 g

Explanations:
* Cang Zhu, Xiang Fu, Zhi Ke and Hou Po are used to eliminate damp, promote the qi circulation in the chest, and harmonize the middle Jiao.
* Zhi Ban Xia, Xing Ren and Jie Geng eliminate damp-phlegm and regulate the functions of the lung to relieve cough and slight tightness of the chest.
* Fu Ling and Chen Pi are used to activate the spleen, eliminate damp in the body and resolve phlegm in the lung.
* Yu Jin and Hong Hua harmonize the collaterals in the lung and the collaterals connected by the lung so as to promote the qi and blood circulation and prevent blood stagnation.
* Ge Gen ascends clear yang and descends the turbid yin so as to eliminate damp in the spleen and resolve phlegm in the body.

Modifications:

- If there is a headache, add Bai Zhi *Radix Angelicae Dahuricae* 10 g to relieve the headache.
- If there is much emotional disorder, add Chang Pu *Rhizoma Anemonis Altaicae* 10 g and Yuan Zhi *Radix Polygalae Tenuifoliae* 10 g to benefit the heart orifice and regulate the emotions.
- If there is muscle pain, add Qiang Huo *Rhizoma et Radix Notopterygii* 10 g and Sang Zhi *Ramulus Mori Albae* 10 g to relieve the muscle pain.
- If there is much expectoration of white phlegm, add Bai Jie Zi *Semen Sinapis Albae* 10 g and Zhi Ban Xia *Rhizoma Pinelliae Ternatae Preparata* 10 g to eliminate phlegm and relieve cough.
- If there is cough with much diluted phlegm, add Ting Li Zi *Semen Descurainiae seu Lepidii* 10 g to descend the lung-qi and eliminate cold-phlegm.
- If there is obvious loss of smell and taste, add Cang Er Zi *Fructus Xanthii Sibirici* 10 g and Xin Yi Hua *Flos Magnoliae* 10 g to open the nasal orifice and improve smell and taste.
- If there is much nausea, add Sha Ren *Fructus Amomi* 3 g and Zi Su Ye *Folium Perillae Frutescentis* 5 g to harmonize the stomach-qi and relieve the nausea.
- If there is much diarrhea and abdominal swelling, add Huo Xiang *Herba Agastaches seu Pogostemi* 10 g and Shan Yao *Radix Dioscoreae Oppositae* 10 g to eliminate damp and stop diarrhea.

Acupuncture Treatment:

- Neiguan P-6 + Gongsun SP-4, Chize LU-5, Feishu BL-13, Zusanli ST-36, Fenglong ST-40, Sanyinjiao SP-6, Yinlingquan SP-9, Yanglingquan GB-34, and Tanzhong Ren-17.
- An even method is used on Neiguan P-6 + Gongsun SP-4, and a reducing method is used on LU-5, BL-13, ST-40, SP-6, SP-9, and GB-34. An even method is used on Ren-17. A tonifying method is used on ST-36.

Explanations:
- P-6 + SP-4 are used to descend the lung-qi and relieve remaining cough.
- LU-5 and BL-13, the he-sea point of the lung channel and the back-shu point of the lung respectively, eliminate remaining pathogens in the lung and relieve cough and sore throat.
- SP-6 and SP-9, the crossing point of the three yin channels of the foot, and the he-sea point of the spleen channel respectively, ST-40, the luo-connecting point of the stomach channel, and GB-34, the he-sea point of the gallbladder channel, are used to remove toxins, eliminate damp in the body and relieve the body pain.
- Ren-17, the gathering point of the qi, is used with an even method to promote the qi circulation in the chest and restore the physiological function of the lung.
- ST-36, the he-sea point of the stomach channel, is used to tonify the zheng-qi, and activate the spleen and stomach so as to improve strength of the body.

Modifications:
- If there is much headache, add Shenting DU-24 to relieve the headache.
- If there is much emotional disorder or insomnia, add the Extra Anmian and Extra Sishencong to calm the shen, regulate the emotions and improve sleeping.
- If there is muscle pain, add Waiguan SJ-5 and Zulinqi GB-41 to harmonize the yangwei channel, regulate the Shaoyang channel and relieve the muscle pain.
- If there is much expectoration of white phlegm, add Zhongfu LU-1, the front-mu point of the lung, to eliminate phlegm and relieve cough.
- If there is cough with much diluted phlegm, add Taiyuan LU-9 to descend the lung-qi and eliminate cold-phlegm.
- If there is obvious loss of smell and taste, add Yingxiang L.I.-20 and Juliao ST-3 to open the nasal orifice and improve smell and taste.

- If there is much nausea, add Zhongwan REN-12, the front-mu point of the stomach, to harmonize the stomach-qi and relieve the nausea.
- If there is much diarrhea and abdominal swelling, add Tianshu ST-25, the front-mu point of the large intestine, to eliminate damp and stop diarrhea.

6.2.2 Impairment of qi by toxic heat

Cough, shortness of breath, pressure over the chest, aggravation of these symptoms by exertion, low grade fever, nausea, lassitude, fatigue, loose and sticky stools, a red tongue with a white or yellow and greasy coating, and a slippery and thready pulse.

Principle of Treatment:
Activate the spleen, benefit qi, clear heat, remove toxins, and eliminate damp.

Herbal Treatment:
Lian Po Yin-*Coptis and Magnolia Bark Drink.*

Huang Lian *Rhizoma Coptidis* 3 g
Huang Qin *Radix Scutellariae Baicalensis* 10 g
Hou Po *Cortex Magnoliae Officinalis* 10 g
Zhi Mu *Radix Anemarrhenae Asphodeloidis* 10 g
Zhi Zi *Fructus Gardeniae Jasminoidis* 10 g
Sang Ye *Folium Mori Albae* 10 g
Xing Ren *Semen Pruni Armeniacae* 10 g
Cao Guo *Fructus Amomi Tsao-Ko* 3 g
Dang Shen *Radix Codonopsis Pilosulae* 10 g
Bai Zhu *Rhizoma Atractylodis Macrocephalae* 10 g
Fu Ling *Sclerotium Poriae Cocos* 15 g
Yu Jin *Tuber Curcumae* 10 g
Hong Hua *Flos Carthami Tinctorii* 10 g

Zhi Gan Cao *Radix Glycyrrhizae Preparata* 3 g

Explanations:
- Huang Lian, Huang Qin and Hou Po are used to clear heat, remove toxins, eliminate damp and harmonize the middle Jiao. Hou Po could also open the chest and relieve the pressure over the chest.
- Zhi Mu and Zhi Zi are used together to support the above herbs to clear remaining damp-heat and reduce feverish feeling.
- Sang Ye and Xing Ren are used to clear heat in the lung and relieve the cough.
- Cao Guo eliminates damp and removes toxins.
- Dang Shen, Bai Zhu, and Fu Ling are used to activate the spleen, eliminate damp, tonify the zheng-qi and relieve diarrhea.
- Yu Jin and Hong Hua harmonize the collaterals in the lung and the collaterals connected by the lung so as to promote the qi and blood circulation and prevent blood stagnation.
- Zhi Gan Cao tonifies the middle Jiao and harmonizes the prescription.

Modifications:
- If there is a headache, add Bai Zhi *Radix Angelicae Dahuricae* 10 g to relieve the headache.
- If there is much emotional disorder, add He Huan Pi *Cortex Albizziae Julibrissin* 10 g and Fu Shen *Sclerotium Poriae Cocos Paradicis* 10 g to calm the shen and regulate the emotions.
- If there is obvious loss of smell and taste, add Cang Er Zi *Fructus Xanthii Sibirici* 10 g and Xin Yi Hua *Flos Magnoliae* 10 g to open the nasal orifice and improve the smell and taste.
- If there is much expectoration of yellow phlegm, add Zhe Bei Mu *Bulbus Fritillariae Thunbergii* 10 g and Sang Bai Pi *Cortex Mori Albae Radicis* 10 g to eliminate phlegm-heat and relieve cough.
- If there is very poor appetite and much nausea, add Jiao Mai Ya *Fructus Hordei Vulgaris Germinantus* 10 g and Sha Ren

Fructus Amomi 3 g to promote digestion and harmonize the stomach-qi.

- If there is much diarrhea and abdominal swelling, add Ge Gen *Radix Puerariae* 10 g and Cang Zhu *Rhizoma Atractylodis* 10 g to eliminate damp and stop diarrhea.

Acupuncture Treatment:
- Neiguan P-6 + Gongsun SP-4, Chize LU-5, Feishu BL-13, Quchi L.I.-11, Zhongwan REN-12, Fenglong ST-40, Neiting ST-44, Sanyinjiao SP-6, Yinlingquan SP-9, Yanglingquan GB-34, and Zusanli ST-36.
- An even method is applied on P-6 + SP-4, a reducing method is used on LU-5, BL-13, L.I.-11, REN-12, ST-40, ST-44, SP-6, SP-9, and GB-34. A tonifying method is used on ST-36.

Explanations:
- P-6 + SP-4 are used to descend the qi of the lung and stomach, relieve remaining cough and nausea.
- LU-5 and BL-13, the he-sea point of the lung channel and the back-shu point of the lung respectively, eliminate remaining pathogens in the lung and relieve cough and pressure over the chest.
- L.I.-11, the he-sea point of the large intestine channel, ST-44, the ying-spring point of the stomach channel, and SP-6, the crossing point of the three yin channels of the foot, clear heat, reduce fever and remove toxins in the body.
- REN-12, the gathering point of the fu organs and the front-mu point of the stomach, SP-9, the he-sea point of the spleen channel, and GB-34, the he-sea point of the gallbladder channel, are used to eliminate damp in the body, harmonize the middle Jiao and promote digestion.
- ST-36, the he-sea point of the stomach channel, is used to tonify the zheng-qi, and activate the spleen and stomach so as to improve strength of the body.

Modifications:

- If there is much headache, add Extra Yintang or Extra Taiyang to relieve the headache.
- If there is much emotional disorder, add Shaohai HE-3, and Shenmen HE-7 to calm the shen and regulate the emotions.
- If there is obvious loss of smell and taste, add Yingxiang L.I.-20 and Juliao ST-3 to open the nasal orifice and improve the smell and taste.
- If there is much expectoration of yellow phlegm, add Yuji LU-10, the ying-stream point of the lung channel, to eliminate phlegm-heat and relieve cough.
- If there is very poor appetite and much nausea, add Zusanli ST-36, the he-sea point of the stomach channel, to promote digestion and improve appetite.
- If there is much diarrhea and abdominal swelling, add Tianshu ST-25, the front-mu point of the large intestine, to eliminate damp and stop diarrhea.

6.2.3 Obstruction of qi and blood circulation

Stabbing pain in the chest with tightness, shortness of breath, slight asthma, aggravation of above symptoms by exertion, palpitations, restlessness, insomnia, stabbing muscle pain, weakness of limbs, defecation and urination, headache, pale or slight purplish tongue, and a wiry and thready pulse.

Principle of Treatment:
Promote the qi and blood circulation, eliminate damp, and remove toxins.

Herbal Treatment:
Xue Fu Zhu Yu Tang-*Drive out Stasis in the Mansion of Blood Decoction.*

Tao Ren *Semen Pruni Persicae* 10 g
Hong Hua *Flos Carthami Tinctorii* 10 g
Chi Shao Yao *Radix Paeoniae Rubrae* 10 g

Yu Jin *Tuber Curcumae* 10 g
Pu Huang *Pollen Typhae* 10 g
Xing Ren *Semen Pruni Armeniacae* 10 g
Huang Qin *Radix Scutellariae Baicalensis* 10 g
Hou Po *Cortex Magnoliae Officinalis* 10 g
Zhi Ke *Fructus Citri Aurantii* 10 g
Tong Cao *Medulla Tetrapanacis Papyriferi* 5 g
Fu Shen *Sclerotium Poriae Cocos Paradicis* 15 g
Zhu Ling *Sclerotium Polypori Umbellati* 10 g
Chuan Niu Xi *Radix Cyathulae Officinalis* 10 g
Da Fu Pi *Pericarpium Arecae Catechu* 10 g

Explanations:
- Tao Ren, Hong Hua, Yu Jin, Chi Shao Yao and Pu Huang are used to strongly promote the blood circulation, eliminate blood stasis and relieve the stabbing pain in the chest and muscle pain.
- Zhi Ke and Hou Po promote the qi circulation so as to promote the blood circulation.
- Hou Po and Xing Ren are used in combination to eliminate damp and phlegm, regulate the qi in the lung, and descend the lung-qi to relieve the cough and asthma.
- Fu Shen calms shen and improves sleep.
- Huang Qin clears remaining heat in the lung.
- Tong Cao and Zhu Ling are used to promote urination and relieve weak urination.
- Da Fu Pi promotes the qi circulation in the abdomen and relieves weak defecation.
- Chuan Niu Xi promotes blood circulation and induces the blood to move downwards.

Modifications:
- If there is much headache, add Chuan Xiong *Radix Ligustici Wallichii* 10 g to relieve the headache.

- If there is an obvious emotional situation, add He Huan Pi *Cortex Albizziae Julibrissin* 10 g and Long Gu *Os Draconis* 20 g to calm the shen and regulate the emotions.
- If there is obvious loss of smell and taste, add Cang Er Zi *Fructus Xanthii Sibirici* 10 g and Xin Yi Hua *Flos Magnoliae* 10 g to open the nasal orifice and improve the smell and taste.
- If there is too much stabbing pain in the chest, add Dan Shen *Radix Salviae Miltiorrhizae* 10 g and Tan Xiang *Lignum Santali Albi* 5 g to eliminate blood stasis in the chest and relieve the pain.
- If there is depression, add Chai Hu *Radix Bupleuri* 5 g and Bai Shao Yao *Radix Paeoniae Lactiflorae* 10 g to smooth the liver and improve the qi circulation.

Acupuncture Treatment:
- Neiguan P-6 + Gongsun SP-4, Chize LU-5, Taiyuan LU-9, Feishu BL-13, Geshu BL-17, Shaohai HE-3, Fenglong ST-40, Sanyinjiao SP-6, Yinlingquan SP-9, Xuehai SP-10, Yanglingquan GB-34, Tanzhong Ren-17 and Zusanli ST-36.
- An even method is applied on Neiguan P-6 + Gongsun SP-4, a reducing method is applied on LU-5, LU-9, BL-13, BL-17, HE-3, ST-40, SP-6, SP-9, SP-10, GB-34, and Ren-17, and a tonifying method is used on ST-36.

Explanations:
- P-6 + SP-4 are used to descend the lung-qi and relieve remaining cough and asthma. Meanwhile they could promote the qi circulation in the body.
- LU-5 and BL-13, the he-sea point of the lung channel and the back-shu point of the lung respectively, together with Ren-17, the gathering point of the qi, eliminate remaining pathogens in the lung and relieve cough and asthma. Ren-17 also promotes and regulates the qi circulation in the body.
- LU-9, the gathering point of the vessels in the body, SP-6, the crossing point of three yin channels of the foot, together with BL-17, the gathering point of the blood, and SP-10, are used to promote the blood circulation and eliminate blood stasis.

- HE-3, the he-sea point of the heart channel, is applied to promote blood circulation, calm the shen and improve sleeping.
- Since damp is one of the chief pathogenic factors, SP-9, the he-sea point of the spleen channel, ST-40, the luo-connecting point of the stomach channel, and GB-34, the he-sea point of the gallbladder channel, are used to eliminate damp in the body.

Modifications:
- If there is much headache, add Fengchi GB-20 and extra Yintang to relieve the headache.
- If there is an obvious emotional situation, add Xinshu BL-15 and Shenmen HE-7, the back-shu point of the heart and the yuan-source point of the heart channel respectively, to calm the shen and regulate the emotions.
- If there is obvious loss of smell and taste, add Yingxiang L.I.-20 and Juliao ST-3 to open the nasal orifice and improve the smell and taste.
- If there is too much stabbing pain in the chest, add Gongsun P-4 and Yinxi HE-6 to eliminate blood stasis in the chest and relieve the pain.
- If there is depression, add Taichong LIV-3 and Ganshu BL-18, the yuan-source point of the liver channel and the back-shu point of the liver respectively, to smooth the liver and improve the qi circulation.

6.2.4 Deficiency of qi of lung and spleen

Slight shortness of breath, fatigue, poor appetite, weakness, nausea, fullness at the abdomen, loose stools or slight water diarrhea, a pale tongue with white coating, and a slippery, thready, and weak pulse.

Principle of Treatment:
Tonify the qi, activate the spleen and reinforce the lung and relieve damp-phlegm.

Herbal Treatment:
Bu Fei Tang-*Tonify the Lungs Decoction*, plus

Si Jun Zi Tang-*Four Gentlemen Decoction.*

Ren Shen *Radix Ginseng* 5 g
Zhi Huang Qi *Radix Astragali Membranacei Praeparata* 10 g
Wu Wei Zi *Fructus Schisandrae Chinensis* 10 g
Zi Wan *Radix Asteris Tatarici* 10 g
Shu Di Huang *Radix Rhemanniae Glutinosae Praeparata* 10 g
Sang Bai Pi *Cortex Mori Albae Radicis* 10 g
Jiao Bai Zhu *Rhizoma Atractylodis Macrocephalae (grill)* 10 g
Fu Ling *Sclerotium Poriae Cocos* 15 g
Sha Ren *Fructus Amomi* 5 g
Zhi Ban Xia *Rhizoma Pinelliae Ternatae Preparata* 10 g
Chen Pi *Pericarpium Citri Reticulatae* 5 g
Zhi Ke *Fructus Citri Aurantii* 10 g
Yu Jin *Tuber Curcumae* 10 g
Hong Hua *Flos Carthami Tinctorii* 5 g
Zhi Gan Cao *Radix Glycyrrhizae Preparata* 3 g

Explanations:
- The first six herbs, which are the complete ingredients of Bu Fei Tang, are used to tonify lung-qi and relieve cough.
- Ren Shen, Fu Ling, Bai Zhu and Zhi Gan Cao, which are the complete ingredients of Si Jun Zi Tang, are used to tonify the qi of the general body and relieve tiredness.
- Sha Ren promotes digestion and eliminates damp in the middle Jiao.
- Zhi Ban Xia and Chen Pi are used to eliminate remaining phlegm in the lung and damp in the body.
- Zhi Ke promotes the qi circulation and prevents qi stagnation.
- Yu Jin and Hong Hua are used to promote the blood circulation, regulate the collaterals, and relieve the pain.

Modifications:
- If there is severe fatigue, add Dong Chong Xia Cao *clerotium Cordyceps Sinensis* 1 g for infusion and Sheng Ma *Rhizoma Cimicifugae* 6 g to ascend qi and relieve the fatigue.

- If there is obvious emotion, add He Huan Pi *Cortex Albizziae Julibrissin* 10 g and Bai He *Bulbus Lilii* 10 g to regulate the emotions and calm the shen.
- If there is obvious aversion to cold with cold hands and feet, add Gan Jiang *Rhizoma Zingiberis Officinalis* 6 g and Gui Zhi *Ramulus Cinnamomi Cassiae* 10 g to warm the interior and dispel cold.
- If there is too much lower back pain, add Du Zhong *Cortex Eucommiae Ulmoidis* 10 g and Sang Ji Sheng *Ramulus Loranthi* 10 g to tonify the kidney and strengthen the lower back.

Acupuncture Treatment:
- Neiguan P-6 + Gongsun SP-4, Lieque LU-7 + Zhaohai KID-6 with even methods.
- Chize LU-5, Taiyuan LU-9, Feishu BL-13, Geshu BL-17, Pishu BL-20, Zusanli ST-36, Qihai REN-6, Taixi KID-3, Yinlingquan SP-9, and Tanzhong Ren-17.
- A tonifying method is applied on LU-5, LU-9, BL-13, BL-20, ST-36, REN-6, KID-3, SP-9, and Ren-17. An even method is used on Ren-17 and BL-17, a reducing method is applied on SP-9. Moxibustion is used on ST-36 and REN-6.

Explanations:
- P-6 + SP-4 are used to descend the lung-qi and relieve remaining cough.
- LU-7 and KID-6 are used to nourish the qi of the body and relax the chest.
- LU-5, LU-9, and BL-13, the he-sea point, the yuan-source point of the lung channel, and the back-shu point of the lung respectively, together with ST-36, the he-sea point of the stomach channel, in combination with BL-20, the back-shu point of the spleen, and KID-3, the yuan-source point of the kidney channel, and REN-6, the important point to reinforce the body, are all applied in groups to tonify the qi of the body, improve yuan-source qi and the strength of the body and relieve fatigue.

- Ren-17, the gathering point of the qi, and BL-17, the gathering point of the blood, together with SP-9, the he-se point of the spleen channel, are used to promote elimination of qi stagnation, toxins accumulation and damp obstruction in the body.

Modifications:
- If there is severe fatigue, add Sanyinjiao SP-6 and Baihui DU-20 to tonify the qi, ascend the qi and relieve the fatigue.
- If there is an obvious emotional situation, add Xinshu BL-15 and Ganshu BL-18, the back-shu point of the heart and liver respectively, to benefit the heart and liver, regulate the emotions and calm the shen.
- If there is obvious aversion to cold with cold hands and feet, add Guanyuan REN-4 to warm the interior and dispel cold.
- If there is too much lower back pain, add Shenshu BL-23 with moxibustion to tonify the kidney and strengthen the lower back.

6.2.5 Deficiency of qi and yin

Slight shortness of breath, dry cough and less sputum, dry mouth, thirst, fatigue, heart palpitations, excessive sweating, night sweating, poor appetite, low or no fever, dry and scanty tongue coating, slightly red tongue, and a thin, weak, and slight rapid pulse.

Principle of Treatment:
Tonify qi, nourish yin, benefit the lung, and relieve dry cough.

Herbal Treatment:
Sha Shen Mai Men Dong Tang-*Glehnia and Ophiopogonis Decoction.*

Nan Sha Shen *Radix Adenophorae* 10 g
Bei Sha Shen *Radix Glehniae Littoralis* 10 g
Mai Men Dong *Tuber Ophiopogonis Japonici* 10 g
Xi Yang Shen *Radix Panacis Quinque Folii* 10 g
Wu Wei Zi *Fructus Schisandrae Chinensis* 10 g

Xing Ren *Semen Pruni Armeniacae* 10 g
Sang Bai Pi *Cortex Mori Albae Radicis* 5 g
Lu Gen *Rhizoma Phragmitis Communis* 15 g
Dan Shen *Radix Salviae Miltiorrhizae* 10 g
Mu Dan Pi *Cortex Moutan Radicis* 10 g
Tian Hua Fen *Radix Trichosanthis Kirilowii* 10 g
Zhi Gan Cao *Radix Glycyrrhizae Preparata* 3 g

Explanations:
- Nan Sha Shen, Bei Sha Shen, and Mai Men Dong are used to nourish the yin of the lung and kidney, and clear the deficient heat, promote the secretion of body fluid, and relieve the thirst.
- Xi Yang Shen nourishes the qi and yin of the general body, improves appetite, and relieves fatigue. When this herb is used in combination with Wu Wei Zi, they could relieve excessive sweating.
- Xing Ren and Sang Bai Pi are used to clear the remaining heat in the lung and relieve dry cough.
- Dan Shen nourishes the yin of the heart, clears the deficient heat, and improves the function of the heart to house the shen.
- Lu Gen and Tian Hua Fen are used to promote the secretion of body fluid and relieve the thirst.
- Mu Dan Pi clears deficient heat in the body and removes the toxins in the blood.
- Zhi Gan Cao harmonizes the prescription.

Modifications:
- If there is severe fatigue, add Huang Qi *Radix Astragali Membranacei* 10 g to tonify the qi and relieve the fatigue.
- If there is obvious emotion, add He Huan Pi *Cortex Albizziae Julibrissin* 10 g and Bai Zi Ren *Semen Biotae Orientalis* 10 g to smooth the emotions and calm the Shen.
- If there is much dry cough, add Chuan Bei Mu *Bulbus Fritillariae Cirrhosae* 10 g and Bai Bu *Radix Stemonae* 10 g to nourish the lung and stop the cough.

- If there is too much night sweating, add Gui Ban *Plastrum Testudinis* 15 g to nourish the yin and stop night sweating.
- If there is obvious constipation, add Huo Ma Ren *Semen Cannabis Sativae* 10 g to promote the defecation and relieve the constipation.

Acupuncture Treatment:
- Neiguan P-6 + Gongsun SP-4, Lieque LU-7 + Zhaohai KID-6, Chize LU-5, Jingqu LU-8, Shenshu BL-23, Taiyuan LU-9, Feishu BL-13, Zusanli ST-36, Qihai REN-6, Taixi KID-3, Fuliu KID-7, Sanyinjiao SP-6 and Tanzhong Ren-17.
- An even method is applied on P-6 + SP-4, LU-7 + KID-6 and Ren-17.
- A tonifying method is applied on LU-5, LU-8, BL-23, LU-9, ST-36, REN-6, KID-3, KID-7, and SP-6.

Explanations:
- P-6 + SP-4 are used to descend the lung-qi and relieve remaining cough.
- LU-7 and KID-6 are used to nourish the qi of the body and relax the chest.
- LU-5, LU-9, and BL-13, the he-sea point, the yuan-source point of the lung channel, and the back-shu point of the lung respectively, together with ST-36, the he-sea point of the stomach channel, KID-3, the yuan-source point of the kidney channel, in combination with BL-20, the back-shu point of the spleen, are all applied in group to tonify the qi of the body, improve yuan-source qi and the strength of the body and relieve fatigue.
- LU-8, the jing-metal point of the lung channel, BL-23, the back-shu point of the kidney, KID-7, the jing-metal point of the kidney channel, SP-6, the crossing point of three yin channels of the foot, KID-3, the yuan-source point of the kidney channel, together with REN-6, are used to nourish the yin of the lung and kidney and clear the deficient heat in the body.

- Ren-17, the gathering point of the qi, is used to promote elimination of qi stagnation, toxins accumulation and damp obstruction in the body.

Modifications:
- If there is severe fatigue, add Baihui DU-20 to lift the qi and relieve the fatigue.
- If there is an obvious emotional situation, add Qimen LIV-14 and Shenmen HE-7 to smooth the emotions and calm the shen.
- If there is much dry cough, add Shenfeng KID-23 to nourish the yin of the lung and kidney and stop the cough.
- If there is too much night sweating, add Tongli HE-5 and Yinxi HE-6 to nourish the yin and stop night sweating.
- If there is obvious constipation, add Tianshu ST-25 to promote the defecation and relieve the constipation.

7

TCM Treatment of Side Effects of COVID-19 Vaccines

As of 14 May 2021, there have been 160,686,749 confirmed cases of COVID-19 globally, including 3,335,948 deaths.[1] The good news is that vaccines from AstraZeneca, Pfizer/BioNTech (henceforth referred to as simply the Pfizer vaccine), Moderna, and Johnson & Johnson are now available in many countries. Except for the Johnson & Johnson vaccine, which only needs one dose, the rest require two doses. According to official reports, all of these vaccines have high effectiveness in preventing COVID-19. For instance, Pfizer has been shown to be 95% effective.[2] However, some have raised doubts. Peter Doshi, an associate editor of the *British Medical Journal*, has questioned the results of the Pfizer and Moderna vaccine trials.[3] Ideally a pandemic vaccine should be delivered in a single shot in order to vaccinate as many people as promptly as possible. The vaccine should be easy to ship and store, and trigger no

---

[1] World Health Organization (WHO). WHO coronavirus (COVID-19) dashboard. 2021. https://covid19.who.int/?gclid=Cj0KCQiA0rSABhDlARIsAJtjfCcog4ziUoRhw7F Mc63Sbm5sf_y6uSbwc14d7D0EICut7WB9Z91IFzMaAnpeEALw_wcB.

[2] Pfizer and BioNTech conclude phase 3 study of COVID-19 vaccine candidate, meeting all primary efficacy endpoints. *Pfizer.com* (Press Release) 18 November 2020. https://www.pfizer.com/news/press-release/press-release-detail/pfizer-and-biontech-conclude-phase-3-study-covid-19-vaccine.

[3] Peter Doshi. Pfizer and Moderna's "95% effective" vaccines—we need more details and the raw data. *BMJ*. (Press Release) 5 February 2021. https://blogs.bmj.com/bmj/2021/01/04/peter-doshi-pfizer-and-modernas-95-effective-vaccines-we-need-more-details-and-the-raw-data/.

side-effects other than a sore arm. Unfortunately, this is not the case for the Pfizer and Moderna COVID-19 vaccines, at least not yet.[4] Fevers and aches following these jabs are not dangerous but can be intense for some.[5] Short-term pain at the injection site is widespread with both vaccines—roughly 90% of those who received the Moderna vaccine reported pain,[6] as did roughly 80% of those who received the Pfizer vaccine.[7] In both trials, injection-site pain was infrequent in people who received a placebo. In research in the US, FDA analysis showed that neither the Pfizer or Moderna vaccines caused problems that would make emergency use unwarranted.[8]

Fewer than 2% of Pfizer and Moderna vaccine recipients developed severe fevers with a temperature of 39°C to 40°C. However, if the companies win regulatory approval, they aim to supply vaccines to 35 million people globally by the end of December 2020.[9] If 2% of recipients experience severe fever, that equates to 700,000 people, while the other transient side-effects would affect even more people. The independent board that conducted the interim analysis of Moderna's huge trial found that severe side-effects included fatigue (9.7% of participants), muscle pain (8.9%), joint pain (5.2%) and headache (4.5%).[10] These numbers were lower for the Pfizer vaccine,

---

[4] Helen Branswell. Comparing the COVID-19 vaccines developed by Pfizer, Moderna, and Johnson & Johnson, *Stat.* 2 February 2021. https://www.statnews.com/2020/12/19/a-side-by-side-comparison-of-the-pfizer-biontech-and-moderna-vaccines/.

[5] Meredith Wadman. Fever, aches from Pfizer, Moderna jabs aren't dangerous but may be intense for some, *Science.* 18 November 2022. https://www.sciencemag.org/news/2020/11/fever-aches-pfizer-moderna-jabs-aren-t-dangerous-may-be-intense-some.

[6] FDA. FDA briefing document moderna COVID-19 vaccine. 17 December 2020. https://www.fda.gov/media/144434/download.

[7] Karen Kaplan. How the COVID-19 vaccines from Moderna and Pfizer compare head to head, *Los Angeles Times.* 15 December 2020. https://www.latimes.com/science/story/2020-12-15/how-the-covid-19-vaccines-from-moderna-and-pfizer-compare-head-to-head.

[8] *Ibid.*

[9] Meredith Wadman. Public needs to prep for vaccine side effects, *Science.* 27 November 2020, 370(6520): 1022. https://science.sciencemag.org/content/370/6520/1022.

[10] *Ibid.*

which caused severe side-effects of fatigue (3.8% of participants) and headache (2%).[11] Recently, there have been reports of deaths due to this vaccine. Ten people have died after receiving the Pfizer vaccine in Germany, as reported in *Der Spiegel*.[12]

The Pfizer and Moderna COVID-19 vaccines were developed using messenger RNA (mRNA) technology. They prime the immune system to attack the coronavirus by delivering a snippet of the genetic code of the virus. This code, or mRNA, instructs the body to build copies of the spike protein that stud the virus surface. The immune system responds by creating antibodies, which remain on standby until confronted by an actual infection.[13] With reference to the side-effects of these vaccines, Drew Weissman, the immunologist whose research contributed to their development, stated, "We suspect the lipid nanoparticle causes the reactogenicity, because lipid nanoparticles without mRNA in them do the same thing in animals"[14] and "We see production, in the muscle, of inflammatory mediators that cause pain, redness, swelling, fever, flu-like symptoms."[15] Long-term side effects of mRNA vaccines remain theoretical, but include the possibility that patients with autoimmune conditions such as lupus, whose disease is driven by antibodies against their genetic code, could experience flare-ups because of the increase in immune responses induced by the vaccines.[16]

Recently a safety report was released by the Medicines & Healthcare products Regulatory Agency, UK, which was based on detailed analysis of data up to 5 May 2021. At this date, an estimated 11.4 million first doses of the Pfizer/BioNTech vaccine and 23.3 million first doses of the COVID-19 Vaccine AstraZeneca had been administered, and around 8.7 million and 7.5 million second

---

[11] Meredith Wadman. 18 November 2022. *op. cit.*

[12] Ten people die after getting Pfizer vaccine in Germany. *NEWS.ru.* https://news.ru/en/europe/ten-people-die-after-getting-pfizer-vaccine-in-germany/.

[13] Karen Kaplan, *op. cit.*

[14] Meredith Wadman. 27 November 2022. *op. cit.*

[15] Meredith Wadman. 18 November 2022. *op. cit.*

[16] *Ibid.*

doses of the Pfizer/BioNTech vaccine and COVID-19 Vaccine AstraZeneca respectively. An approximate 0.1 million first doses of the COVID-19 Vaccine Moderna have also now been administered. As of 5 May 2021, in the UK, 55,716 Yellow Cards have been reported for the Pfizer/BioNTech vaccine, 167,141 have been reported for the COVID-19 Vaccine AstraZeneca, 1,081 for the COVID-19 Vaccine Moderna and 606 have been reported for an unspecified vaccine.

For the Pfizer/BioNTech vaccine and COVID-19 Vaccine AstraZeneca vaccines, the overall reporting rate is around three to six Yellow Cards per 1,000 doses administered.[17] It shows that the rate of side effects of COVID-19 Vaccine AstraZeneca vaccine is relatively high.

Here the author explores the adverse effects of COVID-19 vaccines from the perspective of Chinese medicine, and their clinical management with Chinese herbs and acupuncture.

7.1 TCM Analysis of Side Effects of COVID-19 Vaccines

From the perspective of TCM, the vaccine side-effects are consistent with an invasion of external pathogenic factors:

- The vaccines enter the body through the skin in the same way as other external pathogenic factors.
- Patients develop flu-like symptoms.
- Symptoms start suddenly.
- Symptoms could occur at different stages, not always at Taiyang stage.
- The symptoms are due to the conflict between zheng-qi and xie-qi.
- Symptoms are mostly temporary.

---

[17] Coronavirus vaccine — summary of Yellow Card reporting. https://www.gov.uk/government/publications/coronavirus-covid-19-vaccine-adverse-reactions/coronavirus-vaccine-summary-of-yellow-card-reporting.

From the perspective of TCM, the injection of a foreign protein into the deltoid muscle often presents as an invasion of external pathogenic factors into the large intestine and small intestine channels, which cross each other at Binao L.I.-14. The large intestine channel of Yangming is regarded as a channel with plenty of qi and blood. The small intestine is paired with the heart and belongs to the fire phase of the Wu Xing (five phases). An invasion of external pathogenic factors into these two channels can thus easily cause an immediate reaction, which is different with that invasion through the skin, nose and throat, and results in a struggle between the wei qi and the invading pathogen. In most cases, the body considers this vaccine as a kind of invasion of toxins or toxic heat, so occurrence of relative high fever is a common symptom due to heavy conflict between the zheng-qi and xie-qi in all patterns. Treatment should thus be given according to precise syndrome differentiation.

According to TCM, these external invasions can be subdivided into their most common presentations: Invasion of wind-cold to the Taiyang, invasion to the Shaoyang, invasion to the Yangming, and invasion of toxic heat, etc.

7.1.1 Invasion of wind-cold to the Taiyang

The signs and symptoms of wind-cold invasion include chills, fever, headache, muscle pain, joint pain, neck pain, slight cough and other symptoms related to the lung, including discomfort or pain in the chest, shortness of breath and difficulty breathing, a tongue with a thin white coating and a tight pulse. These symptoms result from the invasion of wind-cold into the superficial layer of the body, where there is a fight between zheng-qi and xie-qi and the wei (defensive) qi is obstructed. In most cases, the wei qi is sufficient to dispel the wind-cold completely. However, if the wei qi is insufficient or not sufficiently supported by other aspects of physiology such as yuan (original) qi or ying (nutritive) qi, or if there is excess in the body obstructing the function of the zang-fu organs, the wind-cold invasion can enter more deeply, resulting in more severe consequences.

7.1.2 Invasion to the Shaoyang

When Shaoyang is invaded by wind-cold, there could be different signs and symptoms as above, because the Gallbladder and San Jiao could be mainly involved, either the meridians or the internal organs. Since Shaoyang is neither interior nor exterior, it could show alternative chills and fever, headache, dizziness, tinnitus, nausea, bitter tastes in the mouth, poor appetite, loose stool, thin and white coating on the tongue, and a wiry pulse. These signs and symptoms need to be dealt with differently. If the same methods of treatment for the invasion of wind-cold to the Taiyang are applied here, there would be no improvement. The methods to harmonize the Shaoyang and regulate the Gallbladder should be used.

7.1.3 Invasion to the Yangming

When the invasion of wind-cold to the Yangming, this wind-cold could change into wind-heat quickly, leading to a heavy fight between the zheng-qi and xie-qi, which will again show different signs and symptoms. There could be high fever, profuse sweating, thirst, restlessness, headache, red face, red tongue, and a big pulse. At this moment, it is still at the Yangming channel level, not yet at the interior fu organ to form fu syndrome. Here, the treatment should be changed accordingly.

7.1.4 Invasion of toxic heat

When the pathogenic factors invade the body at Taiyang, Shaoyang or Yangming stages, they usually could cause more general symptoms, and the pain at the injection site is not a major complaint. However, if there is invasion of toxic heat, the complaints from the local injection site could often be the main symptoms, such as obvious redness at the injection site with heat, pain and swelling, high fever, headache, thirst, a red tongue with a yellow and dry coating, and a superficial and rapid pulse.

7.1.5 Prolonged chronic illness and weak constitution

When the body is healthy, the zang-fu organs, qi, blood, yin and yang are in a dynamic balance. For healthy people, a vaccine is unlikely to lead to severe reactions or long-term illness. Pre-existing chronic illness and/or constitutional imbalances can make some people more prone to adverse reactions to vaccines. These pre-existing conditions include chronic lung disease, heart disease, diabetes, liver disease, HIV and obesity.[18] Constitutional imbalance can involve excess or deficiency patterns, or a mixture of both. Research has shown that both the Pfizer and Moderna vaccines have good results in people with pre-existing health conditions.[19]

In TCM it is emphasized that it is essential that after an external invasion, any clinical symptoms should disappear completely, indicating that the invading pathogens have been cleared. Any pathogens remaining in the body can bring about long-term illness. When the immediate side-effects of vaccines occur, they usually present as pathology involving Taiyang (invasion of wind-cold), Shaoyang or Yangming (invasion of toxic heat). However, in some cases more severe consequences can occur. The MHRA has undertaken a thorough review into UK reports of an extremely rare specific type of blood clot in the brain, known as cerebral venous sinus thrombosis (REN-ST) occurring together with low levels of platelets (thrombocytopenia) following vaccination with the COVID-19 Vaccine AstraZeneca. It is also considering other blood clotting cases (thromboembolic events) alongside low platelet levels. This ongoing scientific review has concluded that the evidence of a link with COVID-19 Vaccine AstraZeneca is stronger.[20] An anaphylactic reaction or even death is

---

[18]Karen Kaplan. *op. cit.*

[19]*Ibid.*

[20]Medicines and Healthcare Products Regulatory Agency. MHRA issues new advice, concluding a possible link between COVID-19 vaccine AstraZeneca and extremely rare, unlikely to occur blood clots. (Press Release) 7 April 2021. https://www.gov.uk/government/news/mhra-issues-new-advice-concluding-a-possible-link-between-covid-19-vaccine-astrazeneca-and-extremely-rare-unlikely-to-occur-blood-clots.

another severe case. For example, Norwegian health officials say that 23 deaths among the frail and elderly were associated with recent COVID-19 vaccinations.[21] More than half of those who died have been assessed, and the agency involved has stated that those fatalities may be linked to common adverse reactions from the vaccine. Note that these life-threatening situations would involve much more complicated pathology than the patterns presented in this chapter.

7.2 TCM Treatment

7.2.1 Invasion of wind-cold to the Taiyang

Principles of Treatment:
Dispel wind-cold and relieve the exterior.

Herbal Treatment:
Jing Fang Bai Du San-*Schizonepeta and Saposhnikovia Powder to Overcome Pathogenic Influences.*[22]

Jing Jie *Herba seu Flos Schizonepetae Tenuifoliae* 10 g
Fang Feng *Radix Ledebouriellae Divaricatae* 10 g
Qiang Huo *Rhizoma et Radix Notopterygii* 10 g
Gao Ben *Rhizoma et Radix Ligustici* 10 g

---

[21] Adam Smith. 23 died after getting covid shot in Norway. Here's the rest of the story, *The Street,* 17 January 2021. https://www.thestreet.com/latest-news/23-died-after-covid-shot-in-norway-heres-the-rest-of-the-story.

[22] There are of course other herbal formulas which might be used to deal with invasion of wind-cold, such as Ma Huang Tang (Ephedra Decoction), Gui Zhi Tang Cinnamon Twig Decoction) and Qiang Huo Sheng Shi Tang (Notoptergium Decoction to Overcome Damp) Ma Huang Tang is suitable to treat severe symptoms of wind-cold invasion following vaccination, in which there is no sweating, obvious aversion to cold, muscle pain, headache and joint pain, thin and white coating and a tight pulse. Qiang Huo Sheng Shi Tang is used when there is severe sensation of heaviness with pain in the head, muscles and joints, a white and greasy tongue coating and a slippery pulse.

Bai Zhi *Radix Angelicae Dahuricae* 10 g
Dang Gui *Radix Angelicae Sinensis* 10 g
Chuan Xiong *Radix Ligustici Wallichii* 10 g
Zhi Ke *Fructus Citri Aurantii* 5 g
Xing Ren *Semen Pruni Armeniacae* 10 g
Zhi Gan Cao *Radix Glycyrrhizae Preparata* 3 g

Explanations:
- Jing Jie and Fang Feng dispel wind-cold and relieve the exterior symptoms.
- Qiang Huo, Gao Ben and Bai Zhi dispel wind-cold and relieve joint and muscle pain.
- Dang Gui and Chuan Xiong promote the circulation of qi and blood and support zheng-qi to eliminate the pathogenic factors.
- Zhi Ke and Xing Ren regulate qi in the lung.
- Zhi Gan Cao harmonizes the prescription.

In some cases, the patients could have some complaints of severe muscle pain or joint pain with cold sensation, stiffness, and difficulty in joint movement. The mechanism is slightly changed, in which invasion of wind cold is often mixed with damp, leading to occurrence of Bi syndrome. Thus, the above herbal formula and prescription will be insufficient to deal with these complaints and Juan Bi Tang-*Remove Painful Obstruction Decoction* should be applied.

Modifications:
- In case of severe headache, add Man Jing Zi *Fructus Viticis* 10 g to relieve the headache.
- In case of severe muscle pain, add Ji Xue Teng *Caulis Milletiae Reticulatae* 10 g to harmonize the collaterals and relieve the muscle pain.
- In case of severe aversion to cold, add Gui Zhi *Ramulus Cinnamomi Cassiae* 10 g and Zi Su Ye *Folium Perillae Frutescentis* 10 g to dispel external cold.

Acupuncture Treatment:
- Sanjian L.I.-3, Hegu L.I.-4 and Jianyu L.I.-15 with reducing technique promote qi and blood circulation and harmonize the large intestine channel (the location of the injection site).
- Sanjian L.I.-3 is the shu-stream point and can thus treat joint pain; Jianyu L.I.-15 is a point local to the injection site; Hegu L.I.-4, the yuan-source point, dispels wind-cold and relieves pain.
- Waiguan SJ-5, Lieque LU-7 and Fengchi GB-20 promote opening the skin pores and cause sweating to dispel external pathogenic factors.

Modifications:
- In case of a severe headache, add Fengfu DU-16 to relieve the headache.
- In case of severe muscle pain, add Feiyang BL-58, the luo-connecting point, and Jinmen BL-63, the xi-cleft point and intersection of the bladder channel and Yang Wei Mai, to harmonize the collaterals and relieve the muscle pain.
- In case of severe joint pain with stiffness and difficulty in movement, add Yanglingquan GB-34, Fenglong ST-40 and Sanyinjiao SP-6 to benefit the tendons and eliminate damp.
- In case of severe aversion to cold, add Zusanli ST-36 with moxibustion, also on Hegu L.I.-4 and Lieque LU-7, to warm up the body and relieve cold at the superficial layer of the body.

7.2.2 Invasion to the Shaoyang

Principles of Treatment:
Harmonize the Shaoyang and regulate the gallbladder and San Jiao.

Herbal Treatment:
Xiao Chai Hu Tang-*Minor Bupleurum Decoction.*

Chai Hu *Radix Bupleuri* 10 g
Huang Qin *Radix Scutellariae Baicalensis* 10 g
Zhi Ban Xia *Rhizoma Pinelliae Ternatae Preparata* 10 g
Zhi Zi *Fructus Gardeniae Jasminoidis* 10 g

Ren Shen *Radix Ginseng* 5 g
Sheng Jiang *Rhizoma Zingiberis Officinalis Recens* 5 g
Da Zao *Fructus Zizyphi Jujubae* 5 g
Zhi Gan Cao *Radix Glycyrrhizae Preparata* 3 g

Explanations:
- Chai Hu and Huang Qin in combination harmonize the Shaoyang and regulate the San Jiao. Meanwhile, they could eliminate the pathogenic factors.
- Zhi Zi clears heat in the Shaoyang.
- Zhi Ban Xia and Sheng Jiang harmonize the stomach and descend the qi to relieve the nausea and vomiting.
- Ren Shen, Da Zao and Zhi Gan Cao support the zheng-qi and benefit the body.

Modifications:
- In case of severe headache, add Bai Zhi *Radix Angelicae dahuricae* 10 g and Man Jing Zi *Fructus Viticis* 10 g to relieve headache.
- In case of severe nausea and vomiting, add Huang Lian 3 g and Zhu Ru *Caulis Bambusae in Taeniis* 10 g to relieve nausea and vomiting.
- In case of high fever, add Jin Yin Hua *Flos Lonicerae Japonicae* 10 g and Lian Qiao *Fructus Forsythiae Suspensae* 10 g to relieve high fever.
- In case of poor appetite add Bai Zhu *Rhizoma Atractylodis Macrocephalae* 10 g and Mai Ya *Fructus Hordei Vulgaris Germinantus* 10 g to improve appetite.
- In case of chest pain, add Yu Jin *Tuber Curcumae* 10 g and Zhi Ke *Fructus Citri Aurantii* 10 g to relieve chest pain.

Acupuncture Treatment:
- Waiguan SJ-5 + Zulinqi GB-41 with even technique to harmonize the Yangwei mai and Shaoyang channel.
- Yangchi SJ-4, Fengchi GB-20, Jianjing GB-21, Yanglingquan GB-34 and Qiuxu GB-40 with even technique to regulate the Shaoyang channel and promote qi circulation.
- Zhongwan REN-12 and Zusanli ST-36 with even technique to harmonize the stomach, descend qi and relieve nausea and vomiting.

Modifications:
- For a severe headache, add Shuaigu GB-8 and Hegu L.I.-4.
- For hypochondriac pain or distention, add Taichong LIV-3 and Qimen LIV-14 to promote qi circulation.
- For mood changes or depression add Neiguan P-6 and Shenmen HE-7 to regulate the emotions and calm the shen.

7.2.3 Invasion of wind-heat into Yangming

Principles of Treatment:
Clear heat in the Yangming channel and reduce fever.

Herbal Treatment:
Bai Hu Tang-*White Tiger Decoction.*

Sheng Shi Gao *Gypsum Fibrosum* 20 g
Zhi Mu *Radix Anemarrhenae Asphodeloidis* 10 g
Geng Mi *Oryzae Sativae* 10 g
Zhi Zi *Fructus Gardeniae Jasminoidis* 10 g
Huang Lian *Rhizoma Coptidis* 5 g
Zhi Gan Cao *Radix Glycyrrhizae Preparata* 3 g

Explanations:
- Sheng Shi Gao strongly clears heat in the Yangming channel and reduces fever.
- Zhi Mu assists Sheng Shi Gao to clear heat and benefits body fluids to relieve thirst.
- Huang Lian and Zhi Zi strengthen the effect of clearing heat in the Yangming channel and reduce fever.
- Geng Mi protects the stomach from the bitter herbs.
- Zhi Gan Cao harmonizes all the herbs in the prescription.

Modifications:
- For a severe headache, add Bai Zhi *Radix Angelicae dahuricae* 10 g and Man Jing Zi *Fructus Viticis* 10 g.

- In case of severe thirst, add Tian Hua Fen *Radix Trichosanthis Kirilowii* 10 g to benefit the body fluids.
- For severe restlessness due to fever, add Dan Zhu Ye *Herba Lophatheri Gracilis* 10 g to clear heat and relieve restlessness.

Acupuncture Treatment:
- Dazhui DU-14, the meeting point of all the yang channels, together with Erjian L.I.-2, the ying-spring point, Hegu L.I.-4, the yuan-source point, and Quchi L.I.-11, the he-sea point of the large intestine channel clear heat and reduce fever.
- Neiting ST-44, the ying-spring point of the stomach channel, clears heat from the Yangming channel, reduces fever and relieves thirst.

Modifications:
- In case of a severe headache, add Fengchi GB-20.
- In case of severe thirst, add Sanyinjiao SP-6, the intersecting point of the three yin channels of the leg, to benefit body fluids.
- In case of severe restlessness, add Shaohai HE-3, the he-sea and water point of the heart channel, to clear heat.
- In case of difficult defecation, add Tianshu ST-25, the front-mu point of the large intestine, to regulate the large intestine.

7.2.4 Invasion of toxic heat

Principles of Treatment:
Clear heat, remove toxins, reduce swelling, and stop pain.

Herbal Treatment:
Wu Wei Xiao Du Yin-*Five Ingredient Drink to Eliminate Toxins.*

Jin Yin Hua *Flos Lonicerae Japonicae* 10 g
Ye Ju Hua *Flos Chrysanthemi Indici* 10 g
Pu Gong Ying *Herba Taraxaci Mongolici cum Radice* 10 g
Lian Qiao *Fructus Forsythiae Suspensae* 10 g
Zi Bei Tian Kui *Begoniae Herba* 10 g

Zi Hua Di Ding *Herba cum Radice Violae Yedoensitis* 10 g
Huang Lian *Rhizoma Coptidis* 5 g
Huang Qin *Radix Scutellariae Baicalensis* 10 g
Zhi Zi *Fructus Gardeniae Jasminoidis* 10 g
Zhi Gan Cao *Radix Glycyrrhizae Preparata* 3 g

Explanations:
- Jin Yin Hua, Ye Ju Hua, Pu Gong Ying, Lian Qiao, Zi Bei Tian Kui and Zi Hua Di Ding clear heat, remove toxins and reduce swelling.
- Huang Lian and Huang Qin clear heat, remove toxins and prevent invasion of toxic heat further into the body.
- Zhi Zi clears the heat in San Jiao.
- Zhi Gan Cao harmonizes the prescription.

Modifications:
- In case of high fever with redness of the face and thirst, add Shi Gao *Gypsum Fibrosum* 20 g and Zhi Mu *Radix Anemarrhenae Asphodeloidis* 10 g to clear heat and reduce fever.
- In case of a severe headache, add Bai Zhi *Radix Angelicae Dahuricae* 10 g to relieve the headache.
- In case of seizures, add Gou Teng *Ramulus cum Uncis Uncariae* 10 g and Jiang Can *Bombyx Batryticatus* 10 g to arrest the internal wind.
- In case of severe palpitations, add Dan Shen *Radix Salviae Miltiorrhizae* 10 g to clear heat in the heart and calm the shen.

Acupuncture Treatment:
- Erjian L.I.-2, the ying-spring point, Hegu L.I.-4, the yuan-source point, and Quchi L.I.-11, the he-sea point of the large intestine channel respectively, to clear heat in the infection site and body, remove toxins and subside swelling.
- Shaohai HE-3, the he-sea and water point of the heart channel, Sanyinjiao SP-6, the crossing point of the three yin channels of the leg, and Xuehai SP-10, combine to cool the blood and relieve pain and swelling at the injection site.
- Dazhui DU-14, the meeting point of all the yang channels, reduces fever and relieves headache.

Modifications:

- In case of high fever with redness of the face or thirst, add Neiting ST-44, the ying-spring point of the stomach channel, to clear heat from the Yangming channel and reduce fever.
- In case of severe headache, add Fengchi GB-20 to relieve headache.
- In case of severe muscle pain in the general body, add Feiyang BL-58 and Jinmen BL-63 to harmonize the Taiyang collaterals and relieve the muscle pain.
- In case of seizure, add Yanglingquan GB-34 and Taichong LIV-3 to arrest internal wind.
- In case of severe palpitations, add Shaofu HE-8, the ying-spring point of the heart channel, to clear heat and calm the shen.

7.2.5 Patients with chronic illness and/or weak constitution

When COVID-19 vaccines are given to those with chronic illness or constitutional weakness (especially the elderly or patients with auto-immune disease such as lupus), their bodies may fail to deal with the external pathogenic invasion, leading to latent pathogens obstructing their qi and blood circulation. In these patients the principles of treatment are to eliminate excess, tonify deficiency, harmonize qi and blood, and benefit yin and yang. Ideally patients with pre-existing illness or constitutional weakness should carefully attend to their physical wellbeing with TCM treatment for two months before and after vaccination. In this way severe reactions can be prevented.

Herbal Treatment:

- For patients presenting with excess patterns, the herbal formula Yue Ju Wan-*Escape Ju Wan* is recommended. *Yue Ju Wan* consists of Xiang Fu *Rhizoma Cyperi Rotundi*, Chuan Xiong *Radix Ligustici Wallichii*, Cang Zhu *Rhizoma Atractylodis*, Shen Qu *Massa Medica Fermentata* and Zhi Zi *Fructus Gardeniae Jasminoidis*. These combine to eliminate the excess of qi, blood, fire, and phlegm. It can be used to treat patients with pre-existing illness who usually suffer from stagnation of these pathogenic factors. As this single foundation formula is not sufficient to deal with all possible excess, modifications should be made accordingly. For instance, if there is mainly stagnation of qi, the addition of other herbs such as Qing Pi *Pericarpium Citri Reticulatae Viride,* Chen Pi *Pericarpium Citri Reticulatae* and Zhi Shi *Fructus Immaturus Citri Aurantii* should be considered. Depending upon the location of the qi stagnation, herbs that enter the appropriate organs should be added.

- For patients presenting with deficiency patterns the formulas Si Jun Zi Tang-*Four Gentlemen Decoction* and Liu Wei Di Huang Wan-*Six-Ingredient Pill with Rehmannia* can be considered. Although these formulas are used to strengthen and build up the physical condition, they may be insufficient to cover all types of weak constitution. They can therefore be used as a foundation, with appropriate modifications made to tonify qi, blood, yin and yang as appropriate. Attention should be paid to identifying the relevant organs in order to alleviate weakness efficiently.

Acupuncture Treatment:
- For excess patterns, the following acupuncture points should be considered with reducing technique: Hegu L.I.-4, Neiguan P-6, Fengchi GB-20, Yanglingquan GB-34, Gongsun SP-4, Sanyinjiao SP-6, Yinlingquan SP-9, Fenglong ST-40, Taichong LIV-3, Zhongwan REN-12. These points regulate the qi and blood and eliminate excess to remove the blockage in the channels and zang-fu organs. Combination of herbs and acupuncture can bring forth faster and more reliable therapeutic benefits.
- For deficiency patterns, the following points should be considered with tonifying technique: Zusanli ST-36, Sanyinjiao SP-6, Taixi KID-3, Guanyuan REN-4, Ganshu BL-18, Pishu BL-20, and Shenshu BL-23. These points can be used to strengthen qi, blood, yin and yang. Combination of herbs and acupuncture can bring forth faster and more reliable therapeutic benefits.

8

COVID-19 Case Study

During the epidemic of new coronary pneumonia, from December 2020 to June 2021, Professor Peilin Sun instructed a TCM treatment team via WeChat with the purpose of helping some critically ill patients who had been diagnosed with COVID-19 through TCM methods. The below five cases of medical records are a partial summary of more than 100 patients treated.

8.1 Case 1

Female, 56 years old, a TCM practitioner.
Chief complaints: Fever with an aversion to cold, cough and short of breath for six days, with further deterioration over two days.
First consultation: 30 December 2020.

Actual Medical History:
On 22 December 2021, due to catching an external wind and cold, she began to have an intermittent fever of 39°C with a sore throat. She was taking Modified Xiao Chai Hu Tang, but her fever was still not controlled. She later developed a persistent fever, which reached 38.3°C under the armpit, accompanied by symptoms of a urinary tract infection. Her GP first gave her a course of the antibiotic amoxicillin with a dosage of 500 mg three times a day. Yet her fever still persisted. On 28 December, her COVID-19 test was confirmed positive. Her GP then switched to the broad-spectrum antibiotic

amoxicillin clavulanate potassium with a dosage of 625 mg, three times a day, and paracetamol 500 mg every four hours. Her fever persisted. She started to have chest tightness, chest pain, coughing and vomiting with a lot of thin white sputum. She had muscle aches all over the body, short of breath and fatigue. She was drinking a lot of water but still felt thirsty. She had constipation for three days and took a single herb Da Huang which made her have a bowel movement the day before the first consultation. At the same time her husband also suffered from COVID-19 and was hospitalized because of respiratory failure. She was extremely exhausted physically and mentally from worrying about her husband. She struggled with Type 2 diabetes for 18 years and uses daily injections of insulin. Her blood sugar is controlled normally, but it has risen recently. It was necessary to increase the insulin dose to control her blood sugar. Short-acting insulin was increased by two to four units compared to normal doses. Long-acting insulin was 12 units in the morning and four units in the evening before getting sick, increased to 16 units in the morning and 6 to 8 units in the evening when she was sick. The tongue was swollen and red, especially red on both sides, with a deep and wide crack in the center, accompanied by dry thick brown coating.

Past Medical History:
She suffers from Type 2 diabetes for 18 years and is regularly injected with insulin.

TCM Diagnosis:
Cough, due to failure of the lung to disperse and descend, phlegm and dampness are accumulating, heat is flaring causing injury to the body's fluids, Yang ming fu shi syndrome (syndrome of excess of Yangming fu-viscera).

Principle of Treatment:
Rapidly remove heat with urgent application of purgatives, eliminate phlegm and descend the lung-qi.

Herbal Treatment:
Da Cheng Qi Tang-*Major Order the Qi Decoction.*

Prescription 1:
Da Huang *Radix et Rhizoma Rhei* 10 g (decocting later)
Mang Xiao *Mirabilitum* 10 g
(infusion at the end with other already cooked herbal tea for oral taking)
Hou Po *Cortex Magnoliae Officinalis* 10 g
Zhi Shi *Fructus Immaturus CitriAurantii* 10 g
Zhi Mu *Radix Anemarrhenae Asphodeloidis* 10 g
Sang Bai Pi *Cortex Mori Albae Radicis* 10 g
Xing Ren *Semen Pruni Armeniacae* 10 g
Huang Qin *Radix Scutellariae Baicalensis* 10 g
Tian Hua Fen *Radix Trichosanthis Kirilowii* 15 g
Lian Qiao *Fructus Forsythiae Suspensae* 10 g

Above formula is for a one day dose, so she was prescribed a three day dose. One dose divided into two portions, take one portion at 8:00 am, and another portion at 4:00 pm.

To prepare this formula you need to follow these special steps:

1. Put all the main herbs except Da Huang and Mang Xiao in a stainless pot with about 1000 ml of water, soak for half an hour and then decocted in the same water for half an hour. The liquid should reduce by half at this stage.
2. Then, put 10 g Da Huang in the pot and boil for another 5 minutes. After this, drain half of the herb tea (about 250 ml) and add to the infusion half of Mang Xiao 5 g and drink it at 8:00 am.
3. Warm the other half of the tea and infuse with the rest of the Mang Xiao 5 g at 4:00 pm.

Treatment Reaction:
On the first day of taking the first dose, she had watery diarrhea eight times. The body temperature was controlled with a reading of

temperature 36°C under armpit that afternoon. She took the second dose the next day and the body temperature was normal and steady. Shortness of breath and chest tightness began to improve. What was particularly gratifying was that after having a high fever that lasted for eight days, it was seen that neither antipyretics nor antibiotics could control it. However, only two days of TCM herbal medicine rescued a critical situation. She was so happy that she was able to avoid being sent to hospital. Since the fever had been controlled and the Yangming excess syndrome disappeared, there was no need to continue taking the third dose.

Further Treatment:
Second consultation: 1 January 2021.
She was still coughing up a lot of white sticky sputum, also with white sticky sputum in the nasal cavity, mild headache, nausea without vomiting, and shows no body pain.

Prescription 2:
Zi Su Zi *Fructus Perillae Frutescentis* 12 g
Bai Jie Zi *Semen Sinapis Albae* 10 g
Lai Fu Zi *Semen Raphani Sativi* 12 g
Zhe Bei Mu *Bulbus Fritillariae Thunbergii* 10 g
Zhi Mu *Radix Anemarrhenae Asphodeloidis* 10 g
Huang Qin *Radix Scutellariae Baicalensis* 10 g
Hou Po *Cortex Magnoliae Officinalis* 10 g
Zhi Shi *Fructus Immaturus CitriAurantii* 10 g
Qing Pi *Pericarpium Citri Reticulatae Viride* 10 g
Xing Ren *Semen Pruni Armeniacae* 10 g
Zhi Ban Xia *Rhizoma Pinelliae Ternatae Preparata* 10 g
Jiao Bai Zhu *Rhizoma Atractylodis Macrocephalae (grill)* 10 g
Sang Bai Pi *Cortex Mori Albae Radicis* 10 g
Zhi Zi *Fructus Gardeniae Jasminoidis* 10 g
Bai Guo *Semen Ginkgo Bilobae* 10 g
Huang Lian *Rhizoma Coptidis* 5 g
Xiang Ru *Herba Elsholtziae seu Moslae* 10 g

(Ma Huang *Herba Ephedrae* 10 g is preferred, but it was not available
due to EU regulations)

Above formula was one day dose, prescribed doses for five days,
decocted in water, one dose daily, taken twice a day.

Treatment Reaction:
The second prescription was taken on 1 January 2021. Although the
fever has subsided, endophytic heat still needs to be controlled. From
the morning of 2 January 2021, her body temperature was 36.6°C,
and she started to cough and spit yellow phlegm, which gradually
turned into white phlegm during the day. She still had chest pain,
mainly in the right chest and back, with poor physical strength. She
had an aversion to oily food and no appetite. Blood oxygen saturation was 94–96%. On 3 January 2021, her body temperature was
36.4°C, her cough deceased, less white sputum, appetite began to
improve, physical strength improved. She had defecations twice a
day, and her tongue became normal pale instead of red, with a thin
layer of yellow coating. Over the following two days the above symptoms improved further. Blood oxygen saturation was 95–97%, but
her blood sugar still fluctuated greatly. She changed her insulin doses
by the following: short-acting insulin increased by 2 to 4 units compared to normal days. Long-acting insulin was 12 units in the morning and four units at night before illness, increased to 16 units in the
morning and six to eight units at night when sick. Starting on 6
January, she got up in the morning with a body temperature of
36.6°C, coughing a few mouthfuls of yellowish sputum.

Further Treatment:
Third consultation: 6 January 2021

Prescription 3:
Zi Su Zi *Fructus Perillae Frutescentis* 10 g
Lai Fu Zi *Semen Raphani Sativi* 12 g
Zhe Bei Mu *Bulbus Fritillariae Thunbergii* 10 g

Zhi Mu *Radix Anemarrhenae Asphodeloidis* 10 g
Huang Qin *Radix Scutellariae Baicalensis* 10 g
Hou Po *Cortex Magnoliae Officinalis* 5 g
Zhi Shi *Fructus Immaturus CitriAurantii* 5 g
Ju Luo *Citrus tangerina Hort. et Tanaka Cherythrosa Tanaka* 5 g
Gua Lou Pi *Pericarpium Trichosanthis* 10 g
Hong Hua *Flos Carthami Tinctorii* 5 g
Yu Jin *Tuber Curcumae* 10 g
Xing Ren *Semen Pruni Armeniacae* 10 g
Zhi Ban Xia *Rhizoma Pinelliae Ternatae Preparata* 10 g
Fu Ling *Sclerotium Poriae Cocos* 15 g
Jiao Bai Zhu *Rhizoma Atractylodis Macrocephalae (grill)* 10 g
Sang Bai Pi *Cortex Mori Albae Radicis* 10 g
Huang Lian *Rhizoma Coptidis* 5 g
Five days doses, decocted in water, one dose daily, taken twice a day.

Treatment Reaction:
During the period of taking the third prescription, the cough decreased, with only a little white phlegm. Diet and physical strength improved day by day, and stool can be maintained twice a day. On 8 January, she improved further, her spirits were good, body temperature was normal, appetite had recovered, blood oxygen saturation was 98% and she was occasionally fatigued. On 9 January 2021, the cough completely stopped, and everything was basically back to normal.

Explanations:
At the beginning of this case, this patient first had the invasion of wind and cold which weakened the dispersing and descending of the lung-qi, therefore she felt cold and fever, body pain, and had a cough with white sputum. Because she has had diabetes for a long time, this resulted in a severe yin deficiency constitution, therefore her exterior symptom had not been cleared yet. She then quickly developed severe inner heat which was forming Yang Ming Fu Shi syndrome, and the interior heat was consuming body fluids. Based on the principle of treating the secondary symptoms in emergency and taking

into account the main symptoms, *Da Cheng Qi Tang* was selected to enable the purging of fu-organs to eliminate heat, and to take care of the loss of the function of the lung at the same time. Otherwise, if the pyretic pathogenic factor had not been resolved, the lung injury would have become worse. The San Cheng Qi Decoction Syndrome is rarely seen in modern clinical practice, but during the epidemic (especially with this patient due to mistreatment and delay), we can see the evidence of Yang Ming Fu Shi syndrome such as persistent high fever, the brown dry tongue coating etc. Therefore, only *Da Cheng Qi Tang* can get rid of the heat and stop the damage of the yin. The patient's treatment reaction proved that the first prescription is very accurate and prompt. But it is particularly important to identify the essential difference and use of San Cheng Qi Decoction.

Prescription 1:
Da Huang, Mang Xiao, Hou Po, Zhi Shi, which are the whole formula of *Da Cheng Qi Tang*, can powerfully purge pyretic accumulation. Xing Ren can soothe the lung and reduce phlegm. Some of the characteristics of COVID-19 are high fever, shortness of breath, chest pain and tightness, and being anxious, while the sputum color is still white instead of yellow. All these symptoms indicate that the lung had failed in the dispersing and descending of qi, which failed to govern regulation of water passages. Therefore, descending lung-qi is top priority. In addition, the fever doesn't go away. Using Zhi Mu, Huang Qin, Lian Qiao, etc. clear lung heat and reduce temperature, Tian Hua Fen clears heat and promotes fluid, and prevents the soaring blood sugar of diabetes.

Prescription 2:
Zi Su Zi, Bai Jie Zi and Lai Fu Zi, the complete composition of *San Zi Yang Qin Decoction*, aims to cleanse the lung and phlegm, descend lung-qi and relieve cough, preventing Yangming excess syndrome. Since Ma Huang is a contraindicated traditional Chinese medicine in Europe, Xiang Ru is used instead. With reference to the book *Ben Cao Zheng Yi* (Materia Medica Zheng yi): "The smell of Xiang Ru is clear and light, and the quality is light. So, it can reach

the upper body, vent the lung, and reach the body surface to relieve the cold on the surface. It can also go to the lower Jiao, ease the bladder, inducing diuresis to reduce fluid retention". Zhe Bei Mu clears away heat and reduces phlegm, accompanied by Huang Qin, Zhi Mu, Zhi Zi to clear lung heat and eliminate phlegm. Among them, Zhi Mu and Zhi Zi can clear away the damp-heat from lower Jiao and promote urination and have a good effect on urinary tract infection (UTI). Together with Bai Guo, Sang Bai Pi and Xing Ren that descend lung-qi, and phlegm heat that cannot dwell in the lung. Zhi Ban Xia, Hou Po and Zhi Shi dry the damp, reduce phlegm, widen the chest, descend qi, and relieve cough. Especially using Huang Lian to clear heat in Yangming and ensure the passage is unobstructed for eliminating the phlegm pyrexia. Qing Pi reduces chest and hypochondriac pain. Jiao Bai Zhu invigorates the spleen to benefit the lung.

Prescription 3:
During the third consultation the patient has turned from the severe stage to the convalescent stage. Su Zi, Lai Fu Zi and Zhe Bei Mu can eliminate phlegm and relieve cough, Zhi Mu, Huang Qin can relieve lung heat, Xing Ren and Sang Bai Pi descend lung-qi and relieve heat phlegm. In addition, using Hou Po and Zhi Shi relieves pressure in the chest, downward qi, and clear the hollow viscera. Huang Lian can prevent the heat accumulating in the middle Jiao, Zhi Ban Xia and Fu Ling to eliminate phlegm and dampness, and further ensure that the middle Jiao does not accumulate dampness and produce phlegm. In order to prevent the formation of pulmonary fibrosis, use Ju Luo and Gua Lou Pi to activate collaterals of lung, Hong Hua and Yu Jin to activate the blood in the chest and repair the damage in the lung caused by pneumonia. Considering that the patient has had diabetes for many years, Jiao Bai Zhu is used to supplement the spleen in order to nourish the lung.

8.2 Case 2

Male, 44 years old, a chef.

Chief complaints: Fever for five days, cough expectoration of yellow sputum, vomiting, nose bleeding.
First consultation: 21 January 2021.

Actual Medical History:
The patient is obese and addicted to eating fatty food and sweets. He developed weakness and physical discomfort on 17 January 2021 and was treated for the common cold with Lian Hua Qing Wen Capsules. His temperature fluctuated sometimes as high as 39.9°C (ear temperature). His COVID-19 test result was positive on the 20th. The antibiotics and ibuprofen prescribed by the GP had no effect, and his condition became serious. On 21 January 2021, his local TCM doctor consulted Professor Peilin Sun for help.

Past Medical History:
None.

Symptoms at the Time of Consultation:
Headache and body pain, warm hands and feet, low volume of urine and stool, cough with yellowish sputum, no sore throat, alternately hot and cold, sweat and aversion to hot after taking antipyretic drugs. The tongue was stiff, with white thick greasy slightly yellow coating wrapping the entire tongue, tongue tip was red.

TCM Diagnosis:
Cough due to external infection of damp toxins, pulmonary failure of dispersing.

Treatment Principles:
Expel toxins and relieve superficies by cooling combined cooling blood to stop bleeding.

Herbal Treatment:
Modified Huang Lian Jie Du Tang-*Coptidis Decoction for Detoxification.*

Prescription 1:
Huang Qin *Radix Scutellariae Baicalensis* 12 g
Huang Lian *Rhizoma Coptidis* 5 g

Zhi Zi *Fructus Gardeniae Jasminoidis* 10 g
Jie Geng *Radix Platycodi Grandiflori* 10 g
Xing Ren *Semen Pruni Armeniacae* 12 g
Xiang Ru *Herba Elsholtziae seu Moslae* 10 g
(Prefer Ma Huang *Herba Ephedrae* 10 g, but not available due to EU
   regulations)
Zhi Mu *Radix Anemarrhenae Asphodeloidis* 10 g
Shi Gao *Gypsum Fibrosum* 20 g
Zhe Bei Mu *Bulbus Fritillariae Thunbergii* 12 g
Sheng Di Huang *Radix Rehmanniae Glutinosae Recens* 15 g
Xuan Shen *Radix Scrophulariae Ningpoensis* 12 g
Zhu Ru *Caulis Bambusae in Taeniis* 10 g

The above formula is one day dose. Prescribed three days dose. Decocted two-day doses together, divided into six portions, one portion taken every four hours, day and night.

Treatment Reaction:
- 21 January 2021 (day 1) 8:00 pm: His body temperature was 37.5°C before taking the herbal medicine and half an hour later after taking the first portion of the herbal tea the temperature dropped to 37.0°C.
- 22 January 2021 (day 2) 11:00 am: At six o'clock in the morning, his temperature was 37.8°C, and at 10:30 am it was 37.3°C. However, his cough increased after taking the herbal tea. He thought his condition had worsened and refused to take it anymore. Plus waking him up at night to take the herbal tea made him angry. We tried to explain to him that herbal medicine clears away heat and resolves phlegm, cools blood to stop bleeding, it also helps the phlegm in the lung to be discharged and restores the normal function of the lung. Otherwise, the phlegm heat will choke the lung, and the lung will lose the dispersing and descending function, just like drowning, and the consequences will be very serious. After understanding that, he began to take it again. All three doses of herbal medicine were taken every 4 hours within a 36 hour time frame to increase the intensity of treatment.

- 22 January 2021 (day 2) 3:07 pm: The cough was significantly reduced, the stool was normal, and the urine was more than before. Nose bleeding stopped, chest tightness and suffocation disappeared, and physical strength gradually increased.

Further Treatment:
Second consultation: 22 January 2021 (day 2)
At first, he suspected that Chinese herbal medicine was useless, but his condition had improved significantly, and he became very confident. After taking three doses of Chinese herbal medicine overnight day and night for 36 hours continuously, he had an increased appetite and still coughs (but without bloodspots in phlegm). His temperature was 37.2°C at 19:45 and 37.1°C at 22:14. The tongue was red, and the greasy coating started to fade away.

Prescription 2:
Huang Qin *Radix Scutellariae Baicalensis* 6 g
Huang Lian *Rhizoma Coptidis* 3 g
Zhi Zi *Fructus Gardeniae Jasminoidis* 5 g
Jie Geng *Radix Platycodi Grandiflori* 5 g
Xing Ren *Semen Pruni Armeniacae* 6 g
Xiang Ru *Herba Elsholtziae seu Moslae* 5 g
(Ma Huang *Herba Ephedrae* 5 g is preferred, but not available due to
    EU regulations)
Zhi Mu *Radix Anemarrhenae Asphodeloidis* 5 g
Shi Gao *Gypsum Fibrosum* 10 g
Zhe Bei Mu *Bulbus Fritillariae Thunbergii* 6 g
Sheng Di Huang *Radix Rehmanniae Glutinosae Recens* 8 g
Xuan Shen *Radix Scrophulariae Ningpoensis* 8 g
Zhu Ru *Caulis Bambusae in Taeniis* 5 g
Ban Xia *Rhizoma Pinelliae Ternatae Cooked* 5 g
Hou Po *Cortex Magnoliae Officinalis* 5 g

The above herbal formula was given as a concentrated powder to be taken in warm water at a dosage of 5 g, four times a day after meals.

Treatment Reaction:
23 January 2021 (day 3)

- 9:30 am: After taking prescription 2, at 9:00 am his temperature was 36.6°C, coughing with a lot of white sputum without blood-spots, chest tightness disappeared, his nose was no longer bleeding, diarrhea, urine volume increased, and fatigue improved.
- 15:18 pm: Body temperature 36.4°C under the armpit, there are bloodspots in the sputum. (Professor Peilin Sun's note: There is no problem with bloodspots in the sputum. This is caused by phlegm fever. Ask him to eat two pears a day.)
- 18:17 pm: Temperature was 37.0°C. Appetite and physical strength increased, still coughing, sputum no longer had bloodspots, body soreness disappeared.

24 January 2021 (day 4):

- 8:20 am temperature 37.1°C.
- 13:30 pm temperature 36.6°C. Normal appetite, still coughing, the sputum was thick and the color was light yellow, but the volume was less than before, no bloodspots, good spirits, tongue was pale red, thick greasy coating gradually turned yellow and the thickness is gradually thinner.

Further Treatment:
Third consultation: 25 January 2021 (day 5)
The patient felt well, managed to go out for a walk, and his appetite increased. Temperature was 36.3°C, cough and sputum were obviously reduced, stool was formed, tongue was pale red, and the yellow greasy coating gradually faded.

Prescription 3:
Huang Qin *Radix Scutellariae Baicalensis* 6 g
Huang Lian *Rhizoma Coptidis* 3 g
Zhi Zi *Fructus Gardeniae Jasminoidis* 5 g
Jie Geng *Radix Platycodi Grandiflori* 5 g

Xing Ren *Semen Pruni Armeniacae* 6 g
Zhi Mu *Radix Anemarrhenae Asphodeloidis* 5 g
Zhe Bei Mu *Bulbus Fritillariae Thunbergii* 6 g
Sheng Di Huang *Radix Rehmanniae Glutinosae Recens* 8 g
Xuan Shen *Radix Scrophulariae Ningpoensis* 8 g
Zhu Ru *Caulis Bambusae in Taeniis* 5 g
Ban Xia *Rhizoma Pinelliae Ternatae Cooked* 5 g
Hou Po *Cortex Magnoliae Officinalis* 5 g
Fu Ling *Sclerotium Poriae Cocos* 6 g
Cang Zhu *Rhizoma Atractylodis* 6 g
Chao Bai Zhu *Rhizoma Atractylodis Macrocephalae* 6 g

The above herbal formula was given as a concentrated powder to be taken in warm water at a dosage of 5 g, four times a day after meals.

Treatment Reaction:
- 27 January 2021 (day 7): After taking prescription 3, cough and sputum were significantly reduced, and the body temperature was normal. The tongue coating was still yellow and greasy. The patient usually has an irregular diet, and prefers to eat sweet, deep-fried greasy food. He was advised to control his diet.
- 30 January 2021 (day 10): His temperature was 36.1°C, only a little cough at night, appetite has greatly increased, and physical strength has improved. He can walk without wheezing, and the yellow greasy coating had gradually disappeared.

Fourth Consultation:
31 January 2021 (day 11): COVID-19 test had turned negative on this day, and the patient was very happy. He was tested positive on 19 January and negative on 30 January which took only 11 days since he took the herbal treatment. His temperature was 36.1°C, his appetite was normal, occasionally coughed, breathing was normal, and his physical strength returned to the previous level. His takeaway business has also reopened. The patient's appetite recovered, and he began to eat irregularly again, resulting in a bit of yellow and greasy tongue coating.

Prescription 4:
To prevent pulmonary fibrosis in the late stage of COVID-19 pneumonia.

Huang Qin *Radix Scutellariae Baicalensis* 6 g
Huang Lian *Rhizoma Coptidis* 3 g
Zhi Zi *Fructus Gardeniae Jasminoidis* 5 g
Jie Geng *Radix Platycodi Grandiflori* 5 g
Xing Ren *Semen Pruni Armeniacae* 6 g
Zhe Bei Mu *Bulbus Fritillariae Thunbergii* 6 g
Qing Pi *Pericarpium Citri Reticulatae Viride* 3 g
Chen Pi *Pericarpium Citri Reticulatae* 3 g
Ju Luo *Citrus tangerina Hort. et Tanaka C.erythrosa Tanaka* 5 g
Si Gua Luo *Fasciculus Vascularis Luffae* 5 g
Yu Jin *Tuber Curcumae* 5 g
Hong Hua *Flos Carthami Tinctorii* 5 g
Tao Ren *Semen Pruni Persicae* 5 g
Ban Xia *Rhizoma Pinelliae Ternatae Cooked* 5 g
Hou Po *Cortex Magnoliae Officinalis* 6 g
Cang Zhu *Rhizoma Atractylodis* 6 g
Zhu Ru *Caulis Bambusae in Taeniis* 5 g
Zhi Da Huang *Radix et Rhizoma Rhei* 5 g

The above herbal formula was given as a concentrated powder to be taken in warm water at a dosage of 5 g, three times a day after meals.

Treatment Reaction:
After taking prescription 4, the patient followed up on 4 February 2021. The tongue coating improved significantly, no cough and sputum, everything was normal.

Explanations:
This patient was in a critical condition when he consulted Professor Peilin Sun. The syndrome was external infection of damp toxins, and pulmonary failure of dispersing. The condition was complicated due

to inappropriate treatment. Therefore, the pulmonary failure of dispersing and descending function was caused.

Prescription 1:
Huang Qin, Huang Lian, Zhi Zi is the *Huang Lian Jie Du Decoction* that aims to clear away heat and detoxification. Jie Geng, Xing Ren and Xiang Ru (prefer Ma Huang) helps in dispersing and descending the lung to relieve cough. Zhi Mu, Shi Gao works by clearing heat and purging fire. Zhe Bei Mu for clearing heat and resolving phlegm and dispelling stagnation. Sheng Di Huang and Xuan Shen cool the blood to stop bleeding. Zhu Ru clears away heat and reduces phlegm, relieves fidgetiness, and prevents vomiting.

Professor Peilin Sun's note: when the patient is seriously ill, he is very anxious and in a bad mood. We, as doctors, should understand and explain patiently to help him through the difficult time. We should care about him more, allow him to lose his temper and vent emotions.

Prescription 2:
After taking the prescription 1, his tongue coating is much better than when he first consulted us. Moreover, his body temperature has become normal, and his appetite has increased. The next step is asking him to be more active. He still has damp and heat in the middle Jiao which is not urgent but coughing with yellow sputum and shortness of breath are very dangerous. Fortunately, it has been controlled now. Since prescription 1 is effective, prescription 2 keeps the same formula and adds Ban Xia and Hou Po to strengthen the effect of widening the chest, resolving phlegm and protecting the lung. After he finished prescription 2, he still needs to take the herbs because the phlegm heat will not be removed at once, and it will take several weeks to clear. Diarrhea is normal because his phlegm has not been removed completely. Considering that the patient weighed 90 kg, the dose of herb medicine was increased to four times a day, 5 g each time. In just two days, we rescued him from the dangerous situation which explained that accurate diagnosis and treatment will bring good results.

Prescription 3:

The patient is much better, and the tongue coating is much cleaner. In the past few days, it has changed dramatically. He should continue to take herbs powder to prevent pulmonary fibrosis. He needs to pay attention to his diet, so based on prescription 2, prescription 3 removed Xiang Ru, Zhi Mu, Shi Gao, and added Fu Ling, Cang Zhu and Bai Zhu to invigorate the spleen and dissipate the damp.

Prescription 4:

The patient's tongue coating is still a bit yellow and greasy. It is related to his unhealthy diet. At this time, he has entered a recovery period. The focus is on preventing pulmonary fibrosis, so the prescription 4 is based on the prescription 3, but removing Zhi Mu and Fu Ling and adding Qing Pi, Chen Pi, Ju Luo, Si Gua Luo, Yu Jin, Hong Hua and Tao Ren to promote qi & blood circulation and clear collaterals. The prescription 4 also uses Da Huang to clear up his damp-heat of Yangming.

8.3 Case 3

Male, 60 years old, an engineer.
Chief complaints: Fever with headache and sore throat for 12 days, cough for three days.
First consultation: 15 February 2021.

Actual Medical History:

The patient developed a headache, sore throat, and fever on 3 February 2021, and the COVID-19 test was positive two days later. He had been feverish since the onset, and his body temperature was as high as 39.7°C (under the armpit). He had taken a prescription issued by a local TCM practitioner for ten days. The prescription was modified Sang Ju Yin Decoction (Mulberry Leaf and Chrysanthemum Beverage), but he still had repeated low-grade fever. The local TCM doctor is a student of Prof. Peilin Sun, who consulted him for guidance and treatment. Before the onset of illness, the patient was busy with work and often stayed up late.

Symptoms at the Time of First Consultation:
At the consultation he complained of fluctuations in body temperature, alternate attacks of chills and fever, headache and sore throat, cough without sputum, blood oxygen concentration 91%, body temperature 37.6°C (under the armpit). He had been coughing for three days, no stool that day but the stool was mushy the day before. He also suffered belching after each meal. His tongue looked red with a scanty and peeled tongue coating, uneven slight yellow and greasy coating on the back tongue, cracks in the middle.

Past Medical History:
A history of allergic asthma 15 years ago.

TCM Diagnosis:
Cough due to stagnant pathogen of Shaoyang, and the damp-heat epidemic toxins is detained in middle Jiao and lower Jiao.

Principle of Treatment:
Harmonize the Shaoyang, clear heat, eliminate damp, remove toxins, and regulate the middle Jiao.

Herbal Treatment:
Modified Xiao Chai Hu Decoction-*Minor Bupleurum Decoction* and Lian Pu Decoction-*Coptis and Officinal Magnolia Bark Beverage.*

Prescription 1:
Chai Hu *Radix Bupleuri* 10 g
Huang Qin *Radix Scutellariae Baicalensis* 10 g
Zhi Ban Xia *Rhizoma Pinelliae Ternatae cooked* 10 g
Lian Qiao *Fructus Forsythiae Suspensae* 10 g
Zhi Zi *Fructus Gardeniae Jasminoidis* 10 g
Zhi Mu *Radix Anemarrhenae Asphodeloidis* 10 g
Zhe Bei Mu *Bulbus Fritillariae Thunbergii* 10 g

Sang Bai Pi *Cortex Mori Albae Radicis* 10 g
Xing Ren *Semen Pruni Armeniacae* 10 g
Huang Lian *Rhizoma Coptidis* 5 g
Hou Po *Cortex Magnoliae Officinalis* 10 g
Cang Zhu *Rhizoma Atractylodis* 10 g
Dan Dou Chi *Semen Sojae Praeparatum* 10 g
Mu Xiang *Radix Aucklandiae Lappae* 10 g
Zhi Shi *Fructus Immaturus Citri Aurantii* 10 g
Fu Ling *Sclerotium Poriae Cocos* 10 g

For five-day doses.
Put the two days' doses together and decoct for half an hour, then divide into eight portions, and take one portion warm every four hours, day and night.

Treatment Reaction:
15 February 2021 (day 1)

- Loose stools twice before noon, body temperature dropped from 37.8°C to 37.3°C. In the middle of the night, blood oxygen was 91%, no cough, and a slight improvement in sleep.

16 February 2021 (day 2)

- 8:41 am: A thin white coating began to appear on the tongue, but the tongue itself was still very red. The yellow greasy coating started to fade away in the back half of the tongue.
- 10:00 am: His body temperature dropped below 37°C for the first time after onset.
- 12:32 pm: There was no cough, no sputum, no chest tightness, and his appetite had improved. He had a smile for the first time after onset. The blood oxygen concentration increased to 95%.
- 8:37 pm: The patient felt well, with a body temperature of 36.9°C. He only felt a little fatigue, he had hiccups after eating, blood oxygen concentration was 93%, no cough and sputum, no chest

tightness, only shortness of breath while walking, and the tongue coating had improved significantly.

Further Treatment:
Second consultation: 17 February 2021 (day 3)
Body temperature was normal, still a little belching, a slight cough, a small amount of stool formation, fatigue, blood oxygen concentration was 94–96%, the tongue was red, and the coating had changed from very yellow and greasy to scattered and thinned.

Prescription 2:
Chai Hu *Radix Bupleuri* 10 g
Huang Qin *Radix Scutellariae Baicalensis* 10 g
Zhi Ban Xia *Rhizoma Pinelliae Ternatae cooked* 10 g
Lian Qiao *Fructus Forsythiae Suspensae* 10 g
Zhi Zi *Fructus Gardeniae Jasminoidis* 10 g
Zhi Mu *Radix Anemarrhenae Asphodeloidis* 10 g
Zhe Bei Mu *Bulbus Fritillariae Thunbergii* 10 g
Sang Bai Pi *Cortex Mori Albae Radicis* 10 g
Xing Ren *Semen Pruni Armeniacae* 10 g
Huang Lian *Rhizoma Coptidis* 5 g
Hou Po *Cortex Magnoliae Officinalis* 10 g
Cang Zhu *Rhizoma Atractylodis* 10 g
Chen Pi *Pericarpium Citri Reticulatae* 5 g
Mu Xiang *Radix Aucklandiae Lappae* 10 g
Zhi Shi *Fructus Immaturus Citri Aurantii* 10 g
Sheng Di Huang *Radix Rehmanniae Glutinosae Recens* 12 g
Xuan Shen *Radix Scrophulariae Ningpoensis* 10 g
Dan Zhu Ye *Herba Lophatheri Gracilis* 10 g
Fu Ling *Sclerotium Poriae Cocos* 10 g
Zhi Gan Cao *Radix Glycyrrhizae Preparata* 3 g

For five-day doses.
Put two days' doses together and decote for half an hour, then divide into eight portions, and take one portion warm every six hours, day and night.

Treatment Reaction:

- 8:35 pm (day 3): The patient had no fever for two days.
- 10:00 am (day 4): No obvious discomfort, red tongue, yellow greasy coating had basically disappeared.
- 10:00 am (day 5): No short of breath when he went up and down the stairs, Normal tongue coating began to appear, belching stopped.

Further Treatment:

Third consultation: 21 February 2021 (day 7)

The patient's condition was getting better every day and he had no cough. He went for a walk on that day and felt his physical strength had recovered well. His tongue was still red but better than before and the coating was only a bit greasy and yellow at the root of the tongue.

Prescription 3:

Huang Lian *Rhizoma Coptidis* 5 g
Hou Po *Cortex Magnoliae Officinalis* 10 g
Zhi Ban Xia *Rhizoma Pinelliae Ternatae cooked* 10 g
Xing Ren *Semen Pruni Armeniacae* 10 g
Sang Bai Pi *Cortex Mori Albae Radicis* 10 g
Zhe Bei Mu *Bulbus Fritillariae Thunbergii* 10 g
Chuan Bei Mu *Bulbus Fritillariae Cirrhosae* 10 g
Huang Qin Radix *Scutellariae Baicalensis* 10 g
Sheng Di Huang *Radix Rehmanniae Glutinosae Recens* 12 g
Dan Zhu Ye *Herba Lophatheri Gracilis* 10 g
Lian Qiao *Fructus Forsythiae Suspensae* 10 g
Zhi Zi *Fructus Gardeniae Jasminoidis* 10 g
Mu Dan Pi *Cortex Moutan Radicis* 10 g
Dan Shen *Radix Salviae Miltiorrhizae* 10 g

For five-days doses.

Put two days' doses together and decoct for half an hour, then divide into eight portions, and take one portion warm every six hours, day and night.

Treatment Reaction:

22 February 2021: Apart from a little night sweats and slight constipation, no other complaints.

27 February 2021: The patient had no obvious discomfort except occasional night sweats and poor sleep. He had resumed normal work.

Explanations:

The patient had been feverish for nearly 12 days when he came to consult Prof. Peilin Sun. The pathogen was in Taiyang at the beginning of the onset. It was right for the local TCM doctor to use modified Sang Ju Yin Decoction to evacuate the Taiyang pathogen. However later the Taiyang exterior cold syndrome got inside the Shaoyang, phlegm-damp and heat began to appear. So, treatment needed to change accordingly because modified Sang Ju Yin Decoction cannot tackle these two new pathogenesis. Failing to do so, his condition gradually became worse. So, the diagnosis and treatment must be accurate and precise.

Prescription 1:

Chai Hu, Huang Qin, Zhi Ban Xia take the meaning of Xiao Chai Hu Decoction to relieve the pathogen of Shaoyang. Lian Qiao clears heat and toxins, Zhi Zi ventilates the fire of San Jiao, Zhi Mu clears heat and purges fire, nourishes yin and moisturizes dryness. Combination of the three herbs can clear and relieve the pathogen of damp-heat, and unblock the San Jiao. Zhe Bei Mu for heat-resolving phlegm and relieving cough, Sang Bai Pi to relieve lung and asthma, hydration and swelling, Xing Ren to relieve cough and asthma, evacuate the lung meridian wind, cold, phlegm and dampness, and also moisten and relax bowels. The combination of the three herbs was used to protect the lung's descending function; Huang Lian, Hou Po, Zhi Zi and Dan Dou Chi which is Lian Pu Yin Decoction to clear heat and reduce damp, regulate qi and neutralize, remove interior retention of heat-damp. Zhi Shi, Cang Zhu, Mu Xiang, Fu Ling which is Mu Xiang Shun Qi Wan to conduct qi and dissipate damp, invigorated the spleen and stomach. Prescription 1 exactly tackles the pathology by reconciling Shaoyang, focusing on clearing away the damp-heat of the San Jiao, grasping the key pathogenesis of the COVID-19 lung injury, so as to cut off the deterioration of the disease. If there was no precise treatment of Prescription 1 herbal formula, he would have had a very high fever and felt very uncomfortable. Also, his condition would have become very dangerous. It happened exactly as was expected. After one day of taking the prescription 1, the fever was controlled, the yellow greasy tongue coating was significantly reduced, his physical strength continued to recover, and a smile appeared on his face for the first time since the onset of the illness.

Prescription 2:
The patient's condition was obviously relieved after taking the prescription 1, only the red tongue indicated that there is still heat in the lung. If it was not controlled in time, it would have transferred to the Ying Fen (Ying level). Therefore, based on prescription 1, Sheng Di Huang and Xuan Shen were added and used together to clear the heat and toxins before they get into the Ying-level. Plus, Lian Qiao and Dan Zhu Ye are used together to clear the heat (also called "*Tou Re Zhuan Ying*"), promoting qi circulation by relieving Ying Fen, so that the pathogen of entering Ying level could be separated and resolved. In addition, combining Chen Pi, Zhi Gan Cao, Hou Po and Cang Zhu makes Ping Wei San Decoction (Stomach-Calming Powder) to dry damp and promote spleen, promote qi and stomach to relieve damp and stagnation of the spleen.

Prescription 3:
After taking the prescription 2, the patient's condition improved every day, except that the tongue was still a little red. Because the patient's Shaoyang syndrome had disappeared and the middle Jiao obstructed by damp had been resolved, so on the basis of the second prescription, prescription 3 removed Chai Hu, Cang Zhu, Chen Pi, Mu Xiang, Zhi Shi, Xuan Shen, Fu Ling and Zhi Gan Cao, added Chuan Bei Mu to moisturize the lung and relieve cough to prevent chronic cough damage to the lung, added Mu Dan Pi and Dan Shen, combined with Huang Lian, Hou Po, Zhi Ban Xia, Xing Ren, Sang Bai Pi, Zhe Bei

Mu, Huang Qin, Zhi Zi to continue to clear the lung of phlegm heat, Sheng Di Huang, Dan Zhu Ye and Lian Qiao continue to clear the heat. Prescription 3 was to protect his lung and heart, prevent blood heat entering Ying level and causing pulmonary embolism.

8.4 Case 4

Female, 50 years old, a TCM practitioner.
Chief complaints: Aversion to cold, fever, and body pain for ten days.
First consultation: 13 December 2020.

Actual Medical History:
On 3 December 2020, the patient felt numbness in the right arm where the location of the lung meridian is and began to experience aversion to cold late in the night, no loss of smell and taste, and no sore throat. The next day she began to have a fever, which was 37.5–38°C under the armpit. On 5 December 2020 her COVID-19 test was positive. The patient is a TCM practitioner. Because of her body pain, especially on the neck, accompanied by slight sweating, she self-prescribed Guizhi plus Ge Gen Decoction. After taking a single day dose of it, she started to experience whole body pain, so she changed to Xin Jia Decoction, and the condition became worse. The patient began to feel fatigue, lack of appetite, slight cough without sputum and persistent fever. The body temperature was between 38–38.5°C under the armpit, and the fever emerged mostly at night. On the morning of 8 December, she started to have an itchy throat and coughed up a small amount of yellow phlegm. She still had the fever and sweating, and fatigue and anorexia became worse, so she started taking Ginseng Baihu Decoction plus Gui Zhi and Da Huang decoction on the recommendation of a friend. After taking three doses intermittently, her condition became even worse. She started to have chest tightness and shortness of breath. Her blood oxygen concentration is around 95%. The body temperature was normal during the day, while at night it is about 37.5–38°C under the armpits, and she woke up sweating at 4–5 o'clock in the morning. On 12 December 2020 she took Qing Fei Pai Du Decoction plus Sanren

Decoction Chinese medicine concentrated powder, and Xiao Chaihu granules (Minor Bupleurum Decoction) at night to try to control the fever. On 13 December 2020, her condition became serious, so she consulted Professor Peilin Sun for online diagnosis and treatment through a friend.

Symptoms at the Time of First Consultation:
Shallow breathing, cough when taking deep breaths. This coughing came with distending pain in both rib-side, a small amount of thin sputum and very poor appetite. The patient reported that she lost her mother in October 2020 and became a vegan. Also, she is always busy with work and not eating properly, thus her immune system had weakened. The tongue was pale red, with horizontal cracks in the middle, yellow and greasy coating especially thick in the roots. While the pulse was slippery and rapid, both middle parts of the pulse were slightly stronger.

TCM Diagnosis:
Cough due to flaring of damp-heat, accumulation phlegm-heat in the lung, and consumption of body fluid by excessive heat.

Treatment Principles:
Clear away heat, remove damp, descend the lung, resolve phlegm, and promote fluid production at the same time.

Herbal Treatment:
Lian Po Yin-*Coptis and Magnolia Bark Drink.*

Prescription 1:
Huang Lian *Rhizoma Coptidis* 3 g
Hou Po *Cortex Magnoliae Officinalis* 5 g
Sang Bai Pi *Cortex Mori Albae Radicis* 5 g
Zhi Ban Xia *Rhizoma Pinelliae Ternatae Cooked* 5 g
Dan Dou Chi *Semen Sojae Praeparatum* 5 g

Jiao Zhi Zi *Fructus Gardeniae Jasminoidis (grill)* 5 g
Lu Gen *Rhizoma Phragmitis Communis* 5 g
Zhe Bei Mu *Bulbus Fritillariae Thunbergii* 5 g
Chuan Bei Mu *Bulbus Fritillariae Cirrhosae* 5 g
Huang Qin *Radix Scutellariae Baicalensis* 5 g
Gua Lou Pi *Pericarpium Trichosanthis* 5 g
Zhi Mu *Radix Anemarrhenae Asphodeloides* 5 g
Ge Gen *Radix Puerariae* 5 g
Fu Ling *Sclerotium Poriae Cocos* 6 g
Hua Shi *Talcum* 6 g
Gan Cao *Radix Glycyrrhizae Uralensis* 1 g

The above herbal formula was given as a concentrated powder to be taken in warm water at a dosage of two grams, three times a day after meals.

Treatment Reaction:
- 14 December 2020: Patient reported that after taking the above herbal medicine within 24 hours the fever was mostly controlled. She coughed up and vomited a large amount of thin white foamy sputum, coughing ceaselessly, shallow breath, occasionally low fever, numbness in the right arm lung meridian area, slight chest tightness, and poor appetite. Sleep became better, and the sputum was white and not thick.
- 15 December 2020: Patient reported that her body temperature was normal, her blood oxygen increased to 98%, and she kept coughing and vomiting a lot of thin white foamy sputum.

Further Treatment:
Second consultation: 19 December 2020.
After taking prescription 1, the patient had no fever, still coughing with left chest pain when taking a deep breath. Her appetite improved, still had night sweats, and her tongue coating became less yellow and grease.

Prescription 2:
Yu Ping Feng San (Jade-screen powder), San Zi Yang Qin Tang (Three-Seed Filial Devotion Decoction), Wei Jing Tang (Phragmitis decoction) combined with modifications.

Zhi Huang Qi *Radix Astragali Membranacei Praeparata* 5 g
Jiao Bai Zhu *Rhizoma Atractylodis Macrocephalae (grill)* 3 g
Zhi Ban Xia *Rhizoma Pinelliae Ternatae Cooked* 5 g
Qing Pi *Pericarpium Citri Reticulatae Viride* 5 g
Zhe Bei Mu *Bulbus Fritillariae Thunbergii* 5 g
Zhi Shi *Fructus Immaturus Citri Aurantii* 5 g
Hou Po *Cortex Magnoliae Officinalis* 5 g
Zi Su Zi *Fructus Perillae Frutescentis* 5 g
Bai Jie Zi *Semen Sinapis Albae* 5 g
Lai Fu Zi *Semen Raphani Sativi* 5 g
Yi Yi Ren *Semen Coicis Lachryma-Jobi* 5 g
Bai Jiang Cao *Herba cum Radice Patriniae* 5 g
Dong Gua Ren *Semen Benincasae Hispidae* 5 g
Tao Ren *Semen Pruni Persicae* 5 g
Chuan Lian Zi *Fructus Meliae Toosendan* 5 g
Yu Jin *Tuber Curcumae* 5 g

The above herbal formula was given as a concentrated powder to be taken in warm water at a dosage of two grams, three times a day after meals.

Treatment Reaction:
25 December 2020: Patient reported that for three consecutive nights there was no cough and fever, sputum reduced significantly, much less chest pain, able to take deep breaths, and less night sweats.

Further Treatment:
Third consultation: 29 December 2020.
At the third follow-up consultation, the sputum coughed up in the morning was slightly brown and bloodspots, and there was no sputum for the rest of the day. She coughed and had slight chest pain. The COVID-19 test also turned negative on that day.

Prescription 3:
Huang Lian *Rhizoma Coptidis* 3 g
Zhu Ru *Caulis Bambusae in Taeniis* 5 g
Hou Po *Cortex Magnoliae Officinalis* 5 g
Zhi Zi *Fructus Gardeniae Jasminoidis* 5 g
Zhi Ban Xia *Rhizoma Pinelliae Ternatae Cooked* 5 g
Chen Pi *Pericarpium Citri Reticulatae* 3 g
Fu Ling *Sclerotium Poriae Cocos* 5 g
Fu Shen *Sclerotium Poriae Cocos Paradicis* 5 g
Hong Hua *Flos Carthami Tinctorii* 5 g
Yu Jin *Tuber Curcumae* 5 g
Yan Hu Suo *Rhizoma Corydalis* 5 g
Zhe Bei Mu *Bulbus Fritillariae Thunbergii* 5 g
Xing Ren *Semen Pruni Armeniacae* 5 g
Huang Bai *Cortex Phellodendri* 5 g
Cang Zhu *Rhizoma Atractylodis* 5 g
Che Qian Zi *Semen Plantaginis* 5 g

The above herbal formula was given as a concentrated powder to be taken in warm water at a dosage of two grams, three times a day after meals.

Treatment Reaction:
30 December 2021: A small amount of white with rusty sputum was reported, chest pain basically disappeared, and cough of qi inverse was alleviated. The amount of discharge was less, and the color was yellow and thinner. Patient also reported normal stool two times a day. In the following days, the patient improved and recovered completely. A follow up consultation a month later, she was fully recovered without any Long-COVID symptoms.

Explanations:
This case is different from the general cause and pathogenesis of COVID-19, it is a case of grief weakening the lung, causing insufficient lung defending, and allowing damp heat to take the advantage.

At the beginning, if she focused on dispersing the lung-defense and clearing away heat and dampness, it will be easy to tackle the problem. However, she used Guizhi plus Gegen Decoction, Xinjia Decoction and Ren Shen Baihu Decoction etc., which failed to eliminate the symptoms of lung-defense and the damp-heat. Therefore, the exogenous pathogenic factors have gradually deepened which led to phlegm-heat accumulation in the lung, and body fluid consumed by excessive heat. Her exterior syndrome is very short, and the exogenous pathogenic factors enter the interior very quickly straight into the lower Jiao, mostly in the upper and lower Jiao. In the upper Jiao the lung loses descending function, while in the lower Jiao the bladder is dysfunctional and the large intestine conduction is lost, which leads to serious damp-heat accumulated. Neither Guizhi plus Gegen Decoction, Xinjia Decoction and Ren Shen Baihu Decoction can tackle the above pathogenesis, because the cause of her condition was not cold-damp factor, but damp-heat factor. Therefore, Ginseng is not suitable because it will nourish the pathogen and make heat-damp worse. In addition, although the fever in this case is rather a low-grade fever emerging at night which is a distinctive feature of damp-heat fever, combining with diarrhea, thick and greasy tongue coating, and pulse conditions which all point to this pathogenesis. Although the patient's tongue coating is yellow and greasy, especially worse in the root area, the treatment is still focused on controlling the phlegm-heat in the lung. The aim is to protect the lung's descending function, resolve phlegm, and clear heat, otherwise the lung condition will immediately deteriorate.

Prescription 1:
Zhi Ban Xia, Hou Po, Sang Bai Pi, and Zhe Bei Mu descend lung-qi, relieve phlegm, reduce cough, soothe the chest, and alleviate pain. Huang Lian, Huang Qin, Zhi Mu and Gua Lou Pi eliminate heat from the lung. Hua Shi and Gan Cao, which is Liu Yi San-*Six One Powder* together with Ge Gen, Fu Ling, are taking care of the lower Jiao damp-heat. Zhi Zi can wipe out all the San Jiao to clean up the damp and heat. Chuan Bei Mu and Lu Gen to relieve cough and enhance the fluid.

The first prescription considers the following aspects: clearing away heat, removing damp, clearing lung, removing phlegm, and nourishing body fluids. It can not only control damp and heat, but also expel phlegm, and recover the descend function of lung. In the treatment of COVID-19, the main task is to always focus on the excessive pathogen, and to protect the lung and restore the lung's descending function, which is key to prevent it turning into a critical condition.

Prescription 2:
Zhi Huang Qi and Jiao Bai Zhu nourish the lung, invigorate the spleen and reduce phlegm, Zhi Ban Xia and Zhe Bei Mu expel phlegm and relieve cough. Zhi Shi and Hou Po dissipate phlegm and remove distension. Zi Su Zi, Bai Jie Zi and Lai Fu Zi which is San Zi Yang Qin Decoction, warm lung and resolve phlegm, direct qi downward and promote digestion. Yi Yi Ren, Bai Jiang Cao, Dong Gua Ren, Tao Ren, Chuan Lian Zi, Qing Pi and Yu Jin remove phlegm and blood stasis, promote blood circulation, regulate qi and relieve pain. Together with all the other herbal medicine, this prescription supplements the spleen to nourish the lung, restores the yang vitality of the delicate viscera, promotes clearness and reduces turbidity, and removes blood stasis and phlegm.

Prescription 3:
Huang Lian, Zhu Ru and Zhi Zi clear the upper Jiao residual heat, Hou Po descend lung-qi, calming the qi counterflow. Zhi Ban Xia, Chen Pi, and Fu Ling which is Er Chen decoction without Gan Cao which help to remove the phlegm dampness in middle Jiao, Hong Hua, Yu Jin and Yan Hu Suo promote blood circulation, regulate qi and relieve pain. Zhe Bei Mu and Xing Ren relieve cough and asthma by resolve phlegm-heat. Huang Bai and Cang Zhu clear the damp and heat of lower Jiao. Che Qian Zi promotes urination, percolates dampness, dispels phlegm through lower Jiao. Fu Shen calms the shen.

The third prescription still focuses on the upper Jiao phlegm dampness, and considers the lower Jiao, so that the phlegm dampness is drained from the lower Jiao. This prescription considers the patient's qi inversion, chest pain, coughing and phlegm, etc. It looks basically the same as the previous two, but the direction has begun to change.

8.5 Case 5

Male, 37 years old, a chef.
Chief complaints: Cough expectoration of whitish foamy sputum, accompanied by a feeling of gas rushing up toward the thorax for two days.
First consultation: 17 January 2021.

Actual Medical History:
Aversion to cold with fever, sore throat, loss of sense of smell and taste, COVID-19 tested positive ten days ago. He took Xiao Chai Hu granules for the first five days and Lian Hua Qing Wen Capsules for another five days. Although his body temperature became normal, he started to have diarrhea with undigested food in the stool. He kept complaining that his chest was very tight.

Symptoms at the Time of First Consultation:
He complained that cough occurred when lying flat, felt dizziness, spit white foamy sputum, short of breath and wheezing, cold and pain on the left side of the chest, and a feeling of coldness and tightness in the retro-cardiac area. He prefers drinking warm water. The tongue was light purple, with vertical cracks in the middle, and the coating was white with a slightly yellow and greasy coating that is thicker in the middle and back of the tongue.

Past Medical History:
Ten years of peanut-sized cyst in left scrotum with a firmer texture. He had taken Western medicine and traditional Chinese medicine for many years but both had no effect, thus he stopped the medicine a long time ago. He suffers from insomnia with stress for many years, but did not take any medicine.

TCM Diagnosis:
Cough due to exterior tightened by wind-cold, cold fluid retention in the chest, the disperse function of the lung is weakened, the damp transforms into heat which gathers in the middle Jiao.

Principle of Treatment:
Expel wind and cold, disperse lung-qi, warm and resolve cold phlegm, and eliminate damp-heat.

Herbal Treatment:
Modified Xiao Qing Long Tang-*Minor Green Dragon Decoction.*

Prescription 1:
Xiang Ru *Herba Elsholtziae seu Moslae* 5 g
(Prefer Ma Huang *Herba Ephedrae* 5 g, but not available due to EU regulations)
Gan Jiang *Rhizoma Zingiberis Officinalis* 10 g
Bai Jie Zi *Semen Sinapis Albae* 10 g
Yu Jin *Tuber Curcumae* 5 g
Ju Luo *Citrus tangerina Hort.et Tanaka C.erythrosa Tanaka* 5 g
Qing Pi *Pericarpium Citri Reticulatae Viride* 10 g
Chen Pi *Pericarpium Citri Reticulatae* 10 g
Jie Geng *Radix Platycodi Grandiflori* 10 g
Cang Er Zi *Fructus Xanthii Sibirici* 10 g
Zhi Ban Xia *Rhizoma Pinelliae Ternatae Cooked* 15 g
Yi Yi Ren *Semen Coicis Lachryma-Jobi* 15 g
Huang Lian *Rhizoma Coptidis* 5 g
Fu Ling *Sclerotium Poriae Cocos* 10 g
Pei Lan *Herba Eupatorii Fortunei* 10 g
Chao Bai Zhu *Rhizoma Atractylodis Macrocephalae* 10 g
For 3-day doses, decocted in water, one dose per day.

Treatment Reaction:
- 17 January 2021 (day 1): Half an hour after taking half dose of prescription 1, his cough and reversed flow of qi improved significantly,

and he coughed a small amount of white phlegm with a slightly yellow color. He could breathe much better and fell asleep for the first time since onset.

- 18 January 2021 (day 2): There was still shortness of breath, but it had improved significantly, breathing was smoother and deeper than before, stool began to form, cold tightness in the retro-cardiac area disappeared, and white sputum was slightly yellow. Sleep improved significantly and he felt more energetic.

Further Treatment:

Second consultation: 19 January 2021 (day 3)

He has finished the prescription 1. As a result, he has only a slight tightness in the chest, slightly coughing and wheezing, and the sputum was thin and white in the morning, much less than before. The image of the tongue was also improved, the coating was thinner and the yellow and greasy coating was reduced, and the middle crack became shallower as well. Urine and stool were normal.

Prescription 2:

Xiang Ru *Herba Elsholtziae seu Moslae* 5 g

(Prefer Ma Huang *Herba Ephedrae* 5 g, but not available due to EU regulations)

Gan Jiang *Rhizoma Zingiberis Officinalis* 10 g

Bai Jie Zi *Semen Sinapis Albae* 10 g

Zi Su Zi *Fructus Perillae Frutescentis* 10 g

Lai Fu Zi *Semen Raphani Sativi* 10 g

Xing Ren *Semen Pruni Armeniacae* 10 g

Hou Po *Cortex Magnoliae Officinalis* 10 g

Yu Jin *Tuber Curcumae* 10 g

Ju Luo *Citrus tangerina Hort.et Tanaka C.erythrosa Tanaka* 5 g

Jie Geng *Radix Platycodi Grandiflori* 10 g

Zhi Ban Xia *Rhizoma Pinelliae Ternatae Cooked* 12 g

Qing Pi *Pericarpium Citri Reticulatae Viride* 10 g

Chen Pi *Pericarpium Citri Reticulatae* 10 g

Sang Bai Pi *Cortex Mori Albae Radicis* 12 g

Huang Qin *Radix Scutellariae Baicalensis* 10 g

Treatment Reaction:

- 24 January 2021 (day 8): After drinking prescription 3, he felt better every day. He had no reversed flow of qi, only a little cough and sputum when he lies down at night, his sleep improved a lot, and had slight night sweats. We repeated the prescription 3 for another two weeks.
- 4 February 2021 (day 17): He occasionally had reversed flow of qi without coughing. Furthermore, he claimed with joy that the peanut-sized cyst in the scrotum which he had for ten years became much smaller after taking the above three formulas. A month later during a follow-up call, the patient's reported pulmonary symptoms disappeared completely. His sleep became a lot better than before onset. He returned to normal work.

Explanations:

The patient's symptoms were coughing, and expectorating white foamy sputum, his retro-cardiac area is tight and cold, he likes to drink warm water, which indicate the main pathogenesis of the patient is cold phlegm and cold fluid dwelling in the lung, plus external cold. The lung disperse function is blocked, so the treatment key point lies in to restore the lung disperse function. However, the yellowish tongue coating indicates that the exterior pathogens have penetrated to the interior and transformed into heat.

Prescription 1:

Because the condition of COVID-19 is very complicated, we cannot stick to the original formula, so in this case we only used Ma Huang (Xiang Ru) and Gan Jiang without Gui Zhi and Xi Xin of the Xiao Qing Long Decoction because the exterior pathogens has penetrated to the interior and transform into heat but the exterior cold was not resolved. Ma Huang (Xiang Ru) is to remove the cold from the surface, and restore the function of the wei-yang (defending yang). Because the pathogenic qi has entered the interior and transformed to heat, Huang Lian was used to clear heat. In this formula, Ma Huang (Xiang Ru) and Gan Jiang of Xiao Qinglong Decoction are used to release the pathogenic factor of warmth and dissipate the cold fluid retention in the lung. Bai Jie Zi warms the lung and resolve phlegm, promote qi and dispel stagnation. Since the patient had been suffering from the disease for ten days already, Yu Jin, Ju Luo and Qing Pi are used to regulate qi and relieve collaterals to prevent pulmonary fibrosis. Jie Geng promotes the lung, Cang Er Zi cannulate the orifice, Huang Lian clears stagnant heat, Zhi Ban Xia, Chen Pi, Yi Yi Ren, Fu Ling, Chao Ba Zhu invigorate the spleen to remove phlegm, and aromatic Pei Lan eliminate dampness.

Prescription 2:
After the patient takes prescription 1, the yellow and greasy tongue coating has obviously changed, and the exterior cold has been resolved, so on the basis of prescription 1, prescription 2 removed Cang Er Zi, Yi Yi Ren, Huang Lian, Pei Lan, and added Zi Su Zi and Lai Fu Zi to strengthen the function of descending lung-qi, and increase the dosage of Fu Ling to increase the function of invigorate the spleen and promote dampness.

Prescription 3:
At this stage, the patient's internal heat has been removed, and the patient still has the slight symptoms of lung-qi reversal, coughing with sputum. Therefore, based on prescription 2, we removed Huang Qin and added Xuan Fu Hua to descend lung-qi and eliminate phlegm, and by adding Tao Ren and Hong Hua to promote blood circulation, increases the strength to prevent pulmonary fibrosis. Adding Pei Lan invigorates the spleen and resolves phlegm.

9

Generalization of Long COVID

Coronavirus disease 2019 (COVID-19) pandemic has resulted in global healthcare problems and strained health resources. At this moment, the COVID-19 pandemic is still affecting all of us and remains a challenge for all aspects of life. It is now generally accepted that COVID-19 is now recognized as a multi-organ disease with a broad spectrum of manifestations. Similar to post-acute viral syndromes described in survivors of other virulent coronavirus epidemics, there are increasing reports of persistent and prolonged effects after acute COVID-19.[1] We could tentatively call these prolonged effects or symptoms as post COVID-19 syndromes. Post COVID-19 syndromes is an umbrella term for the wide range of consequences, symptoms, feelings, conditions, complaints, or manifestations that are present after infection with SARS-CoV-2, the virus that causes COVID-19 illness.

It is quite normal that when recovering from COVID-19, patients could experience some chronic fatigue, weakness, poor appetite, poor digestion, slight pressure over the chest, headache, insomnia, low tolerance to exercise, and achiness during recovery. It could take a while for the body to recoup from that. In some cases, there can be discovery of some slight or serious damage to the respiratory and cardiac functions (kidneys, gastrointestinal tract, and neurological system, etc). However, some patients could take a decent amount of time and energy to feel that they are perfectly back to their normal

---

[1]Ani Nalbandian, *et al.* Post-acute COVID-19 syndrome. *Nature Medicine.* 2021, 27: 601–615. https://www.nature.com/articles/s41591-021-01283-z.

state prior to their illness, although they have been following good advice from the practitioners, taking medications, and being careful with their diets and emotions. Besides, when a patient tests negative for COVID-19, or positive for antibodies, it does not necessarily mean that their symptoms will cease automatically or in a short period of time.

Persistent symptoms and clinical findings can occur regardless of the severity of acute COVID-19. It means that post-COVID syndrome isn't exclusive to people who went to the hospital or stayed in the ICU due to severe organ damage during their illness. Post-COVID syndrome can be seen in people who went to the ER with concerning symptoms or those who had advanced symptoms that required a brief hospital stay, but it can also occur in people who had mild symptoms and self-treated at home. The important thing to note is that these are people who might not have required care from a specialist during their actual illness, may now benefit from specialized care as these lingering symptoms continue to affect their daily lives.[2] Medical and research communities are still learning about these post-acute symptoms and clinical findings.[3] For instance, NIH, US, launched the initiative in February 2021 to bring together researchers and scientists to identify the causes of these symptoms and the means to prevent and treat them.[4]

Previous SARS follow-up studies have shown that persistent lung diffusion impairment could last for months or even years. Hence, a longitudinal study is needed to describe the natural history of lung's structural and functional abnormality after COVID-19, and to explore the effect of these persistent abnormalities on physical function and

---

[2] Katie McCallum. Post-COVID syndrome: What should you do if you have lingering COVID-19 symptoms? *Houston Methodist on Health*. 19 November 2020. https://www.houstonmethodist.org/blog/articles/2020/nov/post-covid-syndrome-what-should-you-do-if-you-have-lingering-covid-19-symptoms/.

[3] Centers for Disease Control and Prevention (CDC). Post-COVID conditions: Information for healthcare providers. 9 July 2021. https://www.cdc.gov/coronavirus/2019-ncov/hcp/clinical-care/post-covid-conditions.html.

[4] National Institutes of Health (NIH). When-COVID-19-symptoms-linger. 13 August 2021. https://covid19.nih.gov/research-highlights/when-COVID-19-symptoms-linger.

quality of life. Meanwhile, some other sequelae symptoms, such as fatigue, hair loss, dysfunction of smell and taste, sleeping and emotion, etc., should also be studied. Some authors have carried out the largest longitudinal cohort study of hospital survivors with COVID-19 so far to describe the dynamic recovery of health consequences within 12 months after symptom onset. They found that most patients had a good physical and functional recovery during follow-up, and the majority of study participants who were employed before COVID-19 had returned to their original work. The proportion of patients with at least one sequelae symptom decreased from 68% (831/1227) at 6 months to 49%(620/1272) at 12 months ($p < 0.0001$). The decrease was observed in all three subgroups of patients with different disease severity (all $p < 0.0001$). Fatigue or muscle weakness was the most commonly reported symptom at both visits, but the proportion fell from 52%(636/1230) at 6 months to 20%(255/1272) at 12 months ($p < 0.0001$). Many symptoms significantly resolved over time in the total cohort and in all three subgroups—e.g., fatigue or muscle weakness, sleep difficulties, hair loss, smell disorder, and taste disorder (all $p < 0.05$). The proportion of patients with dyspnea, characterized by an mMRC score of 1 or more, slightly increased from 26%(313/1185) at the 6-month visit to 30%(380/1271) at the 12-month visit ($p = 0.014$). Additionally, more patients had anxiety or depression (23% [274/1187] at 6 month vs. 26%[331/1271] at 12-month visit, $p = 0.015$), where mild anxiety or depression was predominant (Appendix p. 22) and only one patient visited the psychological department after discharge. The proportion of patients with 6MWD less than the lower limit of the normal range was 12%(147/1248) at 12 months, which was statistically lower than 14%(174/1254) at 6 months ($p = 0.033$). No significant difference in median 6MWD between 6 months and 12 months was noted. Within 12 months after symptom onset, three of 1,276 patients developed ischemic stroke, and one patient newly developed stable angina pectoris. Sequelae symptoms, lung diffusion impairment, and radiographic abnormalities persisted to 12 months in some patients, especially in patients who were critically ill during a hospital stay. In terms of lung function, 128 discharged patients underwent lung

CT examinations at 6 months. The examination results showed that they all had at least one imaging abnormality. After 12 months, the proportion of moderate and severe patients dropped to 39% and 40%, while the proportion of critically severe patients was still as high as 87%. The current health status in the COVID-19 cohort was still lower than that in the control population. To sum up, most COVID-19 hospital survivors (within a year after acute infection) had a good physical and functional recovery over time, but their current health status was still lower than that in the control population. Lung diffusion impairment and radiographic abnormalities, which attributed to lung epithelial damage, or interstitial or pulmonary vascular abnormalities, were still common in critically ill patients at 12 months. Ongoing longitudinal follow-up is needed to better characterize the natural history and pathogenesis of long-term health consequences of COVID-19. The study has been published in *The Lancet* on 28 August, 2021.[5]

Another recent study, published in *EClinical Medicine, The Lancet* on 15 July 2021 has analyzed responses from 3,762 participants with confirmed (diagnostic/antibody positive; 1,020) or suspected (diagnostic/antibody negative or untested; 2,742) COVID-19 from 56 countries, with illness lasting over 28 days and onset prior to June 2020. They estimated the prevalence of 203 symptoms in ten organ systems and traced 66 symptoms over seven months. We measured the impact on life, work, and return to baseline health. Their findings: for the majority of respondents (>91%), the time to recovery exceeded 35 weeks. During their illness, participants experienced an average of 55.9±25.5 (mean±STD) symptoms, across an average of 9.1 organ systems. The most frequent symptoms after month six were fatigue, post-exertional malaise, and cognitive dysfunction. Symptoms varied in their prevalence over time, and we identified three symptom clusters, each with a characteristic temporal profile. 85.9% of participants (95% CI, 84.8% to 87.0%)

---

[5] Lixue Huang, *et al.* 1-year outcomes in hospital survivors with COVID-19: A longitudinal cohort study. *The Lancet.* 2021, 398(10302): 747–758. https://doi.org/10.1016/S0140-6736(21)01755-4.

experienced relapses, primarily triggered by exercise, physical or mental activity, and stress. 86.7%(85.6% to 92.5%) of unrecovered respondents were experiencing fatigue at the time of survey, compared to 44.7%(38.5% to 50.5%) of recovered respondents. 1,700 respondents (45.2%) required a reduced work schedule compared to pre-illness, and an additional 839(22.3%) were not working at the time of survey due to illness. Cognitive dysfunction or memory issues were common across all age groups (~88%). Except for the loss of smell and taste, the prevalence and trajectory of all symptoms were similar between groups with confirmed and suspected COVID-19. Their interpretation: Patients with Long-COVID reported prolonged, multisystem involvement and significant disability. By seven months, many patients have not yet recovered (mainly from systemic and neurological/cognitive symptoms), have not returned to previous levels of work, and continued to experience significant symptom burden. Overall, these findings suggest that the morbidity of COVID-19 illness has been greatly overlooked. Patients experience multisystem symptoms for over seven months, resulting in significant impact to their lives and livelihoods.[6]

9.1 Definition

The definite term is not yet completely defined, but it refers that when the acute phase of COVID-19 is over, some symptoms related to COVID illness could remain for weeks, months, or longer. At this moment, there are different terminologies used in the academic environment to define these remaining symptoms after COVID-19, such as post-COVID syndrome,[7] post-COVID conditions, Long COVID,[8]

---

[6]Hannah E. Davis, *et al.* Characterizing long COVID in an international cohort: 7 months of symptoms and their impact. *The Lancet-EClinical Medicine.* 2021, 38, 101019. https://doi.org/10.1016/j.eclinm.2021.101019.

[7]Daniel Ayoubkhani, *et al.* Post-covid syndrome in individuals admitted to hospital with COVID-19: Retrospective cohort study. *BMJ.* 2021, 372: n693. https://doi.org/10.1136/bmj.n693.

[8]Centers for Disease Control and Prevention (CDC). Long COVID or post-COVID conditions. Updated 1 September 2021. https://www.cdc.gov/coronavirus/2019-ncov/long-term-effects.html.

post-acute COVID-19 syndrome,[9] post-acute sequelae of SARS-COV-2 infection (PASC),[10] sequelae after COVID-19 infection,[11] chronic sequelae of COVID-19,[12] Long COVID,[13] long-term health consequences of COVID-19,[14] and in Chinese it is called Xin Guan Fei Yan Hou Yi Zheng (new coronary pneumonia sequelae—新冠肺炎后遗症).

In terms of persistence of the post-COVID-19 syndromes, both CDC and the journal *Nature* refer to the syndromes beyond four weeks from the onset of symptoms.[15,16]

However, from a medical point of view, to assess whether a disease will have sequelae after it is cured, it usually takes more than six months after the disease is cured, because the human body has a certain degree of self-repair. In many cases when the body organs are damaged by the disease, after the risk factors are eliminated, the body can repair itself and then return to normal without any sequelae. Probably, this is the reason that many research papers stressed their investigation of post-COVID after six months.[17,18] There are also

---

[9]Ani Nalbandian, *et al. op. cit.*

[10]NIH. *op. cit.*

[11]Jennifer K. Logue, *et al.* Sequelae in adults at 6 months after COVID-19 infection. *JAMA Network.* 2021, 4(2): e210830. doi: 10.1001/jamanetworkopen.2021.0830.

[12]Robert J. Rolfe, *et al.* The emerging chronic sequelae of COVID-19 and implications for North Carolina. *North Carolina Medical Journal.* 2021, 82(1): 75–78. https://doi.org/10.18043/ncm.82.1.75.

[13]Wikipedia. Long COVID. https://en.wikipedia.org/wiki/Long_COVID.

[14]Carlos del Rio, *et al.* Long-term health consequences of COVID-19. *JAMA.* 2020, 324(17): 1723–1724. doi: 10.1001/jama.2020.19719.

[15]Ani Nalbandian, *et al. op. cit.*

[16]CDC. 9 July 2021. *op. cit.*.

[17]Chaolin Huang, *et al.* 6-month consequences of COVID-19 in patients discharged from hospital: A cohort study. *The Lancet.* 2021, 397(10270): 220–232. https://doi.org/10.1016/S0140-6736(20)32656-8.

[18]Maxime Taquet, *et al.* 6-month neurological and psychiatric outcomes in 236,379 survivors of COVID-19: A retrospective cohort study using electronic health records. *The Lancet.* May 2021, 8(5): 416–427. https://doi.org/10.1016/S2215-0366(21)00084-5.

some research which observed post COVID-19 syndromes only after two months,[19,20] or even nine months.[21,22]

9.2 Timeline of Post-acute COVID-19

Acute COVID-19 usually lasts for four weeks from the onset of symptoms, beyond which replication-competent SARS-CoV-2 has not been isolated. Post-acute COVID-19 is defined as persistent symptoms and/or delayed or long-term complications beyond four weeks from the onset of symptoms.[23]

The pandemic of the coronavirus disease 2019 (COVID-19) has provoked a second pandemic, the "long-haulers", i.e., individuals presenting with post-COVID symptoms. We propose that to determine the presence of post-COVID symptoms, symptoms should appear after the diagnosis of SARS-CoV-2 infection. However, this situation faced some problems since not all people infected by SARS-CoV-2 receive such diagnosis.

Based on the relapsing/remitting nature of post-COVID symptoms, some authors proposed the following integrative classifications: potentially infection-related symptoms (up to four to five weeks), acute post-COVID symptoms (from week 5 to week 12), long post-COVID symptoms (from week 12 to week 24), and persistent post-COVID symptoms (lasting more than 24 weeks).

It can be seen from the above figure that the period immediately after the acute phase is called the post-acute period, including post-subacute COVID-19 from week 5 till week 12, and post

---

[19]Mardani Masoud. Post COVID syndrome. *Arch. Clin. Infect. Dis.* 2020, 15: e108819. doi: 10.5812/archcid.108819.

[20]Colin Clapson. Over a fifth of corona patients have symptoms two months on. *flandersnews.be.* 8 November 2020. https://www.vrt.be/vrtnws/en/2020/11/08/over-a-fifth-of-corona-patients-have-symptoms-two-months-on/.

[21]Jennifer K. Logue, *et al. op. cit.*

[22]Berkeley Lovelace Jr. Dr. Fauci says new data suggests "Long" Covid symptoms can last up to 9 months. *CNBC.* 24 February 2021. https://www.cnbc.com/2021/02/24/fauci-says-new-data-suggest-long-covid-symptoms-can-last-up-to-9-months.html.

[23]Ani Nalbandian, *et al. op. cit.*

chronic COVID-19 syndromes, from week 13 up till 6 months or longer.[24]

In the absence of agreed definitions, however, some authors even define post-acute COVID-19 as extending beyond three weeks from the onset of first symptoms.[25]

This timeline is very important to determine the principles of TCM treatment. During the acute phase of COVID-19, the treatment focuses on the elimination of pathogenic factors and supports the Zheng-qi as well as protects the zang-fu organs. But when it is in the post-acute phase, no matter post subacute COVID-19 or post chronic COVID-19, the treatment attention will be different from that in the acute phase since both clinical symptoms and their pathogenesis have been changed. There could be some remaining external pathogenic factors, but the main issues and focuses will be harmonizing the zang-fu organs, rebalancing the qi, blood, yin, and yang. There could be a slight difference in treatment for the phase of post subacute COVID-19 and post chronic COVID-19 because the underlying ethology, pathology, and treatment are not the same.

It is believed in TCM that the longer a disease or some symptoms last, the more complicated pathology will be. The purposes of TCM treatment will examine the patients based upon eight principles, differentiation of six channels, San Jiao and wei, qi, ying, and xue systems to find out the mechanisms and finally help the patients.

---

[24]César Fernández-de-las-Peñas, *et al.* Defining post-COVID symptoms (post-acute COVID, long COVID, persistent post-COVID): An integrative classification. *Int J Environ Res Public Health.* 2021, 18(5): 2621. doi: 10.3390/ijerph18052621.
[25]Trisha Greenhalgh, *et al.* Management of post-acute COVID-19 in primary care. *BMJ.* 2020, 370. https://doi.org/10.1136/bmj.m3026.

9.3 Percentage of Post-acute COVID-19 Syndromes

As far as the percentage of post-COVID syndromes goes, one cohort of individuals with a total of 234 participants show that the study followed up for as long as nine months after illness, with approximately 30% reporting post-COVID symptoms. Overall, 11(6.2%) were asymptomatic, 150(84.7%) were outpatients with mild illness, and 16(9.0%) had moderate or severe disease requiring hospitalization. Hypertension was the most common comorbidity (23[13.0%]). Among participants, it was reported by 17 of 64 patients (26.6%) aged 18 to 39 years, 25 of 83 patients (30.1%) aged 40 to 64 years, and 13 of 30 patients (43.3%) aged 65 years and older. Overall, there were 49 of 150 outpatients (32.7%), 5 of 16 hospitalized patients (31.3%), and 1 of 21 healthy participants (4.8%) in the control group.[26] It can be also observed that the patients above 40 were mostly involved with post-COVID syndromes.

A bidirectional cohort study of patients with confirmed COVID-19 who had been discharged six months later from Jin Yin-tan Hospital (Wuhan, China) between 7 January 2020, and 29 May 2020 was conducted. 76% of patients (1,265 of 1,655) reported at least one symptom at follow-up and a higher percentage was observed in women. Patients who died before follow-up, patients whom follow-up would be difficult because of psychotic disorders, dementia, or re-admission to hospital, those who were unable to move freely due to concomitant osteoarthropathy or immobile before or after discharge due to diseases such as stroke or pulmonary embolism, those who declined to participate, those who could not be contacted, and those living outside of Wuhan or in nursing or welfare homes were all excluded. All patients were interviewed with a series of questionnaires for evaluation of symptoms and health-related quality of life, underwent physical examinations and a six-minute walking test, and received blood tests. A stratified sampling procedure was used to sample patients according to their highest seven-category scale

---

[26]Jennifer K. Logue, *et al. op. cit.*

Fu Ling *Sclerotium Poriae Cocos* 15 g
For 3-day doses, decocted in water, one dose per day.

Further Treatment:
Third consultation: 21 January 2021.
All three doses of prescription 2 have been taken. He occasionally felt tightness in the chest, sometimes gas reversal coughing, less white sputum, a little breathlessness when going up the stairs, a little loose stool, and had better sleep with good spirits. The tongue coating was obviously improved, the yellow and greasy coating disappeared, only the middle and back part was slightly white and greasy.

Prescription 3:
Zhi Shi *Fructus Immaturus Citri Aurantii* 5 g
Xiang Ru *Herba Elsholtziae seu Moslae* 5 g
(Prefer Ma Huang *Herba Ephedrae* 5 g, but not available due to EU
    regulations)
Bai Jie Zi *Semen Sinapis Albae* 5 g
Zi Su Zi *Fructus Perillae Frutescentis* 5 g
Lai Fu Zi *Semen Raphani Sativi* 5 g
Xing Ren *Semen Pruni Armeniacae* 5 g
Hou Po *Cortex Magnoliae Officinalis* 5 g
Yu Jin *Tuber Curcumae* 5 g
Ju Luo *Citrus tangerina Hort.et Tanaka C.erythrosa Tanaka* 3 g
Jie Geng *Radix Platycodi Grandiflori* 5 g
Ban Xia *Rhizoma Pinelliae Ternatae* 6 g
Chen Pi *Pericarpium Citri Reticulatae* 5 g
Qing Pi *Pericarpium Citri Reticulatae Viride* 5 g
Tao Ren *Semen Pruni Persicae* 5 g
Hong Hua *Flos Carthami Tinctorii* 3 g
Sang Bai Pi *Cortex Mori Albae Radicis* 6 g
Fu Ling *Sclerotium Poriae Cocos* 7 g
Pei Lan *Herba Eupatorii Fortunei* 3 g

They are in concentrated powder granules. Take it three times a day, each time 2 g.

during their hospital stay (as 3, 4, and 5–6), to receive pulmonary function test, high-resolution CT of the chest, and ultrasonography. Enrolled patients who had participated in the Lopinavir Trial for Suppression of SARS-CoV-2 in China received severe acute respiratory syndrome coronavirus 2 antibody tests. Multivariable adjusted linear or logistic regression models were used to evaluate the association between disease severity and long-term health consequences.[27]

A study published in *The Lancet Psychiatry* journal reported that amongst 236,379 patients diagnosed with COVID-19, the estimated incidence of a neurological or psychiatric diagnosis in the following six months was 33.62%(95% CI 33.17–34.07) Almost 13% of these patients had never received a neurological or psychiatric diagnosis before.[28]

It can be seen from above that the percentage of the post-COVID syndrome is around 30% to 34%, six to nine months after the first onset of illness of COVID-19.

9.4 Symptoms

American CDC listed the following symptoms as post COVID conditions,[29] including:

- tiredness or fatigue
- difficulty thinking or concentrating (sometimes referred to as "brain fog")
- headache
- loss of smell or taste
- dizziness on standing
- fast-beating or pounding heart (also known as heart palpitations)

---

[27]Chaolin Huang, *et al. op. cit.*

[28]Maxime Taquet, *et al.* May 2021. *op. cit.*

[29]CDC. Updated 1 September 2021. *op. cit.*

- chest pain
- difficulty breathing or shortness of breath
- cough
- joint or muscle pain
- depression or anxiety
- fever
- symptoms that get worse after physical or mental activities

In the waning phase of the pandemic, beginning on 21 April 2020, the Fondazione Policlinico Universitario Agostino Gemelli IRCCS in Rome, Italy, established a post-acute outpatient service for individuals discharged from the hospital after recovery from COVID-19. All patients who met the World Health Organization criteria for discontinuation of quarantine (no fever for three consecutive days, improvement in other symptoms, and two negative test results for severe acute respiratory syndrome coronavirus 2 [SARS-CoV-2] 24 hours apart) were followed up. At enrollment in the study, real-time reverse transcriptase-polymerase chain reaction for SARS-CoV-2 was performed and patients with a negative test result were included.[30]

It could be concluded that there is a big chance that severity of the symptoms during the acute phase of COVID-19 is almost proportional to the severity of the symptoms during the post COVID-19 phase.

A Chinese team carried out probably the largest cohort study with the longest follow-up duration assessing the health consequences of adult patients discharged from hospital and are recovering from COVID-19.

In total, 1,733 of 2,469 discharged patients (between 7 January 2020 and 29 May 2020) with COVID-19 were enrolled after 736 were excluded. It was found that 76% of patients (1,265 of 1,655) reported at least one symptom at follow-up and a higher percentage

---

[30]Angelo Carfì, *et al.* Persistent symptoms in patients after acute COVID-19. *JAMA.* 2020, 324(6): 603–605. doi: 10.1001/jama.2020.12603.

was observed in women (Appendix, pp. 10–11). The risk of presenting at least one symptom among participants with scale 5–6 was higher than those with scale 3 (OR 2.42, 95% CI 1.15–5.08). The most common symptoms after discharge were fatigue or muscle weakness (1,038[63%] of 1,655) and sleep difficulties (437[26%] of 1,655; Table 2). The risk of an mMRC score greater than 1 was significantly higher in participants with scale 5–6 than those with scale 3 (OR 2.15, 95% CI 1.28–3.59). Full details of the EQ-5D-5L questionnaire are presented in the appendix (pp. 12–13). Participants with scale 5–6 had more problems in mobility, pain or discomfort, and anxiety or depression as compared to those with scale 3 (all $p < 0.05$; Table 2). 23%(367 of 1617) of participants reported anxiety or depression at follow-up, which was more common in women (Appendix, pp. 10–11). Compared with participants with scale 3, participants with scale 5–6 presented with shorter walking distance in meters in six minutes (479.0, IQR 434.0–515.5 vs 495.0, 446.0–542.0) and a higher proportion of less than the lower limit of the normal range (LLN). However, no significant difference was observed for participants with scale 4. The proportion of patients with a median six minutes walking distance less than LLN was 24%(103 of 423) for scale 3, 22%(255 of 1153) for scale 4, and 29%(34 of 116) for scale 5–6. They also have found that fatigue or muscle weakness, sleep difficulties, and anxiety or depression were common, even at six months after symptom onset.[31]

In terms of the situation in Belgium, one of the findings of a joint survey by the University of Hasselt, the Dutch Knowledge Centre Ciro, Maastricht University and the Dutch Lung Foundation. Longfonds published on Saturday, 3 October 2020 says that close to six months after being infected with the new coronavirus (COVID-19), more than one in two patients in Belgium and the Netherlands still have six or more health complaints. Questionnaires were sent to 1,005 Belgian and Dutch patients who contracted the virus. Six months after they were infected, just 5% of patients said they no longer felt any symptoms. On the other hand, 91% said they

---

[31] Chaolin Huang, *et al. op. cit.*

still had more than one symptom. The vast majority (86%) were still very tired 165 days after their first symptoms, while 59% still experienced shortness of breath. 36% often felt pressure on their chests, 35% had headaches, and 40% experienced muscle pain. The overwhelming majority, 94%, were not hospitalized for COVID-19 and only had light symptoms. These were relatively young people, with an average age of 48 years. About 86% of respondents said they had been in good health before their infection and 61% said they had not had any chronic illness before.[32] Again, in Belgium, a study, published on 28 February 2021 and carried out by Hasselt University together with three other institutions has confirmed the phenomenon, in which some 30% of people who contracted COVID-19 but did not have to be hospitalized continue to feel ill months later. Doctors have been hearing complaints from patients regarding long-term effects from the virus. The 210 patients questioned varied in ages, the average age of the group was 44. None had underlying causes. Nearly one in three is still sick three months later to the extent that they cannot work or need help to get through daily activities.[33]

Besides the symptoms mentioned above, there are a lot of manifestations related to post-COVID syndromes, such as sleep disorder, hair loss, paralysis, stroke, Parkinson's disease, addiction to alcohol or drugs, as well as skin rashes, including vesicular, maculopapular, urticarial, or chilblain-like lesions on the extremities (so-called COVID toe), etc. Moreover, the damage that occurred during the application of some therapeutic devices or drugs is also included in the post COVID-19 syndromes. For instance, there is some possible

---

[32]Coronavirus health challenges persist six months after infection. *The Brussels Times.* Updated 3 October 2020. https://www.brusselstimes.com/news/belgium-all-news/134061/coronavirus-health-challenges-persist-six-months-after-infection-covid-19-novel-sars-cov-2-belgium-netherlands/.

[33]Coronavirus in Belgium: Your general questions answered. *The Bulletin,* Updated 28 February 2021. https://www.thebulletin.be/coronavirus-belgium-your-general-questions-answered.

physical damage caused by intensive and persistent use of ventilators and sedatives in ICU patients.

Another obvious fact is that there are likely to be tens of thousands of Long COVID patients suffering in silence, sure or unsure that their symptoms, brain fog to night sweats, are connected to Long COVID-19. The largest peer-reviewed international study of "long-haulers" has found that there are more than 200 symptoms associated with Long COVID, spanning ten organ systems. Published on Thursday 15 July 2021 in *The Lancet's* open-access journal *EClinical Medicine*, the study surveyed nearly 3,800 people online, from 56 countries, with confirmed or suspected Long COVID. The vast majority of participants in the study also suffered relapses of their symptoms, with about 52% saying those relapses occurred in an "irregular pattern" and in response to a specific trigger, such as physical or mental activity and stress. About a third of those surveyed who menstruate also said they experienced a relapse in symptoms before or during menstruation.[34]

The plethora of symptoms affecting multiple systems exhibited by post-COVID syndromes suggests the presence of different underlying mechanisms. Classification of post-COVID syndromes according to different systems are another method, including

9.4.1 Damage to the lungs

They are mainly manifested as shortness of breath when the walking/running pace is fast, unable to exercise normally, and even unable to return to previous work. The possible reason could be due to severe lung infections, which developed into pulmonary fibrosis. Some severely ill patients will develop lung fibers after they are cured, which affects their daily lives. In the late stage, lung transplantation is the only option. Moreover, there is currently no specific medicine for pulmonary fibrosis, and the condition is irreversible.

---

[34]Hannah E. Davis, *et al. op. cit.*

9.4.2 Damage to liver and kidney

It has been pointed out that if people with pre-existing liver diseases like chronic Liver disease, cirrhosis, or related complications contract the SARS-CoV-2 virus, they are at a high risk of complications and fatalities. But this virus itself is a potential cause of liver injury as it causes inflammatory reactions impacting the generalized immunity adversely. The inflammation can cause complications to the heart, liver, and lungs. In case of impact on the lungs, if there is no underlying long-standing liver damage, then the inflammatory reaction due to COVID is usually mild. Several studies show an association between liver damage and some of the medications that doctors are using to treat COVID-19. This is especially true in the case of a drug called Tocilizumab.[35]

Researchers at the Yale Liver Centre in New Haven, CT, analyzed liver tests from 1,827 patients with COVID-19. All patients were admitted to Yale-New Haven Health hospitals between 14 March and 23 April 2020. These tests measure levels of enzymes that the liver releases into the bloodstream when it sustains damage. An analysis of data from China suggests that around 15% of hospitalized COVID-19 patients had abnormal liver test results. However, 42–67% of the patients in the Yale study had abnormal tests upon admission to the hospital, depending on which of two enzymes the tests measured. During hospitalization, these figures rose to 62% and 83%, respectively.[36]

It is not abnormal and not the first time that a virus mainly involving the respiratory tract can also involve the kidney, as it has been already reported during the SARS epidemic in 2003. Studies have pointed out that kidney damage is common in people with new

---

[35]Sushmita Panda. COVID-19 potential cause of liver injury. *The Sunday Guardian Live*. Updated 17 April 2021. https://www.sundayguardianlive.com/news/covid-19-potential-cause-liver-injury.

[36]James Kingsland. COVID-19 liver damage may be more common than previously thought. *The Medical News Today*. Updated 12 August 2020. https://www.medicalnewstoday.com/articles/covid-19-liver-damage-may-be-more-common-than-previously-thought.

COVID-19 infections. The paper *Caution on Kidney Dysfunctions of 2019-nCoV Patients* mentions that 2019-nCoV shares a common cellular mechanism with the severe acute respiratory syndrome-associated coronavirus (SARS-CoV). They surveyed a previous retrospective case study on SARS which showed that acute renal impairment was uncommon in SARS but carried formidably high mortality rate (91.7%, 33 of 36 cases). Here we report an ongoing case study on kidney functions in 59 patients infected by 2019-nCoV (including 28 diagnosed as severe cases and three deaths). 63% (32/51) of the patients exhibited proteinuria, indicative of renal impairment. 19% (11/59) and 27% (16/59) of the patients had an elevated level of plasma creatinine and urea nitrogen respectively. The computerized tomography (CT) scan showed radiographic abnormalities of the kidneys in 100% (27/27) of the patients. Together, these multiple lines of evidence point to the idea that renal impairment is common in 2019-nCov patients, which may be one of the major causes of the illness by the virus infection and may contribute to multi-organ failure and death eventually.[37]

The incidence of acute kidney injury in patients with COVID-19 infection is about 3–15%; and in patients with severe infection requiring care in the intensive care unit, the rates of acute kidney injury increased significantly from 15% to 50%. Acute kidney injury is an independent risk factor for mortality in COVID-19 patients.[38]

Renal failure is a more important issue, which could greatly increase the mortality rate of patients who need dialysis. When the respiratory function is impaired, oxygen exchange is blocked, other organs will be hypoxic, and the kidneys, which are particularly sensitive to oxygen, often suffer severe functional damage. On the other

---

[37]Zhen Li, *et al.* Caution on kidney dysfunctions of 2019-nCoV patients. *The Medrxiv.* Updated 12 February 2020. https://www.medrxiv.org/content/10.1101/202 0.02.08.20021212v1.

[38]Sreedhar Adapa, *et al.* COVID-19 and renal failure: challenges in the delivery of renal replacement therapy. *J Clin Med Res.* 2020, 12(5): 276–285. doi: 10.14740/jocmr41602020.

hand, renal failure could also cause respiratory problem.[39] Other main reasons for acute renal failure include dehydration, lack of nutrition, insufficient water intake, and low effective blood volume, which makes the kidneys more susceptible to damage. In addition, cytokine storms, use of some medications, or hypotension, etc. can all cause renal failure. If this renal sequelae cannot recover within three months, long-term dialysis is required.

9.4.3 Damage to the brain

In addition to the lungs, liver, and kidneys, studies have also found that many recovered patients have very serious central nervous system sequelae. The neurological study of Huazhong University of Science and Technology on hospitalized patients with new coronary pneumonia showed that more than 30% of the 214 patients had neurological symptoms, which were manifested in three categories: One is central nervous system symptoms such as headache, dizziness, disturbance of consciousness, acute cerebrovascular disease, epilepsy, and loss of memory, etc. The second is the symptoms of the peripheral nervous system, such as decreased sense of taste, decreased sense of smell, and neuralgia etc. The third is skeletal muscle injury.

9.4.4 Damage to cardiovascular and cerebrovascular systems

Complications will be more serious for patients with new coronary disease who have been in the ICU, especially those who have been on a ventilator. They are likely to have problems with their lungs, brain, and heart in the future. Thrombosis may also occur, leading to cerebral infarction, pulmonary infarction, and myocardial infarction.

---

[39]Rajit K. Basu, *et al.* Kidney–Lung cross-talk and acute kidney injury. *Pediatric Nephrology*. 2013, 28: 2239–2248. https://link.springer.com/article/10.1007/s00467-012-2386-3.

9.4.5 Damage to gastrointestinal and skin

The Sixth Affiliated Hospital of Sun Yat-Sen University was informed that the team of Professor Lan Ping of the hospital published a study on "gastrointestinal sequelae 90 days after discharge from the hospital in patients with neo-coronary pneumonia" in the sub-journal *Lancet Gastroenterology & Hepatology of The Lancet*. Studies have found that patients with new coronary pneumonia generally have gastrointestinal sequelae after discharge, including anorexia, nausea, acid reflux and diarrhea. The severity of the disease during hospitalization was not associated with gastrointestinal sequelae after discharge. The new coronavirus symptom research team at King's College London collected information on nearly 12,000 patients with suspected or confirmed new coronavirus and skin rashes through online surveys. It was found that among the respondents who tested positive for the new coronavirus, 17% had skin rash as the first symptom, and 21% had skin rash as the only symptom.

Meanwhile, the following summarizations could be presented when facing a post COVID-19 syndrome.

- The manifestation of post-COVID syndrome is not proportional to the severity of symptoms and age.
- The time of the appearance of post-COVID syndrome is not proportional to the severity of symptoms.
- Even if the symptoms are mild or even recovered, there will be post-COVID syndrome.
- Most patients can have more than two symptoms at the same time.
- The damage could be discovered very late, or even undetected at all.

9.5 Treatment in Modern Medicine

Centers for Disease Control and Prevention (CDC), US, points out that post-COVID conditions also can include the longer-term effects of COVID-19 treatment or hospitalization. Some of these longer-term effects are like those related to hospitalization for other respiratory infections or other conditions. Effects of COVID-19 treatment and hospitalization can also include post-intensive care syndrome (PICS), which refers to health effects that remain after a severe illness. These effects can include weakness and post-traumatic stress disorder (PTSD). PTSD involves long-term reactions to a very stressful event.[40]

Understanding, support, and reassurance from primary care are crucial components of rehabilitation management. T Greenhalgh has discussed the procedures to deal with post-COVID syndrome on the *BMJ*:

After excluding serious ongoing complications or comorbidities, and until the results of long-term follow-up studies are available, patients should be managed pragmatically and symptomatically with an emphasis on holistic support while avoiding over-investigation.[41] Fever, for example, may be treated symptomatically with paracetamol or non-steroidal anti-inflammatory drugs. Monitoring functional status in post-acute COVID-19 patients is not yet an exact science. A post COVID-19 functional status scale has been developed pragmatically but not formally validated,[42] though a simplified version of this is reproduced in the supplementary material.

Referral to a specialist rehabilitation service does not seem to be needed for most patients, who can expect a gradual, if sometimes protracted, improvement in energy levels and breathlessness, aided by careful pacing, prioritization, and modest goal setting. In our experience, most but not all patients who were not admitted to the

---

[40]CDC. Updated 1 September 2021. *op. cit.*

[41]Gemelli Against COVID-19 Post-Acute Care Study Group. Post-COVID-19 global health strategies: The need for an interdisciplinary approach. *Aging Clin Exp Res.* 2020, 32(8): 1613–1620. doi: 10.1007/s40520-020-01616-x pmid:32529595.

[42]Klok FA, *et al.* The post-COVID-19 functional status scale: A tool to measure functional status over time after COVID-19. *Eur Respir J.* 2020, 56: 2001494. doi: 10.1183/13993003.01494-2020 pmid:32398306.

hospital recover well with four to six weeks of light aerobic exercise (such as walking or pilates), gradually increasing in intensity to tolerable levels. Those returning to employment may need support to negotiate a phased return.[43]

9.6 General TCM Aspects of Post COVID-19 Syndromes

9.6.1 TCM views on conventional medical managements

- The effectiveness of home isolation and symptomatic treatment after confirmation of COVID-19.
- The guidance of TCM in theory and practice.
- The limitations of TCM symptomatic treatment.
- Possibility of integration of Chinese and Western medicine.

9.6.2 Pathogenesis

- Damage to the lungs

  - The lung controls the qi.
  - The lung disperses the qi and descends the qi.
  - The main propaganda and subduing.
  - The lung opens into the skin.
  - This is the upper source of water.
  - The lung reacts as the Prime Minister in the body.
  - The lung restricts the liver, being the Mother organ of the kidney.

- Effect on qi and blood

  - The lung influences the production, distribution, and circulation of qi and blood.

---

[43] Trisha Greenhalgh, *et al. op. cit.*

- Damage to the organ and tissue

    - The pathogenic changes could cause damage to different zang-fu organs, meridians, tissues, and five sense organs.

9.6.3 Pathogenic features of post-COVID syndromes

- Incomplete elimination of external pathogenic factors.
- Latent pathogenic factors in the body.
- Damage to the zang-fu organs.
- Obstruction of qi and blood circulation.
- Disharmony of the meridians.
- Disturbance to the heart and shen.

9.6.4 Principle of treatment

- Strengthen the zheng-qi and eliminate the pathogens.
- Adjust zang-fu organs.
- Benefit the qi and blood.
- Smooth the meridians.
- Regulate the heart and calm the shen.

9.6.5 Treatment focus

- Treatment based on syndrome differentiation is the foundation of treatment.
- Treatment to restore the physiological functions of the lung in dispersing and descending is the core of the treatment.
- The interaction of five elements should be taken into account.
- The preventive intervention of treatment should be emphasized.
- A combination of herbal treatment and acupuncture and moxibustion is encouraged.

9.6.6 Precautions of the herbal treatment

- Personalized prescription is advised.
- Be careful in using a fixed and standard prescription.

- Prescriptions should be modified according to the reaction of the treatment.
- Climate, geographical location, and disease at different stages should be analyzed.
- Eliminating the pathogenic factors is the main purpose.
- Avoid overly big prescriptions with the various directions of treatment.

9.6.7 Precautions of the acupuncture treatment

- Application of eight confluence points should be emphasized.
- Frequently using yuan-source, front-mu, and back-shu points.
- Skillfully understanding the five-shu theory and their indications.
- The points to calm the shen should be added.
- Attention should be paid to needle manipulations.

10

Meridian Palpation Treatment for COVID-19 and Long COVID Conditions

Meridian palpation is a differential system based on theories from the *Huang Di Nei Jing* (Yellow Emperor's inner classic), *Shang Han Lun* (Discussion of cold-induced disorders) and Nan Jing (Classic of Difficulties), by introducing a quantitative rating method in palpation on points of different meridians to enable precise evaluation on the different degree of connection between different meridians and the key pathology of the patient's main condition. Through clinical experience, this method of differentiation greatly improves clinical results and deepens the practitioner's understanding of the pathology of the disease. It is especially helpful when treating acute emergency or complex and stubborn conditions, for example those presenting with a mixture of exterior and interior, deficiency and excess, and cold and heat pathology. COVID-19, both at its acute and the Long-COVID stage, provides a perfect live example.

10.1 Method of the Meridian Palpation Differentiation

In this method a numerical rating system is used to assess the meridians and obtain differentiation based on the rating of the assessment. The method requires that the therapist applies an even pressure to points along the meridian pathways on both sides of the body, usually the five shu-stream points and other characteristic points relevant to the specific condition of the patient. The points are given by the patient a numerical rating from 0 to 10 according to their sensitivity to pressure. The higher the number is, the more pronounced the pathology association with the meridian in question will be. Pathology is differentiated between the left and right side of the body. The general rules for differentiation are as follows: higher/stronger signs on the left side of the body are the indication of the differentiation for yin, blood, cold, damp and phlegm; the right side of the body are the indication of the differentiation for yang, qi and heat and fire. In addition, hollowness indicates deficiency, while tightness and puffiness indicate excess and stagnation. Following this quantitative rating, the meridian/s that is most associated with the presenting pathology can be identified and the illness can be analyzed.

10.2 Application of Meridian Palpation in COVID-19 Setting

10.2.1 Interrogation

It is useful to find as much information as possible on the affected meridians related to the presenting major symptoms. To achieve this efficiently, we suggest focusing on the following three major aspects.

10.2.1.1 *Location of the relevant main symptom*

The body location where the main symptom presents strongly implies the possible problematic meridian. The meridians passing the relevant location both superficially and interiorly need to be examined.

10.2.1.2 *Features and characteristic patterns of the symptom*

This includes information related to five-element connections: specific onset time associated with aggravation and relief, circumstance for aggravation and relief, preference to warmth or cold, rest or exercises, reaction to pressure, difference between day and night on specific symptoms, or body temperature and sweat, or pain and so on.

10.2.1.3 *Information associated with constitution and overall, eight principle differential diagnosis*

The interrogation therefore shall be extensive to include questions to cover both the states of the six yin organs, and the symptoms related to six yang meridians. Only by a thorough interrogation, can we propose a complete list of meridians for palpation.

10.2.2 Pulse reading

It is to follow the conventional method.

10.2.3 Tongue reading

It is to follow the conventional method.

10.2.4 Inspection of body surface and meridians

It is to inspect the skin changes: color, heap or dip on the affected area and the pathway of relevant meridians. Different colors indicate different nature of illness. White or pale color implies deficiency of blood and qi, red the heat or fire, blue or purple the stagnation of qi or blood. Dip of surface implies the deficiency. Heap of surface implies the excess.

10.2.5 Touching/sensing

It is to touch by checking temperature, sensing texture along the meridians. Sensation by touch can help enforce the understanding of the changes in the local area/meridian. A cold sensation indicates the cold accumulated in the relevant area/meridian, while hot sensation shows the heat stagnation. Puffiness is usually a sign for damp and phlegm accumulation—the thicker, the more severe. Wetness or clamminess indicates the damp or qi deficiency. Smooth and delicate sensation on the surface point, like the Yuan-source point, is usually a sign for deficiency of the relevant yin meridians.

10.2.6 Palpation

It is to sense, by pressing into the points, the resistance and pains, and hollowness of the relevant affected meridian. Take note of the ratings on the sensitivity and hollowness upon pressure on the points if applicable.

10.2.6.1 *Rating of pain/sensitivity upon pressure*

By applying a standard pressure on the meridian to pick up the most painful/sensitive one point on each meridian, we can then ask the patient to rate the sensitivity by number between 0 (no pain) and 10 (most painful), note down in a form of "n/10", and take down the nature of pain upon pressure if applicable.

- A sharp, stabbing pain indicates excess, such as qi stagnation, fire, phlegm, damp, blood stasis, blood heat, or heat-dominated yin deficiency.
- An ache or bruised pain indicates deficiency, especially blood deficiency and yin deficiency, or some cases of qi deficiency or yang deficiency. But severe qi and yang deficiency do not usually present any tenderness or pain, often only with hollowness.
- A bruised pain mixed with sharp pain indicates a mixture of deficiency and excess, very common in clinical signs.

10.2.6.2 *Rating of hollowness upon pressure*

Level of hollowness on the meridian pathway indicates the level of deficiency on relevant meridians/organs. It is often noted in the form of "+", from 1 "+" to 3 "+" s. Changes of meridian hollowness includes the following aspects.

- The opening of the meridian point or the pathway of the meridian becomes widened. In general, the normal diameter of point or width of the meridian path are not wider than the width of an index fingertip. If it is wider than an index fingertip, it is then considered as deficiency. Wider or hollower points on the left side is more of yin and blood deficiency, while the right is more of qi and yang deficiency.

- A dippy or empty meridian path or wide point is rated into three levels, to be noted by "+".

  - +: feels like balloon filled with water, normal.
  - ++: feels like play-dough, medium deficiency.
  - +++: feels like marshmallow, severe deficiency.

10.2.7 Differential diagnosis by meridian palpation

Meridian palpation differentiation is based on the following framework:

- The left body indicates pathology associated with yin and blood, including yin deficiency, blood deficiency or stasis, or cold and damp.
- The right body indicates pathology associated with yang and qi, including yang deficiency, qi deficiency or stagnation, or heat and fire.
- Skin that feels hot to the touch indicates heat; skin that feels cold indicates cold.
- A point that feels hollow/empty to the touch indicates deficiency; a point that is tight and solid indicates excess and stagnation.
- A point that feels puffy or swollen to the touch indicates damp or phlegm.
- A sharp pain indicates blockage or stagnation, and excess, like qi stagnation, fire, phlegm, damp, blood stasis, blood heat etc.
- A bruised or dull ache is a sign for deficiency, like blood deficiency, qi deficiency, or yang deficiency.
- Severe qi or yang deficiency usually presents only hollowness.
- There could be a mixture of all different signs in reality. Signs of both deficiency and excess may be seen at the same time on one point.

10.2.8 Test treatment, conclusion, and formal treatment

By comparing the palpation result between the two sides of body and between different meridians, and by applying the differentiation principle introduced above, we can distinguish the relevance of different meridians to the pathology of the key symptom, to specify the differentiation on the cold-heat, deficiency-excess pattern. In principle, the higher the meridian is rated, the closer relevance it may be to the key pathology. The relevant meridian and points are therefore referred to as the target for treatment, from which it takes us to the next important step: test treatment.

Test treatment is not only a method of treatment but a key method for precise diagnosis. It is to apply acupressure with circular massage in a certain direction, guided by the following four principles on point decision to gain a more in-depth analysis for the final treatment. This is especially useful when there is a complicated condition involving multiple sensitized meridians. It particularly works well in the case that the improvement of a patient's key symptom can be quantitatively measured on site.

10.2.9 Final treatment

Finally, the points that can relieve the symptom with immediate effect through test treatment, are believed to be the closely related ones in association with the pathology of the presenting symptom and are the points to be used for further formal treatment. The differentiation of the condition is thereafter derived from the same result, so is the treatment principle by means of needles, acupoint massage, Guasha, moxibustion or herbal remedy whichever is convenient and applicable.

10.3 Strategy of Meridian Selection and Point Decision

Test treatment serves as the core step of meridian palpation diagnosis, as it provides us with an efficient approach for a precise answer to the direct cause of the key symptoms and promises immediate and effective results from the treatment. Here is a list of points recommended for meridian palpation check, which are most often sensitized according to the clinical observation.

On six yang meridians:

- Bladder meridian: Points from Kunlun BL-60 to Shugu BL-65.
- Gallbladder meridian: Points from Zulinqi GB-41 to Xiaxi GB-43, sometimes Qiuxu GB-40, Yanglingquan GB-34.
- Stomach meridian: Points from Chongyang ST-42 to Neiting ST-44, sometimes Zusanli ST-36, Shangjuxu ST-37, Fenglong ST-40.
- San Jiao meridian: Points from Waiguan SJ-5, Yemen SJ-2 to Zhongzhu SJ-3.
- Large intestine meridian: Points from Quchi L.I.-11, Sanjian L.I.-3 to Hegu L.I.-4, sometime Shousanli L.I.-10.
- Small intestine meridian: Points from Houxi SI-3 to Yanglao SI-6.

On six yin meridians:

- Liver meridian: Points from Xingjian LIV-2 to Taichong LIV-3, Ququan LIV-8, sometimes Ligou LIV-5.
- Spleen meridian: Points from Taibai SP-3 to Gongsun SP-4, Sanyinjiao SP-6, Yinlingquan SP-9, Xuehai SP-10.
- Kidney meridian: Points from Rangu KID-2 to Zhaohai KID-6, Yingu KID-10.
- Lung meridian: Points from Chize LU-5 to Yuji LU-10, sometimes Taiyuan LU-9, Lieque LU-7.
- Heart meridian: Points from Shaohai HE-3, Tongli HE-5 to Shaofu HE-8.
- Pericardium meridian: Points from Quze P-3, Neiguan P-6 to Laogong P-8.
- On secondary pathology: Points from Yinlingquan SP-9, Xuehai SP-10, Fenglong ST-40 to Sanyinjiao SP-6, sometimes Geshu BL-17.

10.3.1 Procedure of test treatment and the point decision

In meridian palpation treatment, the conclusive diagnosis is based on the rating result. In general, the highest rated meridian is believed to be in highest relevance to the key pathology of the patient's main condition. However, in many complicated cases especially with multiple complaints, the highest rated meridian may not be in line with the prime symptom presented. Upon this, the test treatment can provide a more in-depth interpretation on the ratings and provide a better approach for a precise diagnosis. The basic rules for testing by acupressure method is to apply clockwise massage for reducing effect and anti-clockwise massage for strengthening effect. Clockwise massage often applies to conditions of most exterior patterns in yang meridians and excessive patterns in yin meridians. Anti-clockwise massage applies to conditions of interior deficiency with most yin meridians and a few of the yang meridians with nutritive qi deficiency.

To start with the test, we usually select the point on the highest rated meridian to test its effect by doing circular massage in a specific direction according to the presumed differential diagnosis from the initial palpation rating. After massaging the point, ask the patient to report if there is a change in the targeted symptom. Note down the outcome then move on to the second highest rated meridian for the test, repeat the process until the symptom is fully alleviated by the test, or until tests on all possible meridians are completed. A quantitative measurement on the improvement of symptoms is strongly recommended to achieve a precise differentiation efficiently. Here is an example. A patient with Long-COVID presents chest pain and shortness of breath. From meridian palpation, Zulinqi GB-41 on the left is rated 9/10 (implying exterior cold stuck in Gallbladder meridian), Kunlun BL-60 on the left is also 9/10 (implying exterior cold stuck in bladder meridian), Xiangu ST-43 on the right is 8/10 (implying some heat buildup in stomach meridian). It will be very useful if we can choose the accurate meridian(s) for treatment with higher precision, on which the test treatment is valuable to pin-point the target for final treatment. Prior to the start of the test treatment, ask the patient to rate and take down the level of chest pain and shortness of breath by a number out of 10 (in a form of "n/10", pain 8/10, breathing 9/10). Then apply clockwise massage (as a reducing method) on the sensitized point of each meridian by 50 circles respectively on bladder, gallbladder and stomach meridian. After massaging each point, ask the patient to measure the chest pain level and difficulty level of breathing and note down the number by 1–10. The result with a confirmed reduction of measurement number on symptoms is deemed as effective. In the end, Zulinqi GB-41 is the most effective point to relieve the both symptoms by dropping the pain to 4/10 and breathing to 3/10, Xiangu ST-43 helps some chest pain by dropping to 1/10, while Kunlun BL-60 holds the least effect for both symptoms. We then decide to use GB and ST meridians as the treatment target despite bladder meridian showing a highest rating.

10.3.2 The four main principles for point selection on test treatment

The purpose of test treatment is to provide a shifting approach in order to precisely allocate the meridian in direct relevance to the pathology of the presented symptom. These four principles in test treatment are to be followed as below.

10.3.2.1 *Principle 1: No pain, no treatment*

The highly sensitive point is usually the most efficient point for diagnosis as well as treatment. For most cases, select the highest rated point(s) to start with the test treatment. However, this principle must apply only to the most relevant point in pathology. Sometimes the less sensitive meridian point may be selected, in the case that the highest rated point does not show significant effect. Obviously, the latter can only be applied after testing on the highest one initially. Reducing or enforcing methods are applied for points accordingly in association with differentiation of the symptom.

10.3.2.2 *Principle 2: No hollowness, no treatment*

This principle applies mainly to the hollowness of the six yin meridians. However, in some chronic and relapsing cases the yang meridians may be included too. Rating of "++" and above is deemed as the positive sign for diagnosis of deficiency. Only select the point with positive

"++" and above that is believed in direct relation to the pathology of the targeted symptom. The hollowness and high sensitivity on one point may present together (for example yin deficiency) although they shall be separately considered. In many cases, this principle is in concert with principle 4: "If there is no effect on sensitized point, balance on its coupled meridian". This refers to a situation when testing on the yang meridian does not show satisfactory results, turning to its corresponding yin meridian may secure a better effect. Method on the hollow point usually is enforced by anti-clockwise massage.

10.3.2.3 *Principle 3: No response/effect no treatment*

Effectiveness is the ultimate purpose for point decision. If the stimulation on the point does not prove effective for the targeted symptom, the point will be taken as irrelevant to the final treatment. By comparison on the quantifiable measurement on level of severity of the relevant symptom before and after the test treatment, this method can greatly enhance a precise identification on the potential pathology of the illness in relation to the meridians. The following fundamental test treatment procedure demonstrates exactly what principle 3 aims to achieve.

- Step one: Ask the patient to rate the symptom to be measured in the test treatment beforehand, then select highly sensitized points to apply clockwise massage on points of yang meridians (in most of the cases) or anti-clockwise on the yin meridians with deficiency. Note that some special points on yin meridians may be treated by clockwise massage, depending on the point's nature and function (for example those aiming to clean heat (ying-spring point of the meridian), move blood (Xuehai SP-10) or reduce damp (Yinlingquan SP-9)).
- Step two: Give up on the point if no effect/response was achieved after the test massage. Carry on the procedure on the second rated point and so on, until the point(s) that brings on major immediate improvement is found. Complete the whole process on all possible meridians till the symptom is reduced by as much as possible (usually until a drop in rating of the symptom to under 2/10 is

achieved). At the end, only select the points with good response for final treatment and give up on the points that do not have a positive reaction in the test.

10.3.2.4 *Principle 4: If there is no effect on the sensitized point, balance on its coupled meridian*

This principle involves a very important up-ladder approach in meridian palpation treatment following the principle 3, that gives a further resolution to the condition that a seemingly relevant point does not have satisfactory effect.

This principle in practice refers to two situations:

- When there is a sensitized point on a meridian (usually the yang meridian), but the improvement of targeted symptom is not satisfactory from working on it, then switch to balance/stimulate on the relevant coupled meridian (usually by strengthening the corresponding yin meridian). This can often improve the treatment effect to a greater extent.
- When there is no apparent sensitized point on the meridian that is believed to be closely-related to the pathology of the targeted symptom by differentiation, strengthening on its coupled yin meridian can usually help increase the effect immediately. This quite often happens in the case that the qi within a yang meridian is too weak to present a raised sensitivity on the point. Therefore, instead of working on the low sensitivity yang meridian, strengthen the coupled yin meridian. By giving rise to the qi of the yin meridian, the qi level of the yang meridian will be stronger too. The increase of qi improves the targeted symptom consequently. The yin meridian point is taken for formal treatment then.

In summary, a successful meridian palpation treatment relies on a well-organized interrogation, careful tongue reading and in-depth pulse reading, following the guidance of meridian selection to make a list of potential meridians in relevance to the key symptoms of the patient. Then, through the thorough meridian palpation procedure by the four principles of point decision, finally choose the right points for a formal treatment. A fast-acting, profoundly effective, and reliable treatment will be secured.

10.4 Understanding COVID-19 by Meridian Palpation

10.4.1 COVID-19 infection and its complexity in view of meridian palpation system

Although versatile in presenting symptoms, the COVID-19 associated conditions are viewed through the viewpoint of meridian palpation as a holistic system by a much deeper and wider insight. COVID-19 associated conditions can provide a much deeper and wider understanding.

10.4.1.1 *The disease has a logical line of development in TCM understanding*

This is an exterior condition initially involving yang meridians, which then develops internally under the influence of constitution dominated by interior yin organs expressed on yin meridians. Its prognosis and recovery are also affected by the secondary pathological result that involves damp, phlegm, blood stasis etc. Therefore, a complete reading over the pathology of COVID-19 associated illnesses shall be composed of these three elements: yang meridian illness, yin meridian illness, and secondary pathology.

10.4.1.2 *Yang meridians are believed to be more related to the immunity function of the body*

Based on its nature of five elements, each yang meridian has different susceptibility toward the EPFs. In summary, bladder meridian is more prone to cold, gallbladder meridian more to wind, stomach meridian more to damp, small intestine meridian more to heat, large intestine meridian more to heat-induced dryness. Once the EPFs (which normally starts with cold) invades into the yang meridians it then follows a route of Taiyang-Shaoyang-Yangming, progresses further into the body, and finally settles into the yin organs (Ling Shu Spirit, Axis Chapter 76, Wei Qi Xing, *The Movement of Defensive qi*). The raised sensitivity of points on relevant yang meridians gives answers to the success of diagnosis and treatment.

10.4.1.3 *The state of qi-blood-yin-yang*

The state of qi-blood-yin-yang within the interior yin organs (internal constitution) determines the strength of ying/nutritive-qi and wei/defensive qi in the yin meridian and its relevant coupled yang meridian, and therefore influences their susceptibility to the EPFs. A weak yin organ can make the progress from the invasion into exterior yang meridian much more severe and challenging. The raised sensitivity or hollowness on points of the yin meridians is the key for success of diagnosis and treatment.

10.4.1.4 *The pathological product*

The pathological products including damp, phlegm, blood stasis, commonly as the consequence from a prolonged process of the infection, are also the factors to greatly affect the recovery quality of the post-stage. Treatment toward these will help improve the progress of recovery (of course based on a strong and substantial foundation of the constitution of qi, blood, yin and yang within the internal organs). A precise differentiation on the complicated pathology (for example between phlegm or damp, blood heat or blood stasis, damp-heat or damp-cold), can be distinguished by comparison on the sensitivity of different points between different meridians and between the left and right sides of the body.

10.4.2 Interpretation on common clinical presentations of COVID-19 infection and diagnostic advice on meridian palpation

The common symptoms discussed here came from the list from NHS website (https://www.nhs.uk/conditions/coronavirus-covid-19/

long-term-effects-of-coronavirus-long-covid/). The relevant analysis and suggestion here provide the readers a wider range view on where to check for the most possible meridians for a more profound differentiation. The overall principle on selecting the point for treatment is finding a pronounced point that is highly sensitive in palpation and effective in test treatment. This is the point to be used in treatment. In meridian palpation treatment with meridian palpation differentiation, there is not such a point that is "useful in theory" or "said to be magical". The point to be selected must be highly sensitive and/or highly effective in test treatment. Therefore, there is no fixed formula for treatment point selection for any conditions we discuss in this chapter. In this sense, instead of giving individual advice on points for each of the listed conditions, we mainly focus on the explanation of relevant pathology in relation to individual meridians. During the differential procedure, the test treatment is highly recommended for cases where symptoms are present and treatment outcome can be measured instantly. In cases with symptoms that do not present at the time of consultation or have non-applicable test treatment, a treatment strategy under the differentiation derived from the rating of sensitivity and hollowness on individual meridians shall then be followed.

10.4.2.1 *Fatigue*

- Yang meridian illness: Consistent disturbance on any yang meridians as a result from the external invasion of virus and the continuous fighting state due to the disturbance within the yang meridians can be a key factor that exhausts and depletes the body. Therefore, all three yang meridians shall be checked. Diagnosis on these patterns is straightforward. The highly sensitized points on relevant meridians are the direct evidence for the diagnosis.

- Yin meridian illness: Because of the depleting impairment from the infection, it is understandable to see overall energy decline within the body, especially with the yin organs. The most important thing is to identify which organ is the leading one that was most affected by the virus and needs immediate treatment so that we can help speed up and support the recovery of the body. Among all the yin organs, the spleen, lung, heart and kidney are the most common organs to be affected. Their meridians hence need palpation check.

- Secondary pathology: Damp is the most possible factor of secondary pathology to cause tiredness. Besides, Fenglong ST-40 may be sensitive when there is phlegm pathology.

10.4.2.2 *Shortness of breath, chest pain or tightness*

- Yang meridian: Shaoyang, gallbladder and San Jiao meridians, are the most common yang meridians related to chest and breathing function. To confirm the diagnosis, be aware of other characteristic symptoms of Shaoyang syndrome. Yangming, stomach and large intestine meridians may also affect breathing, considering their meridian connection to the chest, but with more digestive symptoms like stomach pain or acid reflux or constipation etc. Taiyang, bladder meridian may affect the chest and breathing function by restricting muscles on the upper back, causing shortness of breath and tightness of chest or pain.
- Yin meridian: Taiyin, lung meridian, are directly related to the chest and breathing function. Spleen, liver, heart, kidney, and pericardium meridians pass the chest either internally or externally on the chest cage, and therefore may contribute to the restriction of movement of chest cage or the breathing function.
- Secondary pathology: Damp, fluid-yin, phlegm are the most common factors to be related to the pathology. Yinlingquan SP-9 is the diagnostic point for damp and fluid-yin, Fenglong ST-40 is the one for phlegm. Key to success in diagnosis and treatment is to find the high sensitivity on points and work accordingly.

10.4.2.3 *Brain fog*

The problem with memory and concentration is believed to do with the reduced function of the Brain. But in TCM pathology within the meridian palpation system, the blockage of meridians or weakness of meridians leading to failure to transport sufficient qi, blood and essential nutrients into the head can both cause symptoms like memory loss or brain fog. All meridians linking the head superficially or internally can play a role in it.

- Yang meridians: All Yang meridians travel onto the head. Different Yang meridians may differ in accompanied symptoms, but meridian palpation with quantifiable rating on relevant points increases the accuracy of differentiation.
- Yin meridians: Shaoyin kidney meridian has branches joining the Du channel and entering the brain, and therefore affects the ability of clear thinking, memory, and concentration. Taiyin spleen meridian is responsible for lifting clear-qi to the head to support the functions of all sense-orifices. Deficiency of spleen or kidney or blockage on their meridians can lead to declining function of the brain. Jueyin liver meridian goes to the vertex of head, and headaches with vision disturbance or vomit may happen with the Jueyin associated pathology. However when compared to the Shaoyin and Taiyin meridians, the chance of foggy and concentration with liver meridian is less. Differentiation depends on the sensitivity increase on relevant meridians and test treatment can help clarify directly.
- Secondary pathology: Phlegm and damp are sticky forms of body fluid and is a pronounced consequence with COVID-19 infection, because of spleen and lung impairment. When the accumulation of these blocks the pathway of clear qi into the brain to affect the transmissions of the nerve system, the memory, concentration difficulty, or even more severe psycho-neurological conditions like delirium may arise.

10.4.2.4 *Difficulty sleeping*

Insomnia presents in different patterns including the difficulty to fall asleep, shallow, and frequently broken sleep, early waking, dream disturbed sleep. Despite the diversity of clinical presentations, overall pathology of sleeplessness is a state of disturbed shen and hun. Any factor that causes shen and/or hun to be over-excited or unsettled, will cause insomnia. The relevant meridian signs detectable by meridian palpation routine serve as the confirming evidence for a conclusion. The meridian palpation differentiation enables us to efficiently figure out which is the closest problematic meridian associated with the disturbance of shen and hun and of course guides us to treat accordingly.

- Yang meridians: Shaoyang San Jiao and gallbladder meridian are respectively in charge of the time between 9:00–11:00am and 11:00pm–1:00am, when the shen is supposed to switch off for sleep. People having difficulty falling asleep around the time, is highly possible having excess heat or other pathological disturbance within the two meridians. It is important to point out that Shaoyang pathology is usually related to acute insomnia, due to their immediate connection to shen and hun. Yangming stomach and large intestine meridian with acute heat may disturb sleep and mental state by stirring up heart fire via meridian connection. Stomach deficiency, paired with SP meridian, although not directly related to shen or hun, serve as a key role in maintaining profound sleep. Zusanli ST-36 and Sanyinjiao SP-6 are usually selected for chronic insomnia with apparent spleen and heart blood deficiency featuring shallow and early waking sleep.
- Yin meridians: Heart, liver, pericardium and kidney meridians are closely related to shen and hun. The differentiation and selection of points for treatment depend on the sensitivity of points on individual meridians. The higher the sensitivity, the closer the relation to insomnia pathology.
- Secondary pathology: Phlegm, and blood stasis shall be considered. Apart from the increased sensitivity on Fenglong ST-40 and Xuehai SP-10, Geshu BL-17, we also look for characteristic signs on tongue and pulse for diagnostic reference.

10.4.2.5 *Heart palpitations*

We shall be aware that the palpitation is not limited to the pathology of heart only. From the viewpoint of meridian palpation, any meridian that passes by or is linked to the heart or pericardium can all play a role in the occurrence of palpitation if it is in trouble.

- Yang meridians: Shaoyang gallbladder and San Jiao meridians both pass the diaphragm and connect to heart or pericardium via various levels of connection. In addition, the gallbladder and San Jiao meridians are paired with liver and pericardium meridians, and both are closely linked to emotional disturbance. Thus, palpitation along with unsettled emotions, like panic, anxiety, depression, or frustration, could indicate the possibility of gallbladder and San Jiao meridians. Also, divergent of Yangming stomach meridian connects to the heart, and therefore may affect the heart's function to cause palpitation.
- Yin meridians: Shaoyin heart, kidney meridians both have connection with the heart, and directly affect the function of heart. Jueyin liver meridian by meridian connection to Jueyin pericardium, through diaphragm and rib side, can cause tightness of chest and breathing problems too. It usually presents with stress or frustration associated causes.
- Secondary pathology: Phlegm and blood stasis serve as the pronounced pathology factors after a long period of suffering or following a critical phase of severe illness, which involves complex or prolonged treatments.

10.4.2.6 *Dizziness*

It reflects the impairment related to body balancing. In meridian palpation system, look for the connections to affect the neck, inner ears, and eyeball movement, by which the blockage or impairment of the relevant meridian(s) leads to muscle spasm or weakening, yin-fluid or phlegm retention, accumulation of inflammation, or disorders of blood supply into the brain. Overall, any meridian that travels to the head, connects to eyes, and ears, and reaches the neck may all have a potential to disturb the body balancing function. In addition, although not as often, vertigo may occur with COVID-19 infection, the understanding of pathology and treatment are similar.

- Yang meridian: All three yang meridians can have a play in the pathology and need full meridian palpation check.
- Yin meridian: All yin meridians do not reach the head by their own main pathways. They link to head by the divergent paths linking their pairing yang meridians. Among the three Yin meridians Jueyin liver meridian joins the Du mai reaching the vertex of head, via internal connection to the back of eyes. Liver pathology is the most common yin meridian associated with dizziness, which is often interpreted as "hypertension" and so on. Shaoyin kidney meridian joins Du mai along the spine into the brain, pathology of kidney therefore can incur brain illnesses like dizziness, however usually with a more chronic and deficient setting.
- Secondary pathology: When phlegm and damp blocks the "clear orifices" (清窍 Qing-qiao), the spleen is not able to transport the clear yang/qi to support the function of head and brain, and protect it from attacks by wind, causing dizziness. This is from the same origin as "brain fog" of Taiyin spleen deficiency and damp-phlegm root.

10.4.2.7 *Pins and needles*

The symptom of pins and needles is usually a sign reflecting the insufficiency of qi and blood within the relevant meridians. All three yang and three yin meridians, damp and phlegm or blood stasis could all act as the possible cause. Regarding the pins and needles with fingers and toes, a definition on which tendino-muscular channel (Jing-jin 经筋) is responsible for which fingers/toes are relevant to allocate the meridian in trouble. The tendino-muscular channel of each meridian system is a wider area to cover the muscles and tendons on the body. We often find that the corresponding areas of each individual meridian system is cross-lapping with the neighboring meridians.

10.4.2.8 *Joint pain*

The COVID-19 infection is a trigger that stirs up inflammation in association with auto-immune disorders all over the body. Therefore, not only joints are attacked, but all body parts can be affected. Because the immunity disorder apparently involves more yang meridian disturbance, all yang meridians in principle need palpating check. One important fact is that the involved yang meridians are not only limited to the ones nearest to the affected joint or muscles (especially in those cases with multiple locations of pains), considering this is a systematic disorder. The best treatment result comes from the right selection of meridian(s) with the highest sensitivity. A good test treatment procedure will help increase the efficacy and accuracy of the treatment, and requires testing the effect of associated yang meridian on joints and its corresponding yin meridian. If there are noticeable signs of swelling or deformity on the relevant joint(s), we also need to investigate the causes of damp, phlegm, and blood stasis. Obviously, the sensitivity rating on the corresponding points for these pathologies will enable us to make clear conclusions efficiently.

10.4.2.9 *Depression and anxiety*

People with post-viral syndrome often suffer from depression and anxiety long after the subsidence of the infection. Being different states of emotional disorder, they are generally believed to be related to the disturbance of heart shen. However, it is worth mentioning that any factor to cause disturbance or weakening of any spirits associated with five yin organs (Shen-Hun-Po-Yi-Zhi), can lead to the changes of pattern of rational thinking and proper emotional expression. The thought shall not be constricted to the fixed stereotype of diagnostic patterns. Exploration into yang meridian, yin meridian patterns and secondary pathology will prove to be more effective.

- Yang meridian: Since Shaoyang gallbladder meridian is linking the liver, and Shaoyang San Jiao meridian linking the pericardium, these two meridians are the most common yang meridians associated with emotional disorders. In addition, Yangming stomach and large intestine meridians do not directly cause emotional disorders, but their meridian distribution can lead to chest or stomach discomfort such as tightening or butterfly feeling of upper abdomen, which can be conceived as some anxiety associated experience. Wind-cold attacking Yangming and Taiyang can also cause tiredness. In some severe cases, this can present as over-whelming sleepiness and struggling to wake up in the morning, which can be confusing as a feature of depression.

- Yin meridian: Shaoyin heart and kidney meridians contribute directly to the disorders of heart-shen. Jueyin liver meridian directly affects the liver-hun. Jueyin PC meridian, due to its special role in direct connection with the heart, liver and kidney Ming-men, is usually in the cross-over position to reflect either one or all of the three organs' pathology. To reach a precise differentiation for following treatment, the diagnosis usually falls on the highest rated meridian among liver, heart, kidney and pericardium meridians.
- Secondary pathology: As mentioned in previous discussion, damp and phlegm may cause brain-fog or exhaustion, which may be conceived as depression. In severe cases, blood stasis may play a part too.

10.4.2.10 *Tinnitus and earaches*

The conditions related to ears are very much closely affected by the meridians nearby the ears. All three yang meridians have a connection to the ears, among which the Shaoyang Gallbladder and San Jiao and Taiyang small intestine meridians are the closest ones. However, in many cases, Yangming large intestine and stomach meridians can also play a key role, because their meridian connections affect the lower jaw and stern-cleido-mastoid muscle. Taiyang bladder merid-ian has its tendino-muscular channel spreading behind the ears, and therefore can cause tension on the cervical spine then further affect ears too. While all the yin meridians interact with their coupled yang meridians, in many cases when the yang meridian has weaker effect in test treatment, it could be very helpful to adjust the coupled yin meridian, by which the ear problem may be further improved. Among all the six pairs of meridians, Jueyin liver + Shaoyang gallbladder and Shaoyin kidney + Taiyang bladder, Taiyin lung + Yangming large intestine meridians are the most common meridian pairs that cause ear problems.

The secondary pathology like phlegm and damp/yin-fluid, can also play a part in the occurrence of tinnitus and earache, but they always serve as accompanying factors. The inclusion of the relevant points in treatment for ears relies on strictly whether stimulation on the point shows a definite effect through the test treatment.

10.4.2.11 *Feeling sick, diarrhea, stomach aches, loss of appetite*

These symptoms are closely related to digestive function. The solution to these symptoms is to investigate what meridians pass the surface and inside of the abdomen. For yang meridians, stomach, large intestine, gallbladder and San Jiao meridians travel past the stomach, and the large intestine, small intestine, San Jiao and gallbladder meridians also reach the Intestines. For yin meridians, the lung meridian starts from middle Jiao stomach, then reaches down to large intestine. Heart, liver, kidney, and spleen meridians also have connections with stomach and intestines. Damp associated point Yinlingquan SP-9 may be highly active in these cases. The efficiency for a precise diagnosis relies on the test treatment by the yang-yin meridian pairing order. The point that reduces the symptom is used for treatment and the pathology this point represents is hereof considered as the differential pattern.

10.4.2.12 *A high temperature, cough, headache, sore throat, change to sense of smell or taste*

Although these symptoms do not hold significance for precise diagnosis, they can still provide clues for possible problematic meridians. The high temperature reflects the disorders of all yang meridians. Therefore all three yang meridians should be checked on patients with high temperature. The most common meridians that can cause cough and sore throat are those passing the throat and chest, therefore Shaoyang gallbladder, San Jiao, Yangming large intestine, stomach, and lung, heart, liver, kidney, and spleen meridians need to be checked. The meridians that reach the head can all cause headaches, although the affected area may vary according to the pathways of relevant meridians. The most widely accepted guidance for allocating the meridian regarding headache area, is that the forehead headache is related to Yangming, temporal headache Shaoyang and back and top of headache Taiyang. However, this guidance is not adequate to cover the precise distribution of the meridian route and sometimes leads to false judgement. For example, the Taiyang bladder meridian starts from the inner corner of eyes and the beginning of the eyebrows then up over the forehead to reach the vertex of head. Therefore, center-front headache may be related to the BL meridian. Same idea applies to gallbladder meridian as the Yangbai GB-14 stays above the eyebrow on forehead, the front headache above eyebrows can be related to the gallbladder meridian, and not strictly exclusive to the Yangming. Vice versa, Yangming stomach and large intestine meridians reach the corner of the forehead across to the temporal area. When there is little effect by using the Shaoyang meridian point to treat temporal headache, we shall consider the Yangming meridians. The selection of meridian and point follows the similar principle as that for brain fog or memory loss and even emotional disorders like anxiety and depression.

10.4.2.13 *Skin rashes*

Unlike the general impression that considers skin diseases as "blood-heat", a precise differentiation by meridian palpation enables us to look more deeply and widely into the actual pathology of skin disorders. The COVID-19 associated skin rashes can occur on any stage of the infection, and therefore may involve all yin and yang meridians.

- Yang and yin meridian illness: Taiyang bladder meridian usually is related to wind-cold attack. When damp-cold dominates the condition, it usually reflects as the involvement of Yangming stomach meridian, featuring the blisters and discharges on skin lesions. The damp cold condition can linger and develop deeper into Taiyin spleen either as an initial or following factor. When heat dominates the condition, it usually represents the involvement of Yangming large intestine meridian. When large intestine pathology develops deeper, it then can enter Taiyin lung, Shaoyin heart and kidney or Jueyin liver and pericardium depending on the severity of yin being depleted. Involvement of Shaoyang gallbladder and San Jiao meridians, according to my personal observation, is often an indicator for auto-immune disorders. Meridian sensitivity rating provides accuracy on differential diagnosis.

• Secondary pathology: Damp-heat or cold, blood-heat or blood stasis, and phlegm can all play a role at different stages of the illness, however usually not at the earliest.

All in all, through the analysis on the possible pathology of COVID-19 and its connection with individual meridians and characteristic points, the outline framework here on differential diagnosis by meridian palpation can enable practitioners to comprehend deeper on the occurrence, development, and prognosis of COVID-19, and therefore achieve more efficient success in treatment.

10.5 Case Study

Female, age 52, office clerk.
Chief complaints: Chest oppression and shortness of breath for 12 months.
First consultation: 2 March 2021.

This lady started having breathing difficulties and chest symptoms following the COVID-19 infection in March 2020. She suffers from constant chest tightness with difficulty of breathing (which gets worse when inhaling), wakened by the shortness of breath and chest pain several times a night. Chest X-ray exams did not indicate anything positive in her lung. Other symptoms include constant fatigue, brain fog, headache all over the head, dull ache in ears, dry and rough feeling in eyes, morning sneezing and running nose, mucus and phlegm in throat, poor memory and concentration, and dry mouth. Tongue: puffy with teeth marks and light purple in color, white greasy coating, and sublingual veins are not obvious.

Result of meridian palpation rating:

Yang Meridian:
- GB: Zulinqi GB-41, L=R 8/10; ST: Chongyang ST-42, L=R 8/10; SJ: Waiguan SJ-5, L=R 7/10.
- Yin meridian, LU: Chize LU-5, L=R 6/10; LIV: Taichong LIV-3, L=R 9/10; KID: Zhaohai KID-6, L=R 9/10; P: Quze P-3, L=R 8/10.
- Secondary pathology, Yinlingquan SP-9, R 9/10; Fenglong ST-40, L=R 8/10.

TCM Diagnosis:
- Invasion of wind-cold on Shaoyang and Yangming, with some heat conversion.
- Formation of deficient heat in the liver, kidney and pericardium.
- Accumulation of damp-heat and phlegm-heat.

Test Treatment Procedure:
A pre-treatment rating of 8/10 for the prime symptom (breathlessness and chest oppression) is noted, carried out the following steps, and asked to re-rate after each step.

1. Reduce (clockwise massage) on Zulinqi GB-41, breathing better 7/10.
2. Enforce (anticlockwise massage) on Taichong LIV-3, breathing no change.
3. Reduce on Taichong LIV-3, breathing 6/10.
4. Enforce on Taixi KID-3, breathing 5/10.
5. Reduce on Quze P-3, breathing 5/10, but start spitting phlegm.
6. Reduce on Waiguan SJ-5, breathing 4-5/10, but pulsating on ear and head.
7. Reduce on Quchi L.I.-11, breathing 3/10.
8. Enforce on Chize LU-5, no change but triggered more phlegm, shaking hands with numbness on fingers.
9. Reduce on Chize LU-5, breathing 2/10.
10. Reduce on Yinlingquan SP-9, no change.
11. Reduce on Fenglong ST-40, breathing 0-1/10.

Explanations:
The result of the test treatment exactly reflects a clear picture of the pathology:

- Yang meridian, blockage of cold and heat in gallbladder, San Jiao, large intestine meridians.
- Yin meridians, stagnation on liver, lung, with deficiency of kidney-yin.
- Secondary pathology, phlegm accumulation.

Therefore, a self-treatment plan by acupressure is given to the patient:

- Enforcing on Taixi KID-3, reducing methods on Taichong LIV-3 and Chize LU-5.
- Reducing on Fenglong ST-40.
- Reducing on Quchi L.I.-11, Waiguan SJ-5, Zulinqi GB-41.

The patient feedback's the next morning stated: the breathing difficulty subsided before bedtime straight after the massage, a "miracle" since she fell ill. She felt so much better.

After about a total of four months of acupressure self-treatment, we are pleased to see that the patient has achieved about 80% recovery, and she is not suffering from night chest oppression when going to bed or waking up with chest pain anymore. After 16 months on sick leave, she is now going back to work, and regained her confidence and hope for a normal life as was taken for granted before the illness.

11

TCM Treatment of Long COVID

11.1 Fatigue

As millions of patients have been infected by SARS-CoV-2 virus, a vast number of individuals complain about some continuing symptoms even months after the onset of the infection. During Long COVID, concern has been raised that SARS-CoV-2 has the potential to trigger a post-viral fatigue syndrome. Fatigue is a normal part of the body's physiological reaction and response to fighting a viral infection such as COVID-19. Fatigue is likely to continue for some time, e.g., a couple of weeks, after the infection has cleared. Fatigue could make the patients sleep more, feel unsteady on the feet, make standing for long periods difficult, as well as affect the ability to remember and concentrate.

There are various main complaints during Long COVID (fatigue is one of them) and the quality of life could be markedly affected by fatigue. It usually appears in combination with shortness of breath, and insomnia. Besides, fatigue significantly impacts the depression scale. In this way, fatigue may identify a group worthy of further study and early intervention.

A study published in the *Journal of the American Medical Association* found that of 143 COVID-19 patients at a hospital in Rome, 87% still had at least one coronavirus symptom two months later, while more than half reported ongoing fatigue.[1] In terms of

---

[1] Ashley Zlatopolsky. Can chronic fatigue syndrome be treated? Rochester-based doctor is trying to find an answer. *The Detroit News.* 30 November 2020. https://eu.detroitnews.com/story/life/2020/11/30/rochester-based-doctors-research-links-chronic-fatigue-syndrome-covid-19/6462044002/.

persistent fatigue following SARS-CoV-2 infection and its relationship with the severity of initial infection, some research confirmed that fatigue following SARS-CoV-2 infection is common and independent of the severity of initial infection. This study examined the prevalence of fatigue in individuals who recovered from the acute phase of COVID-19 illness using the Chalder Fatigue Score (CFQ-11). The research further examined potential predictors of fatigue following COVID-19 infection, evaluating indicators of COVID-19 severity, markers of peripheral immune activation and circulating pro-inflammatory cytokines. Out of the 128 participants (49.5 ± 15 years; 54% female), more than half reported persistent fatigue (67/128; 52.3%) at a median of 10 weeks after initial COVID-19 symptoms. There was no association between COVID-19 severity (need for in-patient admission, supplemental oxygen, or critical care) and fatigue following COVID-19. Additionally, there was no association between routine laboratory markers of inflammation and cell turnover (leukocyte, neutrophil or lymphocyte counts, neutrophil-to-lymphocyte ratio, lactate dehydrogenase, C-reactive protein) or pro-inflammatory molecules (IL-6 or sCD25) and fatigue post-COVID. Females and those with a pre-existing diagnosis of depression/anxiety were over-represented in those with fatigue. The findings demonstrate a significant burden of post-viral fatigue in individuals with previous SARS-CoV-2 infection after the acute phase of COVID-19 illness. This study highlights the importance of assessing those recovering from COVID-19 for symptoms of severe fatigue, irrespective of the severity of initial illness.[2]

There are striking similarities to myalgic encephalomyelitis, also called chronic fatigue syndrome, that are linked to viral and autoimmune pathogenesis. In both disorders, neurotransmitter receptor antibodies against ß-adrenergic and muscarinic receptors may play a key role. One study found similar elevation of these autoantibodies in both patient groups. Extracorporeal apheresis using a special filter

---

[2] Liam Townsend, *et al.* Persistent fatigue following SARS-CoV-2 infection is common and independent of severity of initial infection. *PLOS ONE.* 2020, 15(11): e0240784. https://doi.org/10.1371/journal.pone.0240784.

seems to be effective in reducing these antibodies in a significant way, clearly improving the debilitating symptoms of patients with chronic fatigue syndrome. Therefore, such form of neuropheresis may provide a promising therapeutic option for patients with post-COVID syndrome.[3] However, this method is not yet well accepted everywhere in the hospital.

As to the treatment to combat fatigue during Long COVID, there are no concrete medications available at this moment, other than life cases, such as to avoid going for intense workouts, ensuring following a proper sleep cycle, having a nutritious diet, hydrating sufficiently and having a proper sleep, etc.

11.1.1 TCM understanding of Long COVID associated fatigue

A significant proportion of COVID-19 patients are suffering from prolonged Post-COVID-19 Fatigue Syndrome, with characteristics typically found in Myalgic Encephalomyelitis/Chronic Fatigue Syndrome (ME/CFS). One researcher tried to demonstrate a clear pathophysiological explanation for the patients suffering from prolonged Post-COVID-19 Fatigue Syndrome. A novel paradigm for Post-COVID-19 Fatigue Syndrome is developed from a recent unifying model for ME/CFS. SARS-CoV-2, in common with the triggers (viral and non-viral) of ME/CFS, is proposed to be a physiologically severe stressor, which could be targeting a stress-integrator within the Brain: the hypothalamic paraventricular nucleus (PVN). It is proposed that inflammatory mediators, released at the site of COVID-19 infection, would be transmitted as stress-signals via humoral and neural pathways, which overwhelm this stress center. In genetically susceptible people, an intrinsic stress threshold is suggested to have exceeded, causing ongoing dysfunction to the hypothalamic PVN's complex neurological circuitry. In this compromised state, the hypothalamic

---

[3] Stefan R. Bornstein, *et al.* Chronic post-COVID-19 syndrome and chronic fatigue syndrome: Is there a role for extracorporeal apheresis? *Mol Psychiatry.* 2022, 27: 34–37. https://doi.org/10.1038/s41380-021-01148-4.

PVN might then be hypersensitive to a wide range of life's ongoing physiological stressors. This could result in the reported post-exertional malaise episodes and more severe relapses, in common with ME/CFS, that perpetuate an ongoing disease state. When a certain stress tolerance level is exceeded, the hypothalamic PVN can become an epicenter for microglia-induced activation and neuroinflammation, affecting the hypothalamus and its proximal limbic system, which would account for the range of reported ME/CFS-like symptoms.[4]

However, fatigue is considered differently in TCM—it could be caused by the following etiologies with different pathologies.

11.1.1.1 *Accumulation of damp-phlegm*

Prolonged persistence of external factors in the body due to incomplete elimination of external cold-damp or damp-heat, improper medical treatment, lack of life care during COVID-19, constitutional overweight or accumulation of damp-phlegm in the body, etc., could cause dysfunction of the spleen and stomach with transportation and transformation, leading to formation and accumulation of damp there. This situation could lead to dysfunction of the spleen and stomach in the production of qi and blood, and fatigue occurs. Accumulation of damp varies in damp-phlegm, cold-damp, and damp-heat.

11.1.1.2 *Emotional disorders*

Emotional stress or frustration during or after COVID-19 could cause stagnation of liver-qi. Overthinking could bring about the stagnation of heart-qi, and over-sadness could lead to stagnation of lung-qi. Moreover, over-worry could result in the stagnation of spleen-qi, and over-anxiety and fear could damage the kidney, bringing about

---

[4] Angus Mackay. A paradigm for post-covid-19 fatigue syndrome analogous to ME/CFS. *Front. Neurol.* 2021. 12: 701419. doi: 10.3389/fneur.2021.701419.

disturbance to kidney-qi. All these conditions may cause disorder in qi circulation.

Since the liver dominates the free flow of qi in the body, it can help digestion and transportation of qi to the spleen and stomach. In case of stagnation of liver-qi due to emotional dysfunction, there could be a disorder of ascending and descending functions in the body, especially the spleen and stomach, resulting in fatigue and depression.

11.1.1.3 *Deficiency of qi and yang*

Prolonged persistence of COVID-19 could cause consumption of qi, blood, yin and yang of the body, leading to deficiency of qi and yang of the spleen and stomach, deficiency of qi and yang of the heart or kidney, deficiency of qi and yin of the lung and kidney, or deficiency of yin of the liver, etc.

When there is a deficiency of qi and yang of the spleen and stomach, there would be fatigue, loss of appetite, cold hands and feet, aversion to cold, loose stools or diarrhea, and abdominal swelling, etc.

The heart is a fire organ according to the Five Elements theory. Deficiency of qi and yang of the heart could cause the failure of the spleen and stomach to be warmed and stimulated, thus the transportation and transformation of the spleen and stomach will be impaired, causing fatigue with palpitations, insomnia, and loss of appetite.

11.1.1.4 *Deficiency of blood and yin*

When there is a deficiency of yin of the lung, there would be fatigue, dry cough, slight pressure in the chest, and dry throat, etc. If there is a deficiency of the yin of the liver, there could be fatigue, headache, dry eyes, dizziness, hypochondriac pain and distention, etc.

The kidney is an organ, which contains both yin and yang. kidney-yang could also warm the spleen in physiology. In case of deficiency of kidney-yang (qi), the spleen will not be properly warmed and supported, the physiological functions of the spleen will be impaired, causing fatigue with lower back pain and weakness, hair loss, poor memory, etc.

11.1.2 TCM treatment of Long COVID-associated fatigue

Although there are various causes for fatigue in TCM, detailed differentiation of symptoms and signs should be made to identify the main causative factors. Sometimes, there is a combination of more than two pathogenic factors in one syndrome, and they should be treated accordingly.

11.1.2.1 *Accumulation of damp-phlegm*

Fatigue, lassitude, heaviness of the four limbs and body, heaviness in the head, difficulty to think and concentrate, poor appetite, nausea, vomiting, swollen epigastric region and abdomen, loose stool, white and greasy coating on the tongue, and a slippery and wiry pulse.

Principle of Treatment:
Eliminate damp, resolve phlegm, activate the spleen, and improve appetite.

Herbal Treatment:
Ping Wei San-*Calm the Stomach Powder,* plus
Xiang Sha Liu Jun Zi Tang-*Six Gentlemen Decoction with Aucklandia and Amomum.*

Cang Zhu *Rhizoma Atractylodis* 10 g
Hou Po *Cortex Magnoliae Officinalis* 10 g
Chen Pi *Pericarpium Citri Reticulatae* 5 g
Xiang Fu *Rhizoma Cyperi Rotundi* 10 g
Sha Ren *Fructus Amomi* 3 g
Zhi Ban Xia *Rhizoma Pinelliae Ternatae Preparata* 10 g
Fu Ling *Sclerotium Poriae Cocos* 12 g
Huo Xiang *Herba Agastaches seu Pogostemi* 10 g
Bai Zhu *Rhizoma Atractylodis Macrocephalae* 10 g

Qiang Huo *Rhizoma et Radix Notopterygii* 10 g
Shen Qu *Massa Medica Fermentata* 15 g
Jiao Gu Ya *Fructus Oryzae Sativae Germinantus (grill)* 15 g
Zhi Gan Cao *Radix Glycyrrhizae Preparata* 3 g

In case of cold-damp, add Gui Zhi *Ramulus Cinnamomi Cassiae* 10 g and Gan Jiang *Rhizoma Zingiberis Officinalis* 6 g.
In the case of damp-heat, add Huang Lian *Rhizoma Coptidis* 5 g and Zhi Zi *Fructus Gardeniae Jasminoidis* 10 g.

Explanations:
- Cang Zhu, Hou Po, Chen Pi, and Zhi Gan Cao, the complete composition of Ping Wei San, eliminate damp, resolve phlegm, activate the spleen, and improve appetite.
- Bai Zhu, Fu Ling, Zhi Gan Cao, Zhi Ban Xia, Chen Pi, Huo Xiang, Xiang Fu and Sha Ren, the main compositions of Xiang Sha Liu Jun Zi Tang, activate the spleen and stomach, eliminate damp, resolve phlegm, harmonize the middle Jiao, relieve diarrhea, promote qi circulation, and improve the appetite.
- Qiang Huo eliminates damp in the muscle and relieves the heaviness of the muscles.
- Shen Qu and Jiao Gu Ya are used to promote digestion and improve appetite.
- Gui Zhi and Gan Jiang warm the spleen and stomach and eliminate cold in the body.
- Huang Lian and Zhi Zi clear heat and eliminate damp in the middle Jiao.

Herbal Remedy:
Xiang Sha Liu Jun Wan-*Six Gentlemen Pill with Aucklandia and Amomum.*

Acupuncture Treatment:
- Hegu L.I.-4, Neiguan P-6, Taichong LIV-3, Zhongwan REN-12, Liangmen ST-21, Tianshu ST-25, Zusanli ST-36, Fenglong ST-40, Sanyinjiao SP-6, and Yinlingquan SP-9.

- A tonifying method is applied on ST-36 and SP-6, and a reducing method is applied on the rest of these points.
- In case of cold-damp, add moxa on REN-12, ST-36, and SP-9.
- In case of damp-heat, add Yanglingquan GB-34 and Dadu SP-2.

Explanations:
- L.I.-4 and LIV-3, the yuan-source point of the large intestine channel and the liver channel respectively, promote the qi circulation in the body and relieve qi stagnation caused by the accumulation of damp-phlegm.
- P-6, the luo-connecting point of the pericardium channel, regulates qi circulation in the chest and abdomen, harmonizes the stomach, descends stomach-qi, and improves appetite.
- REN-12, the front mu point of the stomach and the gathering point of the fu organs in the body, Fenglong ST-40, the luo-connecting point of the stomach channel, and SP-9, and the he-sea point of the spleen channel respectively, eliminate damp and resolve phlegm in the body.
- ST-25, the front collecting point of the large intestine, together with ST-21 are able to promote digestion and transportation in the large intestine.
- ST-36, the he-sea point of the stomach channel, and SP-6, the crossing point of the three yin channels of the feet, tonify and activate the spleen and stomach and improve the appetite.
- Moxa on REN-12, ST-36 and SP-9 could warm the internal organs and eliminate cold.
- GB-34, the he-sea point of the gallbladder channel, and SP-2, the ying-spring point of the spleen channel clear heat and eliminate damp.

11.1.2.2 *Stagnation of qi*

Fatigue, depression, headache, tension at the neck, fullness of the chest, insomnia, hypochondriac pain and distention, poor appetite, belching, acid regurgitation, slight depression, headache, insomnia, aggravation of above situations when being nervous, irregular menstruation for women, sometimes irritable, thin and white coating on the tongue, and a wiry pulse.

Principle of Treatment:
Smooth the liver, promote qi circulation, calm the shen and improve sleep.

Herbal Treatment:
Xiao Yao San-*Rambling Powder.*

Chai Hu *Radix Bupleuri* 10 g
Bai Shao Yao *Radix Paeoniae Lactiflorae* 15 g
Zhi Ke *Fructus Citri Aurantii* 10 g
Dang Gui *Radix Angelicae Sinensis* 10 g
Chuan Xiong *Radix Ligustici Wallichii* 10 g
Xiang Fu *Rhizoma Cyperi Rotundi* 10 g
Chuan Lian Zi *Fructus Meliae Toosendan* 10 g
Fu Shen *Sclerotium Poriae Cocos Paradicis* 12 g
Yuan Zhi *Radix Polygalae Tenuifoliae* 10 g
Bai Zhu *Rhizoma Atractylodis Macrocephalae* 10 g
Chen Pi *Pericarpium Citri Reticulatae* 5 g
Sha Ren *Fructus Amomi* 3 g

Explanations:
- Chai Hu and Bai Shao Yao smooth the liver and relieve qi stagnation in the liver.
- Zhi Ke, Xiang Fu, and Chuan Lian Zi promote qi circulation and relieve qi stagnation and pain in the body.
- Dang Gui and Chuan Xiong nourish the liver-blood, benefit the liver, and relieve spasms in the liver.
- Fu Shen and Yuan Zhi smooth emotions, regulate and calm the shen, and improve sleep.
- Bai Zhu, Chen Pi and Sha Ren activate the spleen and stomach, promote the qi circulation in the middle Jiao and improve the appetite.

Herbal Remedy:
Xiao Yao Wan-*Rambling Pill.*

Acupuncture Treatment:
- Neiguan P-6 + Gongsun SP-4, Hegu L.I.-4, Shaohai HE-3, Shenmen HE-7, Tanzhong REN-17, Fengchi GB-20, Sanyinjiao SP-6, Yanglingquan GB-34, Taichong LIV-3, Zhangmen LIV-13, Xinshu BL-15, and Ganshu BL-18.
- Even method is applied on P-6 + SP-4, and a reducing method is applied on the rest of the points.

Explanations:
- The combination of P-6 + SP-4 promotes the qi circulation in the body, regulates the Yinwei channel and Chong channel, and improves appetite.
- L.I.-4, the yuan-source point of the large intestine channel, REN-17, the gathering point for the qi in the body, LIV-3, the yuan-source point of the liver channel, BL-18, the back-shu point of the liver, GB-34, the he-sea point of the gallbladder channel, and GB-20 promote the qi circulation in the body, smooth the liver, improve emotions, and relieves pain and headache.
- SP-6, the crossing point of the three yin channels of the feet, and LIV-13, the front-mu point of the spleen, activate the spleen and improve appetite.
- HE-3 and HE-7, the he-sea point and the yuan-source point of the heart respectively, BL-15, the back-shu point of the heart, calms the shen, improves emotions and benefits sleep.

11.1.2.3 *Deficiency of qi and yang*

Fatigue, weakness, cold hands and feet, aversion to cold, loss of appetite, tastelessness in the mouth, weight loss, low voice, dislike to speak, spontaneous sweating, loose stools or diarrhea, sleepiness, pale tongue, thin and white coating with some tooth marks on the tongue, and a thready, weak, and slow pulse.

If there is a deficiency of qi and yang of the heart, there could be palpitations, superficial sleep, and a weak feeling of heartbeat, etc.

If there is a deficiency of qi and yang of the kidney, there would be lower back pain, weakness of the knees, frequent urination, or aggravation of urine incontinence, poor memory, shortness of breath by slight exertion, etc.

Principle of Treatment:
Tonify qi, warm yang, activate the spleen and improve appetite.

Herbal Treatment:
Fu Zi Li Zhong Tang-*Prepared Aconite Pill to Regulate the Middle,* plus
Shen Ling Bai Zhu San-*Ginseng, Poria and Atractylodis Macrocephalae Powder.*

Zhi Fu Zi *Radix Lateralis Aconiti Carmichaeli Praeparata* 6 g
Gan Jiang *Rhizoma Zingiberis Officinalis* 5 g
Gui Zhi *Ramulus Cinnamomi Cassiae* 10 g
Zhi Dang Shen *Radix Codonopsis Pilosulae Praeparata* 10 g
Zhi Huang Qi *Radix Astragali Membranacei Praeparata* 10 g
Bai Zhu *Rhizoma Atractylodis Macrocephalae* 10 g
Fu Ling *Sclerotium Poriae Cocos* 12 g
Shan Yao *Radix Dioscoreae Oppositae* 10 g
Zhi Gan Cao *Radix Glycyrrhizae Preparata* 5 g

In case of deficiency of qi and yang of the heart, add Rou Gui *Cortex Cinnamomi Cassiae* 5 g.
In case of deficiency of qi and yang of the kidney, add Ba Ji Tian *Radix Morindae Officinalis* 10 g and Xian Mao *Rhizoma Curculiginis Orchioidis* 10 g.

Explanations:
• Zhi Fu Zi, Gui Zhi and Gan Jiang warm yang and qi, eliminate cold and strengthen the body.

- Zhi Dang Shen, Bai Zhu, Fu Ling, and Zhi Gan Cao activate the spleen, tonify the spleen-qi and the general body, and improve appetite.
- Zhi Huang Qi and Shan Yao activate the spleen, tonify spleen-qi, and lift the qi to the head.
- Rou Gui warms the heart-yang and strengthens heart-fire.
- Ba Ji Tian and Xian Mao warm the kidney, eliminate interior cold and strengthen the back.

Herbal Remedy:
Li Zhong Wan-*Decoction (Pill) to Regulate the Middle*, or Si Jun Zi Wan-*Four Gentlemen Decoction*.

Acupuncture Treatment:
- Zusanli ST-36, Taibai SP-3, Shenmen HE-7, Guanyuan REN-4, Qihai REN-6, Taixi KID-3, Baihui DU-20, Xinshu BL-15, Pishu BL-20, and Shenshu BL-23.
- A tonifying method is applied to the first three points.
- Moxibustion could be applied on REN-4, REN-6, and ST-36.

Explanations:
- ST-36, the he-sea point of the stomach channel, SP-3, the yuan-source point BL-20, the back-shu point of the spleen, activate the spleen and stomach, and tonify qi of the general body.
- REN-4 and REN-6 tonify the yuan-qi in the body, warm yang, eliminate interior cold and strengthen the body.
- HE-7 and BL-15, the yuan-source point and the back-shu point of the heart respectively, tonify qi and yang of the heart and strengthen the heart.
- KID-3, the yuan-source point of the kidney channel, BL-23, the back-shu point of the kidney, warms the kidney, tonifies qi and yang of the kidney and eliminates interior cold.
- DU-20 lifts qi and yang to the head and relieves fatigue.
- Moxibustion warms the qi and yang of the body and eliminates interior cold.

11.1.2.4 *Deficiency of yin*

Fatigue, slight headache, restlessness, insomnia, night sweating, nervousness, thirst, dry mouth, eyes, throat and stool, the hot sensation of the chest, palms and soles, poor appetite, dry stool, red tongue, thin and scanty tongue coating, and a deep, thready, weak, and slightly rapid pulse.

Principle of Treatment:
Nourish the yin, clear deficient heat, benefit the body fluid and relieve the tiredness.

Herbal Treatment:
Sheng Mai San-*Generate the Pulse Powder.*

Ren Shen *Radix Ginseng* 10 g
Mai Men Dong *Tuber Ophiopogonis Japonici* 10 g
Wu Wei Zi *Fructus Schisandrae Chinensis* 10 g
Sheng Di Huang *Radix Rehmanniae Glutinosae Recens* 10 g
Shu Di Huang *Radix Rhemanniae Glutinosae Praeparata* 12 g
Mu Dan Pi *Cortex Moutan Radicis* 10 g
Han Lian Cao *Herba Ecliptae Prostratae* 10 g
Nu Zhen Zi *Fructus Ligustri Lucidi* 10 g
Gou Qi Zi *Fructus Lycii* 10 g
Tian Hua Fen *Radix Trichosanthis Kirilowii* 10 g
Bai Zhu *Rhizoma Atractylodis Macrocephalae* 10 g
Fu Ling *Sclerotium Poriae Cocos* 12 g
Zhi Gan Cao *Radix Glycyrrhizae Preparata* 3 g

In case of deficiency of lung-yin, add Chuan Bei Mu *Bulbus Fritillariae* 10 g and Zi Wan *Radix Asteris Tatarici* 10 g.
In case of deficiency of heart-yin, add Dan Shen *Radix Salviae Miltiorrhizae* 10 g and Yuan Zhi *Radix Polygalae Tenuifoliae* 10 g.
In case of deficiency of liver-yin, add Chuan Lian Zi *Fructus Meliae Toosendan* 10 g and Wu Mei *Fructus Pruni Mume* 10 g.

Explanations:

- Ren Shen, Mai Men Dong and Wu Wei Zi, the complete composition of Sheng Mai San, nourish the yin of the body. Meanwhile, they can also tonify the qi of the body. They are the main herbs in this prescription to relieve fatigue.
- Sheng Di Huang and Mu Dan Pi nourish the yin and clear the deficient heat in the body.
- Ren Shen, Bai Zhu, Fu Ling, and Zhi Gan Cao, the complete composition of Si Jun Zi Tang, activate the spleen and tonify the qi in the body so as to promote the production of yin in the body.
- Shu Di Huang, Gou Qi Zi, Nu Zhen Zi and Han Lian Cao tonify the kidney, nourish the yin and benefit the jing.
- Tian Hua Fen promotes the production of body fluid and relieves thirst.
- Chuan Bei Mu and Zi Wan nourish the lung-yin and relieve dry cough.
- Dan Shen and Yuan Zhi benefit the heart and calm the shen.
- Chuan Lian Zi and Wu Mei benefit the liver and relieve the spasm in the liver.

Herbal Remedy:
Sheng Mai San (Wan)-*Generate the Pulse Powder (Pill)*.

Acupuncture Treatment:

- Lieque LU-7 + Zhaohai KI-6, Chize LU-5, Taiyuan LU-9, Shenmen HE-7, Feishu BL-13, Zusanli ST-36, Sanyinjiao SP-6, Taixi KID-3, Zhaohai KID-6, Yingu KID-10, Qihai REN-6 and Shenshu BL-23.
- An even method is applied on LU-7 + KID-6, and a tonifying method is applied on the rest of the points.

Explanations:

- LU-7 + KID-6 are used to nourish the yin of the general body and relieve dryness and deficient heat.
- LU-5 and LU-9,the he-sea point and the yuan-source point of the lung channel respectively, and BL-13, the back-shu point of the

lung, nourish the yin of the lung, consolidate the skin and restore the physiological functions of the lung.

- ST-36, SP-6, REN-6, KID-3, KID-6, KID-10, and BL-23 tonify the spleen and stomach, benefit the yin of the kidney and strengthen the whole body.
- HE-7, the yuan-source point of the heart channel, tonifies the heart, regulates the shen and relieves night sweating.

11.2 Breathlessness

Most people who have coronavirus disease 2019 (COVID-19) recover completely within a few weeks. But some patients, even those who had mild cases of the disease continue to experience symptoms after their initial recovery. It has been noticed that older people and people with many serious medical conditions are the most likely to experience lingering COVID-19 symptoms, but even young and otherwise healthy people can feel unwell for weeks to months after infection. Fatigue and breathlessness are among the continuing and debilitating symptoms being reported by people with COVID-19 months, or even more than one year after the onset of the disease and after they have been declared to have recovered. One study, published in *JAMA (The Journal of the American Medical Association)* on 9 July 2020, shows that a high proportion of individuals still reported dyspnea (43.4%), which is the second complaint besides fatigue (53.1%).[5]

Breathlessness, sometimes called shortness of breath and known clinically as dyspnea, is one of the hallmark symptoms of COVID-19. It is characterized by difficulty breathing deeply or feeling as if unable to get enough air into the lungs. Some patients describe it as feeling "puffed", "winded" or like breathing through a straw. The chest may feel too tight to inhale or exhale fully. The patient needs to take greater effort to perform each shallow breath, which could

---

[5]Angelo Carfì, *et al. op. cit.*

happen when being active or resting. It can come on gradually or suddenly. The feeling of shortness of breath may continue for a while after COVID-19, and that is a normal part of the recovery process.

Some daily activities, such as brisk walking, running into the bathroom, doing heavy physical work or simply being stressed, could make people feel breathless, especially among older patients. High intensity or strenuous workouts, extremely humid and high temperatures, and high altitudes can all cause shortness of breath. Anxiety can also lead to changes in the breathing rate and pattern. Unlike many other conditions that can cause shortness of breath, breathlessness can persist or even quickly escalate in people with COVID-19. Some lung damage caused by COVID-19 may slowly and fully heal. But in other cases, patients who suffered from severe cases of COVID-19 may face chronic lung problems, this is because these lung injuries may cause the formation of scar tissue known as pulmonary fibrosis. Scarring further stiffens the lungs and makes it harder to breathe. Since COVID-19 is an acute viral infectious disease with a relatively short course, the probability of causing pulmonary fibrosis to develop is relatively low, especially in mild cases, most of which will not develop pulmonary fibrosis (PPF). However, in severe and critically ill cases, pulmonary fibrosis may occur. One report analyzed the CT images of more than 60 patients with COVID-19 when they were admitted to the hospital and before they were discharged. According to the standard of *"New Coronavirus Pneumonia Diagnosis and Treatment Plan (Trial Seventh Edition)"* issued by The National Health Commission on 3 March 2020,[6] the incidence of pulmonary fibrosis was as high as 70% on patients with ordinary types of COVID-19 after inflammation, and presence of pulmonary fibrosis was 100% when patients with severe type were discharged.

---

[6] Interpretation of "new coronavirus pneumonia diagnosis and treatment plan (trial seventh edition)" (《新型冠状病毒肺炎诊疗方案 (试行第七版)》解读) http://www.nhc.gov.cn/yzygj/s7652m/202003/a31191442e29474b98bfed5579d5af95.shtml.

80% of patients still suffer from shortness of breath after being discharged.[7]

When breathlessness occurs on its own, it usually rules out COVID-19. However, when it happens suddenly with other key symptoms, such as fever, cough, loss of smell, and tastes, the likelihood of having an infection with SARS-CoV-2 increases. PCR could confirm the infection quickly. The Center for Disease Control and Prevention (CDC) Trusted Source pointed out symptoms may differ with the severity of the disease. For example, shortness of breath is more commonly reported among people who are hospitalized with COVID-19 than among people with the milder symptoms (non-hospitalized patients)[8].

11.2.1 TCM's understanding of Long COVID-associated breathlessness

The main pathologies of Long COVID-associated breathlessness is dysfunctions of the lung in dispersing or descending the lung-qi due to various causative factors.

11.2.1.1 *Incomplete elimination of external pathogenic factors*

When these hospitalized or non-hospitalized COVID-19 patients are not treated timely or properly, their pathogenic factors will not be eliminated, causing stagnation and latent accumulation in the body, which results in some constant disturbance to the body. Since the common causative etiologies are an invasion of cold-damp or damp-heat, the lung could be one of the main affected organs. Disorder of

---

[7]Zhan Xi, *et al.* Current status and thinking of pulmonary fibrosis after inflammation of new coronavirus pneumonia. *Chinese Journal of Tuberculosis and Respiratory* (中华结核和呼吸杂志). 2020, 43(9): 728–732. doi: 10.3760/cma.j.cn112147-20200317-00359.

[8]Centers for Disease Control and Prevention (CDC). Symptoms of COVID-19. Updated 22 February 2021. https://www.cdc.gov/coronavirus/2019-ncov/symptoms-testing/symptoms.html.

the lung in may cause failure of the dispersing or descending the qi, leading to stagnation of qi in the chest, thus breathlessness occurs.

11.2.1.2 *Accumulation of damp-phlegm*

Either invasion of cold-damp or invasion of damp-heat to the spleen or stomach, or San Jiao, may cause dysfunction of the spleen and stomach in digestion, transportation, and transformation, resulting in the formation of damp-phlegm internally, which could eventually cause a mixture of external damp with internal damp. In this condition, it could result in blockage of the yang-qi or clear-qi in the body. When it is accumulated in the chest or lung, it may cause breathlessness. Besides, disturbance to the San Jiao by external damp could also lead to dysfunction of the San Jiao in distributing water and yang-qi, aggravating accumulation of damp-phlegm in the body. In turn, this situation could cause blockage of the yang in the chest or the qi in the lung, thus breathlessness happens.

11.2.1.3 *Stagnation of qi*

Accumulation of damp, improper health care and treatment, being emotionally upset or disturbed during COVID-19, unsolved emotional disorders before COVID-19, etc., could lead to retardation of qi circulation. When there is the occurrence of qi stagnation, it could also block the chest or the lung, bringing about breathlessness. It is a rule in TCM that qi circulation leads to blood circulation and blood stagnation aggravates qi stagnation. When there is qi stagnation for a while, there could be stagnation of blood, thus forming stagnation of qi and blood at the same time. Blood stagnation often presents in some severe types of COVID-19.

11.2.1.4 *Deficiency of qi*

Prolonged persistence of COVID-19 could cause consumption of qi, leading to deficiency of qi in the body. It may affect different zang-fu organs, such as the lung, spleen, and kidney, etc.

Deficiency of lung-qi could lead to weakness of the lung in dispersing and descending the qi, resulting in breathlessness. Since the spleen is considered as the Earth Element, which produces the Metal Element according to the Five Elements theory in TCM, thus deficiency of spleen-qi could eventually lead to weakness of the lung, and result in breathlessness. Moreover, the respiration function of the lung needs to be held by the kidney. In case of deficiency of kidney-qi, it could cause the failure of the lung in performing its physiological functions, dysfunction of the lung happens. In this condition, breathlessness appears.

11.2.2 TCM treatment of Long COVID-associated breathlessness

11.2.2.1 *Incomplete elimination of external pathogenic factors*

Breathlessness, slight cough, expectoration of diluted whitish phlegm or slight yellow phlegm, or even dry cough, pressure over the chest with heaviness, sensitivity to weather changes, slight muscle pain and headache, a thin, white greasy or slight mixture of white and yellow greasy coating on the tongue, and a tight and slippery pulse.

Principle of Treatment:
Eliminate pathogenic factors, disperse the lung-qi, descend the lung-qi, and relieve the breathlessness.

Herbal Treatment:
Xing Su San-*Apricot Kernel and Perilla Leaf Powder.*

Xing Ren *Semen Pruni Armeniacae* 10 g
Zhi Ban Xia *Rhizoma Pinelliae Ternatae Preparata* 10 g
Jie Geng *Radix Platycodi Grandiflora* 10 g
Zi Su Ye *Folium Perillae Frutescens* 10 g
Qiang Huo *Rhizoma et Radix Notopterygii* 10 g

Hou Po *Cortex Magnoliae Officinalis* 10 g
Gua Lou Pi *Pericarpium Trichosanthis* 10 g
Zhi Ke *Fructus Citri Aurantii* 10 g
Hong Hua *Flos Carthami Tinctorii* 10 g
Yu Jin *Tuber Curcumae* 10 g
Chen Pi *Pericarpium Citri Reticulatae* 5 g
Fu Ling *Sclerotium Poriae Cocos* 12 g

Explanations:
* Xing Ren, Jie Geng and Zhi Ban Xia disperse the lung-qi, eliminate phlegm, and relieve the cough.
* Hou Po, Yu Jin, Gua Lou Pi, and Zhi Ke are used to relax the chest, promote the qi circulation in the chest, descend the lung-qi, and relieve the breathlessness.
* Qiang Huo and Zi Su Ye promote sweating, relieve some external symptoms, and alleviate muscle pain and heaviness.
* Chen Pi and Fu Ling are used to activate the spleen and eliminate damp in the spleen.
* Hong Hua promotes blood circulation and prevents blood stagnation.

If it is allowed in some countries, then it is suggested to add Ma Huang *Herba Ephedrae* 10 g into the prescription to disperse and descend the lung-qi, relieve cough, and alleviate breathlessness.

Herbal Remedy:
Qiang Huo Sheng Shi Tablets-*Notopterygium Tablets to Overcome Damp Tablets.*

Acupuncture Treatment:
* Neiguan P-6 + Gongsun SP-4, Hegu L.I.-4, Waiguan SJ-5, Lieque LU-7, Chize LU-5, Tanzhong REN-17, Fenglong ST-40, Sanyinjiao SP-6, Yinlingquan SP-9, Taichong LIV-3, Qimen LIV-14.
* Even method is applied on P-6 + SP-4, and a reducing method is applied on the rest of the points.

Explanations:
- The combination of P-6 + SP-4, one group of the eight confluence points, promotes the qi circulation, and relaxes the chest to relieve breathlessness.
- SJ-5, the luo-connecting point of the San Jiao, ST-40, the luo-connecting point of the stomach channel, SP-6, the crossing points of the three yin channels of the foot, and SP-9, the he-sea point of the spleen channel, regulate the San Jiao, eliminate damp-phlegm in the body and activate the spleen and stomach.
- LU-7, and LU-5, the luo-connecting point and the he-sea point of the lung channel respectively, disperse and descend the lung-qi, restore the physiological functions of the lung, and relieve cough and breathlessness.
- L.I.-4, the yuan-source of the large intestine channel, LIV-3, the yuan-source of the liver channel, LIV-14, the front-mu point of the liver, and REN-17, the confluence point for the qi in the body, promote the qi circulation, and relieve breathlessness.

11.2.2.2 *Accumulation of damp-phlegm*

Breathlessness, slight cough, expectoration of sticky whitish phlegm or slight yellow phlegm, pressure over the chest with heaviness, nausea, poor appetite, loose stool or diarrhea, heaviness in the head with foggy feeling, lassitude, tiredness, white and greasy coating on the tongue, with a wiry and slippery pulse.

Principle of Treatment:
Eliminate damp-phlegm, disperse lung-qi, descend lung-qi, and relieve breathlessness.

Herbal Treatment:
Ban Xia Hou Po Tang-*Pinellia and Magnolia Bark Decoction,* plus Cang Fu Dao Tan Tang-*Atractylodes-Poria Phlegm-Dissipating Decoction.*

Hou Po *Cortex Magnoliae Officinalis* 10 g
Zhi Ban Xia *Rhizoma Pinelliae Ternatae Preparata* 10 g
Xing Ren *Semen Pruni Armeniacae* 10 g
Zi Su Zi *Fructus Perillae Frutescentis* 10 g
Sheng Jiang *Rhizoma Zingiberis Officinalis Recens* 5 g
Cang Zhu *Rhizoma Atractylodis* 10 g
Xiang Fu *Rhizoma Cyperi Rotundi* 10 g
Tian Nan Xing *Rhizoma Arisaematis* 10 g
Gua Lou Pi *Pericarpium Trichosanthis* 10 g
Zhi Ke *Fructus Citri Aurantii* 10 g
Fu Ling *Sclerotium Poriae Cocos* 12 g
Chen Pi *Pericarpium Citri Reticulatae* 5 g

Explanations:
- Hou Po, Xing Ren and Zi Su Zi resolve phlegm, descend the lung-qi, relieve the cough and breathlessness.
- Tian Nan Xing, Zhi Ban Xia, Chen Pi, Fu Ling, and Sheng Jiang disperse the lung-qi, eliminate phlegm, and relieve cough.
- Cang Zhu eliminates damp-phlegm and activates the spleen.
- Xiang Fu, Gua Lou Pi and Zhi Ke promote the qi circulation in the chest and relieve the blockage of the chest by damp-phlegm.

Herbal Remedy:
Cang Fu Dao Tan Wan-*Atractylodes-Poria Phlegm-Dissipating Decoction*.

Acupuncture Treatment:
- Neiguan P-6 + Gongsun SP-4, Hegu L.I.-4, Kongzui LU-6, Lieque LU-7, Chize LU-5, Zhongwan REN-12, Tanzhong REN-17, Fenglong ST-40, Sanyinjiao SP-6, Yinlingquan SP-9, Taichong LIV-3, Qimen LIV-14.
- An even method is applied on P-6 + SP-4, and a reducing method is applied on the rest of the points.

Explanations:
- The combination of P-6 + SP-4 promotes the qi circulation and relaxes the chest to relieve breathlessness.
- REN-12, the gathering point of the fu organs in the body, ST-40, SP-6 and SP-9 activate the spleen and stomach and eliminate damp-phlegm in the body.
- LU-6, the xi-cleft point of the lung channel, LU-7, and LU-5 disperse and descend the lung-qi, restore the physiological functions of the lung, and relieve cough and breathlessness.
- L.I.-4, LIV-3, LIV-14, and REN-17 promote the qi circulation and relieve breathlessness.

11.2.2.3 *Stagnation of qi*

Breathlessness, fullness of the chest with distending pain, difficulty with breathing out, depression, unstable emotions, headache, stiffness, and pain at the neck, insomnia, fullness of hypochondriac regions, irritability, nervousness, poor appetite, thin and white coating on the tongue, and a wiry and thready pulse.

Principle of Treatment:
Harmonize the liver, smooth emotions, promote qi circulation, and relieve the breathlessness.

Herbal Treatment:
Xiao Yao San-*Rambling Powder.*

Chai Hu *Radix Bupleuri* 10 g
Bai Shao Yao *Radix Paeoniae Lactiflorae* 15 g
Zhi Ke *Fructus Citri Aurantii* 10 g
Gua Lou Pi *Pericarpium Trichosanthis* 10 g
Yu Jin *Tuber Curcumae* 10 g
Hou Po *Cortex Magnoliae Officinalis* 10 g
Dang Gui *Radix Angelicae Sinensis* 10 g

Fu Shen *Sclerotium Poriae Cocos Paradicis* 12 g
Bai Zhu Rhizoma *Atractylodis Macrocephalae* 10 g
Duan Long Gu *Os Draconis (calcin)* 15 g
Yuan Zhi *Radix Polygalae Tenuifoliae* 10 g

Explanations:
- Chai Hu and Bai Shao Yao smooth the liver and relieve qi stagnation in the liver.
- Zhi Ke and Yu Jin promote the qi circulation in the body and regulate emotions.
- Dang Gui nourishes the liver-blood and benefits the liver.
- Hou Po and Gua Lou Pi promote the qi circulation in the chest and relieve the fullness in the chest.
- All these herbs are used to promote and regulate the qi circulation in the liver and chest to relieve qi stagnation and breathlessness.
- Bai Zhu activates the spleen and eliminates damp in the body.
- Fu Shen, Duan Long Gu and Yuan Zhi smooth the emotions, regulate the shen and improve sleep.

Herbal Remedy:
Xiao Yao Wan-*Rambling Pill.*

Acupuncture Treatment:
- Neiguan P-6 + Gongsun SP-4, Hegu L.I.-4, Lieque LU-7, Chize LU-5, Tanzhong REN-17, Fengchi GB-20, Jianjing GB-21, Sanyinjiao SP-6, Taichong LIV-3, Qimen LIV-14, Xinshu BL-15 and Ganshu BL-18.
- An even method is applied on P-6 + SP-4, and a reducing method is applied on the rest of the points.

Explanations:
- The combination of P-6 + SP-4 promotes the qi circulation and relaxes the chest to relieve breathlessness.
- LU-7, LU-5, and REN-17 disperse and descend the lung-qi, relieve the qi stagnation in the chest, and improve breathlessness.
- L.I.-4 promotes the qi and blood circulation in the body and relieves pain and headache.

- SP-6, the crossing points of the three yin channels of the foot, GB-20, GB-21, LIV-3, LIV-14, BL-15 the back-shu point of the heart, and BL-18 the back-shu point of liver, calm the shen, smooth the liver, promote the qi circulation, and relieve breath-lessness.

11.2.2.4 *Stagnation of blood*

Stabbing chest pain at a fixed location (radiating to the back), the fullness of chest, shortness of breath, palpitations, purplish or ecchymoses on the tongue, and an unsmooth or wiry pulse.

Principle of Treatment:
Promote the circulation of blood, eliminate stagnant blood, and sedate pain.

Herbal Treatment:
Xue Fu Zhu Yu Tang-*Drive out Stasis in the Mansion of Blood Decoction,* plus
Dan Shen Yin-*Saliva Decoction.*

Tao Ren *Semen Pruni Persicae* 10 g
Hong Hua *Flos Carthami Tinctorii* 10 g
Chi Shao Yao *Radix Paeoniae Rubrae* 10 g
Dang Gui *Radix Angelicae Sinensis* 10 g
Shu Di Huang *Radix Rhemanniae Glutinosae Praeparata* 10 g
Dan Shen *Radix Salviae Miltiorrhizae* 12 g
Chuan Xiong *Radix Ligustici Wallichii* 10 g
Yan Hu Suo *Rhizoma Corydalis* 10 g
Tan Xiang *Lignum Santali Albi* 3 g
Xiang Fu *Rhizoma Cyperi Rotundi* 10 g
Zhi Ke *Fructus Citri Aurantii* 10 g
Yu Jin *Tuber Curcumae* 10 g

Explanations:
- Tao Ren, Hong Hua, Dang Gui, Chi Shao Yao, Chuan Xiong, and Shu Di Huang, the complete composition of Tao Hong Si Wu Tang,

promote blood circulation, eliminate blood stasis, and relieve pain.

- Dan Shen and Tan Xiang promote blood circulation and relieve the blood stasis in the heart.
- Zhi Ke, Xiang Fu, Yu Jin, and Yan Hu Suo promote qi circulation, eliminate blood stasis, and relieve pain.

Herbal Remedy:
Tao Hong Si Wu Tang tablet-*Four Substance (Things) Decoction Pill with Safflower and Peach Pit.*

Acupuncture Treatment:
- Neiguan P-6 + Gongsun SP-4, Hegu L.I.-4, Kongzui LU-6, Lieque LU-7, Chize LU-5, Tanzhong REN-17, Ximen P-4, Sanyinjiao SP-6, Taichong LIV-3, Xinshu BL-15, and Geshu BL-17.
- An even method is applied on P-6 + SP-4, and a reducing method is applied on the rest of the points.

Explanations:
- The combination of P-6 + SP-4 promotes the qi circulation, relaxes the chest, relieves breathlessness, and relieves the chest pain.
- LU-6, LU-7, LU-5, REN-17 and P-4 disperse and descend the lung-qi, harmonize the collaterals, relieve the stagnation in the chest, and improve breathlessness.
- L.I.-4 and LIV-3 promote the qi circulation in the body and relieve pain and headache.
- SP-6, BL-15 and BL-17 promote blood circulation and relieve breathlessness.

11.2.2.5 *Deficiency of qi*

Breathlessness which gets worse after exertion, difficulty in breathing in, slight cough, no expectoration of phlegm, tiredness, dizziness, palpitations, poor memory, timidness, pale complexion, pale tongue with a thin and white coating, and a thready and weak pulse.

Principle of Treatment:
Tonify qi, activate the spleen, and reinforce the kidney.

Herbal Treatment:
Bu Fei Tang-*Tonify the Lungs Decoction,* plus
Si Jun Zi Tang-*Four Gentlemen Decoction.*

Zhi Dang Shen *Radix Codonopsis Pilosulae Praeparata* 10 g
Zhi Huang Qi *Radix Astragali Membranacei Praeparata* 10 g
Bai Zhu *Rhizoma Atractylodis Macrocephalae* 10 g
Shu Di Huang *Radix Rhemanniae Glutinosae Praeparata* 12 g
Wu Wei Zi *Fructus Schisandrae Chinensis* 10 g
Zi Wan *Radix Asteris Tatarici* 10 g
Sang Bai Pi *Cortex Mori Albae Radicis* 10 g
Fu Ling *Sclerotium Poriae Cocos* 12 g
Zhi Gan Cao *Radix Glycyrrhizae Preparata* 3 g

Explanations:
- Zhi Dang Shen, Bai Zhu, Fu Ling, and Zhi Gan Cao, the complete composition from Si Jun Zi Tang, activate the spleen and tonify the qi in the body.
- Zhi Huang Qi, Wu Wei Zi, and Zi Wan tonify the qi in the lung and benefit the lung.
- Sang Bai Pi descends the lung-qi and relieves the breathlessness.
- Shu Di Huang tonifies the kidney and benefits the lung.

Herbal Remedy:
Bu Zhong Yi Qi Wan-*Tonify the Middle and Augment the Qi Decoction.*

Acupuncture Treatment:
- Neiguan P-6 + Gongsun SP-4, Zhongfu LU-1, Chize LU-5, Taiyuan LU-9, Tanzhong REN-17, Zusanli ST-36, Sanyinjiao SP-6, Taixi KID-3, Qihai REN-6, Feishu BL-13, and Shenshu BL-23.

- An even method is applied on P-6 + SP-4, and a tonifying method is applied on the rest of the points. Moxibustion could be applied on ST-36, KID-3, and REN-6.

Explanations:
- The combination of P-6 + SP-4 promotes the qi circulation, relaxes the chest, relieves breathlessness, and relieves chest pain.
- LU-1, the front-mu point of the lung, LU-5, the he-sea point of the lung channels, and LU-9, the yuan-source point of the lung channel, and BL-13, the back-shu point of the lung, tonify the qi of the lung and restore the physiological functions.
- REN-17, ST-36, SP-6, REN-6, KID-3, and BL-23 tonify the qi of the spleen and kidney and support the lung-qi to relieve breathlessness.
- Moxibustion warms the qi and dispel cold in the body.

11.3 Joint Pain

As the number of patients recovering COVID-19 are increasing, different types of Long COVID are coming to the fore. At this moment, clinicians and scientists are still in the process of fully discovering consequences of COVID-19. Joint pain is one of the most common complaints among Long COVID patients. One research, published in JAMA (*The Journal of the American Medical Association*) on 9 July 2020, points out that a high proportion of individuals (27.3%) still reported joint pain, which is the third complaint from Long COVID besides fatigue (53.1%) and dyspnea (43.4%).[9]

A joint is any place in the body where two or more bones meet and allow for movement. Joints are formed by fibrous connective tissues that hold the bones together, and pieces of cartilage that provide cushioning and slip between the bones. Many people will experience joint pain at some points in their life, and mostly these kind of joint pain are not serious and will improve or get better quickly. But in some cases, joint pain could be more serious. For instance, the

---

[9]Angelo Carfì, *et al. op. cit.*

inevitable wearing down of cartilage and bone tissue over time for most patients over the age of 50, and patients who have some joint pain or joint stiffness due to rheumatoid arthritis, knee pain caused by a torn meniscus, etc. However, joint pain during Long COVID should not be thought simply as a normal part of aging or physical damage. It is important to pay close attention to identify the symptoms and signs to find out their etiologies, and take steps to prevent them from worsening, since TCM believes that joint pain could be caused by a wide variety of etiologies and pathologies.

For some individuals, their joint pain becomes obvious, long lasting, and even bizarre, which impacts their quality of life. They start to seek medical attention and imaging investigation. Joint pain due to Long COVID could cause swelling, stiffness, and muscle weakness of the joints somewhere in the body, such as shoulder, back, or any part of the body. Sometimes, multiple joints and muscles could be affected at the same time. Joint pain and muscle weakness can lead to difficulties when performing activities such as standing, climbing the stairs, gripping objects with the hands, or lifting the arms above the head. Some people have a widespread aching that come and go for a while, while some people have odd or altered feelings, such as numbness, pins and needles or weakness in the arms or legs.

In general, the main clinical features of joint pain during Long COVID include:

- Pain in joints, which may be sharp or stabbing, constant or occasional.
- Stiffness in joints, especially when waking up in the morning.
- Swelling in joints, with possible redness or hotness in the skin around the joint.
- Reduced range of joint motion.
- Difficulty in getting up when sitting or lying down.
- Weakness in the joint with difficulty in walking and some movement.
- Fatigue and insomnia.
- Emotional stress that could cause aggravation of joint pain sometimes.

In modern medicine, COVID-19 may lead to rheumatoid arthritis flares, autoimmune myositis or "COVID toes". For the exact causes for joint pain, there could be a clear explanation for some cases, but there is also a possibility that abnormalities could be confirmed by blood or imaging tests. In COVID-19, mostly drugs for treating rheumatoid arthritis were used to deal with joint pain. Therefore, many people, including clinicians, think that patients who recovered from COVID are safe from arthritis, but some rheumatologists are seeing many patients who have started suffering from arthritis from the Long COVID phase.[10] Some radiologists also tried to explain the cause and mechanism of joint pain. A new Northwestern Medicine study has confirmed the causes of these symptoms through radiological imaging. It illustrates that the COVID virus can trigger the body to attack itself in different ways, which may lead to rheumatological issues that require lifelong management. The study is a retrospective review of data from patients who presented to Northwestern Memorial Hospital between May 2020 and December 2020.[11]

11.3.1 TCM understanding of Long COVID-associated joint pain

According to TCM, most cases of joint pain fall under the category of Bi syndromes, which covers various conditions. For instance, qi or blood are somehow blocked by various pathogenic factors, such as cold, damp, heat, and stasis, which could cause retardation of qi and blood circulation freely through the meridian pathways of the body. Alternatively, it could be that qi and blood are deficient, in which the joint and meridians around the joints are not properly nourished, thus joint pain occurs.

---

[10] Chaitanya Deshpande. Long-term post Covid joint pain could be arthritis: Experts. *The Times of India*. Updated 9 July 2021. https://timesofindia.indiatimes.com/city/nagpur/long-term-post-covid-joint-pain-could-be-arthritis-experts/articleshow/84246127.cms.

[11] Northwestern University. Radiological images confirm "COVID-19 can cause the body to attack itself". 17 February 2021. https://www.eurekalert.org/news-releases/731722.

During TCM differentiation, efforts should be made to find out whether a problem stems from external or internal factors, or a mixture of these two factors at the same time. However, the main cause for joint pain of Long COVID is incomplete disappearance of wind, cold and damp. Above all, TCM has its typical way of analysis of joint pain.

Joint pain in TCM could include the following three stages:

- superficial stages
- tissues stages
- internal organ stages

The primary factors for joint pain at superficial stages are an invasion of wind, cold and damp at the same time, which can be the cause of the blockage, causing pain, numbness, and impaired movement of the joints. Due to the predominance of three pathogenic factors, the superficial stage of joint pain could be again subdivided into wind Bi, cold Bi and damp Bi.

- Wind Bi: joint pain is not fixed, and it can be wandering in different joints in different areas.
- Cold Bi: joint pain with stiffness that improves with the application of heat and feels worse when it gets cold. It is accompanied by reduced circulation and pale skin.
- Fixed Bi: the joint feels heavy, sore, and swollen and the pain is in a definite spot.

When superficial Bi syndromes last too long, or preexisting heat in the body, there would be the formation of heat, leading to heat Bi.

- Heat Bi: the joints are red, swollen, and inflamed, and joint pain improves with cold application and feels worse when it gets hot.

When superficial Bi syndromes are not kept under control in time, they may develop into the tissue stages, including skin Bi, muscle Bi, vascular Bi, tendon Bi, and bone Bi. Occurrence of joint pain due to

Long COVID are mostly caused by muscle Bi or tendon Bi. Internal organ Bi usually is not involved.

The main pathologies of Long COVID-associated joint pain include the following.

11.3.1.1 *Incomplete elimination of external pathogenic factors*

Invasion of cold-damp or damp-heat to the body could cause various damage, also including the damage to the meridians, muscles, tendons, and joints. When these pathogenic factors are not eliminated in time or completely, they accumulate in these tissues, resulting in joint pain due to stagnation of qi and blood with dysfunction in the joint, and joint pain occurs.

11.3.1.2 *Accumulation of damp in the body*

Invasion of cold-damp or damp-heat to the spleen and stomach may cause dysfunction in transportation and transformation, resulting in the formation of damp internally. Thus, there is a mixture of external damp and internal damp, which could block the qi and blood circulation in the body. In TCM, joints, tendons and muscles are related to certain zang-fu organs. When these organs are disturbed with the stagnation of qi and blood, joints could also be affected, and joint pain happens.

11.3.1.3 *Stagnation of qi and blood*

Accumulation of damp, disharmony of cold and heat, improper health care and treatment, emotional stress or disturbance due to Long COVID are factors that could lead to retardation of qi or blood circulation, which could block the joints and muscle around the joints, and joint pain appears. When there is qi stagnation for a while, there could be stagnation of blood, thus forming stagnation of qi and blood at the same time, resulting in severe joint pain.

11.3.1.4 *Deficiency of qi and blood*

Prolonged persistence of COVID-19 could cause consumption of qi and blood, leading to deficiency of qi and blood in the body, especially kidney-qi and liver-blood, which could lead to dysfunction of the bones and tendons, and joint pain may occur eventually.

11.3.2 TCM treatment of Long COVID-associated joint pain

Conventional treatment in modern medicine for joint pain mainly focuses on alleviating pain with NSAIDs, analgesics and corticosteroids, or by reducing inflammation with injectable medications. In some cases, though, these medications aren't enough to control pain and many of these medications also come with possible side effects. TCM methods, including herbs and acupuncture, have been applied to keep the joint tissues strong and healthy, subside swelling, control pain and prevent further damage for centuries. Besides, it can also be used to deal with some joint pain that is unexplained by modern medical science.

11.3.2.1 *Incomplete elimination of external pathogenic factors*

Joint pain (which is sensitive to wind, cold and damp weather), wandering pain or fixed pain, severe pain in nature, heaviness of the joints, muscle pain, headache, lower back pain, insomnia, poor appetite, a thin, white, and greasy tongue coating, and a wiry and tight pulse.

Principle of Treatment:
Eliminate external pathogenic factors and harmonize the collaterals.

Herbal Treatment:
Fang Feng Tang-*Saposhnikovia Decoction.*

Fang Feng *Radix Ledebouriellae Divaricatae* 10 g
Qiang Huo *Rhizoma et Radix Notopterygii* 10 g

Du Huo *Radix Angelicae Pubescentis* 10 g
Ma Huang *Herba Ephedrae* 6 g
Ge Gen *Radix Puerariae* 10 g
Qin Jiao *Radix Gentianae Macrophyllae* 10 g
Dang Gui *Radix Angelicae Sinensis* 10 g
Chuan Xiong *Radix Ligustici Wallichii* 10 g
Fu Ling *Sclerotium Poriae Cocos* 15 g
Sang Ji Sheng *Ramulus Loranthi* 10 g
Zhi Gan Cao *Radix Glycyrrhizae Preparata* 6 g

In case of local redness and hotness due to damp-heat, remove Qin Jiao *Radix Gentianae Macrophyllae* and Ma Huang *Herba Ephedrae*, and add:

- Huang Bai *Cortex Phellodendri* 10 g
- Cang Zhu *Rhizoma Atractylodis* 10 g

Explanations:
- Fang Feng, Qin Jiao, Ge Gen, Qiang Huo and Du Huo dispel remaining wind, cold and damp, harmonize the collaterals and relieve the joint pain.
- Ma Huang opens the superficial portions of the body, dispel wind, cold and damp, regulate lung-qi and blood vessels, and relieve joint pain.
- Dang Gui and Chuan Xiong promote qi and blood circulation and relieve joint pain.
- Fu Ling activates the spleen and stomach and eliminates damp in the body.
- Sang Ji Sheng strengthens the tendons and relieves joint pain.
- Zhi Gan Cao harmonizes the herbs in the prescription.
- Huang Bai and Cang Zhu eliminate damp, clear heat, and subside swelling.

Herbal Remedy:
Qiang Huo Sheng Shi Tablets-*Notopterygium Tablets to Overcome Damp.*

Acupuncture Treatment:
- Waiguan SJ-5 + Zulinqi GB-41, Shenmai BL-62 + Houxi SI-3, Hegu L.I.-4, Lieque LU-7, Fenglong ST-40, Sanyinjiao SP-6, Yinlingquan SP-9, Taichong LIV-3 and Yanglingquan GB-34.
- The xi-cleft points, luo-connecting points, and yuan-source points from some affected channels, together with some local Ah Shi points, should be applied accordingly.
- Moxibustion should be used on SP-9, GB-34, and some local Ah Shi points.
- Even method is applied on SJ-5 + GB-41, BL-62 + SI-3, and a reducing method is applied on the rest of the points. A reducing method is applied on selected xi-cleft points, luo-connecting points, and yuan-source points.
- If there is local redness and hotness around the affected joints, add Quchi L.I.-11 and ying-spring point from affected channels.

Explanations:
- The combination of SJ-5 + GB-41, and BL-62 + SI-3, two groups of the eight confluence points, harmonize and invigorate Yangwei, Dai, Yangqiao and Du channels and promote the qi circulation to relieve joint pain.
- LU-7, the luo-connecting point of the lung channel, opens the skin pores to eliminate the remaining pathogenic factors, disperses the lung-qi, and restores the physiological functions of the lung.
- L.I.-4, the yuan-source of the large intestine channel, LIV-3, the yuan-source of the liver channel, promotes the qi circulation and relieves the pain in the body.
- GB-34, the influential point of the tendons in the body, relaxes the tendons and relieves joint pain.
- ST-40, the luo-connecting point of the stomach channel, SP-6 and SP-9, the crossing point of three yin channels of the foot and the he-sea point of the spleen channel respectively, eliminate damp in the body, promote blood circulation and relieve joint pain.
- The xi-cleft points, luo-connecting points, and yuan-source points from some affected channels, together with some local Ah Shi points, promote the qi and blood circulation and relieve the joint

pain. Without these points, the acupuncture effect to relieve joint pain is limited.

- Moxibustion warms the channels and collaterals and eliminates cold.
- L.I.-11 and the ying-spring points from affected channels could clear heat and subside swelling.

11.3.2.2 *Accumulation of damp-phlegm*

Joint pain with heaviness and swelling, limitation of joint movement, stiffness in the joints, heaviness of the body, nausea, poor appetite, loose stool or diarrhea, heaviness in the head with foggy feeling, lassitude, tiredness, white and greasy coating on the tongue, and a wiry and slippery pulse.

Principle of Treatment:
Eliminate damp phlegm, harmonize the collateral, promote qi circulation, and relieve joint pain.

Herbal Treatment:
Juan Bi Tang-*Remove Painful Obstruction Decoction.*

Qiang Huo *Rhizoma et Radix Notopterygii* 10 g
Qin Jiao *Radix Gentianae Macrophyllae* 10 g
Chuan Niu Xi *Radix Cyathulae Officinalis* 10 g
Wu Jia Pi *Cortex Acanthopanacis Gracilistyli Radicis* 10 g
Dang Gui *Radix Angelicae Sinensis* 10 g
Chuan Xiong *Radix Ligustici Wallichii* 10 g
Sang Zhi *Ramulus Mori Albae* 30 g
Hou Po *Cortex Magnoliae Officinalis* 10 g
Cang Zhu *Rhizoma Atractylodis* 10 g
Fu Ling *Sclerotium Poriae Cocos* 15 g
Chen Pi *Pericarpium Citri Reticulatae* 5 g
Gui Zhi *Ramulus Cinnamomi Cassiae* 10 g
Mu Xiang *Radix Aucklandiae* 6 g
Zhi Gan Cao *Radix Glycyrrhizae Preparata* 3 g

In case of local redness and hotness due to damp-heat, remove Qin Jiao *Radix Gentianae Macrophyllae* and Gui Zhi *Ramulus Cinnamomi Cassiae*, and add

- Huang Bai *Cortex Phellodendri* 10 g
- Cang Zhu *Rhizoma Atractylodis* 10 g

Explanations:
- Qiang Huo, Qin Jiao and Wu Jia Pi eliminate damp in the channels and collaterals and relieve joint pain.
- Chuan Niu Xi eliminates damp in the collaterals, strengthens the tendons, and relieves joint pain.
- Sang Zhi induces the effects of the herbs to the collaterals and relieves the joint pain.
- Dang Gui and Chuan Xiong promote the circulation of blood and sedate joint pain.
- Gui Zhi warms the channels and promotes blood circulation in the collaterals.
- Mu Xiang promotes the circulation of qi in the middle Jiao, resolves damp and relieves diarrhea.
- Hou Po, Cang Zhu, Fu Ling and Chen Pi activate the spleen and stomach and eliminate damp in the body.
- Zhi Gan Cao harmonizes the herbs in the prescription.
- Huang Bai and Cang Zhu eliminate damp, clear heat, and subside swelling.

Herbal Remedy:
Shen Ling Bai Zhu Wan-*Ginseng, Poria and Atractylodis Macrocephalae Pill.*

Acupuncture Treatment:
- Waiguan SJ-5 + Zulinqi GB-41, Shenmai BL-62 + Houxi SI-3, Hegu L.I.-4, Zhongwan REN-12, Fenglong ST-40, Taibai SP-3, Sanyinjiao SP-6, Yinlingquan SP-9, Taichong LIV-3 and Yanglingquan GB-34.
- The xi-cleft points, luo-connecting points, and yuan-source points from some affected channels should be selected accordingly.

- Moxibustion should be used on SP-9, GB-34, and some local Ah Shi points.
- Even method is applied on SJ-5 + GB-41, BL62 + SI3, and a reducing method is applied on the rest of the points. A reducing method is applied on selected xi-cleft points, luo-connecting points, and yuan-source points.
- If there is local redness and hotness around the affected joints, add Quchi L.I.-11 and ying-spring point from affected channels.

Explanations:
- The combination of SJ-5 + GB-41, and BL-62 + SI-3, two groups of the eight confluence points, harmonize and invigorate Yangwei, Dai, Yangqiao and Du channels and promote the qi circulation to relieve joint pain.
- L.I.-4, the yuan-source of the large intestine channel, LIV-3, the yuan-source of the liver channel, promote the qi circulation and relieve the pain in the body.
- GB-34, the influential point of the tendons in the body, relaxes the tendons and relieves joint pain.
- REN-12, the gathering point of the fu organ, ST-40, SP-6 and SP-9 eliminate damp in the body, promote blood circulation and relieve joint pain.
- The xi-cleft points, luo-connecting points, and yuan-source points from some affected channels, together with some local Ah Shi points, promote the qi and blood circulation and relieve the joint pain.
- Moxibustion warms the channels and collaterals and eliminates cold.
- L.I.-11 and the ying-spring points from affected channels could clear heat and subside swelling.

11.3.2.3 *Stagnation of qi and blood*

Wandering joint pain or stabbing joint pain with fixed location, swelling and limitation of joint movement, stiffness in the joints, aggravation of joint pain at night, insomnia, the fullness of hypochondriac regions, irritability, nervousness, poor appetite, thin and white coating on the tongue, and a wiry and thready pulse.

Principle of Treatment:
Smooth the liver and emotions, promote the qi circulation, and relieve the breathlessness.

Herbal Treatment:
Shu Jing Huo Xue Tang-*Relax the Channels and Invigorate the Blood Decoction.*

Qiang Huo *Rhizoma et Radix Notopterygii* 10 g
Chuan Xiong *Radix Ligustici Wallichii* 10 g
Dang Gui *Radix Angelicae Sinensis* 10 g
Chi Shao Yao *Radix Paeoniae Rubrae* 10 g
Cang Zhu *Rhizomz Atractylodis* 10 g
Chuan Niu Xi *Radix Cyathulae Officinalis* 10 g
Bai Zhi *Radix Angelicae Dahuricae* 10 g
Chen Pi *Pericarpium Citri Reticulatae* 5 g
Fu Ling *Sclerotium Poriae Cocos* 12 g
Ru Xiang *Gummi Olibanum* 10 g
Mo Yao *Resina Commiphorae Myrrhae* 10 g
Ji Xue Teng *Caulis Milletiae Reticulatae* 10 g
Wei Ling Xian *Radix Clematidis* 10 g
Zhi Gan Cao *Radix Glycyrrhizae Preparata* 3 g

Explanations:
- Qiang Huo, Bai Zhi, Wei Ling Xian and Ji Xue Teng eliminate damp in the body and collaterals, relax the tendons and relieve joint pain.
- Dang Gui, Chuan Xiong, Chi Shao Yao, Ru Xiang and Mo Yao promote qi and blood circulation, eliminate blood stasis, and relieve joint pain.
- Cang Zhu, Fu Ling and Chen Pi activate the spleen, regulate the middle Jiao and eliminate damp in the body.

- Chuan Niu Xi promotes blood circulation and relieves joint pain.
- Zhi Gan Cao harmonizes the herbs in the prescription.

Herbal Remedy:
Shu Jing Huo Xue Wan-*Relax the Channels and Invigorate the Blood Pill.*

Acupuncture Treatment:
- Waiguan SJ-5 + Zulinqi GB-41, Shenmai BL-62 + Houxi SI-3, Hegu L.I.-4, Taiyuan LU-9, Tanzhong REN-17, Yanglingquan GB-34, Sanyinjiao SP-6, Taichong LIV-3, Xinshu BL-15 and Geshu BL-17.
- The xi-cleft points, luo-connecting points, and yuan-source points from some affected channels should be selected accordingly.
- Even method is applied on SJ-5 + GB-41, BL-62 + SI-3, and a reducing method is applied on the rest of the points. A reducing method is applied on selected xi-cleft points, luo-connecting points, and yuan-source points.

Explanations:
- The combination of SJ-5 + GB-41, and BL-62 + SI-3, two groups of the eight confluence points, harmonize and invigorate Yangwei, Dai, Yangqiao and Du channels and promote the qi circulation to relieve joint pain.
- L.I.-4, the yuan-source of the large intestine channel, LIV-3, the yuan-source of the liver channel, REN-17, the influential point for the qi in the body, promote the qi circulation and relieve the pain.
- GB-34, the influential point of the tendons in the body, relaxes the tendons and relieves joint pain.
- LU-9, the influential point for the vessels in the body, SP-6, the crossing point of three yin channels of the food, BL-15, the back-shu point of the heart, and BL-17, the influential point for the blood, promote blood circulation, eliminate blood stasis, and relieve joint pain.
- The xi-cleft points, luo-connecting points, and yuan-source points from some affected channels, together with some local Ah Shi points, promote the qi and blood circulation and relieve the joint pain.

11.3.2.4 *Deficiency of qi and blood*

Slight joint pain with stiffness which becomes worse with physical movement, weakness of joints during movement, tiredness, dizziness, palpitations, poor appetite, lower back pain, pale complexion, pale tongue with a thin and white coating, and a thready and weak pulse.

Principle of Treatment:
Tonify qi, benefit blood, strengthen the tendons and reinforce the kidney.

Herbal Treatment:
Du Huo Ji Sheng Tang-*Angelica Pubescentis and Taxillus Decoction.*

Du Huo *Radix Angelicae Pubescentis* 10 g
Fang Feng *Radix Ledebouriellae Divaricatae* 10 g
Qin Jiao *Radix Gentianae Macrophyllae* 10 g
Sang Ji Sheng *Ramulus Loranthi* 10 g
Du Zhong *Cortex Eucommiae Ulmoidis* 10 g
Huai Niu Xi *Radix Achyranthis Bidentatae* 10 g
Shu Di Huang *Radix Rhemanniae Glutinosae Praeparata* 15 g
Bai Zhu *Rhizoma Atractylodis Macrocephalae* 10 g
Shan Yao *Radix Dioscoreae Oppositae* 10 g
Fu Ling *Sclerotium Poriae Cocos* 12 g
Rou Gui *Cortex Cinnamomi Cassiae* 5 g
Chuan Xiong *Radix Ligustici Wallichii* 10 g
Bai Shao Yao *Radix Paeoniae Lactiflorae* 10 g
Dang Gui *Radix Angelicae Sinensis* 10 g
Zhi Gan Cao *Radix Glycyrrhizae Preparata* 3 g

Explanations:
- Du Huo, Fang Feng and Qin Jiao eliminate some remaining pathogenic factors and relieve joint pain.
- Sang Ji Sheng, Du Zhong and Huai Niu Xi strengthen the tendons and lower back, benefit kidney-jing and relieve joint pain.

- Dang Gui, Shu Di Huang and Bai Shao Yao tonify liver-blood and kidney-jing to strengthen the tendons and bones in the body.
- Bai Zhu, Shan Yao and Fu Ling activate the spleen and stomach, eliminate damp and tonify the qi in the body.
- Rou Gui warms the channels and relieves cold in the body.
- Chuan Xiong promotes blood circulation and relieves joint pain.
- Zhi Gan Cao harmonizes the herbs in the prescription.

Herbal Remedy:
Ren Shen Zai Zao Wan-*Ginseng Recreating Pill.*

Acupuncture Treatment:
- Waiguan SJ-5 + Zulinqi GB-41, Shenmai BL-62 + Houxi SI-3, Yanglingquan GB-34, Zusanli ST-36, Sanyinjiao SP-6, Qihai REN-6, Taixi KID-3 and Shenshu BL-23.
- The xi-cleft points, luo-connecting points, and yuan-source points from some affected channels should be selected accordingly.
- Moxibustion should be used on ST-36, REN-6, GB-34, and some local Ah Shi points.
- Even method is applied on SJ-5 + GB-41, BL-62 + SI-3, and a tonifying method is applied on the rest of the points. A reducing method is applied on selected xi-cleft points, luo-connecting points, and yuan-source points.

Explanations:
- The combination of SJ-5 + GB-41, and BL-62 + SI-3, two groups of the eight confluence points, harmonize and invigorate Yangwei, Dai, Yangqiao and Du channels and promote the qi circulation to relieve joint pain.
- GB-34, ST-36, SP-6, REN-6, KID-3 and BL-23 tonify liver-blood, benefit the tendons, strengthen the bones, and reinforce kidney-jing.
- Moxibustion warms the channels and collaterals, eliminates internal colds, and supports yang-qi.
- The xi-cleft points, luo-connecting points, and yuan-source points from some affected channels, together with some local Ah Shi

points, promote the qi and blood circulation and relieve the joint pain.

11.4 Chest Pain

Chest pain refers to discomfort or pain between the neck and upper abdomen, which can be sharp, distending, dull or stabbing, and can happen in short bursts or be continuous. A small proportion of patients with COVID-19 can experience significant chest pains, which are mostly brought on by breathing deeply, coughing, sneezing, physical movements, or emotions. Patients with severe COVID-19 are more likely to report trouble breathing or chest pain than people with mild illness.

Although many viral infections are self-limiting and making people feel unwell for only a few days before clearing up, this SARS-CoV-2 infection is not just causing pneumonia. In some patients it could attack many other different systems in the body, e.g., the heart and blood vessels, the brain, and the kidneys. With high efficacy of COVID-19 vaccines, the initial efforts concentrated on saving the lives of the tens of thousands of people have shifted to the raised awareness of persistence and extremely debilitating COVID problems. Those suffering from it describe a varying combination of overlapping symptoms and chest pain is one of the most common symptoms experienced during Long COVID. One research published in JAMA (*The Journal of the American Medical Association*) on 9 July 2020, points out that worse quality of life was observed among 44.1% of patients and a high proportion of individuals still reported chest pain (21.7%), which is the fourth complaint from Long COVID besides fatigue (53.1%), dyspnea (43.4%) and joint pain (27.3%).[12]

Chest pains are most likely to occur alongside other symptoms. When clustered with a lot of severe symptoms, such as high fever, cough, shortness of breath, abdominal pains and confusion, chest pain is a clear sign for hospitalization, particularly in older people.

---

[12]Angelo Carfì, *et al. op. cit.*

In milder cases, chest pain usually appears alongside headaches, shortness of breath, and fatigue.

Chest pain during Long COVID is usually not life threatening since it may present for the first time after COVID infection or during Long COVID (likely caused by the virus directly affecting the muscles and lungs). However, some cases of chest pain might be related to potentially serious heart or lung conditions, such as a heart attack or pulmonary embolism. When experiencing a sudden chest pain (which persists for more than 15 minutes), together with nausea, vomiting, sweating, shortness of breath, or loss of consciousness, immediate medical examinations should be taken.

According to some scientific studies, the virus that causes COVID-19 is thought to enter the heart, lungs, and other tissues through an angiotensin converting enzyme 2 (ACE2), which causes damage to these tissues. Researchers speculate that once the virus is in the heart and lungs, it can release molecules called cytokines that promote inflammation. These molecules can cause injury to the heart or inflammation of the lungs.

Therefore, COVID-19 chest pain occurs. Chest pain is most common in patients with severe COVID-19 infection and is found to be about three times more common in patients who die of the disease than in survivors.[13] One study of adult patients who recently recovered from COVID-19 suggested that 60% of them had myocarditis, regardless of how severe their COVID symptoms were during the infection.[14] Mechanisms of microvascular disease in COVID-19

---

[13] Lin-Man Weng, *et al.* Pain symptoms in patients with coronavirus disease (COVID-19): A literature review. *J Pain Res.* 2021, 14: 147–159. doi: 10.2147/JPR.S269206.

[14] Valentina O. Puntmann, *et al.* Outcomes of cardiovascular magnetic resonance imaging in patients recently recovered from coronavirus disease 2019 (COVID-19). *JAMA Cardiol.* 2020, 5(11): 1265–1273. doi: 10.1001/jamacardio.2020.3557.

include endothelial injury with endothelial dysfunction and micro-vascular inflammation and thrombosis.[15,16]

In fact, chest pain of Long COVID could also be non-specific/non-cardiac chest pain, which is the term that is used to describe pain in the chest that is not caused by heart disease. In most people, non-cardiac chest pain is related to a problem with the esophagus, such as gastroesophageal reflux disease. Other causes include muscle or bone problems, stomach problems, stress, anxiety, and depression.

Treatment for chest pain of Long COVID in modern medicine depends on the underlying causes, in which NSAIDs are often applied.

11.4.1 TCM understanding of Long COVID-associated chest pain

In TCM, the chest belongs to the upper Jiao, storing the chest yang, heart and lung. Physiologically, the heart controls blood and blood vessels and houses the shen, and the lung governs respiration and regulates the upper source of water in the body. Functional coordination of the heart and lungs maintains the normal circulation of qi and blood, clear-yang in the chest and water distribution in the body.

Chest pain of Long COVID is considered chest Bi syndrome. Bi means obstruction of qi and blood with pain, distension, or another complaint.

Chest Bi can be caused by various pathogenic factors, such as invasion of cold-damp or damp-heat with a pestilent toxin to the heart and lung, dysfunction of the spleen and stomach with the formation of damp-phlegm, emotional disturbance, debility after COVID-19, ageing, weak constitution, and lack of daily life care, etc.

---

[15]Zsuzsanna Varga, *et al*. Endothelial cell infection and endotheliitis in COVID-19. *The Lancet.* 2020, 395: 1417–1418.

[16]Charles J. Lowenstein and Scott D. Solomon. Severe COVID-19 is a microvascular disease. *Circulation.* 2020, 142: 1609–1611. doi: 10.1161/CIRCULATIONAHA.120.050354.

This leads to obstruction of chest yang by damp-phlegm, stagnation of qi and blood, or deficiency of qi or yang of the heart and kidney. In some severe cases, there could be retention of fluid in the heart and lung. The above pathogenesis may coexist, and when they do, the conditions become more complicated.

11.4.1.1 *Incomplete elimination of external pathogenic factors*

COVID-19 is mainly caused by the invasion of cold-damp or damp-heat with a pestilent toxin to the body, especially the lung and heart. When the zheng-qi is sufficient, or the treatment is proper and in time, these pathogenic factors could be eliminated completely. Otherwise, they could cause stagnation and latent accumulation in the body, resulting in disturbance and obstruction of the chest-yang, or the qi and blood in the chest, and chest Bi syndrome occurs. When there is a disorder of the lung in dispersing or descending the qi, there could be stagnation of qi in the chest, thus chest Bi syndrome happens with cough, shortness of breath. When there is a disorder of the heart in regulating the blood circulation and blood vessels, there would be chest bi with palpitations, restlessness, and insomnia, etc.

11.4.1.2 *Accumulation of damp-phlegm*

During COVID-19, a disorder of San Jiao in water regulation and yuan-qi distribution, dysfunction of the spleen and stomach in digestion, transportation and transformation, disharmony of cold and heat in the body, poor function of the intestine, bladder, and gallbladder, etc., could cause the formation of damp-phlegm internally, which may block the chest-yang, causing chest Bi.

11.4.1.3 *Emotional disturbance*

Being emotionally upset or disturbed during COVID-19, having unsolved emotional disorders before COVID-19, etc., could lead to retardation of qi circulation. It is believed in TCM that qi circulation leads to blood circulation and blood stagnation aggravates qi stagnation. When there is qi stagnation for a while, there could be stagnation of blood, thus forming stagnation of qi and blood at the same time. Stagnation of qi and blood could show different manifestations. Blood stagnation often presents in some severe cases of chest pain of Long COVID.

11.4.1.4 *Deficiency of qi and yang*

Prolonged persistence of COVID-19, especially in old and weak patients, lack of post COVID care for daily life and diet, overstrain, etc., could cause consumption of qi, leading to deficiency of qi or even yang, bringing about the formation of deficient cold and stagnation in the different zang-fu organs, such as the lung, heart, spleen and kidney.

Deficiency of lung-qi could lead to weakness of the lung in dispersing and descending the qi. Deficiency of qi and yang of the heart could cause disorder of the blood circulation and contraction of the blood vessels. Deficiency of qi or yang of the spleen could eventually lead to the formation of cold-damp and weakness of the lung. Deficiency of qi or yang of the kidney could cause the failure of the lung in performing its physiological functions, dysfunction of the lung happens. All the above conditions may result in chest pain from Long COVID.

11.4.2 TCM treatment of Long COVID-associated chest pain

11.4.2.1 *Blockage of the chest-yang by external pathogenic factors*

Persistence of chest pain since the onset of COVID-19 (which is aggravated by cold), oppression over the chest, palpitation or even dyspnea, coldness of limbs, white and greasy tongue coating, and a tense and slippery pulse.

Principle of Treatment:
Expel cold, eliminate damp, activate stagnated yang, and relieve chest pain.

Herbal Treatment:
Gua Lou Xie Bai Ban Xia Tang-*Trichosanthis Fruit, Chinese Garlic and Pinellia Decoction.*

Gua Lou Pi *Pericarpium Trichosanthis* 12 g
Xie Bai *Bulbus Allii Macrostemi* 10 g
Zhi Ban Xia *Rhizoma Pinelliae Ternatae Preparata* 10 g
Qiang Huo *Rhizoma et Radix Notopterygii* 10 g
Rou Gui *Cortex Cinnamomi Cassiae* 5 g
Dan Shen *Radix Salviae Miltiorrhizae* 12 g
Chuan Xiong *Radix Ligustici Wallichii* 10 g
Xing Ren *Semen Pruni Armeniacae* 10 g
Yu Jin *Tuber Curcumae* 10 g
Chen Pi *Pericarpium Citri Reticulatae* 5 g

Explanations:
• Gua Lou Pi and Xie Bai open and relax the chest, promote qi circulation, and relieve chest pain.
• Qiang Huo dispels remaining pathogenic factors and relieves chest pain.
• Zhi Ban Xia and Xing Ren eliminate phlegm in the lung, disperse and descend the lung-qi and relieve cough.
• Rou Gui warms the channels and dispels cold in the chest to relieve the blockage in the chest.
• Yu Jin and Chen Pi promote qi circulation and relieve chest pain.
• Dan Shen and Chuan Xiong promote blood circulation and relieve chest pain.

Herbal Remedy:
Qiang Huo Sheng Shi Tablets-*Notopterygium Tablets to Overcome Damp.*

Acupuncture Treatment:
- Neiguan P-6 + Gongsun SP-4, Hegu L.I.-4, Lieque LU-7, Chize LU-5, Ximen P-4, Tanzhong REN-17, Fenglong ST-40, Sanyinjiao SP-6, Yinlingquan SP-9, Taichong LIV-3, Qimen LIV-14. Some local Ah Shi points as well.
- An even method is applied on P-6 + SP-4, and a reducing method is applied on the rest of the points.

Explanations:
- The combination of P-6 + SP-4, one group of the eight confluence points, promotes the qi circulation, and relaxes the chest to relieve chest pain.
- LU-7, and LU-5, the luo-connecting point and the he-sea point of the lung channel respectively, disperse and descend the lung-qi, restore the physiological functions of the lung, and relieve cough and chest pain.
- P-4, the xi-cleft point of the pericardium channel, L.I.-4, the yuan-source of the large intestine channel, LIV-3, the yuan-source of the liver channel, LIV-14, the front-mu point of the liver, and REN-17, the confluence point for the qi in the body, together with the local Ah Shi points, relax the chest, promote qi circulation and relieve chest pain.
- ST-40, the luo-connecting point of the stomach channel, SP-6, the crossing points of the three yin channels of the foot, and SP-9, the he-sea point of the spleen channel, regulate the San Jiao, eliminate damp-phlegm in the body, activate the spleen and stomach and relieve chest pain.

11.4.2.2 *Accumulation of damp-phlegm*

Chest pain, pressure over the chest with heaviness, heaviness in the head with foggy feeling, slight cough with expectoration of sticky whitish phlegm, lassitude, nausea, poor appetite, loose stool or diarrhea, tiredness, white and greasy coating on the tongue, and a wiry and slippery pulse.

Principle of Treatment:
Eliminate damp-phlegm, promote qi circulation, and relieve chest pain.

Herbal Treatment:
Ban Xia Hou Po Tang-*Pinellia and Magnolia Bark Decoction*, plus Cang Fu Dao Tan Tang-*Atractylodes-Poria Phlegm-Dissipating Decoction.*

Hou Po *Cortex Magnoliae Officinalis* 10 g
Zhi Shi *Fructus Immaturus Citri Aurantii* 10 g
Zhi Ban Xia *Rhizoma Pinelliae Ternatae Preparata* 10 g
Xing Ren *Semen Pruni Armeniacae* 10 g
Zi Su Zi *Fructus Perillae Frutescentis* 10 g
Cang Zhu *Rhizoma Atractylodis* 10 g
Xiang Fu *Rhizoma Cyperi Rotundi* 10 g
Gua Lou Pi *Pericarpium Trichosanthis* 10 g
Chuan Xiong *Radix Ligustici Wallichii* 10 g
Zhi Ke *Fructus Citri Aurantii* 10 g
Yu Jin *Tuber Curcumae* 10 g
Fu Ling *Sclerotium Poriae Cocos* 12 g
Chen Pi *Pericarpium Citri Reticulatae* 5 g
Sheng Jiang *Rhizoma Zingiberis Officinalis Recens* 5 g

Explanations:
- Hou Po, Xing Ren and Zi Su Zi resolve phlegm, descend the lung-qi, and relieve chest pain.
- Zhi Shi, Gua Lou Pi and Cang Zhu eliminate damp-phlegm, promote qi circulation, and relieve chest pain.
- Xiang Fu, Chuan Xiong, Yu Jin and Zhi Ke promote the qi circulation in the chest and relieve the blockage of the chest by damp-phlegm.
- Zhi Ban Xia, Fu Ling, Chen Pi and Sheng Jiang disperse the lung-qi, eliminate phlegm and relieve cough.

Herbal Remedy:
Cang Fu Dao Tan Wan-*Atractylodes-Poria Phlegm-Dissipating Pill.*

Acupuncture Treatment:
- Neiguan P-6 + Gongsun SP-4, Hegu L.I.-4, Kongzui LU-6, Lieque LU-7, Chize LU-5, Ximen P-4, Tanzhong REN-17, Fenglong ST-40, Sanyinjiao SP-6, Yinlingquan SP-9, Taichong LIV-3, Qimen LIV-14.
- An even method is applied on P-6 + SP-4, and a reducing method is applied on the rest of the points.

Explanations:
- The combination of P-6 + SP-4 promotes the qi circulation and relaxes the chest to relieve chest pain.
- ST-40, SP-6 and SP-9 activate the spleen and stomach and eliminate damp-phlegm in the body.
- LU-6, the xi-cleft point of the lung channel, LU-7, and LU-5 disperse and descend the lung-qi, restore the physiological functions of the lung, and relieve cough and chest pain.
- P-4, L.I.-4, LIV-3, LIV-14, and REN-17 promote the qi circulation in the chest and relieve chest pain.

11.4.2.3 *Stagnation of qi*

Chest pain, fullness of the chest with distending pain, difficulty in breathing out, depression, unstable emotions, headache, stiffness of neck with some pain, insomnia, fullness of hypochondriac regions, irritability, nervousness, poor appetite, swollen feeling in the abdomen, thin and white coating on the tongue, and a wiry and thready pulse.

Principle of Treatment:
Harmonize the liver, smooth emotions, promote qi circulate, and relieve chest pain.

Herbal Treatment:
Xiao Yao San-*Rambling Powder.*

Chai Hu *Radix Bupleuri* 10 g
Bai Shao Yao *Radix Paeoniae Lactiflorae* 15 g

Zhi Ke *Fructus Citri Aurantii* 10 g
Gua Lou Pi *Pericarpium Trichosanthis* 10 g
Yu Jin *Tuber Curcumae* 10 g
Gui Zhi *Ramulus Cinnamomi Cassiae* 10 g
Hou Po *Cortex Magnoliae Officinalis* 10 g
Dang Gui *Radix Angelicae Sinensis* 10 g
Fu Shen *Sclerotium Poriae Cocos Paradicis* 12 g
Bai Zhu *Rhizoma Atractylodis Macrocephalae* 10 g
Duan Long Gu *Os Draconis (calcin)* 15 g
Yuan Zhi *Radix Polygalae Tenuifoliae* 10 g

Explanations:
- Chai Hu and Bai Shao Yao smooth the liver and relieve qi stagnation in the liver.
- Zhi Ke and Yu Jin promote the qi circulation in the body and regulate emotions.
- Dang Gui nourishes the liver-blood and benefits the liver.
- Hou Po and Gua Lou Pi promote the qi circulation and eliminate damp-phlegm in the chest and relieve the fullness in the chest.
- All the above herbs are used to promote and regulate the qi circulation in the liver and chest and relieve chest pain.
- Gui Zhi promotes blood circulation in the heart and invigorates blood circulation in the chest.
- Bai Zhu activates the spleen and eliminates damp in the body.
- Fu Shen, Duan Long Gu and Yuan Zhi smooth emotions, regulate the shen, and improve sleep.

Herbal Remedy:
Xiao Yao Wan-*Rambling Pill.*

Acupuncture Treatment:
- Neiguan P-6 + Gongsun SP-4, Hegu L.I.-4, Lieque LU-7, Chize LU-5, Ximen P-4, Tanzhong REN-17, Fengchi GB-20, Sanyinjiao SP-6, Taichong LIV-3, Qimen LIV-14, Xinshu BL-15 and Ganshu BL-18. Some local Ah Shi points on the chest could be selected.

- An even method is applied on P-6 + SP-4, and a reducing method is applied on the rest of the points.

Explanations:
- The combination of P-6 + SP-4 promotes the qi circulation and relaxes the chest to relieve breathlessness.
- LU-7, LU-5, and REN-17 disperse and descend the lung-qi, relieve the qi stagnation in the chest, and relieve chest pain.
- L.I.-4 promotes the qi and blood circulation in the body and relieves pain and headache.
- GB-20 and BL-15 calm the shen and improve the emotions.
- L.I.-4, P-4, SP-6, LIV-3, LIV-14 and BL-18, together with some local Ah Shi points, smooth the liver, promote the qi circulation, and relieve chest pain.

11.4.2.4 *Stagnation of blood*

Stabbing chest pain with a fixed location radiating to the back, fullness of the chest, shortness of breath, palpitations, purplish or ecchymoses on the tongue, and an unsmooth or wiry pulse.

Principle of Treatment:
Promote the circulation of blood, eliminate stagnant blood, and sedate chest pain.

Herbal Treatment:
Xue Fu Zhu Yu Tang-*Drive out Stasis in the Mansion of Blood Decoction.*

Tao Ren *Semen Pruni Persicae* 10 g
Hong Hua *Flos Carthami Tinctorii* 10 g
Chi Shao Yao *Radix Paeoniae Rubrae* 10 g
Dang Gui *Radix Angelicae Sinensis* 10 g
Shu Di Huang *Radix Rhemanniae Glutinosae Praeparata* 10 g
Dan Shen *Radix Salviae Miltiorrhizae* 12 g

Chuan Xiong *Radix Ligustici Wallichii* 10 g
Yan Hu Suo *Rhizoma Corydalis* 10 g
Tan Xiang *Lignum Santali Albi* 3 g
Xiang Fu *Rhizoma Cyperi Rotundi* 10 g
Zhi Ke *Fructus Citri Aurantii* 10 g
Yu Jin *Tuber Curcumae* 10 g

Explanations:
- Tao Ren, Hong Hua, Dang Gui, Chi Shao Yao, Chuan Xiong, and Shu Di Huang, the complete composition of Tao Hong Si Wu Tang, promote blood circulation, eliminate blood stasis, and relieve the pain.
- Dan Shen and Tan Xiang promote blood circulation and relieve the blood stasis in the heart.
- Zhi Ke, Xiang Fu, Yu Jin and Yan Hu Suo promote qi circulation, eliminate blood stasis, and relieve chest pain.

Herbal Remedy:
Tao Hong Si Wu Tang tablet-*Four Substance (Things) Decoction Pill with Safflower and Peach Pit.*

Acupuncture Treatment:
- Neiguan P-6 + Gongsun SP-4, Lieque LU-7 + Zhaohai KID-6, Hegu L.I.-4, Kongzui LU-6, Chize LU-5, Tanzhong REN-17, Ximen P-4, Sanyinjiao SP-6, Taichong LIV-3, Xinshu BL-15 and Geshu BL-17. Some local Ah Shi points should be applied at the same time.
- An even method is applied on P-6 + SP-4 and LU-7 + KID-6, and a reducing method is applied on the rest of the points.

Explanations:
- The combination of P-6 + SP-4, and LU-7 + KID-6 promote the qi circulation, relaxes the chest, and relieves chest pain.
- LU-6, LU-5, REN-17, and P-4 disperse and descend the lung-qi, harmonize the collaterals, relieve the stagnation in the chest and relieve chest pain.

- L.I.-4 and LIV-3 promote the qi circulation in the body and relieve pain.
- SP-6, BL-15, and BL-17, together with the local Ah Shi points, promote blood circulation, eliminate blood stasis, and relieve breathlessness.

11.4.2.5 *Deficiency of qi and yang*

Slight chest pain with cold sensation which often becomes worse by exertion, difficulty in breathing in, slight cough, no expectoration of phlegm, tiredness, dizziness, palpitations, poor memory, timidness, pale complexion, pale tongue with a thin and white coating, and a thready and weak pulse.

Principle of Treatment:
Tonify qi, warm the heart and reinforce the kidney.

Herbal Treatment:
Zhi Gan Cao Tang-*Honey-Fried Licorice Decoction,* plus
You Gui Wan-*Restore the Right Pill.*

Zhi Gan Cao *Radix Glycyrrhizae Preparata* 10 g
Gui Zhi *Ramulus Cinnamomi Cassiae* 10 g
Shu Di Huang *Radix Rhemanniae Glutinosae Praeparata* 12 g
E Jiao *Gelatinum Corii Asini* 10 g
Wu Wei Zi *Fructus Schisandrae Chinensis* 10 g
Zhi Dang Shen *Radix Codonopsis Pilosulae Praeparata* 10 g
Zhi Huang Qi *Radix Astragali Membranacei Praeparata* 10 g
Shan Yao *Radix Dioscoreae Oppositae* 10 g
Du Zhong *Cortex Eucommiae Ulmoidis* 10 g
Xian Mao *Rhizoma Curculiginis Orchioidis* 10 g
Fu Ling *Sclerotium Poriae Cocos* 12 g

Explanations:
- Zhi Gan Cao and Gui Zhi warm the heart, eliminate cold in the chest, and regulate the heart vessels.

- Zhi Dang Shen, Bai Zhu, Fu Ling, Wu Wei Zi and Zhi Huang Qi activate the spleen and tonify the qi in the body.
- Shan Yao, Du Zhong and Xian Mao warm the kidney, tonify the kidney-yang and strengthen the lower back.
- Shu Di Huang and E Jiao tonify blood and benefit the heart.

Herbal Remedy:
You Gui Wan-*Restore the Right Pill.*

Acupuncture Treatment:
- Neiguan P-6 + Gongsun SP-4, Lieque LU-7 + Zhaohai KID-6, Taiyuan LU-9, Tanzhong REN-17, KID-23, KID-24, Zusanli ST-36, Sanyinjiao SP-6, Taixi KID-3, Qihai REN-6, Feishu BL-13 and Shenshu BL-23.
- An even method is applied on P-6 + SP-4, and LU-7 + KID-6, and a tonifying method is applied on the rest of the points. Moxibustion could be applied on ST-36, KID-3 and REN-6.

Explanations:
- P-6 + SP-4, and LU-7 + KID-6 promote the qi circulation, relax the chest, and relieve chest pain.
- LU-9, the yuan-source point of the lung channel and the influential point for the vessels, and BL-13, the back-shu point of the lung, tonify the qi of the lung and restore the physiological functions.
- ST-36 and SP-6 tonify the qi of the spleen and activate the spleen.
- KID-3 and BL-23 tonify the qi of the kidney and strengthen the lower back.
- REN-17, KID-23 and KID-24, together with the local Ah Shi point, promote the qi circulation and relieve chest pain.
- REN-6 tonifies the qi of the general body and eliminates cold in the body.
- Moxibustion warms the qi and dispels cold in the body.

11.5 Headache

The so-called Long COVID is a set of symptoms that accompanies the patient for months after initial discharge from the hospital. These symptoms include muscle fatigue, moderate breathlessness, persistent headache, the feeling of a foggy head, and the development of psychiatric disorders. In general, the quality of life of at least half of the patients who come out of the COVID-19 syndrome, both mild and severe, shows a markedly worsening despite having passed a difficult physical and psychological test.[17] Although headache does not represent a prognostic picture for the evolution of COVID-19, it must always be taken into consideration as a possible chronic sequelae of the infection.[18]

During the acute phase, headache associated with COVID-19 is a frequent symptom. Headaches can persist after COVID-19 resolution. Pathophysiological, its migraine-like features may reflect an activation of the trigeminovascular system by inflammation or direct involvement of SARS-CoV-2, a hypothesis supported by concomitant anosmia.[19]

One study shows that headache was the most frequent first symptom of COVID-19, described by 128 (27.9%) of the patients who reported headache, followed by fever in 109 (23.1%), cough in 60 (13.1%), and asthenia in 32 (7.0%).[20] However, headache is also one of the most common symptoms being experienced by those with lingering issues related to the coronavirus or the patients with Long COVID-19. It could continue for weeks or even months after being tested positive for COVID-19 even for people who had only a mild case of COVID-19.

One and half years after the outbreak of coronavirus disease 2019 (COVID-19), referrals for persistent headache associated with

---

[17]Willi S, *et al.* COVID-19 sequelae in adults aged less than 50 years: A systematic review. *Travel Med Infect Dis.* 2021, 40: 101995. doi: 10.1016/j.tmaid.2021.101995.
[18]Paolo Martelletti, *et al.* Long-COVID headache, *SN Compr Clin Med.* 2021, 3, 1704–1706. doi: 10.1007/s42399-021-00964-7.
[19]Edoardo Caronna, *et al.* Headache: A striking prodromal and persistent symptom, predictive of COVID-19 clinical evolution. *Cephalalgia.* 2020, 40(13): 1410–1421. https://doi.org/10.1177/0333102420965157.
[20]David García-Azorín, *et al.* Frequency and phenotype of headache in COVID-19: A study of 2194 patients. *Sci Rep.* 2021, 11: 14674. https://doi.org/10.1038/s41598-021-94220-6.

COVID-19 have become increasingly common in outpatient headache clinics. It is important to take into consideration that this term may include a spectrum of clinically different headache types. Some cases could show migraine-like headaches in individuals with a history of mild or severe COVID-19 infection. Any complaint of headache highlights the importance of a careful evaluation when assessing the complexities of "Long COVID" headache, as well as the need to further investigate the different underlying pathophysiological mechanisms. One research identified 9,573 studies, 28 peer-reviewed studies and 7 preprints. The sample was 28,438 COVID-19 survivors (12,307 females; mean age: 46.6, SD: 17.45 years). The methodological quality was high in 45% of the studies. The overall prevalence of post-COVID headache was 47.1% (95% CI 35.8–58.6) at onset or hospital admission, 10.2% (95% CI 5.4–18.5) at 30 days, 16.5% (95% CI 5.6–39.7) at 60 days, 10.6% (95% CI 4.7–22.3) at 90 days, and 8.4% (95% CI 4.6–14.8) at more than 180 days after onset/ hospital discharge. Headache as a symptom at the acute phase was more prevalent in non-hospitalized (57.97%) than in hospitalized (31.11%) patients. Time trend analysis showed a decreased prevalence from the acute symptoms' onset to all post-COVID follow-up periods which was maintained afterwards. This meta-analysis concluded that the prevalence of post COVID headache ranged from 8% to 15% during the first six months after SARS-CoV-2 infection.[21]

Headache during Long COVID could be sharp or dull, slight or severe, constant or intermittent, usually occurring at the forehead, vertex or occipital region. Sometimes, skull-pounding headaches with around-the-clock pain are separated only by periods of agonizing and extreme spikes.

In daily practice, it is not always easy to find a clear etiology or cause behind the headache. Brain scans of those with persistent headaches tend to be normal. Besides, such a headache is often just one of many symptoms experienced by COVID-19 long-haulers. Many also report fatigue, shortness of breath, painful joints, and chest

---

[21]César Fernández-de-las-Peñas, *et al.* Headache as an acute and post-COVID-19 symptom in COVID-19 survivors: A meta-analysis of the current literature. *Eur J Neurol.* 2021, 28(11): 3820–3825. https://doi.org/10.1111/ene.15040.

pain, etc. Thus, it could be concluded that a symptomatic treatment by using a painkiller is not a real solution to relieve headache together with other accompanying symptoms. TCM treatment based upon syndrome differentiation could be an ideal option.

11.5.1 TCM understanding of Long COVID-associated headache

All the six Yang Channels are going through the head area. Besides, Du channel and liver channel also have their connection or distribution on the head. The kidney is the important organ to produce marrow and the brain is the sea of marrow. The spleen transforms the essence of food into qi and blood, which nourishes the brain. Lung disperses qi to all the parts of the body, including the head. Heart dominates blood circulation and is in charge of mental activity. Moreover, blood is the basic energetic source for the physiological activity of the brain. Disorders in one of these channels or internal organs during Long COVID will influence the qi and blood circulation in the head, leading to headache.

11.5.1.1 *Incomplete elimination of external pathogenic factors*

COVID-19 is mainly caused by the invasion of cold-damp or damp-heat with a pestilent toxin to the body, especially the lung and heart. When these pathogenic factors are not eliminated completely or in time, they could cause stagnation and latent accumulation in the body, resulting in disturbance and obstruction of the channels and collaterals, as well as clear-yang, or the qi and blood or internal zang-fu organs, headache occurs.

11.5.1.2 *Emotional disturbance*

The liver plays an important role in emotional activities. It regulates qi circulation and stores blood. Stress, resentment and frustration during COVID-19 may cause retardation of liver-qi circulation, stagnation of liver-qi occurs. Once stagnation of liver-qi is formed, it may influence the physiological functions in the head, thus there would be stagnation of qi and blood, and headache occurs. This kind of headache is quite often seen in daily practice.

Qi is a kind of yang energy, which should be in the state of constant movement. In case of prolonged persistence of liver-qi stagnation, it may cause gradual formation of liver-fire. Moreover, anger and too much stress may accelerate this process of fire formation. Fire is characterized by uprising and burning. When there is formation of liver-fire in the body, it may rise to the head, disturbing qi and blood circulation and burning the channels on the head, causing headache. It is usually accompanied by distending of the head, redness of face and eyes, swelling of eyes, nervousness, irritability, insomnia, bitter taste in the mouth, red tongue with a thin and yellow coating, and a rapid and wiry pulse.

Headache caused by stagnation of liver-fire is usually located at temple areas of the head or whole head.

Prolonged persistence of flaring of liver-fire may cause hyperactivity of liver-yang, leading to the occurrence of severe headache or migraine.

11.5.1.3 *Accumulation of damp-phlegm*

The spleen has a function to transport and TCM. Invasion of external damp to the spleen and stomach, or improper diets during COVID-19 (such as overeating of sweet, fatty, greasy, and pungent food as well as indulgence in alcoholic drinks), may cause the physiological function of the spleen and stomach to be impaired, resulting in accumulation of damp-phlegm in the body. When the head is blocked by damp-phlegm, clear-yang, or qi and blood would fail to rise and Turbid qi would fail to descend, qi and blood circulation in the head is stagnant, causing headache.

11.5.1.4 *Deficiency of qi and blood*

The spleen is the acquired source for qi and blood production, thus dysfunction of the spleen and stomach during COVID-19, or overconsumption of qi and blood during sickness would cause deficiency of qi and blood, causing the head to be under-nourished, and a headache appears. Improper diets and eating too little during COVID-19 may cause the poor function of the spleen in transportation and transformation, impairing qi and blood production, and forming deficiency of qi and blood.

11.5.2 TCM treatment of Long COVID-associated headache

To understand the key points for the differentiation for headache, special attention should be paid to the quality, the location of the headache and other factors, which may alleviate or aggravate the headache. For instance, a dull pain indicates deficiency condition, while a sharp pain indicates an excess condition according to the eight principles perspective. A headache with the feeling of heaviness is usually caused by the accumulation of damp-phlegm, a headache with distending feeling is a type of pain with "swollen", "throbbing", "bursting" and "pulsating" sensation. This kind of headache is usually caused by a disorder of the liver.

A headache with stabbing, fixed in one place and aggravation of pain at night or before menstruation indicates stagnation of blood. A headache with the sensation of emptiness of the head indicates Deficiency of qi and blood.

11.5.2.1 *Disturbed head by external wind-damp*

Slight headache with heavy sensation, feeling of the head to be wrapped with a piece of cloth, aggravation of the headache when exposed to cold and humid weather, lassitude, slight general body pain with heavy sensation, fatigue, thin, white, and greasy coating on the tongue, and a slippery and superficial pulse.

Principle of Treatment:
Dispel wind, eliminate damp, harmonize the collaterals, and relieve headache.

Herbal Treatment:
Qiang Huo Sheng Shi Tang-*Notopterygium Decoction to Overcome Dampness.*

Qiang Huo *Rhizoma seu Radix Notopterygii* 10 g
Du Huo *Radix angelicae Pubescentis* 10 g
Gao Ben *Rhizoma Radix Ligustici* 10 g
Fu Ling *Sclerotium Poriae Cocos* 15 g
Chuan Xiong *Rhizoma Ligustici Chuanxiong* 10 g
Fang Feng *Radix Ledebouriellae* 6 g
Ban Xia *Rhizoma Pinelliae Praeparata* 10 g
Man Jing Zi *Fructus Viticis* 10 g
Zhi Gan Cao *Radix Glycyrrhizae Preparata* 3 g

Explanations:
- Qiang Huo, Du Huo and Fang Feng can dispel wind, eliminate cold-damp from the upper parts of the body so as to relieve remaining external pathogenic factors.
- Chuan Xiong expels wind, promotes qi and blood circulation, and relieves headache.
- Gao Ben and Man Jing Zi dispel wind-damp and relieve headache.
- Ban Xia and Fu Ling are used to dry damp, eliminate phlegm and harmonize the middle Jiao.
- Zhi Gan Cao coordinates the effects of the other herbs in the recipe.

Herbal Remedy:
Qiang Huo Sheng Shi Pian-*Notopterygium Tablets to Overcome Dampness.*

Acupuncture Treatment:
- Hegu L.I.-4, Lieque LU-7, Waiguan SJ-5, Zhigou SJ-6, Fengchi GB-20, Sanyinjiao SP-6, Extra Yintang and Ashi points on the head.
- A reducing method is applied on all these points.

Explanations:

- L.I.-4, the yuan-source point of the large intestine channel, and GB-20, the crossing point of the foot Shaoyang and Yangwei channels, dispel wind-damp, regulate qi circulation, and relieve headache.
- LU-7, the luo-connecting point of the lung channel, promotes the qi circulation, eliminates damp in the upper Jiao and relieves headache.
- Extra Yintang relieves headache symptomatically.
- SJ-5 and SJ-6 dispel wind-damp, harmonize the collaterals and relieve headache.
- SP-6, the crossing point of three yin channels of the foot, promotes qi circulation and eliminates damp.
- Ashi points are used to regulate qi circulation, harmonize the local collateral and relieve headaches.

11.5.2.2 *Stagnation of liver-qi*

Headache with pressure and tension sensation (which starts or gets worse under stress or emotional disturbance), depression, painful neck, distension and pain in the hypochondriac region, insomnia, irregular menstruation, poor appetite or overeating, thin and white tongue coating, and a wiry pulse.

Principle of Treatment:
Smooth the liver, promote qi circulation, calm the shen and relieve headache.

Herbal Treatment:
Xiao Yao San-*Rambling Powder.*

Chai Hu *Radix Bupleare* 10 g
Dang Gui *Radix Angelicae Sinensis* 10 g
Bai Shao Yao *Radix Paeoniae Lactiflorae* 10 g
Bai Zhu *Rhiizoma Areactylodis Macrocephalae* 10 g

Fu Ling *Sclerotium Poriae Cocos* 15 g
Chuan Xiong *Rhizoma Ligustici Chuan Xiong* 10 g
Huang Qin *Radix Scutellariae Baicalensis* 10 g
Bo He *Herba Menthae Haplocalycis* 3 g
Man Jing Zi *Fructus Viticis* 10 g
Zhi Gan Cao *Radix Glycyrrhizae Preparata* 3 g

Explanations:
* Chai Hu regulates and promotes liver-qi circulation and relieve qi stagnation in the liver.
* Bai Shao Yao and Dang Gui are used to nourish blood in the liver, harmonize and smooth the liver, and relieve headache and hypochondriac pain.
* Chuan Xiong regulates liver-qi and relieves headaches.
* Bai Zhu and Fu Ling strengthen the spleen and stomach and improve the appetite.
* Huang Qin and Bo He clear internal heat resulting from the stagnation of liver-qi and prevent further formation of liver-fire.
* Man Jing Zi relieves headaches.
* Zhi Gan Cao harmonizes the actions of the other herbs.

Herbal Remedy:
Xiao Yao Wan-*Rambling Pill.*

Acupuncture Treatment:
* Waiguan SJ-5 + Zulinqi GB-41, Hegu L.I.-4, Shuaigu GB-8, Extra Yintang, Extra Taiyang, Fengchi GB-20, Jianjing GB-21, Taichong LIV-3, Qimen LIV-14, Neiguan P-6, Sanyinjiao SP-6, Extra Sishencong.
* An even method is applied on SJ-5 + GB-41, and a reducing method is applied on these points.

Explanations:
* SJ-5 + GB-41 is a combination to harmonize Shaoyang channels, benefit the gallbladder and relieve headaches.

- L.I.-4 and LIV-3, the yuan-source point of the large intestine channel and the liver channel respectively, and LIV-14, the front-mu point of the liver, smooth the liver, regulate the qi circulation in the body and relieve liver-qi stagnation. Meanwhile, they could relieve headaches.
- P-6, the luo-connecting point of the pericardium channel, regulates qi circulation and calms the shen.
- Extra Sishencong calms the shen, improves sleep and regulates emotion.
- SP-6, the crossing point of the three yin channels of the foot, promotes the smooth qi and blood circulation in the liver and in the head to relieve headache.
- GB-8, GB-20 and GB-21 regulate the collateral of the gallbladder channel, smooth the emotions, relieve the neck tension, and promote qi circulation in the head to relieve headache.
- Extra Yintang and Extra Taiyang, the local points, relieve headaches.

11.5.2.3 *Flaring up of liver-fire*

Persistent headache with sharp pain or distending pain, redness of eyes, irritability, bitter taste in the mouth, restlessness, insomnia, irregular menstruation, poor appetite, deep yellow urine, constipation, red tongue, and a rapid and wiry pulse.

Principle of Treatment:
Reduce liver-fire, clear heat, calm the shen and relieve headache.

Herbal Treatment:
Long Dan Xie Gan Tang-*Gentiana Longdancao Decoction to Drain the Liver.*

Long Dan Cao *Radix Gentianae Anomalae* 10 g
Huang Qin *Radix Scutellariae Baicalensis* 10 g
Zhi Zi *Fructus Gardenniae* 10 g

Ze Xie *Rhizoma Alismatis* 12 g
Chuan Xiong *Rhizoma Lagustici Chuanxiong* 10 g
Xia Ku Cao *Spica Prunellae* 10 g
Che Qian Zi *Semen Plantaginis* 10 g
Dang Gui *Radix Angelicae Sinensis* 10 g
Sheng Di Huang *Radix Rehmanniae Glutinosae* 12 g
Chai Hu *Radix Bupleuri* 10 g
Man Jing Zi *Fructus Viticis* 10 g
Zhi Gan Cao *Radix Glycyrrhizae Preparata* 3 g

In case of hyperactivity of liver-yang, add Gou Teng *Ramulus cum Uncis Uncariae* 10 g and Tian Ma *Rhizoma Gastrodiae Elatae* 10 g.

Explanations:
- Long Dan Cao, Huang Qin, Xia Ku Cao and Zhi Zi clear heat in the liver, reduce liver-fire and relieve headaches.
- Dang Gui, Chuan Xiong and Chai Hu promote liver-qi circulation, smooth the liver, and relieve headache.
- Ze Xie and Che Qian Zi promote urination and induce fire out of the body through urination.
- Sheng Di clears heat and nourishes the yin of the liver and kidney.
- Man Jing Zi relieves headaches.
- Zhi Gan Cao harmonizes the actions of the other herbs.
- Gou Teng and Tian Ma calm the liver, suppress liver-wind, and relieve headache.

Herbal Remedy:
Long Dan Xie Gan Wan-*Gentiana Longdancao Pill to Drain the Liver.*

Acupuncture Treatment:
- Waiguan SJ-5 + Zulinqi GB-41, Zhongfeng LIV-4, Shaohai HE-3, Shaofu HE-8, Shuaigu GB-8, Fengchi GB-20, Jianjing GB-21, XiaxiGB-43, Baihui DU-20, Xingjian LIV-2, Qimen LIV-14, Sanyinjiao SP-6 and Extra Tai Yang.
- An even method is applied on SJ-5 + GB-41, and a reducing method is applied on the rest of the points.

Explanations:

- A combination of SJ-5 + GB-41 harmonizes the Shaoyang channels, benefits the gallbladder, and relieves headaches.
- L.I.-4 and LIV-14, the yuan-source point of the large intestine channel and the front-mu point of the liver, smooth the liver, regulate the qi circulation in the body and relieve liver-qi stagnation. Meanwhile, they could relieve headaches.
- LIV-2 and GB-43, the ying-spring point of the liver channel and gallbladder channel respectively, DU-20, clear heat, reduce liver-fire and relieve headache.
- HE-3 and HE-8, the he-sea point and the ying-spring point of the heart channel respectively, clear heat in the heart, calm the shen and smooth the liver as well.
- GB-8, GB-20 and GB-21 regulate the collateral of the gallbladder channel, smooth the emotions, relieve the neck tension, and promote qi circulation in the head to relieve headache.
- SP-6, the crossing point of the three yin channels of the foot, promotes the smooth qi and blood circulation in the liver and in the head to relieve headache.
- Extra Taiyang, the local point, relieves headaches.

11.5.2.4 *Stagnation of Blood*

Prolonged persistence of stabbing headache with a fixed location, aggravation of headache at night, before or during menstruation, dark and purplish menstruation with clots, history of physical trauma and other cerebral diseases, insomnia, purplish tongue or purplish spots on the tongue, and a thready or unsmooth pulse.

Principle of Treatment:
Promote circulation of blood, eliminate blood stasis, and relieve headache.

Herbal Treatment:
Tong Qiao Huo Xue Tang-*Open the Portals and Quicken the Blood Decoction.*

Chuan Xiong *Rhizoma LiGustici Chuanxiong* 10 g
Chi Shao Yao *Radix Paeoniae Rubra* 10 g
Dang Gui *Radix angelicae Sinensis* 10 g
Dan Shen *Radix Salviae Miltiorrhizae* 10 g
Hong Hua *Flos Carthami* 10 g
Xiang Fu *Rhizoma Cyperi* 10 g
Qing Pi *Pericarpium Citri Reticulatae Viride* 5 g
Zhi Qiao *Fructus Aurantii* 10 g
Bai Zhi *Radix Angelicae Dahuricae* 10 g
Man Jing Zi *Fructus Viticis* 10 g

Explanations:
- Chuan Xiong, Chi Shao Yao, Dan Shen and Hong Hua promote blood circulation and eliminate blood Stasis. Besides, Chuan Xiong is a very good herb to induce the other herbs to reach the head to treat headaches.
- Dang Gui promotes blood circulation and harmonizes the blood so as not to harm the blood by using blood-circulating herbs.
- Since qi circulation promotes blood circulation, some herbs to promote qi circulation are prescribed here as well, such as Qing Pi, Zhi Qiao and Xiang Fu.
- Bai Zhi and Man Jing Zi, which are used together with Chuan Xiong and Dang Gui to relieve headaches.

Herbal Remedy:
Yan Hu Suo Zhi Tong Pian-*Corydalis Pain Relief Tablet.*

Acupuncture Treatment:
- Hegu L.I.-4, Fengchi GB-20, Neiguan P-6, Taiyuan LU-9, Shaohai HE-3, Shenmen HE-7, Geshu BL-17, Sanyinjiao SP-6, Taichong LIV-3, Qimen LIV-14 and Ashi points on the head.
- A reducing method is applied to these points.

Explanations:
- Qi is the guide for blood. L.I.-4 and LIV-3, the yuan-source point of the large intestine channel and the liver channel respectively,

regulate qi circulation to lead to blood circulation and relieve headache.

- GB-20, the crossing point of foot Shaoyang and Yangwei channels, some local Ah Shi points on the head, promote qi and blood circulation in the head and relieve headache.
- SP-6, the crossing point of three yin channels of the foot, and BL-17, the influential point of blood, promote blood circulation, eliminate blood stasis, and relieve headache.
- HE-3, HE-7 and LU-9, the influential point of the vessel in the body, calm the shen, regulate emotions, promote blood circulation, and relieve headache.
- P-6, the luo-connecting point of the pericardium channel, and LIV-14, the front-mu point of the liver, regulate qi circulation, smooth the liver, and promote blood circulation.

11.5.2.5 *Blockage of the clear-yang by damp-phlegm*

Headache with heavy sensation, dizziness, the fullness of the chest and epigastric region, nausea, vomiting, poor appetite, casting of phlegm, diarrhea, white and greasy coating on the tongue, and a slippery or wiry and slippery pulse.

Principle of Treatment:
Activate the spleen, eliminate damp, resolve phlegm, harmonize the collaterals, and sedate headache.

Herbal Treatment:
Ban Xia Bai Zhu Tian Ma Tang-*Pinellia, Atractylodes Macrocephala and Gastrodia Decoction.*

Ban Xia *Rhizoma Pinelliae* 10 g
Bai Zhu *Rhizoma Atractylodis Macrocephalae* 10 g
Tian Ma *Rhizoma Gastrodiae* 10 g
Cang Zhu *Rhizoma Atractylodis* 10 g
Hou Po *Cortex Magnoliae Officinalis* 10 g
Fu Ling *Sclerotium Poriae Cocos* 15 g

Chen Pi *Pericarpium Citri Reticulatae* 5 g
Bai Ji Li *Fructus Tribulli Terrestris* 10 g
Man Jing Zi *Fructus Viticis* 10 g
Zhi Gan Cao *Radix Glycyrrhizae Preparata* 3 g

Explanations:
- Ban Xia and Chen Pi dry damp, resolve phlegm in middle Jiao and relieve nausea.
- Fu Ling and Bai Zhu activate the spleen and eliminate damp.
- Tian Ma, Bai Ji Li and Man Jing Zi calm the liver, eliminate damp in the head and relieve headache and dizziness.
- Cang Zhu and Hou Po eliminate damp-phlegm in the body and relieve nausea and diarrhea.
- Zhi Gan Cao harmonizes the functions of other herbs.

Herbal Remedy:
Ban Xia Bai Zhu Tian Ma Pian-*Pinellia, Atractylodes Macrocephala and Gastrodia Tablet.*

Acupuncture Treatment:
- Waiguan SJ-5 + Zulinqi GB-41, Hegu L.I.-4, Shuaigu GB-8, Fengchi GB-20, Jianjing GB-21, Touwei ST-8, Extra Taiyang, Extra Yintang, Zhongwan REN-12, Taichong LIV-3, Fenglong ST-40, Sanyinjiao SP-6, Yinlingquan SP-9 and Ashi points on the head.
- An even method is applied on SJ-5 + GB-41, and a reducing method is applied on the rest points.

Explanations:
- SJ-5 + GB-41 could regulate the shaoyang channels and relieve headaches and dizziness.
- GB-20 and GB-21 smooth the tension at the neck, promote the qi circulation in the gallbladder channel and relieve headache.
- L.I.-4 and LIV-3, the yuan-source point of the large intestine channel and liver channel respectively, promote qi circulation, calm the liver, and relieve headache.

- GB-8, ST-8, Extra Taiyang and Extra Yintang, as well as some local Ah Shi points on the head, promote qi circulation, eliminate damp-phlegm in the head and relieve headache.
- REN-12, the front-mu point of the stomach and the influential point for the fu organs, SP-6, the crossing point of three yin channels of the foot, and SP-9, the he-sea point of the spleen channel, activate the spleen, eliminate damp-phlegm, and relieve nausea and diarrhea.

11.5.2.6 *Deficiency of qi*

Headache after COVID-19, empty sensation in the head, aggravation of headache after physical exertion, fatigue, general weakness, pale complexion, aversion to cold, cold hands, shortness of breath, spontaneous sweating, loose stools, poor appetite, low voice, thin and white coating on the tongue, pale tongue, tooth marks on tongue, and a slow and deep pulse.

Principle of Treatment:
Activate the spleen and stomach, tonify qi and relieve headache.

Herbal Treatment:
Bu Zhong Yi Qi Tang-*Tonify the Middle and Augment the Qi Decoction.*

Dang Shen *Radix Codonopsis Pilosulae* 10 g
Bai Zhu *Rhizoma Atractylodis Macrocephalae* 10 g
Fu Ling *clerotium Poriae Cocos* 15 g
Huang Qi *Radix Astragali Membranacea* 10 g
Chen Pi *Pericarpium Citri Reticulatae* 5 g
Gan Jiang *Rhizoma Zingiberis Officinalis* 5 g
Mu Xiang *Radix Aucklandiae* 10 g
Sha Ren *Fructus Amomi* 3 g
Man Jing Zi *Fructus Viticis* 10 g
Zhi Gan Cao *Radix Glycyrrhizae Praeparata* 3 g

Explanations:
- Dang Shen, Bai Zhu, Fu Ling and Zhi Gan Cao, known as Si Jun Zi Tang-Four Gentlemen Decoction, activate the spleen and stomach, tonify spleen-qi and relieve general fatigue and weakness.
- Huang Qi tonify spleen-qi and lift-up the qi to the head to benefit it.
- Chen Pi, Mu Xiang and Sha Ren harmonize stomach-qi and promote appetite.

Herbal Remedy:
Bu Zhong Yi Qi Wan-*Tonify the Middle and Augment the Qi Pill.*

Acupuncture Treatment:
- Baihui DU-20, Shenting DU-24, Extra Yintang, Zusanli ST-36, Taibai SP-3, Sanyinjiao SP-6, Qihai REN-6, Pishu BL-20 and Weishu BL-21.
- A tonifying method is applied on these points. Moxibustion should be applied on REN-6 and ST-36.

Explanations:
- ST-36, the he-sea point of the stomach channel, and SP-3, the yuan-source point of the spleen channel, BL-20 and BL-21, the back-shu point of the spleen and stomach respectively, activate the spleen and stomach, tonify qi and promote digestion.
- REN-6, and SP-6, the crossing point of the three yin channels of the foot, tonify qi and blood at the same time and strengthen the body to relieve general fatigue and weakness.
- DU-20, DU-24 and Extra Yintang lift up qi to the head and relieve headache.
- Moxibustion promotes the yang-qi movement, benefits the body, and relieves the weakness and cold in the body.

11.5.2.7 *Deficiency of blood*

Headache after COVID-19, a hollow sensation in the head, aggravation of headache after physical exertion and alleviation of headache by rest, dizziness, hair loss, palpitations, listlessness, insomnia, pale complexion, irregular menstruation in women, poor appetite, dry skin or stools, pale tongue with a thin and white coating, and a thready and weak pulse.

Principle of Treatment:
Tonify blood, relieve weakness and sedate headache.

Herbal Treatment:
Si Wu Tang-*Four Substances Decoction.*

Shu Di Huang *Radix Rehmanniae Praeparatae* 15 g
Dang Gui *Radix Angelicae Sinensis* 10 g
Bai Shao *Radix Paeoniae Alba* 10 g
Chuan Xiong *Rhizoma Ligustici Chuanxiong* 10 g
Tian Ma *Rhizoma Gastrodiae Elatae* 10 g
Bai Ji Li *Fructus Tribulli Terrestris* 10 g
Man Jing Zi *Fructus Viticis* 10 g
Zhi Gan Cao *Radix Glycyrrhizae Preparata* 3 g

Explanations:
- Shu Di Huang, Dang Gui, Bai Shao and Chuan Xiong benefit kidney-jing, tonify and nourish blood, and relieve headache.
- Tian Ma and Bai Ji Li benefit the head and relieve headaches.
- Man Jing Zi relieves headache.

Herbal Remedy:
Gui Pi Wan-*Restore the Spleen Pill.*

Acupuncture Treatment:
- Zusanli ST-36, Sanyinjiao SP-6, Taichong LIV-3, Ququan LIV-8, Taixi KID-3, Yingu KID-10, Xuanzhong GB-39, Baihui DU-20, Shenmen HE-7, Extra Taiyang and Extra Yintang.
- An even method is applied on LIV-3, Extra Taiyang and Extra Yintang.
- A tonifying method is applied on the rest points.

Explanations:

- ST-36, the he-sea point of the stomach channel, and SP-6, the crossing point of three yin channels of the foot, activate the spleen and stomach, tonify qi and blood and relieve headache.
- Since kidney-jing and blood share the same origin and benefit each other constantly, some points should be used to tonify kidney-jing to tonify blood. KID-3, the yuan-source point of the kidney channel, LIV-8 and KID-10, the he-sea point of the liver channel and kidney channel respectively, tonify blood and jing at the same time, relieve the general fatigue and weakness so as to relieve headache.
- GB-39, the influential point for marrow, benefits blood and relieves blood deficiency.
- DU-20, Extra Taiyang and Extra Yintang benefit the head, harmonize the collateral and relieve headache.
- LIV-3, the yuan-source point of the liver channel, and HE-7, the yuan-source point of the heart channel, promote qi and blood circulation, calms the shen, improves sleep and relieves headache.

11.6 Myalgia

The World Health Organization (WHO) estimates that approximately 1.7 billion people around the world have a musculoskeletal condition. This is a group of conditions that affect the muscles and bones and may cause body aches.[22] But myalgia in Long COVID is something different.

Long COVID refers to a variety of symptoms affecting different organs reported by people who contracted the coronavirus disease 2019 (COVID-19) infection. To date, there have been no robust estimates of the incidence and co-occurrence of Long COVID features, their relationship to age, sex, or severity of infection, and the extent to which they are specific to COVID-19. Therefore, some experts started a study on this subject. They believe that Long COVID clinical

---

[22]World Health Organization (WHO). Musculoskeletal health. 14 July 2022. https://www.who.int/news-room/fact-sheets/detail/musculoskeletal-conditions.

features occurred and co-occurred frequently and showed some specificity to COVID-19, though they were also observed after influenza. Different Long COVID clinical profiles were observed based on demographics and illness severity.[23]

Myalgia is a common symptom in patients with viral infections such as influenza. Since novel coronavirus disease 2019 (COVID-19) is also a viral infection, myalgia also occurs. One study reviews that myalgia reflects generalized inflammation and cytokine response and can be the onset symptom of 36% of patients with COVID-19.[24]

Another study investigated the association between COVID-related myalgia experienced by patients at hospital admission and the presence of Long COVID symptoms. A case-control study including patients hospitalized due to COVID-19 between 20 February and 31 May 2020 was conducted. Patients reporting myalgia and patients without myalgia at hospital admission were scheduled for a telephone interview seven months after hospital discharge. Hospitalization and clinical data were collected from medical records. A list of post-COVID symptoms with attention to musculoskeletal pain was evaluated. Anxiety and depressive symptoms, and sleep quality were likewise assessed. Out of a total of 1,200 hospitalized patients with COVID-19, 369 with and 369 without myalgia at hospital admission were assessed 7.2 months (SD 0.6) after hospital discharge. A greater proportion ($p = 0.03$) of patients with myalgia at hospital admission (20%) showed ≥3 post-COVID symptoms when compared with individuals without myalgia (13%). A higher proportion of patients presenting myalgia (odds Ratio 1.41, 95% confidence interval 1.04–1.90) exhibited musculoskeletal Long COVID pain when compared to those without myalgia. The prevalence of musculoskeletal Long

---

[23] Maxime Taquet, *et al.* Incidence, co-occurrence, and evolution of long-COVID features: A 6-month retrospective cohort study of 273,618 survivors of COVID-19. *PLOS MEDICINE.* September 2021, 18(9): e1003773. https://doi.org/10.1371/journal.pmed.1003773.

[24] Giuseppe Lippi, *et al.* Myalgia may not be associated with severity of coronavirus disease 2019 (COVID-19). *World J Emerg Med.* 2020, 11(3): 193–194. doi: 10.5847/wjem.j.1920-8642.2020.03.013.

COVID pain in the total sample was 38%. Fifty percent of individuals with preexisting musculoskeletal pain experienced a worsening of their symptoms after COVID-19. No differences in fatigue, dyspnea, anxiety/depressive levels, or sleep quality were observed between myalgia and non-myalgia groups. The presence of myalgia at hospital admission was associated with preexisting history of musculoskeletal pain (OR 1.62, 95% confidence interval 1.10–2.40). In conclusion, myalgia at the acute phase was associated with musculoskeletal pain as long-term post-COVID sequelae. In addition, half of the patients with preexisting pain conditions experienced a persistent exacerbation of their previous syndromes.[25] But one examination shows that myalgia is only 3.24% based upon the data from 81 million patients including 273,618 COVID-19 survivors.[26]

As a matter of fact, people can expect that myalgia may disappear or improve a lot by taking some painkillers, but it is not always the case this time during COVID-19 and Long COVID. Besides, there are so many questions that arise during COVID-19 and Long COVID, such as why is the common myalgia caused by COVID-19 longer and more severe than myalgia of other viral infections? Myalgia and fatigue in patients with COVID-19 may be longer in duration than other viral infections and may be unresponsive to conventional painkillers? What is the mechanism of myalgia caused by COVID-19? Is there an effective treatment for myalgia during Long COVID? Both scientists and medical practitioners are doing their best to find these answers to the above questions, and something has been done so far. For instance, according to one observation that when viral load is reduced with virus treatment, muscle pain may decrease. In addition to the classic mechanisms of myalgia known in viral infections, COVID-19 can cause musculoskeletal pain with

---

[25] César Fernández-de-las-Peñas, *et al.* Myalgia as a symptom at hospital admission by severe acute respiratory syndrome coronavirus 2 infection is associated with persistent musculoskeletal pain as long-term post-COVID sequelae: A case-control study. *PAIN.* 2021, 162(12): 2832–2840. doi: 10.1097/j.pain.0000000000002306.
[26] Angelo Carfì, *et al. op. cit.*

completely different mechanisms. Lactate dehydrogenase (LDH) increases when the virus damages muscles and other tissues. Due to both increased LDH and anaerobic glycolysis, lactate levels may increase excessively. Cytosolic PH may decrease more. Muscle pain may increase further due to increased lactate levels, low pH, and low oxygen levels. It is necessary to eliminate the cause of hypoxia for treatment in this pain type. Painkillers may not be effective. When the virus load decreases, the oxygenation of erythrocytes increases, and muscle lactate level decreases. Pain can disappear with virus treatment.[27] However, the authors did not propose any concrete treatment.

Myalgia due to COVID-19 can feel like a dull, aching sensation in the muscles that may limit mobility or energy. This sensation could affect one or several body parts and may range from mild to severe, typically occurring with other symptoms. In the most serious cases, myalgia could interfere with or prevent daily activities and tasks. The types of myalgia a person experiences may vary by age. When myalgia occurs with other symptoms (for instance, trouble breathing, persistent chest pain, inability to stay conscious, or confusion), drinking plenty of fluids and resting will not be usually sufficient to support recovery. Some patients may not benefit from taking over-the-counter medications, such as ibuprofen, a nonsteroidal anti-inflammatory drug, to reduce body and muscle aches.

11.6.1 TCM understanding of Long COVID-associated myalgia

According to TCM, most cases of myalgia fall under the category of Bi syndromes, which covers various conditions. It may occur with joint pain, tiredness, and insomnia. The main pathologies of myalgia in TCM are due to stagnation of qi or blood in some tissues, such as channels or collaterals, muscles, or tendons, or in the internal

---

[27]Adem Kucuk, *et al.* Can COVID-19 cause myalgia with a completely different mechanism? A hypothesis. *Clin Rheumatol.* 2020, 39(7): 2103–2104. doi: 10.1007/s10067-020-05178-1.

zang-fu organs. There could be a deficiency of qi and blood due to the prolonged persistence of COVID. The remaining external pathogenic factors—accumulation of damp in the body, emotional disturbance, deficiency of qi and blood—are the common causative factors. Besides, TCM pays special attention to the relationship between muscles and the spleen.

TCM divides myalgia into three different stages, such as:

- superficial stages
- tissues stages
- internal organ stages

This way, attention to analysis and treatment could be more focused on eliminating the causative factors, restoring the pathological changes and relieving pain.

During myalgia in the superficial stage, the primary factors are the remaining external pathogenic factors, mainly wind, cold and damp at the same time. Due to the predominance of these three pathogenic factors, the superficial stage of myalgia could again be subdivided into wind Bi, cold Bi and damp Bi.

- Wind Bi: body pain is not fixed, and it can be wandering in different joints in different areas.
- Cold Bi: body pain with stiffness that improves with the application of heat and feels worse when it gets cold.
- TCM: the body feels heavy, sore, and swollen and the pain is at a definite spot.

It is also possible that in the long duration of the above situations, or preexisting heat in the body, there would be the formation of heat, leading to heat Bi.

- Heat Bi: body pain with burning sensation, redness and swelling at a certain place on the body, the body pain improves with the application of cold and feels worse when it gets hot.

When superficial Bi syndromes are not under control in time, myalgia could develop into muscle Bi, or involve different tissues in the body, such as vascular Bi, tendon Bi, and bone Bi. Internal organ Bi usually is not involved.

The main pathologies of Long COVID-associated myalgia include the following.

11.6.1.1 *Remaining external pathogenic factors*

Invasion of cold-damp or damp-heat to the body could cause various damage, including the damage to the meridians, muscles, and tendons. It has been noticed that COVID-19 in most cases could cause infection in the respiratory tract and digestive tract, leading to fever, cough, muscle pain, nausea, or diarrhea. In TCM, these manifestations are very important, because they show that the lung and spleen are mainly involved. The lung opens into the skin and the spleen opens into the muscles. When these external pathogens are not eliminated completely, they may accumulate in the different parts of the body, leading to stagnation of qi and blood in the channels, collaterals, tissues and even the internal zang-fu organs, and eventually myalgia occurs.

11.6.1.2 *Accumulation of damp in the body*

Incomplete elimination of cold-damp or damp-heat may cause damage to the spleen and stomach, resulting in dysfunction in transportation and transformation, and formation of damp happens internally. Pre-existing medical conditions, lack of life care, overeating of fatty and greasy food, or even improper treatment during COVID-19, such as an overdose of antibiotics, intake of too many painkillers, or other chemical drugs, carelessness in diet, etc., may all cause weakness or damage to the spleen and stomach, resulting in retardation of transportation and transformation of the spleen and stomach, and damp-phlegm appears. When damp-phlegm blocks the qi and blood circulation and damages the smooth circulation in the channels and collaterals in the muscles, myalgia happens.

11.6.1.3 *Emotional disturbance*

Being emotionally upset, anxiety, over worrying, and sad prior to or during COVID-19 or Long COVID could lead to retardation of qi or blood circulation, which could block qi and blood movement and damage the smooth circulation in the channels and collaterals in the muscles, causing myalgia.

11.6.1.4 *Deficiency of qi and blood*

Prolonged persistence of COVID-19 could cause consumption of qi and blood, leading to deficiency of qi and blood in the body, especially kidney-qi and liver-blood, which could lead to failure of the muscles to be nourished properly, and myalgia occurs eventually.

11.6.2 TCM treatment of Long COVID-associated myalgia

In most cases, myalgia never appears as an individual complaint but occurs mostly with some other symptoms. Conventional treatment in modern medicine for myalgia mainly focuses on alleviating pain with NSAIDs, analgesics or reducing inflammation with injectable medications. As mentioned above, they did not work as promised, and in some cases, though, these medications aren't enough to control pain, and many of these medications also bear some possible side effects. The drug discovery model of "one-compound-one-target" has failed, and recently switched to the "multi-target approach" for developing and designing agents to target various intracellular constituents and signaling pathways.[28]

TCM has been widely used in the treatment of inflammatory diseases. During the coronavirus disease 2019 (COVID-19) epidemic, acupuncture has been practiced and used as a complementary treatment for COVID-19 both in China and overseas. One study paper systematically revealed the multi-target mechanisms of acupuncture

---

[28]Dhanya Sunil, *et al*. Multi-target directed indole based hybrid molecules in cancer therapy: An up-to-date evidence-based review. *Curr Top Med Chem*. 2017, 17(9): 959–985. doi: 10.2174/1568026616666160927150839.

therapy for COVID-19 through text mining, bioinformatics, network topology, etc. The findings suggested that acupuncture treatment of COVID-19 was associated with suppression of inflammatory stress, improving immunity, and regulating the nervous system function, including activation of neuroactive ligand-receptor interaction, calcium signaling pathway, cancer pathway, viral carcinogenesis, Staphylococcus aureus infection, etc.[29]

11.6.2.1 *Remaining external pathogenic factors*

Myalgia after COVID-19 especially at the upper parts of the body, sensitivity to wind, cold and damp weather, wandering pain or fixed pain, or severe pain in nature, heaviness of the body, sometimes headache or diarrhea, insomnia, poor appetite, thin, white, and greasy tongue coating, and a wiry and tight pulse.

Principle of Treatment:
Eliminate external pathogenic factors and harmonize the collaterals.

Herbal Treatment:
Qiang Huo Sheng Shi Tang-*Notopterygium Decoction to Overcome Damp.*

Qiang Huo *Rhizoma et Radix Notopterygii* 10 g
Du Huo *Radix Angelicae Pubescentis* 10 g
Fang Feng *Radix Ledebouriellae* 10 g
Chuan Xiong *Rhizoma Ligustici Chuanxiong* 10 g
Bai Zhi *Radix Angelicae Dahuricae* 10 g
Cang Zhu *Rhizoma Atractylodis* 10 g
Ge Gen *Radix Puerariae* 10 g
Ji Xue Teng *Caulis Milletiae Reticulatae* 15 g
Fu Ling *Sclerotium Poriae Cocos* 15 g
Sang Zhi *Ramulus Mori Albae* 10 g
Zhi Gan Cao *Radix Glycyrrhizae Preparata* 6 g

---

[29]Zhenzhen Han, *et al. op. cit.*

In case of local redness and hotness due to damp-heat, add Huang Bai *Cortex Phellodendri* 10 g.

Explanations:
* Qiang Huo and Du Huo dispel remaining wind, cold and damp, harmonize the collaterals and relieve the body pain.
* Fang Feng and Bai Zhi promote sweat, eliminate external pathogenic factors, and relieve myalgia.
* Cang Zhu, Ge Gen and Fu Ling eliminate damp in the muscles and resolve phlegm in the body.
* Chuan Xiong, Sang Zhi and Ji Xue Teng promote the qi and blood circulation in the channels and collaterals and relieve myalgia.
* Zhi Gan Cao harmonizes the herbs in the prescription.
* Huang Bai eliminates damp, clears heat, and subsides swelling.

Herbal Remedy:
Qiang Huo Sheng Shi Tang Tablets-*Qiang Huo Overcome Wind Decoction Tablet.*

Acupuncture Treatment:
* Waiguan SJ-5 + Zulinqi GB-41, Shenmai BL-62 + Houxi SI-3, Hegu L.I.-4, Lieque LU-7, Fenglong ST-40, Sanyinjiao SP-6, Diji SP-8, Yinlingquan SP-9, Taichong LIV-3, Yanglingquan GB-34 and some local Ah Shi points.
* Moxibustion should be used on SP-9, GB-34, and some local Ah Shi points.
* An even method is applied on SJ-5 + GB-41, BL-62 + SI-3, and a reducing method is applied on the rest of the points.
* If there is local redness and hotness around the affected joints, add Quchi L.I.-11 and ying-spring point from the affected channels.

Explanations:
* The combination of SJ-5 + GB-41, BL-62 + SI-3, and two groups of the eight confluence points, harmonize and invigorate Yangwei, Dai, Yangqiao and Du channels and promote the qi circulation to relieve myalgia.

- LU-7, the luo-connecting point of the lung channel, L.I.-4, the yuan-source of the large intestine channel, and LIV-3, the yuan-source of the liver channel, open the skin pores to eliminate the remaining pathogenic factors, promote the qi circulation and relieve myalgia.
- GB-34, the influential point of the tendons in the body, relaxes the tendons and relieves stiffness of the joints.
- ST-40, the luo-connecting point of the stomach channel, SP-6 and SP-9, the crossing point of three yin channels of the foot and the he-sea point of the spleen channel respectively, eliminate damp in the body, regulate the middle Jiao and digestion, and relieve myalgia.
- SP-8, the xi-cleft point of the spleen channel, harmonizes collaterals and relieves myalgia.
- Moxibustion warms the channels and collaterals and eliminates cold.
- L.I.-11 clears heat and subsides swelling.

11.6.2.2 *Accumulation of damp-phlegm in the spleen*

Myalgia after COVID-19, heaviness and swelling of the muscles, limitation of body movement, stiffness in the limbs, heaviness of the body, nausea, poor appetite, loose stool or diarrhea, heaviness in the head with foggy feeling, lassitude, tiredness, white and greasy coating on the tongue, and a wiry and slippery pulse.

Principle of Treatment:
Eliminate damp, resolve phlegm, activate the spleen and stomach, and relieve myalgia.

Herbal Treatment:
Cang Fu Dao Tan Tang-*Atractylodes-Poria Phlegm-Dissipating Decoction.*

Cang Zhu *Rhizoma Atractylodis* 10 g
Xiang Fu *Rhizoma Cyperi Rotundi* 10 g
Mu Xiang *Radix Aucklandiae Lappae* 10 g

Zhi Ban Xia *Rhizoma Pinelliae Ternatae* 10 g
Chen Pi *Pericarpium Citri Reticulatae* 5 g
Fu Ling *Sclerotium Poriae Cocos* 15 g
Huo Xiang *Herba Agastaches seu Pogostemi* 10 g
Hou Po *Cortex Magnoliae Officinalis* 10 g
Chuan Xiong *Rhizoma Ligustici Chuanxiong* 10 g
Wu Jia Pi *Cortex Acanthopanacis Gracilistyli Radicis* 10 g
Gui Zhi *Ramulus Cinnamomi* 10 g
Zhi Gan Cao *Radix Glycyrrhizae Preparata* 3 g

In case of swelling of the muscle with local redness and hotness due to damp-heat, remove Gui Zhi *Ramulus Cinnamomi Cassiae* and Wu Jia Pi *Cortex Acanthopanacis Gracilistyli Radicis*, and add Huang Lian *Rhizoma Coptidis* 5 g.

Explanations:
- Cang Zhu, Zhi Ban Xia, Chen Pi, Fu Ling, Hou Po and Huo Xiang eliminate damp, resolve phlegm, harmonize the middle Jiao, and relieve nausea and diarrhea.
- Xiang Fu, Mu Xiang and Chuan Xiong promote qi circulation, relieve the blockage in the muscles by damp-phlegm and sedate myalgia.
- Wu Jia Pi and Gui Zhi warm the muscles, eliminate damp-phlegm, and relieve myalgia.
- Zhi Gan Cao harmonizes the herbs in the prescription.
- Huang Lian clears heat, eliminates damp, subsides swelling and relieves myalgia.

Herbal Remedy:
Shen Ling Bai Zhu Wan-*Ginseng, Poria and Atractylodis Macrocephalae Pill.*

Acupuncture Treatment:
- Waiguan SJ-5 + Zulinqi GB-41, Shenmai BL-62 + Houxi SI-3, Hegu L.I.-4, Zhongwan REN-12, Fenglong ST-40, Taibai SP-3,

Sanyinjiao SP-6, Diji SP-8, Yinlingquan SP-9, Taichong LIV-3 and Yanglingquan GB-34.
- Moxibustion should be used on SP-9, GB-34, REN-12, ST-40, and some local Ah Shi points.
- An even method is applied on SJ-5 + GB-41, BL-62 + SI-3, and a reducing method is applied on the rest of the points.

If there is local redness and hotness around the affected muscles, add Quchi L.I.-11 and ying-spring point from the affected channels.

Explanations:
- The combination of SJ-5 + GB-41, and BL-62 + SI-3, two groups of the eight confluence points, harmonize and invigorate Yangwei, Dai, Yangqiao and Du channels and promote the qi circulation to relieve myalgia.
- L.I.-4, the yuan-source of the large intestine channel, LIV-3, the yuan-source of the liver channel, promotes the qi circulation and relieves myalgia.
- GB-34, the influential point of the tendons, relaxes the tendons and relieves joint pain.
- REN-12, the gathering point for the Fu organ, ST-40, SP-3, SP-6 and SP-9 eliminate damp in the body, harmonize the middle Jiao, promote digestion and relieve joint pain.
- SP-8, the xi-cleft point of the spleen channel, promotes the qi and blood circulation and relieves myalgia.
- Moxibustion warms the channels and collaterals, eliminates cold and strengthens the body.
- L.I.-11 and the ying-spring points from affected channels clear heat and subside swelling.

11.6.2.3 *Stagnation of qi and blood*

If there is a predominance of qi stagnation, there could be myalgia with wondering nature, depression, headache, the fullness of the chest and abdomen, tension at the neck and head, painful eyes, insomnia, irregular menstruation in women, irritability, nervousness, poor appetite, loose stool or constipation, thin and white tongue coating, and a wiry and deep pulse.

If there is a predominance of blood stagnation, there could be myalgia with a stabbing sensation at a fixed location, stiffness in the joints, aggravation of myalgia at night, insomnia, thin and white coating on the tongue, purplish tongue, and a wiry and unsmooth pulse.

Principle of Treatment:
Smooth the liver, calm the emotions, promote the qi and blood circulation, and relieve body pain.

Herbal Treatment:
Xiao Yao San-*Rambling Powder.*

Chai Hu *Radix Bupleare* 10 g
Dang Gui *Radix Angelicae Sinensis* 10 g
Bai Shao Yao *Radix Paeoniae Lactiflorae* 10 g
Bai Zhu *Rhiizoma Areactylodis Macrocephalae* 10 g
Fu Shen *Sclerotium Poriae Cocos Paradicis* 15 g
Chuan Xiong *Rhizoma Ligustici Chuan Xiong* 10 g
Yan Hu Suo *Rhizoma Corydalis* 10 g
Chuan Lian Zi *Fructus Meliae Toosendan* 10 g
Zhi Qiao *Fructus Citri Aurantii* 10 g
Hong Hua *Flos Carthami Tinctorii* 10 g
Ji Xue Teng *Caulis Milletiae Reticulatae* 10 g
Zhi Shi *Fructus Immaturus Citri Aurantii* 10 g
Zhi Gan Cao *Radix Glycyrrhizae Preparata* 3 g

Explanations:
- Chai Hu and Bai Shao Yao smooth the liver, promote liver-qi circulation, and relieve qi stagnation in the liver.
- Chuan Lian Zi, Zhi Ke and Zhi Shi promote qi circulation in the body and relieve myalgia.
- Dang Gui, Chuan Xiong, Hong Hua and Yan Hu Suo promote blood circulation, eliminate blood stasis, and relieve myalgia.

- Ji Xue Teng harmonizes the collaterals and relieves myalgia.
- Fu Shen calms shen and improves sleep.
- Bai Zhu strengthens the spleen and stomach and improves the appetite.
- Zhi Gan Cao harmonizes the actions of the other herbs.

Herbal Remedy:
Xiao Yao Wan-*Rambling Pill.*

Acupuncture Treatment:
- Waiguan SJ-5 + Zulinqi GB-41, Hegu L.I.-4, Taichong LIV-3, Qimen LIV-14, Neiguan P-6, Sanyinjiao SP-6, Diji SP-8, Geshu BL-17, Taiyuan LU-9, Shaohai HE-3 and Shenmen HE-7.
- An even method is applied on SJ-5 + GB-41, and a reducing method is applied on these points.

Explanations:
- The combination of SJ-5 + GB-41 harmonizes Shaoyang channels, benefits the gallbladder, and relieves myalgia.
- L.I.-4 and LIV-3, the yuan-source point of the large intestine channel and the liver channel respectively, and LIV14, the front-mu point of the liver, smooth the liver, regulate the qi circulation in the body and relieve liver-qi stagnation so as to relieve myalgia.
- P-6, the luo-connecting point of the pericardium channel, regulates qi circulation and calms the shen.
- SP-6, the crossing point of the three yin channels of the foot, LU-9, the influential point of the vessels, HE-3 and HE-7, the he-sea point and the yuan-source point of the heart channel respectively, BL-17, the influential point of blood, promote the smooth qi and blood circulation in the body, calm the shen and relieve myalgia.
- SP-8, the xi-cleft point of the spleen channel, harmonizes the collaterals in the muscles and relieves myalgia.

11.6.2.4 *Deficiency of qi and blood*

Slight myalgia which goes up and down, aggravation of the pain by physical movement, weakness of the body, fatigue, dizziness, pale complexion, palpitations, poor appetite, shortness of breath, lower back pain, poor memory, pale tongue with a thin and white coating, and a thready and weak pulse.

Principle of Treatment:
Tonify qi, benefit blood, strengthen the muscle and relieve the pain.

Herbal Treatment:
Shi Quan Da Bu Tang-*All-Inclusive Great Tonifying Decoction.*

Shu Di Huang *Radix Rhemanniae Glutinosae Praeparata* 15 g
Dang Gui *Radix Angelicae Sinensis* 10 g
Chuan Xiong *Rhizoma Ligustici Chuanxiong* 10 g
Bai Shao Yao *Radix Paeoniae Lactiflorae* 10 g
Ren Shen *Radix Ginseng* 5 g
Bai Zhu *Rhizoma Atractylodis Macrocephalae* 10 g
Fu Ling *Sclerotium Poriae Cocos* 15 g
Shan Yao *Radix Dioscoreae Oppositae* 10 g
Huang Qi *Radix Astragali Membranacei* 10 g
Rou Gui *Cortex Cinnamomi Cassiae* 5 g
Zhi Gan Cao *Radix Glycyrrhizae Preparata* 3 g

Explanations:
- Ren Shen, Bai Zhu, Fu Ling and Zhi Gan Cao, the complete composition of Si Jun Zi Tang, tonify qi, activate the spleen, improve appetite, and relieve fatigue.
- Shu Di Huang, Dang Gui, Bai Shao Yao and Chuan Xiong, the complete composition of Si Wu Tang, tonify blood, benefit kidney-jing and nourish the muscles.
- Huang Qi lifts qi and benefits the energy in the body.
- Rou Gui warms the channels and relieves cold in the body.

Herbal Remedy:
Ren Shen Zai Zao Wan-*Ginseng Recreating Pill.*

Acupuncture Treatment:

- Waiguan SJ-5 + Zulinqi GB-41, Shenmai BL-62 + Houxi SI-3, Yanglingquan GB-34, Zusanli ST-36, Sanyinjiao SP-6, Diji SP-8, Qihai REN-6, Taixi KID-3 and Shenshu BL-23.
- Moxibustion should be used on ST-36, REN-6 and KID-3.
- An even method is applied on SJ-5 + GB-41, BL-62 + SI-3, and SP-8, and a tonifying method is applied on the rest of the points.

Explanations:

- The combination of SJ-5 + GB-41, and BL-62 + SI-3, harmonizes and invigorates Yangwei, Dai, Yangqiao and Du channels and promotes the qi circulation to relieve myalgia.
- GB-34, ST-36, SP-6, REN-6, KID-3 and BL-23 tonify qi and blood, as well as kidney-jing, benefit the tendons and strengthen the body.
- Moxibustion warms the channels and collaterals, eliminates internal cold. and supports yang-qi. It can also relieve myalgia.
- SP-8, the xi-cleft point of the spleen channel, promotes qi and blood circulation and relieves myalgia.

11.7 Cough

Physiologically, coughing is a normal and important defense mechanism of the body to protect the lung and get rid of anything that irritates them. During COVID-19, viral infections could leave patients with a cough because the lung has been irritated. Coughing could be non-productive, but sometimes people may have a cough with phlegm. This should gradually disappear during the recovery.

Globally, cough is the most commonly reported symptom in acute COVID-19 infection. Between 50–80% of those infected report a dry persistent cough.[30] Cough is one of the most common

---

[30]Hasan Israfil, *et al.* Clinical characteristics and diagnostic challenges of COVID-19: An update from the global perspective. *Front Public Health.* 2021, 8: 567395. doi: 10.3389/fpubh.2020.567395.

presenting symptoms of COVID-19, along with fatigue, joint pain, shortness of breath, and loss of taste and smell, etc. Cough can persist for weeks or months after SARS-CoV-2 infection, but not being sure exactly how long after coronavirus will patients still have a cough can be frustrating at times. When cough happens in acute COVID-19, it is often accompanied by fatigue and headaches. It often comes together with symptoms like a sore throat, chest pain, shortness of breath, hoarseness, and loss of smell. Cough may be associated with different symptoms amongst hospitalized adult patients and non-hospitalized individuals, e.g., cough, fever and shortness of breath are the three most common features amongst hospitalized adult patients, while cough, fever and myalgia were the most common symptoms amongst non-hospitalized individuals. Both dry (58%) and productive (25%) coughs have been described in the literature.[31]

Whilst recovering quickly from COVID-19, some may have ongoing symptoms. For instance, some of these patients may continue to experience an irritating cough for some time. Over time, a cough can develop into a cycle, where excessive coughing causes irritation and inflammation, which worsens the cough. A cough because of Long COVID is highly likely to occur alongside throat dryness, expectoration of slight sputum or an non-productive cough, and it becomes aggravated by physical activities or exposure to cold weather. Pressure over the chest and throat pain may also occur at the same time. Cough is not limited to people who were seriously unwell or hospitalized when they first caught the virus.

Moreover, a cough is no longer the most common reported symptom during Long COVID.

One review showed that patients may experience symptoms related to any system in the body, including respiratory, neurological, and gastroenterological symptoms. This pooled data demonstrated

---

[31] Government of Canada. COVID-19 signs, symptoms and severity of disease: A clinician guide. https://www.canada.ca/en/public-health/services/diseases/2019-novel-coronavirus-infection/guidance-documents/signs-symptoms-severity.html.

that the ten most commonly reported symptoms in Long COVID are fatigue, shortness of breath, muscle pain, cough, headache, joint pain, chest pain, an altered sense of smell, diarrhea and altered taste.[32]

As these clinical symptoms of Long COVID are new medical conditions, we are still trying to understand it gradually.

In terms of the prevalence of Long COVID cough, in a pooled analysis, one study found that the estimated prevalence of persistent cough was 18% (95% CI 12–24%; I2 = 93%) in 14 studies of hospitalized patients (follow-up duration ranged from six weeks to four months).[33] One multicenter study examined prevalence data and associated risk factors of Long COVID cough one year after hospital discharge in COVID-19 survivors, in which the individuals who recovered from COVID-19 at three public hospitals in Madrid (Spain) were enrolled. The patients were systematically asked about the presence of respiratory symptoms, e.g., fatigue, dyspnea, chest pain, and cough after hospital discharge. Clinical and hospitalization data were collected from hospital records. Overall, 1,950 patients (47% women, mean age: 61, SD: 16 years) were assessed at 11.2 months (SD 0.5) after hospital discharge. Just 367(18.8%) were completely free of any respiratory post-COVID-19 symptoms. The prevalence of long-term cough, chest pain, dyspnea, and fatigue were 2.5%, 6.5%, 23.3%, and 61.2%, respectively. Clinical and hospitalization factors were not associated with long-term Long COVID cough. In conclusion, the prevalence of Long COVID cough one year after SARS-CoV-2 infection was 2.5% in subjects who had survived hospitalization

---

[32]Olalekan Lee Aiyegbusi, *et al.* Long COVID: Symptoms experienced during infection may predict lasting illness. *Down to Earth.* 28 July 2021. https://www.downtoearth.org.in/blog/health/long-covid-symptoms-experienced-during-infection-may-predict-lasting-illness-78146.

[33]Woo-Jung Song, *et al.* Confronting COVID-19-associated cough and the post-COVID syndrome: Role of viral neurotropism, neuroinflammation, and neuroimmune responses. *The Lancet Respir Med.* 2021, 9(5): 533–544. https://doi.org/10.1016/S2213-2600(21)00125-9.

for COVID-19. No clear risk factor associated to long-term post-COVID cough was identified.[34]

In a recent prospective UK cohort study of hospitalized patients with COVID-19, the most common ongoing symptoms were breathlessness (39%), fatigue (39%) and insomnia (24%), with only 11.6% reporting residual cough.[35] Similarly, only 7% of patients ($n = 119$) who had COVID-19 and associated severe pneumonia reported a troublesome chronic cough two months post infection.[36] But despite the high prevalence of cough in the acute infective period, early data indicate that post-viral cough is neither a frequent nor a debilitating residual effect.[37]

Another situation, i.e., pulmonary fibrosis, should be mentioned. After the new coronavirus invades the human body, the lungs are one of the main organs to be attacked. From the previously collected data, it could be seen that many patients have lungs with ground-glass opacity when they visit a doctor, and the degree of lung damage has a lot to do with the patient's severity. If the symptoms are not severe at the time of treatment, the patient's sequelae are also mild and will subside over time. But for severely ill patients, lung damage is more serious, and irreversible situations could appear. Perhaps in the future, coughing and breathing difficulties will follow for a lifetime. Fortunately, it seems that there are not many such patients like this until this moment.

---

[34] César Fernández-de-las-Peñas, *et al.* Prevalence of post-COVID-19 cough one year after SARS-CoV-2 infection: A multicenter study. *Lung.* 2021, 199: 249–253. https://doi.org/10.1007/s00408-021-00450-w.

[35] David T. Arnold, *et al.* Patient outcomes after hospitalisation with COVID-19 and implications for follow-up: Results from a prospective UK cohort. *Thorax.* 2021, 76(4): 399–401. doi: 10.1136/thoraxjnl-2020-216086.

[36] Office for National Statistics. Prevalence of long COVID symptoms and COVID-19 complications. *Office for National Statistics.* 16 December 2020. https://www.ons.gov.uk/news/statementsandletters/theprevalenceoflongcovidsymptomsandcovid19complications.

[37] Peter V. Dicpinigaitis and Brendan J. Canning. Is there (will there be) a post-COVID-19 chronic cough? *Lung.* 2020, 198: 863–865. doi: 10.1007/s00408-020-00406-6.

Although prevalence rates of self-reported Long COVID were greatest in people aged 35 to 69 years, females, those living in the most deprived areas, those working in health or social care, and those with a pre-existing, activity-limiting health condition.[38] Another study also presented a model that successfully predicted whether a person would get Long COVID using only their age, their gender and the number of symptoms reported in the first week.[39] No clear risk factor associated with long-term post-COVID cough was identified. Besides, the prevalence of post-infective cough in non-hospitalized COVID-19 cases is unreported. Many COVID-19 patients are asymptomatic (~40–45%).[40] *Nature* looks at four of the biggest questions that scientists are investigating about the mysterious condition known as Long COVID, pointing out that it is less certain who is most at risk, why it affects only some, and why most of the early prevalence studies looked only at patients who had been hospitalized with acute COVID-19, when in fact, most people with COVID-19 are never ill enough to be hospitalized. Finally, there is the question of what part COVID-19 vaccines might play. Although many of them prevent death and severe illness, scientists do not yet know whether they prevent Long COVID.[41]

Some scientists have tried to explain why cough persists during Long COVID. They hypothesize that the pathways of neurotropism, neuroinflammation, and neuroimmunomodulation through the vagal sensory nerves, which are implicated in SARS-CoV-2 infection, lead to a cough hypersensitivity state. The Long COVID syndrome might also result from neuroinflammatory events in the brain. They also confirmed that although neuromodulators such as gabapentin or

---

[38] Angelo Carfì, *et al. op. cit.*

[39] Carole H. Sudre, *et al.* Attributes and predictors of long COVID. *Nature Medicine.* 2021, 27: 626–631. doi: https://www.nature.com/articles/s41591-021-01292-y.

[40] Daniel P. Oran, *et al.* Prevalence of asymptomatic SARS-CoV-2 infection. *Annals of Internal Medicine.* 2020, 1730(5): 362–367. https://doi.org/10.7326/M20-3012.

[41] Michael Marshall. The four most urgent questions about long COVID. *Nature.* 2021, 594: 168–170. https://doi.org/10.1038/d41586-021-01511-z.

opioids might be considered for acute and chronic COVID-19 cough, they discuss the possible mechanisms of COVID-19-associated cough and the promise of new anti-inflammatories or neuromodulators that might successfully target both the cough of COVID-19 and the post-COVID syndrome.[42] However, in most cases, cough of Long COVID may have no obvious cause.

In terms of the treatment for cough in Long COVID, there is no evidence to support specific treatment or investigation recommendations other than ensuring that acute illness and radiological changes have resolved.[43] The British Thoracic Society do not differentiate between those with persistent cough following COVID-19 and those who present with chronic cough. The first-line management for people with residual cough after COVID-19 infection are the same as the guidelines on the management of cough in adults.[44]

11.7.1 TCM understanding of Long COVID-associated cough

In TCM, it is considered that cough of Long COVID is caused either by incomplete elimination of some external pathogenic factors or disorders of internal organs due to dysfunction of the lung in dispersing the qi.

Cough on one hand is an individual symptom. On the other hand, it's also a symptom indicating the lung is involved during Long COVID.

---

[42]Woo-Jung Song, *et al. op. cit.*

[43]Long Covid: Ongoing cough. *Pulse Today.* 7 June 2021. https://www.pulsetoday. co.uk/clinical-feature/clinical-areas/respiratory/long-covid-ongoing-cough/.

[44]Alyn Morice, *et al.* British thoracic society cough guideline group recommendations for the management of cough in adults. *Thorax.* 2006, 61(Suppl 1): i1–24. doi: 10.1136/thx.2006.065144.

11.7.1.1 *Incomplete elimination of external pathogenic factors*

Invasion of external pathogenic factors with a pestilent toxin to the lung could cause the occurrence of COVID-19. When it is properly treated in time, these external pathogenic factors should be eliminated completely, leaving no further damage to the lung and the lung could also recover gradually in weeks. However, when these pathogenic factors remain in the lung, and causes some disturbance to the lung in dispersing the qi, cough may occur.

11.7.1.2 *Accumulation of damp-phlegm*

Either invasion of cold-damp or invasion of damp-heat to the spleen, stomach, or San Jiao may cause dysfunction of the spleen and stomach in digestion, transportation, and transformation, resulting in the formation of damp-phlegm internally, which could eventually disturb the lung in dispersing the qi, and cough appears.

Obesity, constitutional weakness of the spleen and stomach, or lack of care for daily diet during COVID-19, could cause the production of damp-phlegm in the body. It is held in TCM that the spleen is the production organ of damp-phlegm, and the lung is the container organ of damp-phlegm. During Long COVID, formation of damp-phlegm could become worse due to external invasion and sickness, thus the spleen could submit much more damp-phlegm to the lung, resulting in dysfunction of the lung in dispersing the qi, and cough happens.

11.7.1.3 *Deficiency of qi or yin*

Prolonged persistence of COVID-19 could cause consumption of qi, leading to deficiency of qi in the body, especially the lung-qi. It may affect the lung in dispersing the qi, and cough occurs. Deficiency of qi may also happen in the spleen and kidney, leading to aggravation of lung-qi deficiency. In this case, the cough becomes much worse.

The prolonged persistence of COVID-19 could also cause the consumption of yin in the body. Besides, underlying medical conditions prior to COVID-19 could be add-on effects to cause aggravation of deficiency of yin. When the lung fails to be properly nourished by the yin, the physiological function of the lung in dispersing the qi will be impaired, and cough starts. Of course, deficiency of yin in different organs may also bring about cough due to disharmony between the lung with these associated organs. For instance, deficiency of liver-yin could cause hyperactivity of deficient fire, which eventually attacks the lung to cause cough. Deficiency of kidney-yin could, on the other hand, lead to improper nourishment of the lung by kidney-yin, and cough happens.

11.7.2 TCM treatment of COVID-19-associated cough

A systematic review and meta-analysis done in many trials have shown that TCM combined with conventional therapy in the treatment of mild to moderate COVID-19 was superior to conventional therapy alone. In terms of cough, three trials enrolling 205 patients mentioned cough reduction cases. A fixed-effects model was used due to the lack of significant heterogeneity (I2 = 0%, p = 0.89) Meta-analyses revealed that combination therapy could significantly reduce cough cases [RR = 1.43, 95%CI (1.16, 1.75), p = 0.0006]. Four trials enrolling 482 participants reported TCM symptom score of fever. A random-effects model was used due to the significant heterogeneity (*I2* = 84%, p = 0.0003). The pooled estimate found combination therapy decreased TCM symptom score of coughs [MD = −1.07, 95%CI (−1.29, −0.85), p < 0.00001].[45]

---

[45] Xuqin Du, *et al.* Add-on effect of Chinese herbal medicine in the treatment of mild to moderate COVID-19: A systematic review and meta-analysis. *PLoS ONE.* 2021, 16(8): e0256429. https://doi.org/10.1371/journal.pone.0256429.

11.7.2.1 *Remaining some external pathogenic factors*

Persistence of slight dry cough after COVID-19 or cough with expectoration of some diluted whitish phlegm, occasional nasal discharge, itching in the throat, absence of thirst, slight aversion to cold and muscle pain, headache, thin and whitish coating on the tongue, and a tight pulse.

Principle of Treatment:
Dispel wind, eliminate cold-damp, disperse the lung-qi and relieve cough.

Herbal Treatment:
Xing Su San-*Apricot Kernel and Perilla Leaf Powder,* plus
Zhi Sou San-*Stop Coughing Powder.*

Jing Jie *Herba seu Flos Schizonepetae Tenuifoliae* 5 g
Fang Feng *Radix Ledebouriellae Divaricatae* 5 g
Qiang Huo *Rhizoma et Radix Notopterygii* 10 g
Bai Bu *Radix Stemonae* 10 g
Xing Ren *Semen Pruni Armeniacae* 10 g
Zi Su Zi *Fructus Perillae Frutescentis* 10 g
Zhi Ban Xia *Rhizoma Pinelliae Ternatae Preparata* 10 g
Chen Pi *Pericarpium Citri Reticulatae* 5 g
Fu Ling *Sclerotium Poriae Cocos* 12 g
Jie Geng *Radix Platycodi Grandiflori* 10 g
Zhi Ke *Fructus Citri Aurantii* 10 g

Explanations:
- Jing Jie and Fang Feng are prescribed in low doses because the external pathogenic factors are not so strong anymore. They are applied in combination with Qiang Huo to dispel the remaining pathogens and relieve some external symptoms, such as itching in the throat, occasional nasal discharge, slight aversion to cold and muscle pain, and headache.

- Xing Ren, Jie Geng, Zi Su Zi, Zhi Ban Xia, Fu Ling, and Chen Pi are applied to eliminate phlegm and relieve cough.
- Bai Bu relieves cough.
- Zhi Ke promotes qi circulation and relieves cough.

Herbal Remedy:
Zhi Sou San-*Stop Coughing Powder.*

Acupuncture Treatment:
- Waiguan SJ-5 + Zulinqi GB-41, Hegu L.I.-4, Lieque LU-7, Chize LU-5, Tianzhu BL-10, Feishu BL-13, Fenglong ST-40 and Yinlingquan SP-9.
- An even method is applied on SJ-5 + GB-41, and a reducing method is applied on the rest of the points.

Explanations:
- The combination of SJ-5 + GB-41, one group of the eight confluence points, regulates the Yangwei channel, dispel the remaining pathogenic factors and relieve muscle pain and headache.
- L.I.-4, the yuan-source of the large intestine channel, LU-7, the luo-connecting point of the lung channel, and BL-10 open the skin pores, dispel external pathogenic factors, and relieve cough, muscle pain, and headache.
- LU-5 and BL-13, the he-sea point of the lung channel and back-shu point of the lung respectively, disperse the lung-qi, restore the physiological functions of the lung and relieve cough.
- ST-40 and SP-9, the luo-connecting point of the stomach channel and the he-sea point of the spleen channel respectively, eliminate phlegm and relieve cough.

11.7.2.2 *Accumulation of phlegm-turbidity in the lung*

Cough with profuse white and diluted phlegm after COVID-19 (which is easy to be expectorated), aggravation of cough when taking greasy and fatty food, alleviation of cough when phlegm is expectorated, fullness in the chest and epigastric region, nausea, poor appetite, lassitude, loose stools, whitish and greasy coating on the tongue, and a slippery pulse.

Principle of Treatment:
Eliminate damp-phlegm, activate the spleen, and relieve cough.

Herbal Treatment:
Cang Fu Dao Tan Tang-*Atractylodes-Poria Phlegm-Dissipating Decoction.*

Cang Zhu *Rhizoma Atractylodis* 10 g
Xiang Fu *Rhizoma Cyperi Rotundi* 10 g
Zhi Shi *Fructus Immaturus Citri Aurantii* 10 g
Zhi Ban Xia *Rhizoma Pinelliae Ternatae Preparata* 10 g
Fu Ling *Sclerotium Poriae Cocos* 12 g
Chen Pi *Pericarpium Citri Reticulatae* 5 g
Tian Nan Xing *Rhizoma Arisaematis* 10 g
Xing Ren *Semen Pruni Armeniacae* 10 g
Hou Po *Cortex Magnoliae Officinalis* 10 g
Gua Lou Pi *Pericarpium Trichosanthis* 10 g
Zi Su Zi *Fructus Perillae Frutescentis* 10 g
Sheng Jiang *Rhizoma Zingiberis Officinalis Recens* 5 g

Explanations:
- Zhi Ban Xia, Fu Ling, Chen Pi, and Sheng Jiang, the chief compositions of Er Chen Tang, eliminate damp-phlegm and relieve cough.
- Cang Zhu, Hou Po, Zhi Shi, and Xiang Fu eliminate damp-phlegm, relieve the qi stagnation caused by the accumulation of damp-phlegm.
- Xing Ren, Tian Nan Xing, Gua Lou Pi, and Zi Su Zi resolve phlegm, regulate the lung-qi and relieve cough.

Herbal Remedy:
Er Chen Wan-*Decoction of Two Old (Cured) Drugs*
or

Cang Fu Dao Tan Wan-*Atractylodes-Poria Phlegm-Dissipating Decoction.*

Acupuncture Treatment:
- Neiguan P-6 + Gongsun SP-4, Hegu L.I.-4, Lieque LU-7, Chize LU-5, Feishu BL-13, Zhongwan REN-12, Tanzhong REN-17, Fenglong ST-40, Sanyinjiao SP-6 and Yinlingquan SP-9.
- An even method is applied on P-6 + SP-4, and a reducing method is applied on the rest of the points.

Explanations:
- The combination of P-6 + SP-4 promotes the qi circulation in the chest and abdomen and relieves cough.
- REN-12, the gathering point of the fu organs in the body, ST-40, SP-6, and SP-9 activate the spleen and stomach and eliminate damp-phlegm in the body.
- BL-13, the back-shu point of the lung, LU-7, and LU-5 disperse and descend the lung-qi, restore the physiological functions of the lung, and relieve cough.
- L.I.-4, the yuan-source point of the large intestine channel, REN-17, the gathering point of the qi in the body, promotes the qi circulation and relieves the qi stagnation in the body caused by the accumulation of damp-phlegm.

11.7.2.3 *Accumulation of phlegm-heat in the lung*

Slight cough with slight sticky yellow phlegm after COVID-19, slight fullness of the chest, throat pain occasionally, poor appetite, dry stools, red tongue, slightly yellowish and greasy tongue coating, and a slippery and rapid pulse.

Principle of Treatment:
Clear heat, resolve phlegm, disperse the lung-qi, and relieve cough.

Herbal Treatment:
Qing Jin Hua Tan Tang-*Clear Metal and Transform Phlegm Decoction.*

Sang Bai Pi *Cortex Mori Albae Radicis* 10 g
Huang Qin *Radix Scutellariae Baicalensis* 10 g
Zhi Zi *Fructus Gardeniae Jasminoidis* 10 g
Xing Ren *Semen Pruni Armeniacae* 10 g
Zhe Bei Mu *Bulbus Fritillariae Thunbergii* 10 g
Gua Lou Pi *Pericarpium Trichosanthis* 10 g
Jie Geng *Radix Platycodi Grandiflori* 10 g
Zhi Ban Xia *Rhizoma Pinelliae Ternatae Preparata* 10 g
Fu Ling *Sclerotium Poriae Cocos* 12 g
Chen Pi *Pericarpium Citri Reticulatae* 5 g
Zhi Gan Cao *Radix Glycyrrhizae Preparata* 3 g

Explanations:
- Huang Qin, Sang Bai Pi, and Zhi Zi clear heat in the lungs and relieve coughing.
- Xing Ren, Zhe Bei Mu, and Gua Lou Pi clear and resolve heat-phlegm and relieve cough.
- Zhi Ban Xia, Fu Ling, Chen Pi, and Zhi Gan Cao, the compositions of Er Chen Tang, together with Jie Geng, resolve damp-phlegm and relieve cough.

Herbal Remedy:
Qing Qi Hua Tan Tang Wan-*Clear the Qi and Transform Phlegm Pill.*

Acupuncture Treatment:
- Neiguan P-6 + Gongsun SP-4, Chize LU-5, Lieque LU-7, Yuji LU-10, Feishu BL-13, Hegu L.I.-4, Quchi L.I.-11, Tanzhong REN-17, Fenglong ST-40, Sanyinjiao SP-6 and Yinlingquan SP-9.
- An even method is applied on P-6 + SP-4, and a reducing method is applied on the rest of the points.

Explanations:
- The combination of P-6 + SP-4 promotes the qi circulation in the chest and relieves cough.

- LU-7, LU-5, and LU-10, the luo-connecting point, the he-sea point and the ying-spring point of the lung channel respectively, BL-13, the back-shu point of the lung, disperse the lung-qi, clear heat in the lung, and relieve cough.
- L.I.-4 and L.I.-11, the yuan-source point and the he-sea point of the large intestine channel respectively, clear heat in the body and promote defecation.
- REN-17, the gathering point of the qi in the body, promotes the qi circulation in the body and relaxes the chest.
- ST-40, SP-6, and SP-9, the luo-connecting point of the stomach channel, the crossing point of three yin channels of the foot, and the he-sea point of the spleen channel respectively, activate the spleen and stomach and eliminate damp-phlegm in the body.

11.7.2.4 *Deficiency of lung-qi*

Slight cough during Long COVID, expectoration of slight, whitish, and diluted phlegm, low voice, shortness of breath after exertion, listlessness, aversion to wind, spontaneous sweating, easily catching a common cold, cold hands and feet, thin and whitish tongue coating, pale tongue, and a weak and thready pulse.

Principle of Treatment:
Tonify the lung-qi, resolve phlegm, and relieve cough.

Herbal Treatment:
Bu Fei Tang-*Tonify the Lungs Decoction,* plus
Si Jun Zi Tang-*Four Gentlemen Decoction.*

Zhi Dang Shen *Radix Codonopsis Pilosulae Praeparata* 10 g
Zhi Huang Qi *Radix Astragali Membranacei Praeparata* 10 g
Bai Zhu *Rhizoma Atractylodis Macrocephalae* 10 g
Shu Di Huang *Radix Rhemanniae Glutinosae Praeparata* 12 g
Wu Wei Zi *Fructus Schisandrae Chinensis* 10 g
Zi Wan *Radix Asteris Tatarici* 10 g

Zhi Ban Xia *Rhizoma Pinelliae Ternatae Preparata* 10 g
Sang Bai Pi *Cortex Mori Albae Radicis* 10 g
Fu Ling *Sclerotium Poriae Cocos* 12 g
Zhi Gan Cao *Radix Glycyrrhizae Preparata* 3 g

Explanations:
- Zhi Dang Shen, Bai Zhu, Fu Ling, and Zhi Gan Cao activate the spleen and tonify the qi in the body.
- Zhi Huang Qi, Wu Wei Zi, and Zi Wan tonify the qi of the lung and benefit the lung.
- Sang Bai Pi descends the lung-qi and relieves cough.
- Shu Di Huang tonifies the kidney and benefits the lung.
- Zhi Ban Xia eliminates phlegm and relieves cough.

Herbal Remedy:
Bu Fei Tang-*Tonify the Lungs Decoction.*

Acupuncture Treatment:
- Neiguan P-6 + Gongsun SP-4, Chize LU-5, Taiyuan LU-9, Zusanli ST-36, Sanyinjiao SP-6, Taixi KID-3, Qihai REN-6, Feishu BL-13, and Shenshu BL-23.
- An even method is applied on P-6 + SP-4, and a tonifying method is applied on the rest of the points. Moxibustion could be applied on BL-13, BL-23, ST-36, KID-3, and REN-6.

Explanations:
- The combination of P-6 + SP-4 regulates the qi in the body and relieves cough.
- LU-5, the he-sea point of the lung channels, and LU-9, the yuan-source point of the lung channel, and BL-13, the back-shu point of the lung, tonify lung-qi and restore the physiological functions of the lung.
- ST-36, SP-6, REN-6, KID-3, and BL-23 tonify the qi of the spleen and kidney and support the lung-qi to relieve cough.
- Moxibustion warms the qi and dispels the deficient cold in the body.

11.7.2.5 *Deficiency of lung-yin*

Slightly dry cough or cough with scanty phlegm, phlegm mixed with little blood streaks, thirst, dryness of the throat, night sweating, hotness of the palms and soles, dry stools, red tongue, scanty or peeled tongue coating, and a deep, thready, and rapid pulse.

Principle of Treatment:
Nourish yin, moisten the lung, and relieve cough.

Herbal Treatment:
Sha Shen Mai Men Dong Tang-*Glehnia and Ophiopogonis Decoction.*

Bei Sha Shen *Radix Glehniae Littoralis* 10 g
Mai Men Dong *Tuber Ophiopogonis Japonici* 10 g
Wu Wei Zi *Fructus Schisandrae Chinensis* 10 g
Tian Hua Fen *Radix Trichosanthis Kirilowii* 10 g
Xing Ren *Semen Pruni Armeniacae* 10 g
Chuan Bei Mu *Bulbus Fritillariae Cirrhosae* 10 g
Zi Wan *Radix Asteris Tatarici* 10 g
Di Gu Pi *Cortex Lycii Radicis* 10 g
Sheng Di Huang *Radix Rehmanniae Glutinosae Recens* 10 g
Zhi Mu *Radix Anemarrhenae Asphodeloides* 10 g
Huang Qin *Radix Scutellariae Baicalensis* 10 g

Explanations:
- Bei Sha Shen, Mai Men Dong, and Wu Wei Zi nourish the yin of the lung and relieve cough.
- Chuan Bei Mu, Zi Wan, and Di Gu Pi nourish the yin, clear the heat in the lung, eliminate phlegm in the lung and benefit the lung to relieve cough.
- Sheng Di Huang, Zhi Mu, and Huang Qin are used to clear the remaining deficient heat in the lung and relieve coughing.
- Tian Hua Fen nourishes yin, promotes the secretion of body fluid, and relieves thirst and dryness of the throat.

Herbal Remedy:
Sheng Mai San (Wan)-*Generate the Pulse Powder (Pill).*

Acupuncture Treatment:
- Lieque LU-7 + Zhaohai KID-6, Chize LU-5, Taiyuan LU-9, Feishu BL-13, Zusanli ST-36, Sanyinjiao SP-6, Taixi KID-3, Qihai REN-6, and Shenshu BL-23.
- An even method is applied on LU-7 + KID-6, and a tonifying method is applied to the rest of the points.

Explanations:
- The combination of LU-7 + KID-6 nourishes the yin of the body and clears deficient heat.
- LU-5, the he-sea point of the lung channel, and LU-9, the yuan-source point of the lung channel, and BL-13, the back-shu point of the lung, nourish the yin of the lung, and restore the physiological functions of the lung.
- ST-36, SP-6, KID-3, KID-6, BL-23, and REN-6 activate the spleen and stomach, nourishing the yin of the body to benefit the yin of the lung.

11.8 Loss of Smell and Taste

COVID-19 is a respiratory disease caused by SARS-CoV-2, manifesting a variety of symptoms. The clinical symptoms and their severity may vary from person to person.

In addition to respiratory symptoms, such as fever, cough, myalgia and shortness of breath, loss of the sense of smell or taste can be other types of symptoms in COVID-19. It is an absolute truth that there are so many people who don't realize the importance of smell and taste in our lives until we have lost them. This is particularly the case in COVID-19.

COVID-19 is a global pandemic event and is still not yet under complete control globally. Various papers have proven that loss of smell (otherwise known as olfactory dysfunction or anosmia) and taste (otherwise known as dysgeusia) is one of the clinical symptoms when COVID-19 onsets or there is only loss of smell and taste (LST) even without displaying other symptoms. One effect is that it leaves people vulnerable to dangers such as food poisoning and fire. For instance, people with anosmia are less able to detect spoilt food and smoke.[46] A 2014 study found that people with anosmia were more than twice as likely to experience a hazardous event, such as eating spoilt food, as people without smell loss.[47] For a proportion of people, their smell disappeared suddenly, or the sense of smell was warped, i.e., unpleasant scents have taken the place of normally delightful ones. Thus, early identification of loss of smell and taste is of significance since LST should be used as a diagnostic test for COVID-19.

When COVID-19 broke out in China, several editions of national guidelines on diagnosis and treatment were published. The latest edition, published on 3 March 2020, by the National Health Commission & State Administration of Traditional Chinese Medicine, LST was not included in the diagnostic symptoms.

However, when COVID-19 started its global journey from Italy to Europe in March 2020, the loss or change in sense of smell and/or taste—among all the other early symptoms and signs of the infection—was raising more and more awareness as one of the unique early symptoms of the COVID-19 infection. The UK government was the latest one to recognize this, and the loss or change of taste and/or smell was added onto the renewed guideline for

---

[46]Michael Marshall. COVID's toll on smell and taste: What scientists do and don't know. *Nature*. 2021, 589: 342–343. https://doi.org/10.1038/d41586-021-00055-6.
[47]Taylor S. Pence, *et al.* Risk factors for hazardous events in olfactory-impaired patients. *JAMA Otolaryngol Head Neck Surg.* 2014, 140(10): 951–955. doi: 10.1001/jamaoto.2014.1675.

diagnosis of COVID-19 on 18 May 2020.[48] In comparison, the USA CDC already did so early in April.[49]

The exact percentage varies between studies. Spinato *et al.* reported on *JAMA* on 26 May 2020 that 64.6% of patients had an altered sense of smell or taste, which is higher than two typical symptoms—dry or productive cough (60.4%) and fever (55.5%).[50] One review published on June 2020 compiled data from 8,438 people with COVID-19, and found that 41% had reported experiencing the loss of smell.[51] In another study, published in August 2020, confirmed 96% of the participants had some olfactory dysfunction, and 18% had total smell loss.[52] A recent study published in *Mayo Clinic Proceedings* took a deep dive into how common a loss of smell or taste is in COVID-19. Researchers reviewed results from 24 studies, which represented data from over 8,438 people with a confirmed case of COVID-19. They found that the average prevalence of loss of smell was calculated to be about 41% and the average prevalence for loss of taste was calculated to be about 38.2%. Older age correlated with a lower prevalence of loss of smell or taste. No

---

[48] Gemma Mitchell. UK adds loss of smell to COVID-19 symptoms requiring self-isolation. *Nursing Time.* Updated 18 May 2020. https://www.nursingtimes.net/news/coronavirus/uk-adds-loss-of-smell-to-covid-19-symptoms-requiring-self-isolation-18-05-2020/.

[49] CDC. Updated 22 February 2021. *op. cit.*

[50] Giacomo Spinato, *et al.* Alterations in smell or taste in mildly symptomatic outpatients with SARS-CoV-2 infection. *JAMA.* 2020, 323(20): 2089–2091. doi: 10.1001/jama.2020.6771.

[51] Akosua Adom Agyeman, *et al.* Smell and taste dysfunction in patients with COVID-19: A systematic review and meta-analysis. *Mayo Clin Proc.* 2020, 95(8): 1621–1631. doi: 10.1016/j.mayocp.2020.05.030.

[52] Shima T. Moein, *et al.* Prevalence and reversibility of smell dysfunction measured psychophysically in a cohort of COVID-19 patients. *Int Forum Allergy Rhinol.* 2020, 10(10): 1127–1135. doi: 10.1002/alr.22680.

difference in the prevalence of either symptom was seen in men versus women.[53]

One study found that over a median follow-up period of 200 days, approximately half the men, and 60% of women, had regained less than 80% of their original smell acuity compared to before they contracted the infection. About 60% were finally classified as having smell impairments at follow-up, with about 40% also having an impairment of taste. Conversely, a fifth said they had recovered taste but not smell. Only 3% reported the inverse pattern. This indicates that these sensations are not linked in their impairment and recover separately, with the subjects being able to distinguish them separately. The researchers found that while most participants who had varying extents of anosmia or ageusia during the acute phase reported improvement at follow-up, the final number of subjects who said they had persistent smell abnormalities was higher at this time point than during acute infection.[54]

For most patients with COVID-19, their loss of smell and taste return within weeks. A report by the Center for Disease Control and Prevention (CDC) indicated the duration of loss of smell or taste was 8 days symptoms on 274 patients that had COVID-19 symptoms.[55] This finding is also supported by a smaller study from Europe, in which loss of smell and taste lasted an average of 8.9 days.[56]

But for others, the symptoms of loss of smell or taste are more serious. Evidence is emerging that they may emerge and persist long

---

[53] Akosua Adom Agyeman, *et al. op. cit.*

[54] Liji Thomas, *et al.* Smell abnormalities more common among long-COVID Patients. *News-Medical.* 3 September 2021. https://www.news-medical.net/news/20210903/Smell-abnormalities-more-common-among-long-COVID-Patients.aspx.

[55] Mark W. Tenforde, *et al.* Symptom duration and risk factors for delayed return to usual health among outpatients with COVID-19 in a multistate health care systems network-United States, March–June 2020. *Morbidity and Mortality Weekly Report (Weekly),* 69(30): 993–998. https://www.cdc.gov/mmwr/volumes/69/wr/mm6930e1.htm.

[56] T. Klopfenstein, *et al.* Features of anosmia in COVID-19. *Med Mal Infect.* 2020, 50(5): 436–439. doi: 10.1016/j.medmal.2020.04.006.

after initial COVID-19 infection, causing some profound consequences and severe impact to the quality of life, such as loss of appetite, loss of pleasure in food and eating, weight loss, altered intimacy and an altered relationship to self and others, limited or impaired social engagement, public gatherings, travel, and leisure activities, etc.

Loss of smell with a blocked nose is due to the inability of volatile odor molecules to reach the olfactory mucosa at the top of the nasal cavity. It is often not accompanied by a loss of taste. However, loss of smell and taste in COVID-19 is something different, and they usually appear at the same time. Although the mechanisms are not fully understood, among some scientists there is an emerging consensus that loss of smell occurs when the coronavirus infects cells that support neurons in the nose. A team led by Sandeep Robert Datta at Harvard Medical School in Boston, Massachusetts, found that cells that support sensory neurons in the nose, known as sustentacular cells, are probably what the virus is infecting.[57]

There are some reports showing an abundance of nasal epithelial cells expressing cellular receptors and proteases needed for viral entry, i.e., angiotensin-converting enzyme 2 (ACE-2) and transmembrane serine protease 2 (TMPRSS2). One of the most reliable hypotheses lay the importance of the interaction of SARS-CoV-2 with the ACE2 and TMPRSS2 enzymes. Multiple non-neuronal cell types present in the olfactory epithelium express two host receptors (ACE2 and TMPRSS2 proteases, expressed in the oral mucosa and olfactory cavity), that facilitate SARS-CoV-2 binding, replication, and accumulation.[58] Based on the hypotheses, drugs that potentially modulate the expression and activity of ACE2, ACE inhibitors (ACEI) and angiotensin II receptor blockers (ARB) such as captopril, are advised

---

[57] David H. Brann, *et al.* Non-neuronal expression of SARS-CoV-2 entry genes in the olfactory system suggests mechanisms underlying COVID-19-associated anosmia. *Sci Adv.* 2020, 6(31): eabc5801. doi: 10.1126/sciadv.abc5801.

[58] Sara Ferraro, *et al.* Olfactory and gustatory impairments in COVID-19 patients: Mechanism, clinical characteristics, drug interferences and role in early diagnosis. 2020. Preprint doi: 10.31219/osf.io/hztp9.

to be considered in the management of LST.[59] It was also reported that up to 88% of patients develop anosmia or ageusia, and it was thought to be secondary to the invasion of the olfactory bulb by the virus, suggesting brain involvement.[60]

The most frustrating for LST is that since there is a lack of sufficient research yet, it means few established treatments exist.

Here, its etiologies, pathologies, and mechanisms of loss of smell and taste (LST) are studied, pointing out that disturbed Brain-Shen, impairment of the meridians and dysfunction of the zang-fu organs are direct pathogenesis of LST. TCM management with acupuncture and Chinese herbs are presented accordingly, aiming to establish some strategies to deal with LST practically and effectively. These unique explanations in the treatment illustrate that although LST is a single symptom, it implies a profound and complicated background, which requires a comprehensive treatment in time. If left untreated, LST would cause further disturbance to the quality of the patients and may last quite a long time even COVID-19 is cured clinically.

11.8.1 TCM understanding of Long COVID-associated LST

Although the actual mechanism of LST in Western medicine is not yet clear, TCM's thorough logic analysis of pathology over the whole process of SARS-CoV-2 infection can provide a good interpretation as well as a reliable resolution on the treatment of LST.

COVID-19 is believed in TCM to be mainly the invasion by an epidemic pestilence bearing nature of cold-damp, with toxins into the body, especially at early mild or ordinary stages. Although it follows the same pattern of normal EPFs, it also has its own pandemic characters, showing acute onset, dramatic progress at an unexpected

---

[59]Gemma Mitchell. *op. cit.*

[60]Jerome R. Lechien, *et al.* Olfactory and gustatory dysfunctions as a clinical presentation of mild-to-moderate forms of the coronavirus disease (COVID-19): A multicenter European study. *Eur Arch Otorhinolaryngol.* 2020, 277(8):2251–2261. doi: 10.1007/s00405-020-05965-1.

speed, skipping or overlapping different stages at the same time to cause much higher complexity and mortality than other ordinary exogenous diseases.

11.8.1.1 *Dysfunction of meridians*

According to the statements written in various chapters throughout *Huang Di Nei Jing*, it is believed that when external pathogenic factors-EPF(s) invades the body, the first stage of its process is to hit the skin-cutaneous section. If it is not resolved by the system, it then travels deeper into the collaterals and then channels. If it is still not resolved, it then enters further and finally settles in the zang-fu organs. It is generally accepted that the exterior patterns of any illness are on the level between the skin-cutaneous sections and meridians. This is because the skin-cutaneous sections and collaterals are all meridian oriented sub-systems. By studying the meridian distribution, it could be understood that different meridians, including regular and extraordinary meridians, could be involved and sometimes, several meridians could be involved at the same time. For instance, the bladder meridian starts at the inner corner of both eyes close to the root of the nose and frontal sinus. Cold-damp, which hits the bladder meridian, can cause a blocked nose as well as an impaired sense of smell. At this moment, there are no symptoms that show that the lung is involved, showing symptoms of cough or shortness of breath, etc. Ignoring these symptoms could cause further spreading of the virus and deterioration of the disease. Large intestine and stomach meridians both start or end on the sides of nose wings, close to the sphenoid sinus, thus the suffering of cold-damp attacking both meridians can lead to the LST. Medical intervention and personal care should be taken in time to treat LST. When toxins heat dominates the body in the progress of the disease, there would be LST as well. Again, Yangqiao mai starts from the Shenmai BL-62 of the Taiyang meridian of the lateral heel and runs up the back of the lateral malleolus and up to along the posterolateral side of the chest, through the shoulder and lateral neck, and finally to the corner of the mouth and nose to reach the inner corner of the eye. It meets the foot

Shaoyang meridian at Fengchi GB-20. External invasion of cold-damp could cause dysfunction of Yangqiao mai, leading to stiffness of the body at the lateral aspect with LST. Besides, the following channels (such as the lung, heart, spleen, kidney, liver, Du mai, Ren mai, as well as Chong mai), all have a direct or indirect connection with smell and taste. It would be a mistake to consider that LST is only caused by dysfunction of the lung in dispersing the lung-qi.

11.8.1.2 *Disturbance to the Brain-Shen*

The brain, one of the six extraordinary organs, is also called "the sea of marrow". It states in *Ling Shu (Spiritual Pivot)* in *Huang Di Nei Jing* that "The brain is the sea of marrow, it stretches up to the top of the head, and to the point of Fengfu DU-16". In Chapter 28 of Ling Shu, it also says that "when the up-going qi is insufficient, the brain is not filled, so the ears suffer from hearing noises, the head suffers from being bent, causing dizziness because of affected eye vision". Due to the close connection of the bladder meridian with Du mai and the kidney that feeds directly into the brain, COVID-19 progressing in the bladder meridian may rapidly fall into the brain via the connection of Du mai, Ren mai Chong mai, and kidney meridian. Any unsolved disturbance to these meridians could cause LST in Long COVID.

The brain is the place of Shen's activity, which controls memory, concentration, sight, hearing, and smell. As the *Pi Wei Lun-Discussion on Stomach and Spleen* by Li Dong Yuan (1249) states, the "sense of sight, hearing, smelling, touch, and intelligence all depend on the Brain". Wang Qing Ren in the Qing Dynasty says in his book *Yi Lin Gai Cuo-Correcting the errors in the forest of medicine*: "the nose communicates with the brain and therefore smell depends on the brain".[61] Similarly, when talking about Xin Yi Hua *Flos Magnoliae* in the book *Ben Cao Gang Mu*, Li Shi Zhen says "The nose is through the Heaven and the Heaven is the head".

---

[61] Qingren Wang. *Yi Lin Gai Cuo (Correcting the Errors in the Forest of Medicine)*. Blue Poppy Press. Bilingual edition. Boulder, 2007. p. 45. ISBN-13: 978-1891845390.

Hence, it is clear in TCM that the brain is connected to the senses of sight, hearing, smell, and taste. The brain is believed to be the organ to control sight, hearing, smell, and taste, and it also closely interacts with the zang organs (the heart and kidney) in TCM context. The development of the brain's dysfunction is usually a combination of impairment of the brain at its structure along with disruption of internal organs.

From the vast clinical research on the COVID-19 infected patients, we now believe impairment of the brain (encephalopathy) did happen at a comparatively earlier stage of the infection and may persevere throughout the later and recovery stage. Sufferers reported lack of concentration, poor memory, stress, insomnia, delayed recovery of loss of smell and taste, etc. Loss of smell or taste may be a result of impairment of relevant meridians at the beginning of COVID-19 infection, but once the progress of damage reaches the Brain level, a dedicated treatment for recovering the brain's function in TCM is critical for the recovery of LST. However, the recovery of the brain also depends on the repair and healing of its relevant zang-fu organs.

In addition, to maintain a good function of the brain, spleen-qi needs to rise to the head to nourish the upper orifices, such as eyes, nose, ears, tongue, and mouth. Sufficient spleen-qi rises upwards to carry the clear-yang to irrigate the senses. As *Huang Di Nei Jing*-Su Wen (Simple Questions) states "the clear-yang is Heaven", "The clear-yang exits through the upper orifices" (p. 97), "the clear-Yang is effused through the interstice structures" (p. 98), "the clear-yang (qi) can be effused through them" and "the clear-yang transforms to qi and rises to constitute Heaven".[62]

If the clear-yang is strong and healthy, the senses of seeing, smelling, hearing and tasting would be acute and clear. If there are any disorders of ascending, descending, entering, and exiting of

---

[62] Paul U. Unschuld, *et al. Huang Di Nei Jing Su Wen: An Annotated Translation of Huang Di's Inner Classic–Basic Questions.* University of California Press, California USA. 2011. eBook.

spleen-qi, blocked by cold-damp, the clear-yang will not be lifted towards the head, and these may result in impaired senses, including smell and taste.

11.8.1.3 *Impairment of zang-fu organs*

Invasion of cold-damp with toxins into the meridians always ends in internal zang-fu organs, especially in the case of COVID-19. It initially could impair the lung, spleen and San Jiao via meridians, but quickly fall in further to damage the heart (pericardium), liver and kidney, especially at the severe and critical stage. Therefore, zang-fu organs' dysfunction is an unavoidable procedure in studying the recovery of COVID-19.

The sense of ability to smell and taste all depend on the smooth ascending, descending, entering, and exiting of qi. If qi is obstructed or disrupted, these senses will not be functioning properly. Since the nose is the opening of the lung, TCM stresses the importance of the lung in terms of smell, which means that if lung-qi is healthy and strong, the nose will be opened properly, and the sense of smell will be normal and accurate. If lung-qi is disrupted, the sense of smell may be weak or impaired. The mouth is the opening orifice of the spleen, and the tongue is the opening orifice of the heart. If the qi of the spleen and heart is strong, the sense of taste will be normal and acute. If smelling the qi of the spleen or heart is disrupted, the sense of taste may be weak or impaired.

Although each sense of body is mainly related to a certain zang-fu organ, i.e., vision to the liver, taste to the spleen and heart, smell to the lung and hearing to the kidney, TCM still holds that these internal zang-fu organs are mutually connected and influenced through meridians systems and Mother and Son relationships. Moreover, the physiological function of the heart plays an extreme role in the senses' function. For instance, *Huang Di Nei Jing–Su Wen* says: "when the five qi enter the nose, they are stored by heart and lung. When heart and lung have a disease, the nose is not free as a result".[63] This text implies the relationship between the function of the nose and the lung and heart.

11.8.2 TCM treatment of Long COVID-associated LST

Tailored treatment to help reduce the inflammatory reaction caused by cytokine attacks on the nasal mucosal epithelium or taste buds on the tongue can be a great approach to revert or reduce the symptoms of LST in Western medicine. TCM also has its own strategies for protection and repair on the impairment of CNS in the brain by COVID-19 infection. Relevant involvement of TCM in timely treatment will play an important role in the success of LST recovery. However, TCM treatment for LST during Long COVID is of course based upon the syndrome differentiation, which means symptomatic management of LST due to Long COVID will fail to achieve some expected results.

TCM treatment of LST includes the following strategies.

11.8.2.1 *Promote the function of the meridians*

The olfactory nerve is the nerve fiber that passes through the ethmoid epithelium to the olfactory bulb. The olfactory ability is the characteristic of the olfactory cells in the nasal mucosa. Injury of the nasal mucosa, olfactory bulb, olfactory filaments, or central nervous system connection may affect the olfactory sense. The clinical manifestations are: decreased or loss of sense of smell, inversion of sense of smell, or phantom smell. Taste is transmitted by taste nipples densely spread on the tongue, called taste bud cells, and then excited by the taste center of the cerebral cortex. The entire taste analysis activity is completed by the feedback loop neurohumoral system.

As illustrated above, when LST occurs during Long COVID, the chief TCM treatment attention is focused on eliminating the

---

[63] Paul U. Unschuld, *et al. op. cit.* p. 208.

pathogenic factors and recovering the internal organs. Additionally, methods of calming the shen and opening the clear orifices should be included. Meanwhile, one more technique should also be conducted, that is, using acupuncture and Chinese herbs to promote the qi and blood circulation in the relevant meridians, since our body consists of physical zang-fu organs and meridian structures. Only caring for the zang-fu organs without regulating the meridians would not be able to relief LST.

Like choosing points or herbs to calm the shen and open the clear orifices, differentiation of points and herbs is important here in this situation as well. Without this step, a final sophisticated treatment will not yet be formed.

11.8.2.2 *Symptomatic local treatment*

Yingxiang L.I.-20 and Extra Bitong are considered as the local points, which have the function to open the nose, relieve the blockage and improve the sense of smell. Meanwhile, Dicang ST-4 is a good acupoint to improve the taste to treat loss of taste. Juliao ST-3 could be used to treat both loss of smell and taste. They are punctured with a reducing method. However, those points are only considered as the points for symptomatic treatment, and they are combined with the points to solve the fundamental sickness of Long COVID.

When Chinese herbs are concerned, Cang Er Zi *Fructus Xanthii Sibirici* 10 g and Xin Yi Hua *Flos Magnoliae* 10 g, which have a function to open the nasal orifice and improve the sense of smell, should be added into the herbal prescription to relieve loss of smell. Sha Ren *Fructus Amomi* 5 g or Bai Kou Ren *Fructus Amomi Cardamomi* 5 g, which have a function to resolve damp and improve the sense of taste, could be chosen and added into the herbal prescription.

11.8.2.3 *Auxiliary techniques*

Besides choosing the above local points, moxibustion is also encouraged to be applied. It has the effect to dispel external pathogenic factors, eliminate cold, resolve damp, promote the lung to disperse the qi and the spleen in transportation and transformation. Direct moxa, indirect moxa with ginger, or moxa cones on the needles are all positive methods to improve the therapeutic effect of acupuncture.

Meanwhile, electric acupuncture is also advised to be used. Tense and dispersed waves should be applied in order to relieve the local inflammation so as to improve LST.

11.8.2.4 *Regulation of relevant meridians*

Although both acupuncture points and some Chinese herbs could be applied for symptomatic treatment of LST in Long COVID, blockage in certain meridians is still left untreated. For instance, if the loss of taste is caused by a disorder of Chong mai, and Chong mai is not regulated and harmonized in time, this loss of taste will remain the same. Obtaining a clear identification and differentiation of relevant meridians requires a thorough understanding of acupuncture and herbal medicine.

To improve the qi and blood circulation for the loss of smell and taste during Long COVID, the yuan-source points and luo-connecting points from the relevant involved meridians should be selected on purpose, with extra attention to the following meridians, such as the lung, spleen, stomach, liver, heart, bladder, kidney and large intestine. When these different meridians are impaired, they could show different clinical symptoms and signs rather than only manifesting as a loss of smell and taste. In most cases, impairment of one or two meridians are often seen in the practice, seldom involving different meridians at the same time.

The involvement of extraordinary meridians needs special attention and care. To identify and solve their problems, a unique technique in point combinations and procedures is required.

Here are some explanations and suggestions:

- Du mai

From the crown of the head, the channel descends along the midline of the forehead and nose to its final point, Shui Gou DU-26, at the junction of the upper lip and gum.

One of its secondary branches ascends together with the Chong mai and Ren mai, to pass through the heart, circles the mouth and splits to ascend to the lower border of the two eyes.

Since Du mai is the governor of all the Yang meridians, when Du mai is impaired, there would be headache, dizziness, severe aversion to cold, weak heartbeat, cold hands and feet, blocked nose with loss of smell and taste in Long COVID. Houxi SI-3 + Shenmai BL-62 should be added to open this meridian.

• Ren mai

Ren mai is the Sea of Yin in the body, ascending along the midline of the abdomen and ending at Chengjiang REN-24 below the lower lip. An internal portion of the channel then winds around the mouth, connecting with Shuigou DU-26 and ascending to Chengqi ST-1 just below the eye. When Ren mai is impaired, different zang organs could be disturbed, causing respiratory, cardiological, or water metabolism and digestive disorders, including pressure at the chest, abdominal pain and distention, poor appetite, weakness, tiredness, somnolence, coldness of body, blocked nose with loss of smell and taste in Long COVID. Lieque LU-7 + Zhaohai KI-6 should be added to open this meridian.

• Chong mai

The fourth branch of Chong mai from the chest ascends alongside the throat, curves around the lips and terminates below the eye, reaching the end of the Ren mai. When Chong mai is impaired, it can be typically manifested as qi rushing from the lower abdomen up till the chest, or vomiting, nausea, saliva, or abdominal pain, chest pain, blocked nose with loss of smell and taste in Long COVID. Gongsun SP-4 + Neiguan P-6 should be added to harmonize this meridian.

• Yangqiao mai

After reaching the points at Jianyu L.I.-15 and Jugu L.I.-16, Yangqiao mai then travels to the face and connects with Dicang ST-4, Juliao ST-3, Chengqi ST-1 and Jingming BL-1 where it meets with the BL,

DU and Yinqiao mai. From here it travels over the head and terminates at Fengchi GB-20.

When Yangqiao mai is impaired, there can be numbness, weakness, and spasms at the lateral aspect of the lower limbs, headache, eyes or face pain, loss of smell and taste in Long COVID. Shenmai BL-62 + Houxi SI-3 should be added to regulate this meridian.

As compared to acupuncture, there are fewer choices of Chinese herbs that can help regulate or harmonize different meridians. Nonetheless, it is possible to add some specific herbs to achieve this effect to improve the smell and taste.

• Chuan Xiong *Radix Ligustici Wallichii*
It is an ideal herb to lead the prescription to the head and clear orifice to promote the qi and blood circulation in the meridians.

• Bai Zhi *Radix Angelicae Dahuricae*
It enters the lung, spleen and stomach meridians, having a good function to promote qi circulation in the head. Meanwhile, it dispels cold and damp, relieves headache, opens the nasal orifice, and discharges the phlegm in the nose.

• Jie Geng *Radix Platycodi Grandiflori*
It enters the lung meridian, having a function to disperse the lung-qi, benefit the throat, eliminate phlegm, discharge the pus, and open the nasal orifice.

• Aromatic damp-resolving herbs
One of the main pathogenic factors for this pandemic is an invasion of cold-damp, which cause the failure of the lung to disperse the lung-qi or to descend the lung-qi, and dysfunction of the spleen to transport and transform, as well as impairment of the San Jiao in qi and water distribution.

Aromatic damp-resolving herbs could be applied to treat dysfunction of the spleen, manifested as poor appetite, tiredness, chest tightness, loose stools, or diarrhea, loss of taste, greasy tongue coating, and a slippery pulse, etc. Cang Zhu *Rhizoma Atractylodis*, Huo Xiang *Herba Agastaches seu Pogostemi*, Pei Lan *Herba Eupatorii Fortunei*, Bai Kou Ren *Fructus Amomi Cardamomi*, Cao Guo *Fructus Amomi Tsao-Ko*, Cao Dou Kou *Semen Alpiniae Katsumadai*, etc., are suitable to be applied in the herbal prescription to treat Long COVID with LST. Mostly two to three herbs could be used to improve the function of the spleen and sense of taste at the same time. Moreover, patients should be advised to avoid eating cold and raw food, cold drinks as well as irritable foods such as pepper and mustard.

Loss of smell and taste, which could occur in separation, should be treated properly with acupuncture and Chinese herbs based upon thorough understanding of the etiologies, pathologies, and syndrome differentiation. Without the elimination of its causative factors, resolving the pathological changes, restoration of internal zang-fu organs, and symptomatic treatment of LST will have little effect. However, only focusing on all the above treatments without proper treatment for LST will also have no efficiency to improve this complaint. TCM wisdom can be reflected vividly in this case of Long COVID: treating the causative factors and local sickness at the same moment.

11.8.2.5 *Regulation of internal zang-fu organs*

Loss of smell or taste is an early warning or one of the chief symptoms of COVID-19 in the beginning stage, including middle cases and ordinary cases. These two symptoms may appear separately or in combination together with or without some symptoms from the lung, spleen and San Jiao due to failure of the lung in dispersing the lung-qi, dysfunction of the spleen in transportation and transformation, and disturbance of the San Jiao, etc.

It must be noted that loss of smell and tastes in Long COVID is not a life-threatening case. Alleviating the sense of smell and taste is not the main aim of TCM treatment, but the main target is to restore a patient's qualities. Details about TCM treatment based upon syndrome differentiation could refer to some relevant parts in cough and diarrhea of this book.

Although TCM emphasizes the important role that dysfunction of different zang-fu organs and meridian could cause LST during the TCM treatment, the lung and spleen are always the chief organs to be disturbed or impaired, confirming that more attention and care should be given to the lung and spleen. Methods should be applied to promote the lung and spleen in their physiological functions and relieve the pathological changes in their system. In terms of recovery of the physiological functions of the lung, dispersing the lung-qi is always most important in the recovery of loss of smell, and the spleen in the recovery of loss of taste.

As mentioned above, our physical body is unified, forming one entirety. The lung is closely associated with all the other zang-fu organs, forming a system to mutually promote and assist. In some cases of loss of smell, the lung is not the only organ to be blamed and treated during COVID-19. Sometimes the lung could be the victim due to its impairment by some other organs or other pathogens. Without eliminating this disturbance caused by these pathogens, the lung will not be able to fulfill its task to disperse the qi to obtain a good sense of smell.

The loss of taste in TCM is a condition showing that the spleen is chiefly disturbed or impaired. In fact, this pandemic is mainly caused by the invasion of cold-damp with the toxins, and the spleen is often involved from the very beginning of the case. Besides the loss of taste, there are often cases of sudden loose stool or diarrhea, abdominal distention and pain, poor appetite, and tiredness, supporting the diagnosis that the cold-damp has disturbed the transportation and transformation of the spleen. In some cases, loss of taste is a very early symptom and sign, indicating that the spleen is involved. Thus, it will be very logical that eliminating the cold-damp and activating the spleen in transportation and transformation is the main therapeutic management when loss of taste appears. Only focusing on treating loss of taste without consideration of recovery of the spleen in its physiological function is absolutely an incomplete direction, and even a wrong treatment.

Same as the explanations above about the lung, the spleen is an organ connected with other organs and meridians, influenced by many other factors. Therefore, in order to properly deal with the loss of taste, we also need to perform a careful examination of the whole body. For example, Chong mai or Yinwei mai can be impaired during the ordinary cases of COVID-19 besides the spleen, which could also lead to loss of taste. If these two extra meridians are not properly treated—only treating the spleen for loss of taste—its treatment will certainly fail.

11.8.2.6 *Calm the Brain-Shen and open the clear orifices*

Since the heart is considered as the Emperor, it's in charge of housing the shen. Although smell, taste, hearing, and vision belong to different individual organs, they are all different senses, feelings, and activities of the shen, which are dominated by the heart. Our brain, where clear-yang is situated, is also referred to in TCM as yuan shen (the primary shen). Disturbance or disruption to the clear-yang by cold-damp, toxins, or another pathogen could cause dysfunction of the shen, leading to the limited physiological function of the sense of smell and taste. In this sense, it could be seen that methods to regulate the shen to benefit the brain should be applied to deal with the loss of smell and taste due to COVID-19.

Both the lung and heart are in the chest. The lung is responsible for smooth qi circulation and the heart is responsible for regular blood circulation. Coordination of qi and blood circulation could be maintained when the lung and heart are in a harmonious state. So, to treat loss of smell, the heart also needs to be cared for besides treating the lung.

When there is a remaining cold-damp in the spleen, it is possible to see the loss of taste. According to the Five Elements theory, earth-spleen is the Son of the heart-fire, which means that the heart could also be involved, resulting in dysfunction of the heart in housing the shen, therefore the loss of taste could be aggravated. Thus, it should be encouraged to deal with the spleen and heart at the same time.

There are different acupuncture points and Chinese herbs to regulate the shen. However, it may not be suitable to select all of them at the same time, especially selecting them without differentiation.

In terms of acupuncture points, not every point could calm the shen, benefit the brain, and improve smell and taste at the same time. Shenting DU-24 and Extra Yintang are the exceptions. They can be punctured with reducing methods.

• Shenting DU-24

It could calm the shen, benefit the brain, eliminate cold-damp, and improve the sense of smell and taste.

• Extra Yintang

It is located at the midway between the medial ends of the two eyebrows, which could treat nasal congestion, sinus problems, calm the shen, benefit the brain and relieve headache.

Both points are found along with the Du mai, which is connecting and benefits the brain, regulating the nose and taste, and calming the shen. They also have a very important function to regulate the emotions during Long COVID.

Other points which could have the same functions should be Extra Sishencong and Baihui DU-20, etc. In severe cases of LST, Shuigou DU-26 could also be applied. A reducing method is needed.

Usually, two of these points (preferable to the first two points), could be applied in combination with the points to treat various syndromes of Long COVID, dealing with general situations and local complaints at the same time. This is a typical TCM way of treating any disease. Regardless of LST could lead to further impairment.

Scalp acupuncture is one of the modern micro-system acupuncture techniques which combines Chinese acupuncture needling methods with western medical knowledge on neuroanatomy, physiology, pathology, neurology, to allocate the mirror areas on the scalp to the corresponding zones on the cerebral cortex. It is mainly used for brain-related conditions, including neurological and psychological conditions. In the treatment of LST, sensory area lower 2/5 is selected and stimulated to improve the nose-throat-mouth-tongue area.

There are two different types of Chinese herbs that can be used to calm the shen. Similar to acupuncture, not every herb that calms the shen will benefit the brain and improve the sense of smell and taste at the same time. Chang Pu *Rhizoma Anemonis Altaicae* and Yuan Zhi *Radix Polygalae Tenuifoliae* are the exceptions.

• Chang Pu

It has a function to calm the shen and open the clear orifices, including all the orifices. Besides, it could relieve depression and improve emotional states. Due to invasion of cold-damp, the meridians and orifice of the nose, mouth and tongue are obstructed by damp or turbidity, Alternatively, these orifices could be blocked during the deterioration of Long COVID. Chang Pu could be applied in the prescription to open them and promote the free circulation in these orifices. 10 g to 12 g could be prescribed.

• Yuan Zhi

It has a function to clear phlegm and calm the shen, indicated in the acute invasion of cold-damp, or formation of phlegm-heat in the lung, which blocks the nose or other orifices, resulting in LST. 10 g to 12 g could be prescribed.

These two herbs also have good functions to improve emotions, and relieve anxiety and depression during Long COVID.

11.9 Sicca Syndrome

Coronavirus disease 2019 (COVID-19) is an infectious disease caused by severe acute respiratory syndrome (SARS) associated with coronavirus 2 (SARS-CoV-2). Although most of the infected individuals are asymptomatic, a proportion of patients with COVID-19 develop severe disease with multiple organ injuries.[64] The viral

---

[64]Yu Liu, *et al.* COVID-19 and autoimmune diseases. *Curr Opin Rheumatol.* 2021, 33(2): 155–162. doi: 10.1097/BOR.0000000000000776.

infection caused by SARS-CoV-2 seems to lead to the onset or exacerbation of autoimmune diseases in genetically predisposed patients.[65] For instance, patients with Sicca syndrome may be at an increased risk of contracting COVID-19 due to immunosuppressive medications they may be taking.

Sicca syndrome, also known as Sjogren syndrome, is an autoimmune disease with inflammatory glands and other tissues of the body. When there is an inflammation of the lacrimal glands that produce tears, there would be decreased tears and dry eyes. Inflammation of salivary glands, including the parotid glands, that produce the saliva in the mouth could cause dry mouth, etc. Besides, sicca syndrome is a combination of dry eyes, dry mouth, and another disease, such as rheumatoid arthritis, lupus, scleroderma, or polymyositis. Moreover, about 90% of Sicca syndrome patients are middle aged or older females.

Apart from some systemic symptoms, such as difficulty concentrating, memory lapses, fatigue and myalgia, symptoms of Sicca syndrome during Long COVID include:

- Dry eyes (sometimes, there is burning, itching or gritty feeling as though there is sand in the eyes).
- Dry mouth (sometimes there is the feeling of having cotton in the mouth with difficulty in swallowing or speaking).
- Possible painful, swelling, and stiff joints.
- Persistent dry cough.
- Dry skin.
- Dry vagina.

One study shows that out of a total of 1,772 (0.18%) of patients who were diagnosed with dry mouth, 30% were males and 70% were females. Nine patients (1.01%) were diagnosed with both

---

[65] Francesco Caso, *et al.* Could Sars-coronavirus-2 trigger autoimmune and/or auto-inflammatory mechanisms in genetically predisposed subjects? *Autoimmun Rev.* 2020, 19(5): 102524. doi: 10.1016/j.autrev.2020.102524.

COVID-19 and dry mouth. Most of the patients were adults and 100% of patients with both COVID-19 and dry mouth were adults.[66]

The ACE-2 receptor is abundantly expressed on the epithelial cells of the salivary glands, and when infected by SARS-CoV-2, these receptors are overexpressed.[67] It is speculated that signaling of the ACE-2 receptor by the virus triggers a cascade of inflammatory processes, ending in acute and chronic sialadenitis, causing disruption in salivary secretion and resulting in dry mouth.[68–70]

The diagnosis of Sicca syndrome can be confirmed by a biopsy of an affected gland.

Currently, there is no cure for Sicca syndrome in modern medicine. The treatment of Sicca syndrome is mostly achieved by treating the areas of the body that are involved by the disease and the complications such as infection.

11.9.1 TCM understanding of Long COVID-associated Sicca syndrome

Sicca syndrome is a chronic autoimmune disease prior to COVID-19. During the pandemic, it could have deteriorated. The pathologies of Sicca syndrome during Long COVID include the following.

---

[66]Joseph Katz. Prevalence of dry mouth in COVID-19 patients with and without Sicca syndrome in a large hospital center. *Ir J Med Sci.* 2021, 190(4): 1639–1641. doi: 10.1007/s11845-020-02480-4.

[67]Li Liu, *et al.* Epithelial cells lining salivary gland ducts are early target cells of severe acute respiratory syndrome coronavirus infection in the upper respiratory tracts of rhesus macaques. *J Virol.* 2011, 85(8): 4025–30. doi: 10.1128/JVI.02292-10.

[68]Maryam Baghizadeh Fini. Oral saliva and COVID-19. *Oral Oncol.* 2020, 108: 104821. doi: 10.1016/j.oraloncology.2020.104821.

[69]Chenxing Wang, *et al.* Does infection of 2019 novel coronavirus cause acute and/or chronic sialadenitis? *Med. Hypotheses.* 2020, 140: 109789. doi: 10.1016/j.mehy.2020.109789.

[70]Joseph Katz. *op. cit.*

11.9.1.1 *Remaining of toxic fire*

COVID-19 is mainly caused by the invasion of pestilent toxins mixed with cold-damp or damp-heat to the body, especially the lung and heart. When these pathogenic factors are not eliminated completely or in time, they may become a latent heat or fire in the body. It is held in TCM that the lung is in charge of the skin and opens into the nose, and the heart is in charge of blood and opens into the tongue. Accumulation of heat or fire in the lung and heart could cause dysfunctions of these two organs, resulting in failure of related tissues to be nourished, and Sicca syndrome occurs.

11.9.1.2 *Emotional disturbance*

The liver plays an important role in emotional activities. It regulates qi circulation and stores blood. Overstress, resentment, and frustration during COVID-19 may cause retardation of liver-qi circulation, and stagnation of liver-qi occurs.

Qi belongs to the yang energy, which should be in a state of constant movement. In case of prolonged liver-qi stagnation, it may cause the gradual formation of liver-fire. Fire is characterized by its uprising and burning properties. When there is hyperactivity of liver-fire, there would be Sicca syndrome, showing restlessness, insomnia, palpitations, redness of face and eyes, swelling of eyes, nervousness, irritability, bitter taste in the mouth, red tongue, thin and yellow tongue coating, and a rapid and wiry pulse.

11.9.1.3 *Deficiency of yin and blood*

The prolonged persistence of COVID-19 could also cause the consumption of yin in the body. Besides, underlying medical conditions prior to COVID-19 could be some add-on effects to cause aggravation of deficiency of yin. When the lung fails to be properly nourished by the yin, the physiological function of yin in nourishment will be impaired, and Sicca syndrome starts.

Besides general fatigue as a common sign of deficiency of yin, deficiency of yin in different organs may also bring about different manifestations. For instance, deficiency of lung-yin could cause dry mouth, nose and dry cough. Deficiency of liver-yin could cause dry eyes with possible burning sensation and headache. Deficiency of heart-yin could cause palpitations with red spots on the skin with itching. Deficiency of kidney-yin could, on the other hand, lead to dry mouth, eyes, and vagina.

Since blood and yin share the same origin, deficiency of blood could also cause the formation of yin deficiency gradually. Deficiency of blood could be caused by spleen-qi deficiency and kidney-yin deficiency.

11.9.2 TCM treatment of Long COVID-associated Sicca syndrome

11.9.2.1 *Hyperactivity of toxic fire*

Dryness of mouth and eye with burning sensation, feverish feeling, restlessness, red skin with burning feeling, sleep disorders, joint pain with swelling and hotness, restlessness, palpitations, dream-disturbed sleep, redness of eyes, irritability, bitter taste in the mouth, body pain, constipation, thirst, red tongue, yellow and dry tongue coating, and a rapid and wiry pulse.

Principle of Treatment:
Clear heat, remove toxins, reduce, cool blood, and relieve dryness.

Herbal Treatment:
Huang Lian Jie Du Tang-*Coptis Decoction to Relieve Toxicity.*

Huang Lian *Rhizoma Coptidis* 5 g
Huang Qin *Radix Scutellariae Baicalensis* 10 g
Huang Bai *Cortex Phellodendri* 10 g
Zhi Zi *Fructus Gardenniae* 10 g

Sheng Di Huang *Radix Rehmanniae Glutinosae Recens* 12 g
Mu Dan Pi *Cortex Moutan Radicis* 10 g
Xuan Shen *Radix Scrophulariae Ningpoensis* 10 g
Long Dan Cao *Radix Gentianae Longdancao* 10 g
Xia Ku Cao *Spica Prunellae Vulgaris* 10 g
Ren Dong Teng *Ramus Lonicerae Japonicae* 15 g
Tian Hua Fen *Radix Trichosanthis Kirilowii* 10 g
Zhi Gan Cao *Radix Glycyrrhizae Preparata* 3 g

Explanations:
- Huang Lian, Huang Qin, Huang Bai and Zhi Zi clear heat, remove toxins, subside swelling and relieve pain. When heat and fire are eliminated, the body fluid will be protected, and the dryness of the mouth and eye will be improved.
- Sheng Di Huang, Xuan Shen and Mu Dan Pi clear heat in the body and remove toxins.
- Long Dan Cao and Xia Ku Cao clear heat, remove toxins in the liver and relieve dryness and redness in the eyes.
- Tian Hua Fen benefits the body fluid and relieves dryness in the mouth.
- Ren Dong Teng clears heat in the joints and relieves joint pain and swelling.
- Zhi Gan Cao clears heat, removes toxins, and harmonizes the effects from other herbs in the prescription.

Herbal Remedy:
Huang Lian Jie Du Wan-*Coptis Pill to Relieve Toxicity.*

Acupuncture Treatment:
- Waiguan SJ-5 + Zulinqi GB-41, Lieque LU-7 + Zhaohai KID-6, Hegu L.I.-4, Quchi L.I.-11, Shaohai HE-3, Shaofu HE-8, Fengchi GB-20, Jianjing GB-21, Xiaxi GB-43, Xingjian LIV-2, Sanyinjiao SP-6, Juliao ST-3, Dicang ST-4 and Lianquan REN-23.
- An even method is applied on SJ-5 + GB-41, LU-7 + KID-6, and a reducing method is applied on the other points.

Explanations:

- A combination of SJ-5 + GB-41 harmonizes the Shaoyang channels, benefits the gallbladder, and clears heat in the liver.
- A combination of LU-7 + KID-6 promotes the production of body fluid, regulates the zang-fu organs and relieves dryness of the mouth and eyes.
- L.I.-4 and L.I.-11, the yuan-source point and the he-sea point of the large intestine channel respectively, SP-6, the crossing point of three yin channels of the foot, clear heat, remove toxins and reduce fire in the body. Meanwhile, they can also subside swelling in the joints.
- LIV-2 and GB-43, the ying-spring point of the liver channel and gallbladder channel respectively, GB-20, clear heat and reduce liver-fire, which is good to relieve dryness in the eyes.
- HE-3 and HE-8, the he-sea point and the ying-spring point of the heart channel respectively, clear heat in the heart, calm the shen and improve sleep.
- GB-20 and GB-21 regulate the collateral of the gallbladder channel, smooth the emotions, and relieve the neck tension.
- ST-3, ST-4, and REN-23, regulate the eyes and mouth, promote physiological functions, and relieve dryness in the eyes and mouth.

11.9.2.2 *Deficiency of yin*

Persistence and aggravation of dryness of mouth and eyes after COVID-19, fatigue, occasional dry cough or cough with scanty phlegm, thirst, dryness of the throat, night sweating, blurred vision, lower back pain, dry stools, weakness, red tongue, scanty or peeled coating on the tongue, and a deep, thready, and rapid pulse.

Principle of Treatment:
Nourish yin, promote the production of body fluid, benefit the shen and relieve dryness.

Herbal Treatment:
Sha Shen Mai Men Dong Tang-*Glehnia and Ophiopogonis Decoction.*

Nan Sha Shen *Radix Adenophorae* 10 g
Bei Sha Shen *Radix Glehniae Littoralis* 10 g
Mai Men Dong *Tuber Ophiopogonis Japonici* 10 g
Xi Yang Shen *Radix Panacis Quinque Folii* 10 g
Wu Wei Zi *Fructus Schisandrae Chinensis* 10 g
Mu Dan Pi *Cortex Moutan Radicis* 10 g
Zi Wan *Radix Asteris Tatarici* 10 g
Lu Gen *Rhizoma Phragmitis Communis* 15 g
Tian Hua Fen *Radix Trichosanthis Kirilowii* 10 g
Zhi Gan Cao *Radix Glycyrrhizae Preparata* 3 g

Explanations:
- Nan Sha Shen, Bei Sha Shen, and Mai Men Dong nourish the yin of the lung and kidney and clear the deficient heat, promote the secretion of body fluid, and relieve the thirst and dryness of the mouth.
- Xi Yang Shen and Wu Wei Zi nourish the qi and yin of the general body, improve appetite, and relieve fatigue.
- Zi Wan nourishes lung-yin, clears the remaining heat in the lung and relieves dry cough.
- Mu Dan Pi clears deficient heat in the body and removes the toxins in the blood.
- Lu Gen and Tian Hua Fen promote the secretion of body fluid and relieve thirst and dryness of the mouth.
- Zhi Gan Cao harmonizes the prescription.

Herbal Remedy:
Qi Ju Di Huang Wan-*Lyceum Fruit, Chrysanthemum and Rehmannia Pill.*

Acupuncture Treatment:

- Lieque LU-7 + Zhaohai KID-6, Jingqu LU-8, Taiyuan LU-9, Zusanli ST-36, Qihai REN-6, Taixi KID-3, Fuliu KID-7, Sanyinjiao SP-6, Feishu BL-13, Shenshu BL-23, Juliao ST-3, Dicang ST-4 and Lianquan REN-23.
- An even method is applied on LU-7 + KID-6. A tonifying method is applied to the rest of the points.

Explanations:

- A combination of LU-7 and KID-6 nourishes the qi and yin of the body, promotes the secretion of body fluid, and relieves dryness of the mouth and eyes.
- LU-8, LU-9, and BL-13, the jing-metal point, the yuan-source point of the lung channel, and the back-shu point of the lung respectively, nourish lung-yin, restore the physiological functions of the lung, and relieve dry cough.
- KID-3 and KID-7, the yuan-source point and the jing-metal point of the kidney channel respectively, BL-23, the back-shu point of the kidney, nourish kidney-yin, benefit kidney-jing and relieve weakness and dryness in the mouth and eyes.
- ST-36, the he-sea point of the stomach channel, SP-6, the crossing point of three yin channels of the foot, and REN-6 tonify yin of the general body, promote the secretion of body fluid and relieve dryness in the mouth and eyes.
- ST-3, ST-4, and REN-23, regulate the eyes and mouth, promote physiological functions, and relieve dryness in the eyes and mouth.

11.9.2.3 *Deficiency of blood*

Dryness of mouth and eyes after COVID-19, aggravation of dryness of the mouth and eyes after physical exertion, alleviation of headache when resting, itching on the skin, dryness of the skin and hair, hair loss, slight headache, a hollow sensation in the head, dizziness, palpitations, listlessness, insomnia, pale complexion, irregular menstruation in women, poor appetite, dry skin or stools, pale tongue with a thin and white coating, and a thready and weak pulse.

Principle of Treatment:
Tonify blood, improve weakness and relieve dryness.

Herbal Treatment:
Si Wu Tang-*Four Substances Decoction.*

Shu Di Huang *Radix Rehmanniae Praeparatae* 15 g
Dang Gui *Radix Angelicae Sinensis* 10 g
Bai Shao Yao *Radix Paeoniae Alba* 10 g
Chuan Xiong *Rhizoma Ligustici Chuanxiong* 10 g
Gou Qi Zi *Fructus Lycii* 10 g
Jue Ming Zi *Semen Cassiae* 10 g
Lu Gen *Rhizoma Phragmitis Communis* 15 g
Tian Hua Fen *Radix Trichosanthis Kirilowii* 10 g
Zhi Gan Cao *Radix Glycyrrhizae Preparata* 3 g

Explanations:
- Shu Di Huang, Dang Gui, Bai Shao Yao and Chuan Xiong tonify and nourish the blood, benefit the liver, and relieve dryness.
- Gou Qi Zi and Jue Ming Zi nourish the liver, benefit the eyes, and relieve dryness of eyes.
- Lu Gen and Tian Hua Fen benefit the body fluid and relieve dryness in the mouth.
- Zhi Gan Cao harmonizes the herbs in the prescription.

Herbal Remedy:
Si Wu Pian-*Four Substances Tablets.*

Acupuncture Treatment:
- Zusanli ST-36, Sanyinjiao SP-6, Ququan LIV-8, Taixi KID-3, Yingu KID-10, Xuanzhong GB-39, Shenmen HE-7, Juliao ST-3, Dicang ST-4 and Lianquan REN-23.

- A tonifying method is applied to these points.

Explanations:
- ST-36, the he-sea point of the stomach channel, and SP-6, the crossing point of three yin channels of the foot, activate the spleen and stomach, tonify qi and blood and relieve dryness.
- Since kidney-jing and blood share the same origin and benefit each other constantly, some points should be used to tonify kidney-jing to tonify blood. KID-3, the yuan-source point of the kidney channel, LIV-8 and KID-10, the he-sea point of the liver channel and kidney channel respectively, tonify blood and jing at the same time, improve the general fatigue and weakness and relieve dryness.
- GB-39, the influential point for marrow, benefits blood and relieves blood deficiency.
- ST-3, ST-4, and REN-23, regulate the eyes and mouth, promote physiological functions, and relieve dryness in the eyes and mouth.
- HE-7, the yuan-source point of the heart channel, benefits the shen, improves sleep and relieves dryness in the eye.

11.10 Rhinitis

Rhinitis is a condition, characterized by a nasal obstruction or congestion, runny nose or post-nasal drip, itchy nose, and/or sneezing. It is broadly divided into two types: allergic rhinitis and non-allergic rhinitis. In modern medicine, it is considered that rhinitis may occur before a case of sinusitis or with sinusitis, i.e., a condition where infection or inflammation affects the sinuses.

Although there are many asymptomatic patients with SARS-CoV-2 virus, one of the medical tasks is early recognition and correct diagnosis of COVID-19.

When fever, a dry cough, fatigue, and loss of smell and taste, etc., appear during the pandemic, they could be considered as the main warning symptoms and signs of COVID-19.

However, cold-like symptoms like a runny nose, may sometimes also occur as a chief complaint during COVID-19, and it is possible that COVID-19 symptoms are mistaken to be allergic rhinitis, because the characterized symptoms of COVID-19 may overlap with some symptoms of an allergy. Severe allergies may also cause some tightness in the chest or shortness of breath, especially in patients with asthma. Careful medical examinations and close attention should be paid to exclude a COVID-19 diagnosis.

Some allergic diseases, including asthma, have been defined as risk factors for a poor outcome of coronavirus disease 2019 (COVID-19). In order to investigate the role of allergic rhinitis in the severity of COVID-19, a group of scientists started a study. The study included a case group of 125 randomly selected patients who had been diagnosed with allergic rhinitis who were diagnosed with COVID-19 and a control group of 125 patients without allergic rhinitis who were diagnosed with COVID-19. They concluded that allergic rhinitis did not affect the severity of COVID-19.[71]

Indeed, it could be very difficult to tell the difference between COVID-19 and allergies, especially during an allergy season by solely judging based on a runny nose. For instance, in Italy, the SARS-CoV-2 infection rate peaked between March and April 2020, and it was also the pollen season. Some researchers recognize that although olfactory dysfunction (hyposmia or anosmia) is a major symptom of COVID-19, other nasal manifestations (rhinorrhea and obstruction), similar to those of seasonal allergic rhinitis (AR), are reported as well. From a practical and clinical viewpoint, their data suggest that even though there are some coinciding and potentially confounding features, the nasal symptoms of AR and COVID-19 can be differentiated on clinical grounds. Therefore, in the case of future undesirable COVID-19 outbreaks in concomitance with pollen season, clinicians and patients with AR should be reassured and appropriately taught to recognize and to discriminate between the two conditions.[72]

---

[71]Ali Guvey. How does allergic rhinitis impact the severity of COVID-19?: A case-control study. *Eur Arch Otorhinolaryngol.* 2021, 278(11): 4367–4371. doi: 10.1007/s00405-021-06836-z.

[72]Chiara Bruno, *et al.* Seasonal allergic rhinitis symptoms in relation to COVID-19. *Allergy & Rhinology.* 2020, 11: 1–3. https://doi.org/10.1177/2152656720968804.

Nevertheless, another study showed the same result. Among the 192 who were invited to respond to the questionnaire, 89 responded and 87 questionnaires were analyzed. The consensus was then reported. A two-way ANOVA revealed significant differences in the symptom intensity between COVID-19, the common cold and allergic rhinitis ($p < 0.001$).[73]

Symptoms and signs of COVID-19 include:

- fever or chills
- dry cough
- trouble breathing
- body or muscle aches
- sore throat
- fatigue
- fog in the head
- headache
- loss of taste or smell
- congestion or runny nose
- nausea, vomiting, or diarrhea
- palpitations
- sleep problems
- pinkeye
- skin rash
- emotional disturbance, etc.

On the other hand, common symptoms and signs of rhinitis include:

- runny nose with itching
- dry and tickly cough
- frequent sneezing
- itchy eyes or tearing

---

[73] Jan Hagemann, *et al.* Differentiation of COVID-19 signs and symptoms from allergic rhinitis and common cold: An ARIA-EAACI-GA2 LEN consensus. *Allergy.* 2021, 76(8): 2354–2366. https://search.bvsalud.org/global-literature-on-novel-coronavirus-2019-ncov/resource/en/covidwho-1138080.

- itchy throat
- itchy palate
- congestion in the nose, etc.

When rhinitis during Long COVID lasts too long, it may cause some complications, including:

- sinusitis
- middle ear infections
- nasal polyps
- sleep apnea
- dental overbite

A large-scale study confirmed that allergic rhinitis had a high prevalence in western Europe and is frequently undiagnosed. The prevalence of subjects with clinically confirmable allergic rhinitis ranged from 17% in Italy to 29% in Belgium with an overall value of 23%.[74] One examination demonstrated that there was a decreasing trend of allergic rhinitis in the current pandemic lockdown period in the study ($p < 0.001$), probably because of a decrease in pollution due to lockdown, the increased use of masks, and increased indoor activities.[75]

As far as the prevalence of AR in COVID-19 goes, confirmed data is still missing at this moment. It has been noted that the prevalence of allergic children (30%) and asthmatic children (11.6%) is relatively high in south Lombardy and Liguria, Italy. However, only two allergic children (food allergy and AR) and one child with asthma was discovered in 40 pediatric COVID-19 patients.[76]

---

[74]Vincent Bauchau, *et al.* Prevalence and rate of diagnosis of allergic rhinitis in Europe. *Eur Respir J.* 2004, 24(5): 758–764. doi: 10.1183/09031936.04.00013904.

[75]Abhishek Kishore Dayal, *et al.* Trend of allergic rhinitis post COVID-19 pandemic: A retrospective observational study. *Indian J Otolaryngol Head Neck Surg.* 2022, 74: 50–52. https://doi.org/10.1007/s12070-020-02223-y.

[76]Amelia Licari, *et al.* Allergy and asthma in children and adolescents during the COVID outbreak: What we know and how we could prevent allergy and asthma flares. *Allergy.* 2020, 75(9): 2402–2405. doi: 10.1111/all.14369.

In terms of rhinitis in Long COVID, one study examined 836 children admitted to the hospital and with accurate contact information, the researchers were able to conduct a follow-up survey with 518 children. The median age of the children was about 10 years old. The most common pre-existing comorbidity in this cohort was food allergy (13%, 67/514), followed by allergic rhinitis and asthma (9.7%, 50/514), gastrointestinal problems (9.3%, 48/514), and eczema (8.8%, 45/514).[77]

11.10.1 TCM understanding of Long COVID-associated rhinitis

In most cases, a diagnosis of rhinitis in modern medicine can be established based on the patient's symptoms without any testing. Sometimes, allergy skin tests, blood tests for IgE, laboratory and imaging tests, such as examination of the nasal smear microscopically or even Computed Tomography (CT) scans, are required as well. However, in many cases, no abnormalities will be found, and an anti-allergic drug is given for symptomatic treatment.

In TCM, it is considered that rhinitis of Long COVID is caused either by incomplete elimination of wind-cold, weakness of qi of the lung and spleen and formation of phlegm-heat.

11.10.1.1 *Incomplete elimination of wind-cold*

COVID-19 in TCM is mostly caused by invasion of external pathogenic factors, mainly cold-damp or damp-heat, with a pestilent toxin to the lung. However, invasion of wind-cold is another causative factor.

When it is properly treated in time, wind-cold should be eliminated completely, leaving no further damage to the lung and the nasal orifice. However, when wind-cold becomes latent in the nasal orifice, under the skin, or in the lung, it could cause some constant

---

[77] Ismail M. Osmanov, *et al.* Risk factors for long covid in previously hospitalised children using the ISARIC Global follow-up protocol: A prospective cohort study. *Eur Respir J.* 2021, 58(6). doi: 10.1183/13993003.01341-2021.

disturbance to the lung and these tissues, leading to the occurrence of rhinitis of Long COVID.

11.10.1.2 *Weakness of qi in the lung and spleen*

Prolonged persistence of COVID-19, improper treatment, lack of life care, delayed recovery, constitutional weakness, and pre-existing conditions, etc., could cause consumption of qi, especially in the lung and spleen, leading to weakness or deficiency of qi. When the lung's dispersing ability is weak or impaired, there would be rhinitis of Long COVID. In case of weakness of spleen-qi, the transportation and transformation will be disturbed, resulting in the formation of damp and failure of the nose to nourish. This then causes the nose to be blocked and disturbed, and the occurrence of rhinitis of Long COVID follows.

11.10.1.3 *Formation of phlegm-heat*

Invasion of cold-damp or damp-heat to the lung, spleen, stomach, or San Jiao, may cause dysfunction of these organs, gradually leading to the formation of phlegm-heat. When the nose is blocked by phlegm-heat, the occurrence of rhinitis of Long COVID appears.

Obesity, constitutional weakness of the spleen and stomach, dysfunction of San Jiao, or lack of care for daily diet during COVID-19, could cause the production of damp-phlegm or phlegm-heat in the body. Prolonged persistence of damp-phlegm could cause the formation of heat, leading to the occurrence of damp-heat or phlegm-heat. When the lung and nose are disturbed by phlegm-heat, the physiological functions of the lung and nose will be impaired, and rhinitis of Long COVID appears.

11.10.2 TCM treatment of Long COVID-associated rhinitis

11.10.2.1 *Remaining external pathogenic factors*

Running nose with clear nasal discharge, itching and congestion in the nose, frequent sneezing, itchy eyes or tearing, slight cough, occasional itching in the throat or itchy palate, absence of thirst, slight aversion to cold, slight muscle pain or headache, thin and whitish coating on the tongue, and a superficial pulse.

Principle of Treatment:
Dispel wind, eliminate cold-damp, disperse the lung-qi, and open the nasal orifice.

Herbal Treatment:
Jing Fang Bai Du San-*Schizonepeta and Saposhnikoviae Powder to Overcome Pathogenic Influences,* plus
Cang Er Zi San-*Xanthium Powder.*

Jing Jie *Herba seu Flos Schizonepetae Tenuifoliae* 10 g
Fang Feng *Radix Ledebouriellae Divaricatae* 10 g
Qiang Huo *Rhizoma et Radix Notopterygii* 10 g
Zhi Ke *Fructus Citri Aurantii* 5 g
Jie Geng *Radix Platycodi Grandiflori* 5 g
Bai Zhi *Radix Angelicae Dahuricae* 10 g
Cang Er Zi *Fructus Xanthii Sibirici* 10 g
Xin Yi Hua *Flos Magnoliae* 10 g
E Bu Shi Cao *Herba Gynomorii* 10 g
Shi Chang Pu *Rhizoma Acori Graminei* 10 g

Explanations:
- Jing Jie, Fang Feng and Qiang Huo dispel wind, eliminate cold-damp, and relieve some external symptoms.
- Jie Geng eliminates phlegm and relieves cough.
- Zhi Ke promotes qi circulation and eliminates phlegm.
- Bai Zhi, Cang Er Zi, Xin Yi Hua and E Bu Shi Cao open the nasal orifice and promote the physiological functions of the nose.

Herbal Remedy:
Jing Fang Bai Du Wan-*Schizonepeta and Saposhnikoviae Pill to Overcome Pathogenic Influences,* plus
Cang Er Zi San (Wan)-*Xanthium Powder (Pill).*

Acupuncture Treatment:
- Hegu L.I.-4, Lieque LU-7, Tianzhu BL-10, Feishu BL-13, Yingxiang L.I.-20, Juliao ST-3, Extra Bitong, Extra Yintang, Fenglong ST-40 and Yinlingquan SP-9.
- A reducing method is applied to these points.

Explanations:
- L.I.-4, the yuan-source of the large intestine channel, LU-7, the luo-connecting point of the lung channel, and BL-10 open the skin pores, dispel external pathogenic factors, and relieve cough, muscle pain, and headache.
- BL-13, the back-shu point of the lung, disperses the lung-qi, restores the physiological functions of the lung, and relieves nasal disorders.
- L.I.-20, ST-3, extra Bitong and extra Yintang open the nasal orifice and relieve blockage and itching in the nose.
- ST-40 and SP-9, the luo-connecting point of the stomach channel and the he-sea point of the spleen channel respectively, eliminate phlegm in the body and nose and relieve cough.

11.10.2.2 *Deficiency of qi of the lung and spleen*

Running nose with clear nasal discharge during Long COVID, itching and congestion in the nose, frequent sneezing, itchy eyes or tearing, slight cough with expectoration of slight, whitish, and diluted phlegm, occasional itching in the throat or itchy palate, absence of thirst, slight aversion to cold, listlessness, poor appetite, loose stool, spontaneous sweating, easily catching a common cold, cold hands and feet, thin and whitish coating on the tongue, pale tongue, and a weak and thready pulse.

Principle of Treatment;
Tonify qi of the lung and spleen, resolve phlegm and open the nasal orifice.

Herbal Treatment:
Bu Fei Tang-*Tonify the Lungs Decoction,* plus
Cang Er Zi San-*Xanthium Powder.*

Zhi Dang Shen *Radix Codonopsis Pilosulae Praeparata* 10 g
Zhi Huang Qi *Radix Astragali Membranacei Praeparata* 10 g
Bai Zhu *Rhizoma Atractylodis Macrocephalae* 10 g
Shu Di Huang *Radix Rhemanniae Glutinosae Praeparata* 12 g
Wu Wei Zi *Fructus Schisandrae Chinensis* 10 g
Zhi Ban Xia *Rhizoma Pinelliae Ternatae Preparata* 10 g
Fu Ling *Sclerotium Poriae Cocos* 12 g
Cang Er Zi *Fructus Xanthii Sibirici* 10 g
Xin Yi Hua *Flos Magnoliae* 10 g
E Bu Shi Cao *Herba Gynomorii* 10 g
Zhi Gan Cao *Radix Glycyrrhizae Preparata* 3 g

Explanations:
- Zhi Dang Shen, Bai Zhu, Fu Ling, and Zhi Gan Cao activate the spleen and tonify the qi in the body.
- Zhi Huang Qi and Wu Wei Zi tonify the qi of the lung and benefit the lung.
- Shu Di Huang tonifies the kidney and benefits the lung.
- Zhi Ban Xia eliminates phlegm and relieves cough.
- Cang Er Zi, Xin Yi Hua and E Bu Shi Cao open the nasal orifice and promote the physiological functions of the nose.

Herbal Remedy:
Bu Fei Tang-*Tonify the Lungs Decoction,* plus
Cang Er Zi San Wan-*Xanthium Powder Pill.*

Acupuncture Treatment:
- Neiguan P-6 + Gongsun SP-4, Yingxiang L.I.-20, Juliao ST-3, Extra Bitong, Extra Yintang, Chize LU-5, Lieque LU-7, Taiyuan LU-9, Zusanli ST-36, Sanyinjiao SP-6, Taixi KID-3, Qihai REN-6, Feishu BL-13, and Pishu BL-20.

- An even method is applied on P-6 + SP-4, and a tonifying method is applied on the rest of the points. Moxibustion could be applied on BL-13, BL-20, ST-36, KID-3 and REN-6.

Explanations:
- The combination of P-6 + SP-4 regulates the qi in the body and improves the physiological functions of the lung and spleen.
- Since the lung opens into the nose and the physiological functions of the nose rely greatly upon the lung, LU-7, LU-5 and LU-9, the luo-connecting, the he-sea point and the yuan-source point of the lung channels respectively, and BL-13, the back-shu point of the lung, tonify lung-qi and restore the physiological functions of the lung to promote the functions of the nose and relieve nasal disorders.
- ST-36, SP-6, REN-6, KID-3 and BL-20 tonify the qi of the spleen and kidney and support the lung-qi to improve the general conditions of the body.
- Moxibustion warms the qi and dispels the deficient cold in the body.

11.10.2.3 *Accumulation of phlegm-heat in the lung and nose*

Running nose with slight yellow and sticky phlegm during Long COVID, itching and congestion in the nose, frequent sneezing, itchy eyes or tearing, slight cough with expectoration of slight and yellow phlegm, occasional itching in the throat or itchy palate, occasional thirst, headache, loose stool, sweating, a thin, yellow, and greasy whitish tongue coating, red tongue, and a slippery and rapid pulse.

Principle of Treatment:
Clear heat, resolve phlegm, disperse lung-qi, and open the nasal orifice.

Herbal Treatment:
Qing Jin Hua Tan Tang-*Clear Metal and Transform Phlegm Decoction,*
plus
Cang Er Zi San-*Xanthium Powder.*

Huang Qin *Radix Scutellariae Baicalensis* 10 g
Zhi Zi *Fructus Gardeniae Jasminoidis* 10 g
Xing Ren *Semen Pruni Armeniacae* 10 g
Zhe Bei Mu *Bulbus Fritillariae Thunbergii* 10 g
Jie Geng *Radix Platycodi Grandiflori* 10 g
Zhi Ban Xia *Rhizoma Pinelliae Ternatae Preparata* 10 g
Fu Ling *Sclerotium Poriae Cocos* 12 g
Chen Pi *Pericarpium Citri Reticulatae* 5 g
Bai Zhi *Radix Angelicae Dahuricae* 10 g
Cang Er Zi *Fructus Xanthii Sibirici* 10 g
Xin Yi Hua *Flos Magnoliae* 10 g
E Bu Shi Cao *Herba Gynomorii* 10 g
Zhi Gan Cao *Radix Glycyrrhizae Preparata* 3 g

Explanations:
- Huang Qin and Zhi Zi clear heat in the lungs and relieve coughing.
- Xing Ren, Zhe Bei Mu and Jie Geng clear and resolve heat-phlegm and relieve the blockage in the nose.
- Zhi Ban Xia, Fu Ling, Chen Pi, and Zhi Gan Cao, the compositions of Er Chen Tang, eliminate damp and resolve phlegm in the body.
- Bai Zhi, Cang Er Zi, Xin Yi Hua and E Bu Shi Cao open the nasal orifice and promote the physiological functions of the nose.

Herbal Remedy:
Qing qi Hua Tan Tang Wan-*Clear the qi and Transform Phlegm Pill,*
plus
Cang Er Zi San Wan-*Xanthium Powder Pill.*

Acupuncture Treatment:
- Neiguan P-6 + Gongsun SP-4, Lieque LU-7, Chize LU-5, Yuji LU-10, Hegu L.I.-4, Quchi L.I.-11, Yingxiang L.I.-20, Juliao ST-3,

Extra Bitong, Extra Yintang, Fenglong ST-40, Sanyinjiao SP-6 and Yinlingquan SP-9.
- An even method is applied on P-6 + SP-4, and a reducing method is applied on the rest of the points.

Explanations:
- P-6 + SP-4, one of the point combinations from eight confluence points, regulates the internal organs and clears heat in the body.
- LU-7, LU-5, and LU-10, the luo-connecting point, the he-sea point, and the ying-spring point of the lung channel respectively, disperse the lung-qi, clear heat in the lung, and relieve cough.
- Since the large intestine is the paired Fu organ with the lung, L.I.-4 and L.I.-11, the yuan-source point and the he-sea point of the large intestine channel respectively, are applied here to clear heat in the body, promote defecation and reduce heat in the lung.
- ST-40, SP-6, and SP-9, the luo-connecting point of the stomach channel, the crossing point of three yin channels of the foot, and the he-sea point of the spleen channel respectively, activate the spleen and stomach and eliminate damp-phlegm in the body.
- L.I.-20, ST-3, extra Bitong and extra Yintang, which are all the local points, promote the physiological functions of the nose and open the nasal orifice.

11.11 Red Eyes

Although the new coronavirus, named SARS-CoV-2 virus, majorly spreads through direct contact via droplets from the nose or the mouth during a cough or a sneeze, another way the virus can sneak in is via the eyes, in which the mucous membranes, the surface of the eyes, inner eyelids can all act as possible means for the virus to collect and multiply. This infection usually occurs when touching or rubbing the eyes with fingers that are contaminated with the virus. Eye infection in the early weeks of COVID-19 infection may often be missed out. In some patients, especially asymptomatic ones, red eyes may be the single most important symptom of coronavirus. Therefore, apart from a fever, cough, headache, loss of smell and taste, and muscle pain, eye infection should also be one of the signs to look for.

Red eyes caused by COVID-19, often known as conjunctivitis, is a condition in which the clear layer covering the white part of each eye and the inner lining of each eyelid become inflamed and reddish.

One research showed that of the 38 included patients with clinically confirmed COVID-19, 25 (65.8%) were male, and the mean (SD) age was 65.8 (16.6%) years. Among them, 28 patients (73.7%) had positive findings for COVID-19 on RT-PCR from nasopharyngeal swabs, and out of these, two patients (5.2%) yielded positive findings for SARS-CoV-2 in their conjunctival as well as nasopharyngeal specimens. A total of 12 out of 38 patients (31.6%; 95% CI, 17.5–48.7) had ocular manifestations consistent with conjunctivitis.[78]

Another systematic review and meta-analysis have been performed, confirming that conjunctivitis is the most common ocular manifestations reported in adults. This comprehensive meta-analysis quantifies the existing evidence linking conjunctivitis with COVID-19.[79] One study, published in *BMJ Open Ophthalmology* in November 2020, pointed out that in patients with a positive COVID-19 diagnosis, the three most common new symptoms experienced by participants were photophobia (18%), sore eyes (16%) and itchy eyes (17%). The frequency of sore eyes was significantly higher during COVID-19 state compared with pre-COVID-19 state. 81% of participants who had experienced an eye symptom reported to have suffered from it within two weeks of other COVID-19 symptoms, and 80% reported the eye symptom lasted for less than two weeks.[80]

---

[78]Ping Wu, *et al*. Characteristics of ocular findings of patients with coronavirus disease 2019 (COVID-19) in Hubei Province, China. *JAMA Ophthalmol.* 2020, 138(5): 575–578. doi: 10.1001/jamaophthalmol.2020.1291.

[79]Mashael Al-Namaeh. COVID-19 and conjunctivitis: A meta-analysis. *Ther Adv Ophthalmol.* 2021, 13. https://doi.org/10.1177/25158414211003368.

[80]Shahina Pardhan, *et al*. Sore eyes as the most significant ocular symptom experienced by people with COVID-19: A comparison between pre-COVID-19 and during COVID-19 states. *BMJ Open Ophthalmology*. 2020, 5: e000632. doi: 10.1136/bmjophth-2020-000632.

Viral conjunctivitis can affect both eyes. SARS-CoV-2 patients can present with symptoms of conjunctivitis, including eye redness, ocular irritation, eyelid swelling, a sandy or a gritty feeling in the eye, foreign body sensation, tearing, and chemosis, watery or slightly whitish drainage, etc. These are commonly seen in individuals with severe systemic manifestations, but also possible to be seen in the initial presentation of COVID-19. These symptoms normally last five to seven days. However, if they don't disappear entirely and manifested as Long COVID, some medical care, including TCM, should be introduced.

11.11.1 TCM understanding of Long COVID-associated red eyes

In TCM, it is held that the eyesight is not an isolated phenomenon but is rooted in body totality. The eyes are simultaneously connected to the internal organs and different vessels, and they are constantly nourished by qi, blood, jing and body fluid. Among them, the liver is one of the most important organs. This is because the liver opens into the eye, thus the eye is an outside reflection of the liver. Also, the liver is the main reservoir of blood, and the main components used to form the tears that moisten the eyes. If there is an accumulation of toxins or heat in the blood, deficiency of liver-yin with hyperactivity of deficient fire, or accumulation of damp-heat in the liver, red eyes can occur due to disturbance in the eyes.

11.11.1.1 *Remaining toxins and heat in the blood*

Invasion of external pathogenic factors with a pestilent toxin to the lung and other organs could cause the occurrence of COVID-19. When toxic heat is not eliminated, it may accumulate in the body and affect different body substances, and blood can be involved.

Heat is characterized by uprising and disturbance. When toxic heat is accumulated in the blood, it may circulate with qi, leading to the occurrence of red eyes.

Since blood is closely related to the heart, accumulation of toxic heat in the blood could cause a disturbance to the heart, resulting in insomnia, restlessness, some skin rashes, or aggravation of skin conditions, etc.

11.11.1.2 *Disturbance of the emotions*

Excessive stress, frustration, and anger over a long period of time prior to, during and after COVID-19, could cause depression of the liver-qi, leading to its stagnation. Moreover, prolonged stagnation of qi may cause the formation of liver-fire, triggering a fire that flares up and burns the eyes, and red eyes follow. Alcohol drinking, frequent intake of pungent food could cause aggravation of liver-fire, resulting in severe red eye conditions.

11.11.1.3 *Accumulation of damp-heat in the liver*

Incomplete elimination of damp-heat invasion to the body, generation of heat due to prolonged persistence of cold-damp invasion, or constitutional dam-heat accumulation, and disorder in diet prior to or during COVID-19, may cause obstruction of damp-heat in the liver, leading to the disturbance to the eyes, and red eyes appear. In this case, dietary regulation is extremely important when dealing with red eyes.

11.11.1.4 *Prolonged sickness or weak constitution*

Prolonged persistence of COVID-19, lack of proper medical and life care, or congenital weakness could lead to consumption of the yin in the body, especially in the lung, liver and kidney. When the eyes are not properly nourished by the yin, red eyes appear. Meanwhile, deficiency of yin could cause the formation of deficient fire, bringing about hyperactivity of deficient fire. The uprising of deficient fire to the head could lead to the aggravation of red eyes.

11.11.2 TCM treatment of Long COVID-associated red eyes

In TCM, the careful differentiation of the associated symptoms and root causes is important in treating red eyes effectively. Certain local treatment is always combined with systematic management since local treatment itself is hardly helpful.

11.11.2.1 *Accumulation of toxic heat in the blood*

Persistence of red eyes with swelling, irritation and burning feeling, slight thirst, restlessness, insomnia, skin rashes with fresh red color, dry stool, red tongue, thin and dry coating on the tongue, and a rapid and wiry pulse.

Principle of Treatment:
Cool heat in the blood, remove toxins, subside swelling and relieve red eyes.

Herbal Treatment:
Pu Ji Xiao Du Yin-*Universal Benefit Decoction to Eliminate Toxins.*

Huang Qin *Radix Scutellariae Baicalensis* 10 g
Huang Lian *Rhizoma Coptidis* 5 g
Ban Lan Gen *Radix Isatidis* 10 g
Sang Ye *Folium Mori Albae* 10 g
Sheng Di Huang *Radix Rehmanniae Glutinosae Recens* 12 g
Xuan Shen *Radix Scrophulariae Ningpoensis* 10 g
Chi Shao Yao *Radix Paeoniae Rubrae* 10 g
Lian Qiao *Fructus Forsythiae Suspensae* 3 g
Bo He *Herba Menthae Haplocalycis* 3 g
Qing Xiang Zi *Semen Celosiae Argenteae* 10 g
Jue Ming Zi *Semen Cassiae* 10 g
Gan Cao *Radix Glycyrrhizae* 5 g

Explanations:
- Huang Qin and Huang Lian clear heat in the liver and heart, remove toxins and subside swelling of the eyes to relieve red eyes.
- Ban Lan Gen, Bo He and Lian Qiao clear heat and remove toxins in the upper parts of the body and subside the swelling in the eyes.
- Sheng Di Huang, Xuan Shen and Chi Shao Yao cool heat in the blood and remove toxins in the body.
- Sang Ye, Qing Xiang Zi and Jue Ming Zi clear heat in the eyes and benefit the eyes.
- Gan Cao removes toxins and subsides swelling of the eyes.

Herbal Remedy:
Yin Qiao Jie Du Wan-*Lonicera and Forsythia Pill to Eliminate Toxins.*

Acupuncture Treatment:
- Erjian L.I.-2, Hegu L.I.-4, Quchi L.I.-11, Yuji LU-10, Fengchi GB-20, Sanyinjiao SP-6, Xuehai SP-10, Shaohai HE-3, Xingjian LIV-2, Zanzhu BL-2, and Tongziliao GB-1.
- A reducing method is used on these points.

Explanations:
- L.I.-4 and L.I.-11, the yuan-source point and the he-sea point of the large intestine channel respectively, and GB-20 clear heat, remove toxins and subside the swelling in the eyes.
- L.I.-2 and LU-10, the ying-spring points of the large intestine channel and lung channel respectively, strongly clear heat, eliminate toxins at the upper parts of the body and reduce the swelling in the eyes.
- SP-6 and SP-10, the crossing point of three yin channels of the feet and the he-sea point of the spleen channel respectively, HE-3 and LIV-2, the he-sea point of the heart channel and the ying-spring point of the liver channel respectively, cool heat in the blood, reduce swelling, relieve pain, and subside red eyes.

- BL-2 and GB-1, the local points, clear heat in the eyes and relieve red eyes.

11.11.2.2 *Flaming of liver-fire*

Fresh red eyes with burning sensation, irritation and pain, aggravation of red eyes when nervous, headache, neck pain with depression, stress, a feeling of oppression over the chest, insomnia, a bitter taste in the mouth, a poor appetite, red tongue with a thin and slight yellow coating, and a rapid and a wiry pulse.

Principle of Treatment:
Smooth the liver, circulate qi, harmonize the emotions and relieve red eyes.

Herbal Treatment:
Dan Zhi Xiao Yao San-*Augmented Rambling Powder.*

Mu Dan Pi *Cortex Moutan Radicis* 10 g
Zhi Zi *Fructus Gardeniae Jasminoidis* 10 g
Chai Hu *Radix Bupleuri* 10 g
Dang Gui *Radix Angelicae Sinensis* 10 g
Bai Shao Yao *Radix Paeoniae Lactiflorae* 10 g
Sang Ye *Folium Mori Albae* 10 g
Xia Ku Cao *Spica Prunellae Vulgaris* 10 g
Jue Ming Zi *Semen Cassiae* 10 g
Bo He *Herba Menthae Haplocalycis* 3 g
Zhi Gan Cao *Radix Glycyrrhizae Preparata* 3 g

Explanations:
- Chai Hu regulates and promotes liver-qi circulation and relieves qi stagnation in the liver and eyes.
- Bai Shao Yao and Dang Gui relax the liver, nourish the blood, and strengthen the blood circulation in the liver.
- Mu Dan Pi, Zhi Zi, Sang Ye and Xia Ku Cao clear heat produced in the liver and relieve red eyes.

- Jue Ming Zi and Bo He cool and clear heat in the liver and benefit the eyes.
- Zhi Gan Cao harmonizes the actions of the other herbs in the formula.

Herbal Remedy:
Dan Zhi Xiao Yao Wan-*Augmented Rambling Pill.*

Acupuncture Treatment:
- Xingjian LIV-2, Taichong LIV-3, Qimen LIV-14, Fengchi GB-20, Neiguan P-6, Tanzhong REN-17, Zanzhu BL-2, Tongziliao GB-1, Yanglingquan GB-34, Qiuxu GB-40, Xiaxi GB-43, and Shaofu HE-8.
- A reducing method is used on these points.

Explanations:
- LIV-2 and GB-43, the ying-spring points of the liver channel and gallbladder channel respectively, and GB-20 clear heat, reduce liver-Fire, subside swelling in the eyes and relieve red eyes.
- LIV-3 and LIV-14, the yuan-source point, and the front-mu point of the liver channel respectively, smooth the liver and promote the circulation of the liver-qi.
- P-6, the luo-connecting point of the pericardium channel and the confluence point of the Yinwei channel, and REN-17, the gathering point of the qi in the body, promote the circulation of the liver-qi and regulate the emotions. They also promote the circulation of qi in the heart and spleen.
- GB-34 and GB-40, the he-sea point, and the yuan-source point of the gallbladder channel respectively, harmonize the gallbladder and promote the qi circulation in the liver.
- HE-8, the ying-spring point of the heart channel, reduces heat in the body and heart, calms the shen and relieves restlessness.
- BL-2 and GB-1, the local points, clear heat in the eyes and relieve red eyes.

11.11.2.3 *Accumulation of damp-heat in the liver*

Red eyes with irritation and swelling, tearing, occasional slight yellow sticky discharge, headache, irritability, bitter taste in the mouth, scanty urine, yellow and greasy coating on the tongue, and a wiry, slippery and rapid pulse.

Principle of Treatment:
Clear heat, eliminate damp, reduce fire, and relieve red eyes.

Herbal Treatment:
Long Dan Xie Gan Tang-*Gentiana Longdancao Decoction to Drain the Liver.*

Long Dan Cao *Radix Gentianae Anomalae* 10 g
Huang Qin *Radix Scutellariae Baicalensis* 10 g
Zhi Zi *Fructus Gardeniae Jasminoidis* 10 g
Ze Xie *Rhizoma Alismatis* 10 g
Mu Tong *Caulis Akebiae Trifoliatae* 5 g
Che Qian Zi *Semen Plantaginis* 10 g
Dang Gui *Radix Angelicae Sinensis* 10 g
Sheng Di Huang *Radix Rehmanniae Glutinosae* 10 g
Chai Hu *Radix Bupleuri* 5 g
Gan Cao *Radix Glycyrrhizae Uralensis* 5 g
Jue Ming Zi *Semen Cassiae* 10 g
Qing Xiang Zi *Semen Celosiae Argenteae* 10 g

Explanations:
- When damp-heat accumulates in the liver, the channels and collateral of the liver and gallbladder are obstructed, red eyes occur.
- Long Dan Cao, a herb with a bitter and cold nature entering the liver channel, clears the excessive heat and eliminates damp. It is used as the chief herb in the formula.
- Both Huang Qin and Zhi Zi are bitter and cold in nature. They are used to reduce the fire caused by the accumulation of damp-heat in the liver.

- Ze Xie, Mu Tong and Che Qian Zi eliminate damp-heat and promote urination.
- Dang Gui is used to regulate blood. Sheng Di, clears heat in the blood and body, and Chai Hu, spreads the liver-qi. These three herbs are used to smooth the liver and improve its physiological functions of the liver.
- Gan Cao clears the heat and removes toxins.
- Jue Ming Zi and Qing Xiang Zi clear heat in the eyes, subside swelling and relieve red eyes.

Herbal Remedy:
Long Dan Xie Gan Wan-*Gentiana Longdancao Pill to Drain the Liver.*

Acupuncture Treatment:
- Zhigou SJ-6, Yanglingquan GB-34, Xingjian LIV-2, Qimen LIV-14, Ganshu BL-18, Quchi L.I.-11, Sanyinjiao SP-6, Yinlingquan SP-9, Zanzhu BL-2 and Tongziliao GB-1.
- A reducing method is applied to these points.

Explanations:
- SJ-6 and GB-34 regulate the qi in Shaoyang channels, disperse and reduce damp-heat in San Jiao and gallbladder.
- LIV-2, LIV-14 and BL-18, the ying-spring point, the front-mu point of the liver channel, and the back-shu point of the liver respectively, eliminate damp-heat and restore the physiological functions of the liver.
- L.I.-11, the he-sea point of the large intestine channel, SP-6 and SP-9, the crossing point of three yin channels of the feet, and the he-sea point of the spleen channel respectively, clear heat and eliminate damp in the body.
- BL-2 and GB-1, the local points, clear heat in the eyes and relieve red eyes.

11.11.2.4 *Deficiency of the yin of the liver and kidney*

Red eyes with poor vision, dryness, slight pain and burning in the eyes, dizziness, headache, tinnitus, hair loss, poor memory, slight pain in the hypochondriac region, night sweating, lower back pain, weakness of the knees, dry stools, red tongue with a scanty or peeled coating, and a deep, thready, and rapid pulse.

Principle of Treatment:
Nourish yin, promote the production of body fluids, benefit the eyes, and relieve the red eyes.

Herbal Treatment:
Ming Mu Di Huang Wan-*Improve Vision Pill with Rehmannia.*

Shu Di Huang *Radix Rhemanniae Glutinosae Praeparata* 12 g
Shan Yao *Radix Dioscoreae Oppositae* 10 g
Shan Zhu Yu *Fructus Corni Officinalis* 10 g
Fu Shen *Sclerotium Poriae Cocos Paradicis* 10 g
Mu Dan Pi *Cortex Moutan Radicis* 10 g
Gou Qi Zi *Fructus Lycii* 10 g
Ju Hua *Flos Chrysanthemi Morifolii* 10 g
Dang Gui *Radix Angelicae Sinensis* 10 g
Wu Wei Zi *Fructus Schisandrae Chinensis* 10 g
Chong Wei Zi *Semen Leonuri Heterophylli* 10 g
Jue Ming Zi *Semen Cassiae* 10 g
Chai Hu *Radix Bupleuri* 5 g
Bai Shao Yao *Radix Paeoniae Lactiflorae* 10 g
Zhi Mu *Radix Anemarrhenae Asphodeloidis* 10 g

Explanations:
- Shu Di Huang, Shan Zhu Yu and Shan Yao tonify the liver and kidney and benefit kidney-jing.
- Dang Gui and Wu Wei Zi smooth the liver and tonify liver-yin.
- Chai Hu and Bai Shao Yao regulate liver-qi circulation and promote the physiological functions of the liver.
- Mu Dan Pi and Zhi Mu clear deficient heat in the body.
- Fu Shen calms shen and improves sleep.
- Gou Qi Zi, Ju Hua, Chong Wei Zi and Jue Ming Zi benefit the eyes and relieve red eyes.

Herbal Remedy:
Qi Ju Di Huang Wan-*Lyceum Fruit, Chrysanthemum and Rehmannia Pill.*

Acupuncture Treatment:
- Lieque LU-7 + Zhaohai KID-6, Sanyinjiao SP-6, Taixi KID-3, Yingu KID-10, Ququan LIV-8, Qihai REN-6, Ganshu BL-18, Shenshu BL-23, Zanzhu BL-2, and Tongziliao GB-1.
- An even method is applied on LU-7 + KID-6, and a tonifying method is applied to the rest of the points.

Explanations:
- The combination of LU-7 + KID-6 nourishes the yin of the body and clears deficient heat.
- SP-6, the crossing point of three yin channels of the feet, KID-3 and KID-10, the yuan-source point and he-sea point of the kidney channel respectively, KID-6, and BL-23, the back-shu point of the kidney, together with REN-6, nourish the yin of the body, benefit the yin of the kidney, and relieve deficiency of yin in the kidney.
- LIV-8 and BL-18, the he-sea point of the liver channel and the back-shu point of the liver respectively, nourish the yin of the liver, benefit the eyes, and relieve red eyes.
- BL-2 and GB-1, the local points, clear heat in the eyes and relieve red eyes.

11.12 Sputum Production

The emergent outbreak of COVID-19 infected by SARS-CoV-2 has caused a global pandemic. Overall, fever, fatigue, and a dry cough are the most common symptoms in the acute phase of this infectious disease, and once COVID-19 enters a severe stage, it becomes very difficult to manage when there is profuse sputum production. When Long COVID occurs, increased sputum production could be another one of the annoying symptoms.

Physiologically, the respiratory mucosa functions as a defensive layer against pathogens. The layer can trap an invading pathogen through sticky secretions and then move it out via ciliary action.[81] Thus, mucus secretion is a fundamental mechanism for defense against allergens and pathogens, which causes increases of mucus production in the respiratory tract in nearly every instance of airway inflammation. COVID-19 is no exception. It can be particularly severe and even lethal in COVID-19 due to the formation of mucus plugs. Severe mucoid tracheitis is detected in 33% of COVID-19 autopsies.[82] Transmission of COVID-19 appears to occur primarily through dispersal of droplets generated from the respiratory tract when an infected person talks, coughs, or sneezes. Large amounts of the SARS-CoV-2 virus have been reported in sputum and nasal specimens, which account for the transmission through respiratory droplets.[83]

Studies of CT imaging in the pulmonary parenchymal region of COVID-19 patients have reported a 64% occurrence of pathological fluid in the alveolar sacs which appears multifocal, patchy, or segmented, and is distributed around subpleural areas or along bronchovascular bundles. Increase in sputum volume and mucus hypersecretion associated symptoms are seen in up to 40% of patients. The mucus in these patients is also found to be more viscous than in those with chronic obstructive pulmonary disease (COPD). Lastly, the formation of colloidal mucus plugs is more frequent in these patients. The increase in mucus production and secretion is also likely due to mucus cell metaplasia since pulmonary inflammatory diseases are often associated with

---

[81] Ximena M. Bustamante-Marin and Lawrence E. Ostrowski. Cilia and mucociliary clearance. *Cold Spring Harb Perspect Biol.* 2017, 9(4): a028241. doi: 10.1101/cshperspect. a028241.

[82] Faryal I. Farooqi, *et al.* Airway hygiene in COVID-19 pneumonia: treatment responses of 3 critically Ill cruise ship employees. *Am J Case Rep.* 2020, 21: e926596. doi:10.12659/AJCR.926596.

[83] Mohsin Ali Khan, *et al.* Cytokine storm and mucus hypersecretion in COVID-19: Review of mechanisms. *J Inflamm Res.* 2021, 14: 175–189 https://doi.org/10.2147/JIR.S271292.

excessive mucus secretion.[84] Numerous studies conclude that the recent coronavirus infection causes an allergic reaction in respiratory tract mucosa, which activates mucin secretion and modulates its chemical structure to enable the virus to enter the cells.[85-87] Thereafter, SARS-CoV-2 initiates neutrophil and mucus-mediated inflammatory pathways.[88]

Sputum production or expectoration is the act of coughing up and spitting out the material produced in the respiratory tract. A cough, known as the most common symptom of respiratory disorders, is usually an entirely physiologic voluntary reflex, which serves the functions of defending the respiratory tract against foreign substances and maintaining airway patency by shearing and dislodging the secretions accumulated on the mucosal surface from the air passages. Sputum production with coughing occurs when the respiratory tract secretions are beyond the ability of the mucociliary mechanism to deal with them. Although sputum production with coughing could be seen in many diseases, such as bronchiectasis, a lung abscess, pneumococcal pneumonia or pulmonary oedema, sputum production in Long COVID is completely different from these diseases.

Increased sputum production is often characterized by expectoration of diluted, scanty, whitish phlegm, some itching in the throat with slight pain (it may be painless for some patients) at the same time. It is possible that there could be increased nasal discharge with whitish color, diminished smell or taste, poor appetite, loose stools,

---

[84]Jan Hagemann, *et al. op. cit.*

[85]Sufang Tian, *et al.* Pulmonary pathology of early phase 2019 novel coronavirus (COVID-19) pneumonia in two patients with lung cancer. *J Thorac Oncol.* 2020, 15: 700–704. doi: 10.1016/j.jtho.2020.02.010.

[86]Adam Bernheim, *et al.* Chest CT findings in coronavirus disease-19 (COVID-19): relationship to duration of infection. *Radiology.* 2020, 295(3). https://doi.org/10.1148/radiol.2020200463.

[87]Hind Khairi Khashkhosha *et al.* A hypothesis on the role of the human immune system in COVID-19. *Med Hypotheses.* 2020, 143: 110066. doi: 10.1016/j.mehy.2020.110066.

[88]Alexander P Earhart, *et al.* Consideration of dornase alfa for the treatment of severe COVID-19 acute respiratory distress syndrome. *New Microbes New Infect.* 2020, 35: 100689. doi: 10.1016/j.nmni.2020.100689.

and tiredness, etc. Furthermore, the build-up of mucus can also contribute to other complications found in Long COVID such as venous engorgement, elevation in saliva secretions, mucus in stool, and pulmonary oedema. Once there is a fever and profuse sputum (sputum color turns into yellow and becomes sticky, or there is a mixture of blood streaks in the sputum), some further examinations should be carried out to identify the underlying infection or other causes.

11.12.1 TCM understanding of Long COVID-associated sputum production

It is considered in modern medicine that increased sputum production happens when it is triggered by some allergic or infectious pathogens. However, it also occurs without any demonstrable evidence of disease.

Since mucus consists primarily of water (95%), it is considered in TCM that sputum production of Long COVID is caused by the accumulation of damp-phlegm in some zang-fu organs as well as some tissues and cavities due to various kinds of factors (such as the incomplete elimination of some external pathogens, or dysfunction of some internal organs during COVID-19), leading to the disorder of the water metabolism in the body. Above all, the severity of sputum production during Long COVID is not proportional to the severity of the disease during COVID-19.

11.12.1.1 *Incomplete elimination of external pathogenic factors*

Invasion of external pathogenic factors with a pestilent toxin through the nose, mouth, or membranes to the lung, San Jiao or the spleen and stomach, could cause the occurrence of COVID-19. The main pathogenic factor is damp, either cold-damp or damp-heat, which leads to failure of the lung in dispersing the qi and water, dysfunction of the San Jiao in water distribution, and the spleen and stomach in transportation and transformation, formation of damp-phlegm in the body happens. Mostly, the lung is impaired by this external invasion.

Since the lung is the upper source of water in the body and in charge of the nose and throat, impaired function of the lung in dispersing the lung-qi by damp could bring about the disturbance to the qi dispersing and water regulation, and cough with expectoration of sputum occurs. When COVID-19 in the acute phase is under control, there is a great possibility that the external pathogenic factors are incompletely eliminated, and they could still accumulate somewhere in the lung or its opening orifices—the nose and throat. Therefore, sputum production appears occasionally or permanently.

Remaining external damp in the spleen and stomach will cause further disturbance to the physiological functions of these organs, leading to aggravation and continuation of sputum production, increased saliva production, lack of taste, poor appetite, nausea, and loose stools.

Remaining of the external damp in the San Jiao could cause water retention, leading to the heaviness of the limbs and body, swollen abdomen, and irregular defecation, etc.

11.12.1.2 *Accumulation of damp-phlegm*

Prolonged persistence of external damp in the body, mixed with improper treatment, lack of life care during COVID-19, and constitutional overweight or accumulation of damp-phlegm in the body, etc., could cause blockage and impairment in the different zang-fu organs, resulting in dysfunction of water distribution and metabolism, and increased sputum production happens. When the nose and throat are disturbed, there could be nasal discharge, irritation in the throat, or a slight cough with expectoration of some sputum. When the digestive system is disturbed by damp, there could be nausea, much saliva in the mouth, borborygmus, swollen abdomen, heaviness of the limbs, loose stools with mucus, etc.

11.12.1.3 *Accumulation of damp with stagnation of blood*

Since damp moves together with blood, both the invasion of external damp and formation of internal damp due to dysfunction of zang-fu organ during COVID-19 or Long COVID could cause disturbance to the blood vessels, channels, and collaterals in the body, resulting in retardation of qi and blood circulation. In some severe cases, there could be accumulation of damp with stagnation of blood. This situation could cause a blockage in these tissues in the body, leading to swelling and pain of the vessels (presenting a purplish color with protrusion of the veins on the skin). Sometimes there would be the formation of ulcers or cramps on the limbs.

11.12.1.4 *Deficiency of qi or yang*

Prolonged persistence of COVID-19 could cause consumption of qi and yang of the body, leading to deficiency of qi, such as the lung-qi, heart-qi, spleen-qi and kidney-qi. All these situations could eventually lead to the disorder in water metabolism, thus increasing sputum production due to the formation of damp-phlegm in the body.

When deficiency of qi is not properly controlled, it could cause further damage to the yang of the body, resulting in aggravation of the disorder in water metabolism, retention of water and damp-phlegm.

11.12.2 TCM treatment of Long COVID-associated sputum production

11.12.2.1 *Incomplete elimination of external damp*

Increased sputum production in the nose with whitish discharge, slight persistent cough with expectoration of white and diluted phlegm, itching in the throat, absence of thirst, slight aversion to cold and muscle pain, headache, thin and whitish tongue coating, and a tight pulse.

Principle of Treatment:
Eliminate damp, resolve phlegm, and relieve the external pathogens.

Herbal Treatment:
Xing Su San-*Apricot Kernel and Perilla Leaf Powder,* plus
Cang Er San-*Xanthium Powder.*

Xing Ren *Semen Pruni Armeniacae* 10 g
Zi Su Zi *Fructus Perillae Frutescentis* 10 g
Qiang Huo *Rhizoma et Radix Notopterygii* 10 g
Bai Jie Zi *Semen Sinapis Albae* 5 g
Cang Er Zi *Fructus Xanthii Sibirici* 10 g
Xin Yi Hua *Flos Magnoliae* 10 g
Qian Hu *Radix Peucedani* 10 g
Jie Geng *Radix Platycodi Grandiflori* 5 g
Zhi Ke *Fructus Citri Aurantii* 5 g
Zhi Ban Xia *Rhizoma Pinelliae Ternatae Preparata* 10 g
Fu Ling *Sclerotium Poriae Cocos* 12 g
Chen Pi *Pericarpium Citri Reticulatae* 5 g
Zhi Gan Cao *Radix Glycyrrhizae Preparata* 3 g

Explanations:
- Xing Ren, Zi Su Zi, Qian Hu, Jie Geng and Bai Jie Zi eliminate phlegm and relieve cough.
- Cang Er Zi and Xin Yi Hua open the nasal orifice and eliminate phlegm in the throat.
- Zhi Ban Xia, Fu Ling, Chen Pi and Zhi Gan Cao, which are the complete composition of Er Chen Tang, are applied to eliminate damp and resolve phlegm to assist the above herbs to eliminate phlegm and relieve cough.
- Zhi Ke promotes qi circulation caused by the accumulation of damp-phlegm.
- Qiang Huo dispels the remaining pathogens and relieves some external symptoms, such as itching in the throat, sometimes nasal discharge, slight aversion to cold and muscle pain, and headache.

Herbal Remedy:
Zhi Sou San Granulates-*Stop Coughing Powder.*

Acupuncture Treatment:
- Hegu L.I.-4, Yingxiang L.I.-20, Juliao ST-3, Fenglong ST-40, Yinlingquan SP-9, Lieque LU-7, Chize LU-5, Feishu BL-13, and REN-22.
- A reducing method is applied on the rest of the points.

Explanations:
- L.I.-4, the yuan-source of the large intestine channel, and LU-7, the luo-connecting point of the lung channel, open the skin pores, promote sweating, and relieve some external symptoms.
- ST-40 and SP-9, the luo-connecting point of the stomach channel and the he-sea point of the spleen channel respectively, eliminate damp and resolve phlegm in the body.
- LU-5 and BL-13, the he-sea point of the lung channel and back-shu point of the lung respectively, disperse the lung-qi, restore the physiological functions of the lung and relieve cough and sputum expectoration.
- L.I.-20 and ST-3, the local points from the face, are used to open the nasal orifice, eliminate phlegm, and relieve the blockage in the nose.
- REN-22 is applied to resolve phlegm in the throat and improve breathing.

11.12.2.2 *Accumulation of phlegm-turbidity*

Slight fullness in the chest and epigastric region, occasional shortness of breath with exportation of whitish and sticky phlegm, occasional cough, nausea, vomiting, loose stools, or diarrhea, lassitude, heaviness of the four limbs, dizziness, aggravation of above situations when intaking greasy and fatty food, lassitude, whitish and greasy coating on the tongue, and a slippery pulse.

Principle of Treatment:
Resolve phlegm, activate the spleen, disperse the lung-qi and relieve cough.

Herbal Treatment:
Er Chen Tang-*Decoction of Two Old (Cured) Drugs,* plus
Shen Ling Bai Zhu San-*Ginseng, Sclerotium Poriae Cocos and Atractylodis Macrocephalae Powder.*

Zhi Ban Xia *Rhizoma Pinelliae Ternatae Preparata* 10 g
Fu Ling *Sclerotium Poriae Cocos* 12 g
Chen Pi *Pericarpium Citri Reticulatae* 5 g
Cang Er Zi *Fructus Xanthii Sibirici* 10 g
Bai Jie Zi *Semen Sinapis Albae* 10 g
Dang Shen *Radix Codonopsis Pilosulae* 10 g
Bai Zhu *Rhizoma Atractylodis Macrocephalae* 10 g
Shan Yao *Radix Dioscoreae Oppositae* 10 g
Bai Bian Dou *Semen Dolichoris Lablab* 10 g
Cang Zhu *Rhizoma Atractylodis* 10 g
Hou Po *Cortex Magnoliae Officinalis* 10 g
Zhi Ke *Fructus Citri Aurantii* 5 g
Zhi Gan Cao *Radix Glycyrrhizae Preparata* 3 g

Explanations:
- Zhi Ban Xia, Fu Ling, Chen Pi, and Zhi Gan Cao, the complete compositions of Er Chen Tang, eliminate damp and resolve phlegm.
- Dang Shen, Bai Zhu, Shan Yao, and Bai Bian Dou activate the spleen and stomach and eliminate damp in the body.
- Hou Po, Cang Zhu and Zhi Ke eliminate phlegm, promote qi circulation, and relieve the fullness in the chest and abdomen.
- Cang Er Zi and Bai Jie Zi eliminate phlegm in the lung system and relieve cough.

Herbal Remedy:
Er Chen Wan-*Pill of Two Old (Cured) Drugs,* plus
Shen Ling Bai Zhu Wan-*Ginseng, Poria and Atractylodis Macrocephalae Pill.*

Acupuncture Treatment:
- Neiguan P-6 + Gongsun SP-4, Zhongwan REN-12, Fenglong ST-40, Sanyinjiao SP-6, Yinlingquan SP-9, Hegu L.I.-4, Lieque LU-7, Chize LU-5, Feishu BL-13, Yingxiang L.I.-20, Juliao ST-3 and Tiantu REN-22.

- An even method is applied on P-6 + SP-4, and a reducing method is applied on the rest of the points.

Explanations:
- The combination of P-6 + SP-4 promotes the qi circulation in the chest and abdomen and relieves the fullness in the chest.
- REN-12, the gathering point of the fu organs in the body, ST-40, SP-6, and SP-9 activate the spleen and stomach, eliminate damp, and resolve phlegm in the body.
- LU-7 and LU-5, the luo-connecting point and the he-sea point of the lung channel respectively, and BL-13, the back-shu point of the lung, eliminate phlegm in the lung system, disperse and descend the lung-qi, restore the physiological functions of the lung, and relieve cough.
- L.I.-4, the yuan-source point of the large intestine channel, promotes the qi circulation and relieves the qi stagnation in the body caused by the accumulation of damp-phlegm.
- L.I.-20, ST-3, and REN-22 eliminate phlegm in the nasal orifice and throat.

11.12.2.3 *Mixture of damp with stagnant blood*

Slightly swollen veins in the body or protrusion of some veins after COVID-19 (locally or in the general body), heaviness of the body and four limbs, purplish color of the veins and skin, headache, insomnia, slight edema on the low limbs, loose stool, poor appetite, white and greasy coating on the tongue, purplish tongue, and a wiry and slippery pulse.

Principle of Treatment:
Eliminate damp, promote blood circulation, subside the swelling, and harmonize the collaterals.

Herbal Treatment:
Shu Jing Huo Xue Tang-*Relax the Channels and Invigorate the Blood Decoction.*

Dang Gui *Radix Angelicae Sinensis* 10 g
Chuan Xiong *Radix Ligustici Wallichii* 10 g
Chi Shao Yao *Radix Paeoniae Rubrae* 10 g
Shu Di Huang *Radix Rhemanniae Glutinosae Praeparata* 10 g
Tao Ren *Semen Pruni Persicae* 10 g
Hong Hua *Flos Carthami Tinctorii* 10 g
Qiang Huo *Rhizoma et Radix Notopterygii* 10 g
Cang Zhu *Rhizoma Atractylodis* 10 g
Chuan Niu Xi *Radix Cyathulae Officinalis* 10 g
Wei Ling Xian *Radix Clematidis* 10 g
Ji Xue Teng *Caulis Milletiae Reticulatae* 10 g
Di Long *Lumbricus* 10 g
Pu Huang *Pollen Typhae* 10 g

Explanations:
- Dang Gui, Chuan Xiong, Chi Shao Yao and Shu Di Huang tonify blood and promote blood circulation.
- Cang Zhu and Qiang Huo eliminate damp due to external invasion and internal disorder.
- Tao Ren, Hong Hua, Pu Huang and Chuan Niu Xi promote blood circulation and eliminate blood stasis in the vessels.
- Wei Ling Xian, Ji Xue Teng and Di Long promote blood circulation and harmonize the vessels in the body.

Herbal Remedy:
Shu Jing Huo Xue Wan-*Relax the Channels and Invigorate the Blood Pill.*

Acupuncture Treatment:
- Lieque LU-7 + Zhaohai KID-6, Neiguan P-6 + Gongsun SP-4, Zhongwan REN-12, Fenglong ST-40, Sanyinjiao SP-6, Yinlingquan SP-9, Xuehai SP-10, Hegu L.I.-4, Taiyuan LU-9 and Shenmen HE-7.
- An even method is applied on LU-7 + KID-6, P-6 + SP-4, and a reducing method is applied on the rest of the points.

Explanations:
- The combination of LU-7 + KID-6, and P-6 + SP-4 harmonize the qi circulation in the chest and abdomen, regulate the physiological functions of zang-fu organs, eliminate damp, and harmonize the collaterals.
- REN-12, the gathering point of the fu organs in the body, ST-40, SP-6, and SP-9 activate the spleen and stomach, eliminate damp, and resolve phlegm in the body.
- LU-7 and L.I.-4, the yuan-source point of the large intestine channel, LU-9, the yuan-source point of the lung channel and the gathering point of the vessels in the body, HE-7, the yuan-source point of the heart channel, and SP-10, promote qi and blood circulation and eliminate blood stasis in the vessels.

11.12.2.4 *Deficiency of qi and yang*

During Long COVID, there is a formation of diluted phlegm in the nose and throat which is easy to expectorate, slight cough, shortness of breath especially after slight exertion, aversion to cold, cold hands and feet, frequent urination with clear urine, poor appetite, loose stool, nausea, lower back pain, poor memory and concentration, edema on the legs and ankles, pale tongue, thin and whitish tongue coating, and a weak, thready, and slow pulse.

Principle of Treatment:
Tonify qi, strengthen yang and resolve phlegm.

Herbal Treatment:
Bu Fei Tang-*Tonify the Lungs Decoction,* plus
Li Zhong Wan-*Pill to Regulate the Middle.*

Zhi Dang Shen *Radix Codonopsis Pilosulae Praeparata* 10 g
Zhi Huang Qi *Radix Astragali Membranacei Praeparata* 10 g
Bai Zhu *Rhizoma Atractylodis Macrocephalae* 10 g
Shu Di Huang *Radix Rhemanniae Glutinosae Praeparata* 12 g

Wu Wei Zi *Fructus Schisandrae Chinensis* 10 g
Zi Wan *Radix Asteris Tatarici* 10 g
Gan Jiang *Rhizoma Zingiberis Officinalis* 5 g
Gui Zhi *Ramulus Cinnamomi Cassiae* 10 g
Zhi Ban Xia *Rhizoma Pinelliae Ternatae Preparata* 10 g
Sang Bai Pi *Cortex Mori Albae Radicis* 10 g
Fu Ling *Sclerotium Poriae* Cocos 12 g
Zhi Gan Cao *Radix Glycyrrhizae Preparata* 5 g

Explanations:
- Zhi Dang Shen, Bai Zhu, Fu Ling, and Zhi Gan Cao activate the spleen and tonify the qi in the body.
- Zhi Huang Qi, Wu Wei Zi, and Zi Wan tonify the qi of the lung and benefit the lung.
- Sang Bai Pi descends the lung-qi and relieves cough.
- Shu Di Huang tonifies kidney-qi and benefits the lung.
- Zhi Ban Xia eliminates phlegm and relieves cough.
- Gan Jiang and Gui Zhi warm the middle Jiao and dispel the cold.

Herbal Remedy:
Bu Fei Tang Wan-*Tonify the Lungs Decoction Pill,* plus
Li Zhong Wan-*Pill to Regulate the Middle.*

Acupuncture Treatment:
- Neiguan P-6 + Gongsun SP-4, Taiyuan LU-9, Zusanli ST-36, Fenglong ST-40, Sanyinjiao SP-6, Yinlingquan SP-9, Taixi KID-3, Qihai REN-6, Feishu BL-13, and Shenshu BL-23.
- Even method is applied on P-6 + SP-4, and a tonifying method is applied on LU-9, ST-36, SP-6, KID-3, REN-6, BL-13 and BL-23. A reducing method is applied on ST-40 and SP-9. Moxibustion could be applied on BL-13, BL-23, ST-36, KID-3 and REN-6.

Explanations:
- The combination of P-6 + SP-4 regulates and harmonizes the qi in the body.

- LU-9, the yuan-source point of the lung channel, and BL-13, the back-shu point of the lung, tonify lung-qi and restore the physiological functions of the lung.
- ST-36, SP-6, REN-6, KID-3 and BL-23 tonify the qi of the spleen and kidney and eliminate damp in the body.
- ST-40, the luo-connecting point, and SP-9, the he-sea point of the spleen channel, activate the spleen and eliminate damp-phlegm in the body.
- Moxibustion warms the qi and dispels the deficient cold in the body.

11.13 Loss of Appetite

Coronavirus disease 2019 (COVID-19) could cause a wide range of symptoms and signs, in which fever, dry cough and fatigue are the most common ones. Other symptoms include a loss of smell or taste, shortness of breath, muscle aches, sore throat, headache, or chest pain, etc. But COVID-19 in some cases could also cause gastrointestinal symptoms, including loss of appetite, nausea, vomiting, loose stools or diarrhea. These gastrointestinal symptoms happen either alone or along with other COVID-19 symptoms and sometimes develop before fever and respiratory symptoms.

The study, published in *The American Journal of Gastroenterology*, noted that nearly half of COVID-19 patients enrolled in the study presented digestive symptoms, such as diarrhea and loss of appetite, and cited them as their chief complaints.[89]

According to the researchers, who were part of the Wuhan Medical Treatment Expert Group for COVID-19 in China, patients with digestive symptoms had a longer gap between the onset of symptoms and hospital admission than patients presenting only

---

[89] COVID-19 patients experience loss of appetite, diarrhea and other digestive symptoms. *The Economic Times.* 19 March 2020. https://economictimes.indiatimes.com/magazines/panache/covid-19-patients-experience-loss-of-appetite-diarrhea-and-other-digestive-symptoms/articleshow/74709329.cms?from=mdr.

respiratory symptoms. The scientists said the patients with digestive symptoms were less likely to be cured and discharged than those without them.[90]

In terms of loss of appetite, it is not the same as loss of smell and taste, which is the symptom developing between 2 to 14 days after coronavirus exposure during the acute phase of COVID-19. Unlike digestion issues, fatigue, muscle ache, and the loss of smell and taste is not painful or worrisome. However, it is something that can take the longest time to recover from and plague a patient psychologically, since there is no treatment or medicine available to cure it. On the other hand, loss of appetite is one of the gastrointestinal sequelae, which is defined as a gastrointestinal symptom that is present after discharge but was not present within the month before the onset of COVID-19. According to one study, which was published in journal, *The Lancet Gastroenterology & Hepatology* in May 2021, loss of appetite was one of the primary gastrointestinal sequelae. It showed that 52 of 117 patients (44%) reported gastrointestinal symptoms after discharge at the 90-day telephone interview. Out of the 52 patients, 51 had gastrointestinal symptoms at 90 days after discharge, and one had gastrointestinal sequelae that had resolved by the 90-day follow-up. The most common gastrointestinal sequelae in 117 patients was the loss of appetite (28[24%] patients), nausea (21[18%]), acid reflux (21 [18%]), and diarrhea (17[15%]). Less common gastrointestinal sequelae included abdominal distension (16[14%]), belching (12 [10%]), vomiting (11 [9%]), abdominal pain (eight [7%]), and bloody stools (2 [2%]). None of the 65 patients without gastrointestinal sequelae at 90 days had gastrointestinal symptoms on admission or during hospitalization. Of the 52 patients with gastrointestinal sequelae after discharge, 15 = (29%) had gastrointestinal symptoms on admission and during hospitalization, 34(65%) had such symptoms during hospitalization, and three (6%) had such symptoms only

---

[90]Lei Pan, *et al.* Clinical characteristics of COVID-19 patients with digestive symptoms in Hubei, China: A descriptive, cross-sectional, multicenter study. *Am J Gastroenterol.* 2020, 115(5): 766–773. doi: 10.14309/ajg.0000000000000620.

after discharge. Patients with gastrointestinal sequelae at 90 days were similar in age, sex, body-mass index, and incidence of comorbidities to those without gastrointestinal sequelae, and had similar lengths of hospital stay.[91]

It is normal to experience some loss of appetite and reduced food intake during COVID-19 and its recovery process, and the recovery of appetite can take time. When COVID-19 enters the Long COVID phase, some patients could still suffer mainly from loss of appetite due to a wide variety of conditions, ranging from infection, mental stress, and physical illnesses related to COVID-19. In that case, loss of appetite could take an extensive toll, including a loss of smell or taste, finding it extremely difficult to digest common food items, hating foods they enjoyed before, weight loss, bad metabolism, and bad eating habits, etc. When there is a significant loss of appetite or a loss of appetite that occurs alongside fatigue, headache, abdominal pain and distention, loose stools, or diarrhea, then medical care, including TCM intervention, should be introduced.

11.13.1 TCM understanding of Long COVID-associated loss of appetite

One of the hypotheses is that these gastrointestinal conditions could be because of hypoxia—a condition where one region of the body is affected because of reduced oxygen supply. Decreased blood oxygen saturation is a symptom closely related to severe pneumonia and associated with gastrointestinal sequelae.[92] In modern medicine, the treatment of these gastrointestinal symptoms is the symptomatic use of antacids, antiemetics, and antidiarrheal agents. No special medicine is available for loss of appetite.

---

[91] Jingrong Weng, *et al.* Gastrointestinal sequelae 90 days after discharge for COVID-19. *The Lancet Gastroenterology & Hepatology.* 2021, 6(5): 344–346. doi: 10.1016/S2468-1253(21)00076-5.

[92] Ximena M. Bustamante-Marin and Lawrence E. Ostrowski. *op. cit.*

It is considered in TCM that loss of appetite could be caused by the following etiologies with different pathologies.

11.13.1.1 *Accumulation of damp-phlegm*

Prolonged persistence of external factors in the body due to incomplete elimination of external cold-damp or damp-heat, improper medical treatment, or lack of life care during COVID-19, or constitutional overweight or accumulation of damp-phlegm in the body, etc., could cause dysfunction of the spleen and stomach with transportation and transformation, leading to formation and accumulation of damp there. This leads to the lack of appetite with nausea, much saliva in the mouth, borborygmus, swollen abdomen, heaviness of the limbs, loose stools or diarrhea.

Accumulation of damp varies in damp-phlegm, cold-damp, and damp-heat.

11.13.1.2 *Emotional disorders*

Emotional stress, feeling upset or frustrated during or after COVID-19 could cause stagnation of liver-qi. Over worrying could lead to stagnation of spleen-qi. All these conditions may result in disorder in qi circulation. The liver dominates the free flow of qi in the body, which can help digestion and transportation of the spleen and stomach. In case of stagnation of liver-qi due to emotional dysfunction, there could be a disorder of ascending and descending functions in the body, especially the spleen and stomach, thus loss of appetite happens.

The lung controls the liver according to the Five Elements theory. Prolonged COVID-19 infection could cause stagnation of lung-qi, which could eventually lead to stagnation of liver-qi. The heart is the son organ from the liver. Overthinking could bring about the stagnation of heart-qi, which may cause the influence and impairment of the mother by the son, thus, stagnation of liver-qi follows. All these situations could lead to disharmony between the liver, spleen and stomach, and loss of appetite appears.

11.13.1.3 *Deficiency of qi or yang*

Prolonged persistence of COVID-19 could cause consumption of qi and yang of the body, leading to deficiency of qi and yang of the spleen and stomach, or the qi and yang of the heart or kidney.

When there is a deficiency of qi and yang of the spleen and stomach, there would be loss of appetite, cold hands and feet, aversion to cold, loose stools or diarrhea, and abdominal swelling, etc.

The heart is a fire organ according to the Five Elements theory. Deficiency of qi and yang of the heart could cause the failure of the spleen and stomach to be warmed and stimulated, thus the transportation and transformation of the spleen and stomach will be impaired, and loss of appetite happens.

The kidney is an organ, which contains both yin and yang. kidney-yang could also warm the spleen in physiology. In case of deficiency of kidney-yang (qi), the spleen will not be properly warmed and supported, and the physiological functions of the spleen will be impaired, thus causing loss of appetite.

11.13.2 TCM treatment of Long COVID-associated loss of appetite

Besides TCM treatment, it is encouraged to inform the patients to pay some attention to their diets, such as eating three to four little nourishing meals per day with a well-balanced diet, slight protein-rich products (including good meat, fish, eggs, cheese, beans, and lentils), and energy-rich foods. Milk-based drinks or vegetable soup should be provided, as well as some nourishing snacks/drinks in between until the appetite picks up. However, these patients (who have an accumulation of damp-phlegm in the body) should try to avoid overly sweet and greasy foods. Drinking enough water also prevents dehydration. The food can be served on small plates to make it more appealing. Some aromatic herbs could be added to create a good smell, and a variety of food is advised. In this way, the color, smell, and appearance of food could stimulate the appetite.

11.13.2.1 *Accumulation of damp-phlegm*

Loss of appetite, nausea, vomiting, swollen epigastric region and abdomen, loose stool, heaviness of four limbs, white and greasy coating on the tongue, and a slippery and wiry pulse.

Principle of Treatment:
Eliminate damp, resolve phlegm, activate the spleen, and improve appetite.

Herbal Treatment:
Ping Wei San-*Calm the Stomach Powder*, plus
Xiang Sha Liu Jun Zi Tang-*Six Gentlemen Decoction with Aucklandia and Amomum.*

Hou Po *Cortex Magnoliae Officinalis* 10 g
Cang Zhu *Rhizoma Atractylodis* 10 g
Chen Pi *Pericarpium Citri Reticulatae* 5 g
Xiang Fu *Rhizoma Cyperi Rotundi* 10 g
Sha Ren *Fructus Amomi* 3 g
Zhi Ban Xia *Rhizoma Pinelliae Ternatae Preparata* 10 g
Dang Shen *Radix Codonopsis Pilosulae* 10 g
Fu Ling *Sclerotium Poriae Cocos* 12 g
Bai Zhu *Rhizoma Atractylodis Macrocephalae* 10 g
Shen Qu *Massa Medica Fermentata* 15 g
Jiao Gu Ya *Fructus Oryzae Sativae Germinantus (grill)* 15 g
Zhi Gan Cao *Radix Glycyrrhizae Preparata* 3 g

In case of cold-damp, add Gui Zhi *Ramulus Cinnamomi Cassiae* 10 g and Gan Jiang *Rhizoma Zingiberis Officinalis* 6 g.

In the case of damp-heat, add Huang Lian *Rhizoma Coptidis* 5 g and Zhi Zi *Fructus Gardeniae Jasminoidis* 10 g.

Explanations:
- Hou Po, Cang Zhu, Chen Pi, and Zhi Gan Cao, the complete composition of Ping Wei San, eliminate damp, resolve phlegm, activate the spleen, and improve appetite.

- Dang Shen, Bai Zhu, Fu Ling, Zhi Gan Cao, Zhi Ban Xia, Chen Pi, Xiang Fu and Sha Ren, the complete composition of Xiang Sha Liu Jun Zi Tang, activate the spleen and stomach, eliminate damp, resolve phlegm, promote qi circulation, and improve the appetite.
- Shen Qu and Jiao Gu Ya are used to promote digestion and improve appetite.
- Gui Zhi and Gan Jiang warm the spleen and stomach and eliminate cold in the body.
- Huang Lian and Zhi Zi clear heat and eliminate damp in the middle Jiao.

Herbal Remedy:
Xiang Sha Liu Jun Wan-*Six Gentlemen Pill with Aucklandia and Amomum.*

Acupuncture Treatment:
- Zhongwan REN-12, Liangmen ST-21, Tianshu ST-25, Zusanli ST-36, Fenglong ST-40, Sanyinjiao SP-6, Yinlingquan SP-9, Hegu L.I.-4, Neiguan P-6 and Taichong LIV-3.
- A tonifying method is applied on ST-36 and SP-6, and a reducing method is applied on the rest of these points.
- In case of cold-damp, add moxa on REN-12, ST-36, and SP-9.
- In case of damp-heat, add Yanglingquan GB-34 and Dadu SP-2.

Explanations:
- REN-12, the front mu point of the stomach and the gathering point of the fu organs in the body, ST-40, the luo-connecting point of the stomach channel, and SP-9, and the he-sea point of the spleen channel respectively, eliminate damp and resolve phlegm in the body.
- P-6, the luo-connecting point of the pericardium channel, harmonizes the stomach, descends stomach-qi, and improves appetite.
- L.I.-4 and LIV-3, the yuan-source point of the large intestine channel and the liver channel respectively, promote the qi circulation

in the middle Jiao and relieve the fullness and swelling in the epigastric region and abdomen.

- ST-36, the he-sea point of the stomach channel, and SP-6, the crossing point of the three yin channels of the feet, tonify and activate the spleen and stomach and improve the appetite.
- Moxa on REN-12, ST-36 and SP-9 could warm the internal organs and eliminate cold.
- GB-34, the he-sea point of the gallbladder channel, and SP-2, the ying-spring point of the spleen channel clear heat and eliminate damp.

11.13.2.2 *Disharmony between the liver and stomach*

Loss of appetite, fullness in the chest and epigastric region, belching, acid regurgitation, slight depression, headache, insomnia, aggravation of above situations when being nervous, irregular menstruation for women, occasionally irritable, thin and white coating on the tongue, and a wiry pulse.

Principle of Treatment:
Smooth the liver, promote qi circulation, active digestion, and improve appetite.

Herbal Treatment:
Xiao Yao San-*Rambling Powder*.

Chai Hu *Radix Bupleuri* 10 g
Bai Shao Yao *Radix Paeoniae Lactiflorae* 15 g
Zhi Ke *Fructus Citri Aurantii* 10 g
Dang Gui *Radix Angelicae Sinensis* 10 g
Xiang Fu *Rhizoma Cyperi Rotundi* 10 g
Chen Pi *Pericarpium Citri Reticulatae* 5 g
Sha Ren *Fructus Amomi* 3 g
Bai Zhu *Rhizoma Atractylodis Macrocephalae* 10 g
Shen Qu *Massa Medica Fermentata* 15 g
Jiao Gu Ya *Fructus Oryzae Sativae Germinantus (grill)* 15 g

Fu Shen *Sclerotium Poriae Cocos Paradicis* 12 g
Yuan Zhi *Radix Polygalae Tenuifoliae* 10 g

Explanations:
- Chai Hu and Bai Shao Yao smooth the liver and relieve qi stagnation in the liver.
- Zhi Ke, Xiang Fu, Chen Pi and Sha Ren promote the qi circulation in the middle Jiao and improve the appetite.
- Dang Gui nourishes the liver-blood and benefits the liver.
- Bai Zhu activates the spleen and stomach and improves appetite.
- Shen Qu and Jiao Gu Ya promote digestion and improve appetite.
- Fu Shen and Yuan Zhi smooth emotions, regulate the shen, and improve sleep.

Herbal Remedy:
Xiao Yao Wan-*Rembling Pill.*

Acupuncture Treatment:
- Neiguan P-6 + Gongsun SP-4, Hegu L.I.-4, Tanzhong REN-17, Fengchi GB-20, Sanyinjiao SP-6, Taichong LIV-3, Zhangmen LIV-13, Xinshu BL-15, and Ganshu BL-18.
- An even method is applied on P-6 + SP-4, and a reducing method is applied on the rest of the points.

Explanations:
- The combination of P-6 + SP-4 promotes the qi circulation in the body, regulates the Yinwei channel and Chong channel, and improves appetite.
- L.I.-4, the yuan-source point of the large intestine channel, REN-17, the gathering point of the qi in the body, LIV-3, the yuan-source point of the liver channel, BL-18, the back-shu point of the liver, and GB-20 promote the qi circulation in the body, smooth the liver, improve emotions, and relieves pain and headache.
- SP-6, the crossing point of the three yin channels of the feet, and LIV-13, the front-mu point of the spleen, activate the spleen and improve appetite.

- BL-15, the back-shu point of the heart, calms the shen, and improves emotions.

11.13.2.3 *Deficiency of qi and yang of the spleen*

Loss of appetite, tastelessness in the mouth, weakness, fatigue, weight loss, low voice, not wanting to speak, spontaneous sweating, aversion to cold, cold hands and feet, loose stools or diarrhea, pale tongue, thin and white tongue coating with some tooth marks, and a thready, weak, and slow pulse.

If there is a deficiency of qi and yang of the heart, there could be palpitations, superficial sleep, and a weak feeling of heartbeat, etc.

If there is a deficiency of qi and yang of the kidney, there would be lower back pain, frequent urination, shortness of breath by slight exertion, and weakness of the knees, etc.

Principle of Treatment:
Tonify qi, warm yang, activate the spleen and improve appetite.

Herbal Treatment:
Li Zhong Wan-*Pill to Regulate the Middle,* plus
Shen Ling Bai Zhu San-*Ginseng, Sclerotium Poriae Cocos and Atractylodis Macrocephalae Powder.*

Zhi Dang Shen *Radix Codonopsis Pilosulae Praeparata* 10 g
Gan Jiang *Rhizoma Zingiberis Officinalis* 5 g
Gui Zhi *Ramulus Cinnamomi Cassiae* 10 g
Zhi Huang Qi *Radix Astragali Membranacei Praeparata* 10 g
Bai Zhu *Rhizoma Atractylodis Macrocephalae* 10 g
Fu Ling *Sclerotium Poriae Cocos* 12 g
Shan Yao *Radix Dioscoreae Oppositae* 10 g
Shen Qu *Massa Medica Fermentata* 15 g
Ji Nei Jin *Endothelium Corneum Gigeriae Galli* 10 g
Zhi Gan Cao *Radix Glycyrrhizae Preparata* 5 g

In case of deficiency of qi and yang of the heart, add Rou Gui *Cortex Cinnamomi Cassiae* 3 g and Zhi Fu Zi *Radix Lateralis Aconiti Carmichaeli Praeparata* 6 g.

If there is a deficiency of qi and yang of the kidney, add Ba Ji Tian *Radix Morindae Officinalis* 10 g and Xian Mao *Rhizoma Curculiginis Orchioidis* 10 g.

Explanations:
- Zhi Dang Shen, Bai Zhu, Fu Ling, and Zhi Gan Cao activate the spleen, tonify the spleen-qi and the general body, and improve appetite.
- Gui Zhi and Gan Jiang warm the spleen and eliminate cold in the middle Jiao.
- Zhi Huang Qi and Shan Yao activate the spleen, tonify spleen-qi, and improve appetite.
- Shen Qu and Ji Nei Jin are used to promote digestion and improve appetite.
- Rou Gui and Zhi Fu Zi warm the heart-yang and strengthen heart-fire.
- Ba Ji Tian and Xian Mao warm the kidney, eliminate interior cold and strengthen the back.

Herbal Remedy:
Li Zhong Wan-*Pill to Regulate the Middle*, plus
Shen Ling Bai Zhu Wan-*Ginseng, Sclerotium Poriae Cocos and Atractylodis Macrocephalae Pill*.

Acupuncture Treatment:
- Guanyuan REN-4, Qihai REN-6, Zhongwan REN-12, Zhangmen LIV-13, Zusanli ST-36, Taibai SP-3, Sanyinjiao SP-6, Shenmen HE-7, Taixi KID-3, Xinshu BL-15, Pishu BL-20, and Shenshu BL-23.
- A tonifying method is applied to these points.
- Moxibustion could be applied on REN-4, REN-6, and ST-36.

Explanations:
- REN-4 and REN-6 tonify the yuan-qi in the body, warm yang, eliminate interior cold and strengthen the body.
- ST-36, the he-sea point of the stomach channel, SP-3 and SP-6, the yuan-source point and the crossing point of three yin channels of the feet, LIV-13, the front-mu point of the spleen, BL-20, the back-shu point of the spleen, and REN-12, the front-mu point of the stomach, tonify and activate the spleen and stomach, and improve appetite.
- HE-7 and BL-15, the yuan-source point and the back-shu point of the heart channel and of the heart respectively, tonify qi and yang of the heart and strengthen the heart.
- BL-23, the back-shu point of the kidney, warms the kidney, tonifies qi and yang of the kidney and eliminates interior cold.
- Moxibustion warms qi and yang of the body, eliminates interior cold and improves appetite.

11.14 Sore Throat

A sore throat is quite common, and could be caused by various illnesses ranging from non-serious to life-threatening. If there is an isolated sore throat with no other symptoms, it is typically not something to worry about, because it is often due to irritation from allergies, air pollution, smoking or overuse. But when it occurs with other symptoms, such as cough, fever, muscle aching, and loss of smell and taste, it is highly likely that it is related to COVID-19.

One study examined the prevalence of ENT symptoms in COVID-19 positive patients. A cross sectional study was performed at SRTR GMC AMBAJOGAI (a tertiary care hospital) amongst the patients admitted in COVID-19 isolation ward with a positive RT-PCR report. Among the 180 patients included in the study, 112 patients had one or more ENT related symptoms that included throat pain (47.2%), loss of smell (55.5%), loss of taste (58.8%) and hearing loss (54.44%) along with generalized COVID-19 symptoms. ENT symptoms can be considered as biomarkers for early diagnosis of COVID-19 patients to ensure faster treatment and isolation, and to allow better containment of the disease.[93] COVID-19 related sore throats tend to be relatively mild and last no more than five days. A very painful sore throat that lasts more than five days may be something else such as a bacterial infection.

As the pandemic evolves, some symptoms might persist for a long time in a proportion of patients who recovered from the infection's acute phase. Persistent symptoms may take a toll on the lives of "long haulers". Sore throat is among these persistent symptoms, and patients might experience this COVID-19 symptom even after recovery.

A retrospective cohort study was conducted based on linked electronic health records (EHRs) data from 81 million patients including 273,618 COVID-19 survivors. The incidence and co-occurrence within six months and in the three to six months after COVID-19 diagnosis were calculated for nine core features of Long COVID symptoms that are frequently reported (breathing difficulties/breathlessness, fatigue/malaise, chest/throat pain, headache, abdominal symptoms, myalgia, other pain, cognitive symptoms, and anxiety/depression). The percentage of throat pain was 5.71%.[94]

Although the quality of life was markedly affected by fatigue, shortness of breath, and insomnia in Long COVID, sore throat is also a persistent complaint affecting daily life.

11.14.1 TCM understanding of Long COVID-associated sore throat

The throat relates to the oral cavity and the nose, the stomach and lung, and various channels and collaterals as well as some extraordinary channels, such as Ren channel, Chong channel, etc. If there is a remainder of invasion of the external factors or imbalance in the

---

[93] Saee Savtale, *et al.* Prevalence of otorhinolaryngological symptoms in COVID 19 patients. *Indian J Otolaryngol Head Neck Surg.* 2021, 1–7. doi: 10.1007/s12070-021-02410-5.

[94] Maxime Taquet, *et al.* September 2021. *op. cit.*

stomach or lung, disorders in the channels and collaterals can cause pain in the throat in Long COVID. Nevertheless, a bad diet, excessive smoking, excessive strain, emotional disturbance and constitutional weakness or excess during Long COVID may cause disorders of the stomach, lung, liver or kidney, leading to sore throat.

Although cough is one of the main respiratory symptoms, sore throat and cough could appear in combination or as individual complaints. There are some similarities in the causative factors and mechanisms for both complaints, but they are not the same.

11.14.1.1 *Incomplete elimination of external pathogenic factors*

Invasion of external pathogenic factors with a pestilent toxin to the lung could cause the occurrence of COVID-19 with a sore throat. When it is properly treated in time, these external pathogenic factors should be eliminated completely, leaving no further damage to the lung and sore throat could also recover quickly in a few days. However, when these pathogenic factors are not eliminated completely, they could cause some disturbance to the lung in dispersing the qi, and cause dysfunction of the throat, therefore sore throat occurs. Among these external pathogenic factors, the remaining toxic heat is frequently seen.

11.14.1.2 *Accumulation of damp-phlegm*

Either invasion of cold-damp or invasion of damp-heat to the spleen or stomach, or San Jiao, may cause dysfunction of the spleen and stomach in digestion, transportation, and transformation, resulting in the formation of damp-phlegm internally. This could eventually disturb the lung in dispersing the qi, and block the channels in the throat, thus sore throat happens.

Obesity, constitutional weakness of the spleen and stomach, or lack of care for daily diet during COVID-19, could cause the production of damp-phlegm in the body. During Long COVID, the formation of damp-phlegm could become worse due to external invasion and sickness. When the lung is disturbed in dispersing the qi, and the throat is blocked by damp-phlegm, a sore throat appears.

11.14.1.3 *Disturbance of the emotions*

Excessive stress, frustration, and anger over a long period of time prior to, during and after COVID-19, could cause depression of the liver-qi, leading to its stagnation. Meanwhile, excessive thinking may cause stagnation of the heart-qi, and excessive sadness may suppress the lung, bringing about the stagnation of lung-qi. Once the qi stagnates, it blocks the circulation in the channels in the body and throat, causing a sore throat. Moreover, prolonged stagnation of qi may trigger a fire that flares up and burns the throat. Obviously, a long-standing stagnation of qi may result in the stagnation of blood, also causing a sore throat.

Excessive worrying may cause stagnation of qi in the spleen, impeding the function of the spleen in transportation and transformation, causing damp to form. When damp-phlegm blocks the throat, it causes sore throat.

11.14.1.4 *Formation of internal heat*

Overeating of pungent, sweet, or fatty food, as well as drinking too much alcohol prior to COVID-19, may cause the formation of stomach-fire or damp-heat. When the throat is impaired by these pathogenic factors, it could be impaired or blocked, thus a sore throat happens.

11.14.1.5 *Prolonged sickness or weak constitution*

Prolonged persistence of COVID-19, lack of proper medical and life care, or congenital weakness, could lead to consumption of the yin of the lung and kidney, resulting in hyperactivity of deficient fire, thus the throat fails to be properly nourished, and sore throat follows.

11.14.2 TCM treatment of Long COVID-associated sore throat

In TCM, the careful differentiation of the associated symptoms and root causes is important in treating a sore throat effectively.

11.14.2.1 *Remaining toxic heat*

Persistence of a slight sore throat, slight redness and swelling in the throat, occasional expectoration of slight yellow and sticky phlegm in the throat, slight thirst, dry stool or constipation, red tongue, thin and dry tongue coating, and a rapid and wiry pulse.

Principle of Treatment:
Clear heat, remove toxins, subside swelling and relieve sore throat.

Herbal Treatment:
Pu Ji Xiao Du Yin-*Universal Benefit Decoction to Eliminate Toxins.*

Huang Qin *Radix Scutellariae Baicalensis* 10 g
Huang Lian *Rhizoma Coptidis* 5 g
Xuan Shen *Radix Scrophulariae Ningpoensis* 10 g
Ban Lan Gen *Radix Isatidis* 10 g
Jie Geng *Radix Platycodi Grandiflori* 5 g
Lian Qiao *Fructus Forsythiae Suspensae* 3 g
Ma Bo *Fructißcatio Lasiosphaerae seu Calvatiae* 3 g
Niu Bang Zi *Fructus Ardii Lappae* 10 g
Bo He *Herba Menthae Haplocalycis* 3 g
Gan Cao *Radix Glycyrrhizae* 6 g

Explanations:
- Huang Qin, Huang Lian, Ma Bo, and Ban Lan Gen clear heat and remove the toxins.
- Lian Qiao and Niu Bang Zi dispel remaining external heat and toxins, subside swelling, eliminate phlegm in the throat, and relieve sore throat.

- Xuan Shen, Jie Geng, Bo He and Gan Cao cool heat, subside swelling, eliminate toxins and relieve sore throat.

Herbal Remedy:
Yin Qiao San Pian-*Honeysuckle and Forsythia Powder Tablet,*
or Yin Qiao Jie Du Wan-*Honeysuckle and Forsythia Pill to Relieve Toxicity.*

Acupuncture Treatment:
- Erjian L.I.-2, Hegu L.I.-4, Quchi L.I.-11, Chize LU-5, Yuji LU-10, Fengchi GB-20, Tiantu REN-22, Lianquan REN-23, and Renying ST-9.
- A reducing method is used on these points.

Explanations:
- L.I.-4 and L.I.-11, the yuan-source point, and the he-sea point of the large intestine channel respectively, and GB-20 clear heat, remove toxins and subside swelling in the throat and relieve sore throat.
- L.I.-2 and LU-10, the ying-spring points of the large intestine and lung channel respectively, strongly clear heat, eliminate toxins and reduce the swelling in the throat and sore throat.
- LU-5, the he-sea point of the lung channel, clears heat in the lung and causes the lung-qi to disperse and descend. It is also the water point, which serves to distinguish fire and eliminate toxins to relieve sore throat.
- REN-22, REN-23 and ST-9 reduce swelling, relieve pain, and eliminate the blockage in the throat to diminish sore throat.

11.14.2.2 *Accumulation of damp-phlegm in the throat*

Slight sore throat, always having a feeling of phlegm in the throat, occasional cough with expectoration of sticky or whitish phlegm, aggravation of sore throat and cough when intaking greasy and fatty food, alleviation of cough when phlegm is expectorated, slight fullness in the chest and epigastric region, nausea, poor appetite, loose stools, whitish and greasy coating on the tongue, and a slippery pulse.

Principle of Treatment:
Eliminate damp-phlegm, activate the spleen, relieve the blockage in the throat, and relieve sore throat.

Herbal Treatment:
Cang Fu Dao Tan Tang-*Atractylodes-Poria Phlegm-Dissipating Decoction.*

Cang Zhu *Rhizoma Atractylodis* 10 g
Xiang Fu *Rhizoma Cyperi Rotundi* 10 g
Zhi Shi *Fructus Immaturus Citri Aurantii* 10 g
Zhi Ban Xia *Rhizoma Pinelliae Ternatae Preparata* 10 g
Fu Ling *Sclerotium Poriae Cocos* 12 g
Chen Pi *Pericarpium Citri Reticulatae* 5 g
Tian Nan Xing *Rhizoma Arisaematis* 10 g
Xing Ren *Semen Pruni Armeniacae* 10 g
Hou Po *Cortex Magnoliae Officinalis* 10 g
Zi Su Zi *Fructus Perillae Frutescentis* 10 g
Niu Bang Zi *Fructus Arctii Lappae* 10 g
Jie Geng *Radix Platycodi Grandiflori* 5 g
Zhi Gan Cao *Radix Glycyrrhizae Preparata* 3 g

Explanations:
- Zhi Ban Xia, Fu Ling, Chen Pi, and Zhi Gan Cao, the complete compositions of Er Chen Tang, eliminate damp, resolve phlegm, and relieve general symptoms of damp-phlegm accumulation.
- Cang Zhu, Hou Po, Zhi Shi, and Xiang Fu dry damp, resolve phlegm and relieve the qi stagnation caused by the accumulation of damp-phlegm.
- Xing Ren, Tian Nan Xing, Zi Su Zi, Jie Geng and Niu Bang Zi resolve phlegm in the throat and lung, regulate the lung-qi and relieve sore throat.

Herbal Remedy:
Cang Fu Dao Tan Wan-*Atractylodes-Poria Phlegm-Dissipating Pill.*

Acupuncture Treatment:
- Neiguan P-6 + Gongsun SP-4, Hegu L.I.-4, Lieque LU-7, Chize LU-5, Feishu BL-13, Zhongwan REN-12, Tiantu REN-22, Lianquan REN-23, Renying ST-9, Fenglong ST-40, Sanyinjiao SP-6 and Yinlingquan SP-9.
- An even method is applied on P-6 + SP-4, and a reducing method is applied on the rest of the points.

Explanations:
- The combination of P-6 + SP-4 promotes the qi circulation in the lung, chest and abdomen and relieves sore throat.
- REN-12, the gathering point of the fu organs in the body, ST-40, the luo-connecting of the stomach channel, SP-6, and SP-9, the crossing point of three yin channels of the feet and the he-sea point of the spleen channel respectively, activate the spleen and stomach, eliminate damp-phlegm in the body and relieve the blockage in the throat.
- BL-13, the back-shu point of the lung, LU-7, and LU-5 disperse and descend the lung-qi, restore the physiological functions of the lung, and relieve sore throat.
- L.I.-4, the yuan-source point of the large intestine channel, REN-22, REN-23, and ST-9 promote the qi circulation, relieve the blockage in the throat and relieve sore throat.

11.14.2.3 *Stagnation of liver-qi*

Sore throat with a feeling of spasm and tension in the throat which moves up and down (and is closely related with the emotional situation), a feeling as if there is a plum stone in the throat, depression, stress, a feeling of oppression over the chest, headache, insomnia, a poor appetite, a slightly purplish tongue with a thin coating, and a wiry pulse.

Principle of Treatment:
Smooth the liver, circulate qi, harmonize the emotions and relieve sore throat.

Herbal Treatment:
Xiao Yao San-*Rambling Powder*, plus
Ban Xia Hou Po Tang-*Pinellia and Magnolia Bark Decoction*.

Chai Hu *Radix Bupleuri* 10 g
Dang Gui *Radix Angelicae Sinensis* 10 g
Bai Shao Yao *Radix Paeoniae Lactiflorae* 10 g
Bai Zhu *Rhtzoma Atractylodis Macrocephalae* 10 g
Zhi Ban Xia *Rhizoma Pinelliae Ternatae Preparata* 10 g
Hou Po *Cortex Magnoliae Officinalis* 10 g
Zi Su Zi *Fructus Perillae Frutescentis* 10 g
Fu Ling *Sclerotium Poriae Cocos* 15 g
Bo He *Herba Menthae Haplocalycis* 3 g
Yan Hu Suo *Rhizotna Corydalis* 10 g
Zhi Gan Cao *Radix Glycyrrhizae Preparata* 3 g

Explanations:
- Chai Hu regulates and promotes liver-qi circulation and relieves qi stagnation in the liver and throat.
- Bai Shao and Dang Gui relax the liver, nourish the blood, and strengthen the blood circulation in the liver.
- Bai Zhu, Fu Ling and Sheng Jiang activate the spleen and stomach and eliminate damp-phlegm in the body.
- Yan Hu Suo regulates blood circulation and relieves pain.
- Hou Po and Zi Su Zi promote qi circulation, and eliminate damp-phlegm in the throat and sore throat.
- Bo He cools and clears heat in the liver.
- Zhi Gan Cao harmonizes the actions of the other herbs in the formula.

Herbal Remedy:
Xiao Yao Wan-*Rambling Pill,* or Shu Gan Wan-*Liver-Coursing Pill.*

Acupuncture Treatment:
- Taichong LIV-3, Fengchi GB-20, Neiguan P-6, Zhongwan REN-12, Tanzhong REN-17, Tiantu REN-22, Lianquan REN-23, Renying ST-9.
- A reducing method is used on these points.

Explanations:
- In all kinds of qi stagnation, stagnation of the liver-qi is generally the root cause. So, treatment for the stagnation of qi will be focused on alleviating the stagnation of liver-qi.
- LIV-3, the yuan-source point of the liver channel, fulfills the above function.
- P-6, the luo-connecting point of the pericardium channel and the confluence point of the Yinwei channel, and REN-17, the gathering point for the qi in the body, assist LIV-3 to circulate the liver-qi and regulate the emotions. They also promote the circulation of qi in the heart and spleen.
- GB-20 calms the shen and relieves the spasm and tension in the body.
- REN-12, the gathering point of the fu organs, promotes their physiological function and eliminates damp-phlegm.
- REN-22, REN-23 and ST-9, the local points, regulate the qi circulation, eliminate phlegm in the throat and relieve sore throat.

11.14.2.4 *Hyperactivity of stomach-fire*

Sore throat with obvious redness, swelling and a burning feeling, difficulty in swallowing, aggravation of the pain with smoking, drinking alcohol and eating pungent or highly-flavored food, thirst, constipation, a foul smell from the mouth, bleeding and swollen gums, occasional pus in the throat, a red tongue with a yellow and dry coating, and a rapid pulse.

Principle of Treatment:
Clear heat, promote defecation, reduce the swelling, and relieve sore throat.

Herbal Treatment:
Liang Ge San-*Cool the Diaphragm Powder*.

Jin Yin Hua *Flos Lonicerae Japonicae* 10 g
Lian Qiao *Fructus Forsythiae Suspensae* 10 g
Zhi Zi *Fructus Gardeniae Jasminoidis* 10 g
Huang Qin *Radix Scutellariae Baicalensis* 10 g
Bo He *Herba Mentirne Haplocalycis* 6 g
Niu Bang Zi *Fructus Arctii Lappae* 10 g
Xuan Shen *Radix Scrophulariae Ningpoensis* 10 g
Dan Zhu Ye *Herba Lophatheri* 10 g
Mang Xiao *Mirabilitum* 10 g
Da Huang *Radix et Rhizoma Rhei* 6 g
Lu Gen *Rhizoma Phragmitis* 10 g
Gan Cao *Radix Glycyrrhizae* 6 g

Explanations:
- Yin Hua, Lian Qiao, Zhi Zi and Huang Qin clear lung-heat, eliminate toxins, reduce swelling, and relieve sore throat.
- Bo He benefits the throat and relieves sore throat.
- Dan Zhu Ye and Lu Gen clear heat and promote the production of body fluids so as to benefit the throat and relieve thirst.
- Xuan Shen and Niu Bang Zi clear heat in the body and throat and relieve sore throat.
- Da Huang and Mang Xiao clear stomach-fire and promote defecation.
- Gan Cao clears fire and removes toxins.

Herbal Remedy:
Qing Fei Yi Huo Pian-*Clear the Lungs, Suppress Fire Tablets*.

Acupuncture Treatment:
- Hegu L.I.-4, Quchi L.I.-11, Chize LU-5, Yuji LU-10, Chongyang ST-42, Neiting ST-44, Tiantu REN-22, Lianquan REN-23, and Renying ST-9.

- An even method is used on REN-22, REN-23 and ST-9, and a reducing method is used on the rest of the points.

Explanations:
- L.I.-4 and L.I.-11, the yuan-source point and the he-sea point of the large intestine channel, ST-42 and ST-44, the yuan-source point and the ying-spring point of the stomach channel respectively, clear heat, descend stomach-qi, subside swelling in the throat and relieve sore throat.
- LU-5, the water point and he-sea point, and LU-10, the ying-spring point of the lung channel respectively, clear heat, subside swelling in the throat and relieve sore throat. They can also cause the lung-qi to descend, which is the root treatment for reducing fire in the throat.
- REN-22, REN-23, and ST-9 clear heat in the throat, reduce swelling and relieve sore throat.

11.14.2.5 *Deficiency of lung-yin*

Sore throat with dryness and slight redness, slight difficulty in swallowing, dry cough, or cough with scanty phlegm (occasionally the phlegm is mixed with little blood streaks), thirst, night sweating, hotness of the palms and soles, dry stools, red tongue, scanty or peeled tongue coating, and a deep, thready, and rapid pulse.

Principle of Treatment:
Nourish yin, moisten the lung, and relieve sore throat.

Herbal Treatment:
Sha Shen Mai Men Dong Tang-*Glehnia and Ophiopogonis Decoction.*

Bei Sha Shen *Radix Glehniae Littoralis* 10 g
Mai Men Dong *Tuber Ophiopogonis Japonici* 10 g
Wu Wei Zi *Fructus Schisandrae Chinensis* 10 g
Tian Hua Fen *Radix Trichosanthis Kirilowii* 10 g

Xing Ren *Semen Pruni Armeniacae* 10 g
Chuan Bei Mu *Bulbus Fritillariae Cirrhosae* 10 g
Zi Wan *Radix Asteris Tatarici* 10 g
Di Gu Pi *Cortex Lycii Radicis* 10 g
Sheng Di Huang *Radix Rehmanniae Glutinosae Recens* 10 g
Zhi Mu *Radix Anemarrhenae Asphodeloidis* 10 g
Huang Qin *Radix Scutellariae Baicalensis* 5 g
Yu Hu Die *Oroxylum indicum (L.)Vent* 5 g
Pang Da Hai *Semen Sterculiae Scaphigerae* 10 g

Explanations:
- Bei Sha Shen, Mai Men Dong, and Wu Wei Zi nourish the yin of the lung and relieve dryness in the throat and dry cough.
- Chuan Bei Mu, Zi Wan, and Di Gu Pi nourish yin, clear the heat in the lung, eliminate phlegm in the lung and benefit the lung to relieve sore throat.
- Sheng Di Huang, Zhi Mu, and Huang Qin are used to clear the remaining deficient heat in the lung and relieve sore throat.
- Tian Hua Fen nourishes yin, promotes the secretion of body fluid, and relieves thirst and dryness of the throat.
- Yu Hu Die and Pang Da Hai benefit the throat, subside the swelling and relieve sore throat.

Herbal Remedy:
Sheng Mai San (Wan)-*Generate the Pulse Powder (Pill)*.

Acupuncture Treatment:
- Lieque LU-7 + Zhaohai KID-6. Chize LU-5, Taiyuan LU-9, Tiantu REN-22, Lianquan REN-23, Renying ST-9, Sanyinjiao SP-6, Taixi KID-3, Qihai REN-6 and Shenshu BL-23.
- An even method is applied on LU-7 + KID-6, REN-22, REN-23, and ST-9, and a tonifying method is applied to the rest of the points.

Explanations:
- The combination of LU-7 + KID-6 nourishes the yin of the body and clears deficient heat.

- LU-5 and LU-9, the he-sea point and the yuan-source point of the lung channel respectively, nourish the yin of the lung and restore the physiological functions of the lung.
- SP-6, KID-3, KID-6, BL-23, and REN-6 nourish the yin of the body, benefit the yin of the lung and moisten the throat.
- REN-22, REN-23, and ST-9 benefit the throat, clear the deficient heat in the throat and relieve sore throat.

11.15 Dizziness

Dizziness is often used interchangeably with vertigo, however, strictly speaking, they are slightly different. Dizziness is a feeling of being off-balance, unsteady, lightheaded, or disoriented. Some even have trouble staying balanced or may stagger while walking. Vertigo refers to a typical experience or sensation that makes the environment or room spin. These feelings may make people lose their balance.

The symptoms in a mild case may be greatly relieved by closing the eyes or remaining in a sitting or lying position, while a serious case may be accompanied by nausea, vomiting, tinnitus, sweating and even fainting. Headache is usually not seen.

Most patients who have COVID-19 could recover completely within a few weeks. But patients, even those who had mild or asymptomatic disease, could experience some symptoms after their initial infection. Besides, although COVID-19 is seen as a disease that primarily affects the lung, it can also damage many other organs or systems, including the heart, kidney, and neurological system, etc.

When talking about COVID-19 in the acute phase, people are most likely to think of fever, cough, and shortness of breath. When discussing the most common symptoms of Long COVID, fatigue, shortness of breath, coughing, myalgia, and headache, are primarily mentioned. However, COVID-19 can have many symptoms and Long COVID could have different clinical manifestations. All these symptoms and clinical manifestations can vary from person to person.

While the pulmonary complications have received the most attention, it is the neurological manifestations that are disabling, persistent and common in patients infected with SARS-CoV-2. The entire neural-axis can be involved, resulting in a wide variety of manifestations.[95] One study pointed out that nearly 10–35% patients continue to complain of persistent symptoms most of which are neurological in nature.[96] Although headache and loss of smell or taste are the most common neurological symptoms, dizziness and vertigo are another two neurological symptoms that can happen with COVID-19. One study from October 2020 investigated dizziness and vertigo in people who had contracted COVID-19. Out of the 185 people that responded to a study questionnaire, 34(18.4%) reported experiencing dizziness or vertigo.[97] Another research reviewed 14 studies that described dizziness as a COVID-19 symptom. Across these studies, the percentage of people reporting dizziness ranged from about 4–30%.[98]

It's currently unclear why COVID-19 could cause dizziness or vertigo in Long COVID. Some possible explanations include inflammation from the infection as well as direct infection of nerve tissue. It is mostly considered that the COVID-19 virus impacts the vestibular system, a system containing a sound-sensing spiral cavity, as well as several fluid-filled semicircular canals. In research published in the *International Journal of Audiology*, experts found that COVID-19 may damage the inner ear in several ways. That includes direct viral infection of the inner ear or an autoimmune attack by antibodies or immune cells. This can also include blood clotting that potentially blocks the blood supply to the cochlea or semicircular canals. Any of these can lead to inner ear damage, causing long-term vestibular complaints. The researcher confirmed that the pooled estimate of

---

[95] Avindra Nath, *et al*. Neurological issues during COVID-19: An overview. *Neurosci Lett*. 2021, 742: 135533. doi: 10.1016/j.neulet.2020.135533.

[96] Mark W. Tenforde, *et al. op. cit.*

[97] Pasquale Viola, *et al*. Tinnitus and equilibrium disorders in COVID-19 patients: preliminary results. *Eur Arch Otorhinolaryngol*. 2020: 1–6. doi: 10.1007/s00405-020-06440-7.

[98] Jeyasakthy Saniasiaya, *et al*. Dizziness and COVID-19. *Ear Nose Throat J*. 2020, 100(1): 29–30. doi: 10.1177/0145561320959573.

prevalence based primarily on retrospective recall of symptoms, was 7.2% for rotatory vertigo.[99,100]

It has been confirmed in one study that anxiety and stress can also trigger vertigo attacks,[101] and these two factors are common among the general population during the COVID-19 pandemic. It is still unknown what kind of role these two factors play in this situation.

At this moment, most research is focusing on the prevalence and mechanism of dizziness in COVID-19 or Long COVID, and there is still a lack of accepted medical treatment proposals. Most forms of life care, such as trying to keep a sitting or lying down position, moving carefully, avoiding strong physical activities, etc., are recommended.

11.15.1 TCM understanding of Long COVID-associated dizziness

The causes for dizziness during Long COVID are mostly due to impairment of internal organs by fire, yang, wind, phlegm, damp, or deficiency of qi and blood.

The organs chiefly involved are the liver, spleen and kidney.

11.15.1.1 *Emotional disturbance*

The liver plays an important role in emotional activities. It regulates qi circulation and stores blood. Overstress, resentment, and frustration during COVID-19 may cause retardation of liver-qi circulation, and stagnation of liver-qi occurs. If there is stagnation of liver-qi, it may influence the physiological functions in the head, leading to

---

[99] Ibrahim Almufarrij and Kevin Munro. One year on: An updated systematic review of SARS-CoV-2, COVID-19 and audio-vestibular symptoms. *International Journal of Audiology.* 2021, 60(12): 935–945. https://doi.org/10.1080/14992027.2021.1896793.
[100] National Dizzy and Balance Center. Post-COVID vestibular and neurological symptoms. 17 May 2021. https://www.nationaldizzyandbalancecenter.com/post-covid-vestibular-and-neurological-symptoms/.
[101] Zawn Villines. Is dizziness a symptom of anxiety? *Medical News Today.* 24 July 2020. https://www.medicalnewstoday.com/articles/anxiety-and-dizziness.

stagnation of qi and blood in the head. When the clear-yang in the head is blocked by qi and blood, dizziness occurs.

Qi belongs to yang in the body. In case of prolonged persistence of liver-qi stagnation, especially in those with underlying sickness, it may cause the formation of liver-fire. Moreover, improper diet during COVID-19 may accelerate this process of fire formation. When there is the formation of liver-fire in the body, it may rise to the head, disturbing qi and blood circulation and burning the channels on the head, thus dizziness happens. Besides, prolonged persistence of flaring of liver-fire may cause hyperactivity of liver-yang, leading to the occurrence of severe dizziness. Whenever there is an accumulation of damp in the body, the uprising of liver-qi, fire or yang could stir damp, causing disturbance of the clear-yang by damp, and dizziness forms.

11.15.1.2 *Blockage of clear-yang by damp-phlegm*

COVID-19 is mainly caused by the invasion of cold-damp or damp-heat with a pestilent toxin to the body, especially the lung, heart and spleen. When these pathogenic factors are not eliminated completely or in time, they could cause stagnation and latent accumulation in the spleen, resulting in further disturbance to the ascending and descending functions of the spleen and stomach, and there could be the formation of damp-phlegm internally.

Constitutional weakness, lack of life care during COVID-19, overconsumption of alcoholic drinks and fatty and greasy food, could result in dysfunction of the spleen and stomach in transportation and transformation, and formation of damp-phlegm occurs.

When the head is blocked by damp-phlegm, clear-yang, or qi and blood would fail to rise and turbid qi would fail to descend, and dizziness happens.

11.15.1.3 *Deficiency of qi and blood*

Overconsumption of qi and blood, lack of dietary care or improper treatment during COVID-19 could cause deficiency of qi and blood, leading to failure of the head to be nourished, and dizziness appears.

11.15.2 TCM treatment of Long COVID associated dizziness

11.15.2.1 *Stagnation of liver-qi*

Dizziness, spasm, and tension sensation on the scalp or in the head, aggravation of dizziness under stress or emotional disturbance, depression, painful neck, distension and pain in the hypochondriac region, insomnia, irregular menstruation in women, poor appetite or overeating, thin and white tongue coating, and a wiry pulse.

Principle of Treatment:
Smooth the liver, promote qi circulation, calm the shen and relieve dizziness.

Herbal Treatment:
Xiao Yao San-*Rambling Powder*.

Chai Hu *Radix Bupleare* 10 g
Dang Gui *Radix Angelicae Sinensis* 10 g
Bai Shao Yao *Radix Paeoniae Lactiflorae* 10 g
Bai Zhu *Rhiizoma Areactylodis Macrocephalae* 10 g
Fu Ling *Sclerotium Poriae Cocos* 15 g
Chuan Xiong *Rhizoma Ligustici Chuan Xiong* 10 g
Huang Qin *Radix Scutellariae Baicalensis* 10 g
Bo He *Herba Menthae Haplocalycis* 3 g
Bai Ji Li *Fructus Tribulli Terrestris* 10 g
Ju Hua *Flos Chrysanthemi Morifolii* 10 g
Zhi Gan Cao *Radix Glycyrrhizae Preparata* 3 g

Explanations:
- Chai Hu regulates and promotes liver-qi circulation and relieves qi stagnation in the liver.
- Bai Shao Yao and Dang Gui are used to nourish blood in the liver, harmonize and smooth the liver and relieve tension and spasm in the scalp, headaches, and hypochondriac pain.
- Chuan Xiong regulates liver-qi and relieves headaches.

- Bai Zhu and Fu Ling strengthen the spleen and stomach and improve the appetite.
- Huang Qin and Bo He clear internal heat resulting from the stagnation of liver-qi and prevent further formation of liver-fire.
- Bai Ji Li and Ju Hua smooth the liver and relieve dizziness.
- Zhi Gan Cao harmonizes the actions of the other herbs.

Herbal Remedy:
Xiao Yao Wan-*Rambling Pill.*

Acupuncture Treatment:
- Waiguan SJ-5 + Zulinqi GB-41, Hegu L.I.-4, Tongziliao GB-1, Tinghui GB-2, Shuaigu GB-8, Extra Yintang, Extra Taiyang, Fengchi GB-20, Jianjing GB-21, Taichong LIV-3, Qimen LIV-14, Neiguan P-6, Sanyinjiao SP-6, Extra Sishencong.
- An even method is applied on SJ-5 + GB-41, and a reducing method is applied on the rest of the points.

Explanations:
- SJ-5 + GB-41 is a combination to harmonize Shaoyang channels, benefit the gallbladder and relieve dizziness.
- L.I.-4 and LIV-3, the yuan-source point of the large intestine channel and the liver channel respectively, and LIV-14, the front-mu point of the liver, smooth the liver, regulate the qi circulation in the body and relieve liver-qi stagnation.
- P-6, the luo-connecting point of the pericardium channel, regulates qi circulation, calms the shen and benefits the stomach.
- Extra Sishencong calms the shen, improves sleep and regulates emotion.
- SP-6, the crossing point of the three yin channels of the foot, promotes the smooth qi and blood circulation in the liver and in the head.
- GB-1, GB-2, GB-8, GB-20 and GB-21 regulate the collateral of the gallbladder channel, smooth the emotions, benefit the head, relieve the neck tension, and promote qi circulation in the head to relieve dizziness.

- Extra Yintang and Extra Taiyang, the local points, relieve dizziness.

11.15.2.2 *Flaring-up of liver-fire*

Dizziness, sharp or distending pain in the ear or in the head, redness of eyes, irritability, bitter taste in the mouth, restlessness, insomnia, irregular menstruation in women, poor appetite, deep yellow urine, constipation, red tongue, and a rapid and wiry pulse.

Principle of Treatment:
Reduce liver-fire, clear heat, calm the shen and relieve dizziness.

Herbal Treatment:
Long Dan Xie Gan Tang-*Gentiana Longdancao Decoction to Drain the Liver.*

Long Dan Cao *Radix Gentianae Anomalae* 10 g
Huang Qin *Radix Scutellariae Baicalensis* 10 g
Zhi Zi *Fructus Gardenniae* 10 g
Ze Xie *Rhizoma Alismatis* 12 g
Chuan Xiong *Rhizoma Lagustici Chuanxiong* 10 g
Xia Ku Cao *Spica Prunellae* 10 g
Che Qian Zi *Semen Plantaginis* 10 g
Dang Gui *Radix Angelicae Sinensis* 10 g
Sheng Di Huang *Radix Rehmanniae Glutinosae* 12 g
Chai Hu *Radix Bupleuri* 10 g
Bai Ji Li *Fructus Tribulli Terrestris* 10 g
Ju Hua *Flos Chrysanthemi Morifolii* 10 g
Zhi Gan Cao *Radix Glycyrrhizae Preparata* 3 g

In case of hyperactivity of liver-yang, add Gou Teng *Ramulus cum Uncis Uncariae* 10 g and Tian Ma *Rhizoma Gastrodiae Elatae* 10 g.

Explanations:
- Long Dan Cao, Huang Qin, Xia Ku Cao and Zhi Zi clear heat in the liver, reduce liver-fire and relieve dizziness.

- Dang Gui, Chuan Xiong and Chai Hu promote liver-qi circulation and smooth the liver.
- Ze Xie and Che Qian Zi promote urination and induce fire out of the body through urination.
- Sheng Di clears heat and nourishes the yin of the liver and kidney.
- Bai Ji Li and Ju Hua smooth the liver and relieve dizziness.
- Zhi Gan Cao harmonizes the actions of the other herbs.
- Gou Teng and Tian Ma calm the liver, suppress liver-wind and relieve dizziness.

Herbal Remedy:
Long Dan Xie Gan Wan-*Gentiana Longdancao Pill to Drain the Liver.*

Acupuncture Treatment:
- Waiguan SJ-5 + Zulinqi GB-41, Zhongfeng LIV-4, Shaohai HE-3, Shaofu HE-8, Tinghui GB-2, Shuaigu GB-8, Fengchi GB-20, Jianjing GB-21, Xiaxi GB-43, Baihui DU-20, Xingjian LIV-2, Qimen LIV-14, Sanyinjiao SP-6 and Extra Taiyang.
- An even method is applied on SJ-5 + GB-41, and a reducing method is applied on the rest of the points.

Explanations:
- A combination of SJ-5 + GB-41 harmonizes the Shaoyang channels, benefits the gallbladder, and relieves dizziness.
- L.I.-4 and LIV-14, the yuan-source point of the large intestine channel and the front-mu point of the liver, smooth the liver, regulate the qi circulation in the body and relieve liver-qi stagnation.
- LIV-2 and GB-43, the ying-spring point of the liver channel and gallbladder channel respectively, and DU-20, clear heat, reduce liver-fire and relieve dizziness.
- HE-3 and HE-8, the he-sea point and the ying-spring point of the heart channel respectively, clear heat in the heart, calm the shen and smooth the liver as well.
- GB-2, GB-8, GB-20 and GB-21 regulate the collateral of the gallbladder channel, smooth the emotions, relieve the neck tension, and promote qi circulation in the head to relieve dizziness.

- SP-6, the crossing point of the three yin channels of the foot, promotes the smooth qi and blood circulation in the liver and in the head.
- Extra Taiyang, the local point, relieves dizziness.

11.15.2.3 *Blockage of the clear-yang by damp-phlegm*

Dizziness, a heavy sensation in the head, the fullness of the chest and epigastric region, nausea, vomiting occasionally, poor appetite, casting of phlegm, white and greasy coating on the tongue, and a slippery or wiry and slippery pulse.

Principle of Treatment:
Activate the spleen, eliminate damp, resolve phlegm, harmonize the collaterals, and relieve dizziness.

Herbal Treatment:
Ban Xia Bai Zhu Tian Ma Tang-*Pinellia, Atractylodes Macrocephala and Gastrodia Decoction.*

Ban Xia *Rhizoma Pinelliae* 10 g
Bai Zhu *Rhizoma Atractylodis Macrocephalae* 10 g
Tian Ma *Rhizoma Gastrodiae* 10 g
Cang Zhu *Rhizoma Atractylodis* 10 g
Hou Po *Cortex Magnoliae Officinalis* 10 g
Fu Ling *Sclerotium Poriae Cocos* 15 g
Chen Pi *Pericarpium Citri Reticulatae* 5 g
Bai Ji Li *Fructus Tribulli Terrestris* 10 g
Shi Chang Pu *Rhizoma Acori Graminei* 10 g
Yuan Zhi *Radix Polygalae Tenuifoliae* 10 g
Zhi Gan Cao *Radix Glycyrrhizae Preparata* 3 g

Explanations:
- Ban Xia and Chen Pi dry damp, resolve phlegm in the body and relieve nausea.
- Fu Ling and Bai Zhu activate the spleen and eliminate damp.

- Tian Ma, Bai Ji Li, Shi Chang Pu and Yuan Zhi calm the liver, eliminate damp, and relieve dizziness.
- Cang Zhu and Hou Po eliminate damp-phlegm in the body and relieve nausea.
- Zhi Gan Cao harmonizes the functions of other herbs.

Herbal Remedy:
Ban Xia Bai Zhu Tian Ma Pian-*Pinellia, Atractylodes Macrocephala and Gastrodia Tablet.*

Acupuncture Treatment:
- Waiguan SJ-5 + Zulinqi GB-41, Hegu L.I.-4, Tinghui GB-2, Shuaigu GB-8, Fengchi GB-20, Jianjing GB-21, Touwei ST8, Extra Taiyang, Extra Yintang, Neiguan P-6, Zhongwan REN-12, Taichong LIV-3, Fenglong ST-40, Sanyinjiao SP-6 and Yinlingquan SP-9.
- An even method is applied on SJ-5 + GB-41, and a reducing method is applied on these points.

Explanations:
- SJ-5 + GB-41 could regulate the Shaoyang channels and relieve dizziness.
- GB-20 and GB-21 smooth the tension at the neck, promote the qi circulation in the gallbladder channel and relieve dizziness.
- L.I.-4 and LIV-3, the yuan-source point of the large intestine channel and Liver channel respectively, promote qi circulation, calm the liver, and relieve dizziness.
- GB-2, GB-8, ST-8, Extra Taiyang and Extra Yintang promote qi circulation, eliminate damp-phlegm in the head and relieve dizziness.
- REN-12, the front-mu point of the stomach and the influential point for the fu organs, promotes their physiological functions and eliminates damp-phlegm.
- SP-6, the crossing point of three yin channels of the foot, and SP-9, the he-sea point of the spleen channel, P-6 and ST-40, the luo-connecting point of the pericardium channel and stomach channel respectively, activate the spleen, eliminate damp-phlegm and improve digestion.

11.15.2.4 *Deficiency of qi*

Dizziness after COVID-19, empty sensation in the head, aggravation of dizziness after physical exertion, fatigue, general weakness, pale complexion, aversion to cold, cold hands, shortness of breath, spontaneous sweating, loose stools, poor appetite, low voice, thin and white coating on the tongue, pale tongue with tooth marks, and a slow and deep pulse.

Principle of Treatment:
Tonify qi, activate the spleen and stomach and relieve dizziness.

Herbal Treatment:
Bu Zhong Yi Qi Tang-*Tonify the Middle and Augment the Qi Decoction.*

Dang Shen *Radix Codonopsis Pilosulae* 10 g
Bai Zhu *Rhizoma Atractylodis Macrocephalae* 10 g
Fu Ling *clerotium Poriae Cocos* 15 g
Huang Qi *Radix Astragali Membranacea* 10 g
Chen Pi *Pericarpium Citri Reticulatae* 5 g
Gan Jiang *Rhizoma Zingiberis Officinalis* 5 g
Mu Xiang *Radix Aucklandiae* 10 g
Sha Ren *Fructus Amomi* 3 g
Bai Ji Li *Fructus Tribulli Terrestris* 10 g
Shi Chang Pu *Rhizoma Acori Graminei* 10 g
Zhi Gan Cao *Radix Glycyrrhizae Praeparata* 3 g

Explanations:
- Dang Shen, Bai Zhu, Fu Ling and Zhi Gan Cao, known as Si Jun Zi Tang-Four Gentlemen Decoction, activate the spleen and stomach, tonify spleen-qi and relieve general fatigue and weakness.
- Huang Qi tonify spleen-qi and lift-up the qi to the head to benefit it.
- Chen Pi, Mu Xiang and Sha Ren harmonize stomach-qi and promote appetite.
- Bai Ji Li and Shi Chang Pu resolve damp in the head and relieve dizziness.

Herbal Remedy:
Bu Zhong Yi Qi Wan-*Tonify the Middle and Augment the Qi Pill.*

Acupuncture Treatment:
- Zusanli ST-36, Taibai SP-3, Sanyinjiao SP-6, Qihai REN-6, Pishu BL-20 and Weishu BL-21, Tinghui GB-2, Touwei ST-8, Extra Yintang, Baihui DU-20, Shenting DU-24.
- A tonifying method is applied on these points. Moxibustion should be applied on REN-6 and ST-36.

Explanations:
- ST-36, the he-sea point of the stomach channel, and SP-3, the yuan-source point of the spleen channel, BL-20 and BL-21, the back-shu point of the spleen and stomach respectively, activate the spleen and stomach, tonify qi and promote digestion.
- REN-6, and SP-6, the crossing point of the three yin channels of the foot, tonify qi and blood at the same time and strengthen the body to relieve general fatigue and weakness.
- GB-2 and ST-8 resolve damp in the head and relieve dizziness.
- DU-20, DU-24 and extra Yintang lift-up qi to the headache to benefit the head and relieve dizziness.
- Moxibustion promotes the yang-qi movement, benefits the body and relieves the weakness and cold in the body.

11.15.2.5 *Deficiency of blood*

Dizziness after COVID-19, a hollow sensation in the head, aggravation of dizziness after physical exertion, alleviation of dizziness when resting, dizziness, dry eyes, hair loss, palpitations, listlessness, dry skin and stools, insomnia, pale complexion, irregular menstruation in women, poor appetite, pale tongue, thin and white tongue coating, and a thready and weak pulse.

Principle of Treatment:
Tonify blood, benefit kidney-jing, relieve weakness and relieve dizziness.

Herbal Treatment:
Si Wu Tang-*Four Substances Decoction.*

Shu Di Huang *Radix Rehmanniae Preparata* 15 g
Dang Gui *Radix Angelicae Sinensis* 10 g
Bai Shao *Radix Paeoniae Alba* 10 g
Chuan Xiong *Rhizoma Ligustici Chuanxiong* 10 g
Huang Jing *Rhizoma Polygonati* 10 g
He Shou Wu *Radix Polygoni Multiflori* 10 g
Tian Ma *Rhizoma Gastrodiae Elatae* 10 g
Bai Ji Li *Fructus Tribulli Terrestris* 10 g
Zhi Gan Cao *Radix Glycyrrhizae Preparata* 3 g

Explanations:
- Shu Di Huang, Dang Gui, Bai Shao, Chuan Xiong, Huang Jing and He Shou Wu benefit kidney-jing, tonify and nourish blood and relieve dizziness.
- Tian Ma and Bai Ji Li benefit the head and relieve dizziness.
- Zhi Gan Cao harmonizes the herbs in the prescription.

Herbal Remedy:
Gui Pi Wan-*Restore the Spleen Pill.*

Acupuncture Treatment:
- Zusanli ST-36, Sanyinjiao SP-6, Taichong LIV-3, Ququan LIV-8, Taixi KID-3, Yingu KID-10, Xuanzhong GB-39 and Shenmen HE-7, Tinghui GB-2, Shuaigu GB-8, Baihui DU-20, Extra Taiyang, Extra Yintang.
- An even method is applied on LIV-3, Extra Taiyang and Extra Yintang.
- A tonifying method is applied to the rest points.

Explanations:
- ST-36, the he-sea point of the stomach channel, and SP-6, the crossing point of three yin channels of the foot, activate the spleen and stomach, tonify qi and blood and relieve dizziness.

- Since kidney-jing and blood share the same origin and benefit each other constantly, some points should be used to tonify kidney-jing to tonify blood. KID-3, the yuan-source point of the kidney channel, LIV-8 and KID-10, the he-sea point of the liver channel and kidney channel respectively, tonify blood and jing at the same time, relieve the general fatigue and weakness so as to relieve headache.
- GB-39, the influential point for marrow, benefits blood and relieves blood deficiency.
- DU-20 benefits the head and relieves dizziness.
- GB-2, GB-8, Extra Taiyang and Extra Yintang benefit the head, harmonize the collateral and relieve dizziness.
- LIV-3, the yuan-source point of the liver channel, and HE-7, the yuan-source point of the heart channel, promote qi and blood circulation, calm the shen, improve sleep and relieve dizziness.

11.16 Diarrhea

COVID-19 is a respiratory disease caused by SARS-CoV-2 infection. Although the most common symptoms of COVID-19 are fever, tiredness, a dry cough and myalgia, some patients may develop gastrointestinal symptoms such as diarrhea, loss of appetite, or vomiting even in the absence of other flu-like symptoms.

Diarrhea is the condition characterized by the frequent passage of loose, soft and unformed or watery stools. It could be accompanied by abdominal pain, cramp or distension, nausea, vomiting, poor appetite, weakness, fatigue, and weight loss, etc. Although most cases of acute diarrhea's are self-curing, chronic diarrhea may be a sign of some serious health problems.

Diarrhea isn't a very common symptom of COVID-19. It can be an early sign of COVID-19, starting on the first day of infection and building in intensity during the first week. One finding points out that in some cases, the digestive symptoms, particularly diarrhea, can be the initial presentation of COVID-19. The patient may later or never present with respiratory symptoms or fever.[102] The findings are important because those without classic symptoms of COVID-19, such as fever, dry cough, shortness of breath and myalgia, may go undiagnosed and could potentially spread the illness to others.

The likelihood of having diarrhea increases with age. 10% of children, 21% of adults aged 16–35 and around 30% of adults aged over 35 experience diarrhea during their illness. Only 2% of people who were ill with COVID-19 reported diarrhea as their only symptom.[103] Another systematic review and meta-analysis of 23 published and 6 preprint studies found that approximately 12% of patients with COVID-19 infection reported gastrointestinal symptoms, including diarrhea, nausea, and vomiting.[104] One finding says that diarrhea rate is 34% in the study.[105] Several factors could be responsible for variation in the prevalence of diarrhea in these studies. Documentation of Gastrointestinal (GI) symptoms at the time of hospitalization, high suspicion, and early recognition, and if patients are treated either in an outpatient or inpatient basis, could be responsible for this variation.[106]

Diarrhea usually lasts for an average of two to three days but can last up to seven days in adults in the acute COVID phase. Some

---

[102] Chaoqun Han, *et al.* Digestive symptoms in COVID-19 patients with mild disease severity: Clinical presentation, stool viral RNA testing, and outcomes. *Am J Gastroenterol.* 2020, 115(6): 916–923. doi: 10.14309/ajg.0000000000000664.

[103] ZOE Health Study. Is diarrhea a symptom of COVID-19? 1 April 2021. https://covid.joinzoe.com/post/covid-symptoms-diarrhea.

[104] Sravanthi Parasa, *et al.* Prevalence of gastrointestinal symptoms and fecal viral shedding in patients with coronavirus disease 2019: A systematic review and meta-analysis. *JAMA Netw Open.* 2020; 3(6): e2011335. doi: 10.1001/jamanetworkopen.2020.11335.

[105] Lei Pan, *et al. op. cit.*

[106] Abhilash Perisetti, *et al.* Prevalence, mechanisms, and implications of gastrointestinal symptoms in COVID-19. *Front Med—Gastroenterology.* 2020, 7: 588711. https://doi.org/10.3389/fmed.2020.588711.

people can suffer from ongoing bouts of COVID-related diarrhea, and these are commonly reported in people with Long COVID syndrome. During the survivors' acute COVID-19 phase, a mean of 4.8 months after acute-phase recovery, half had experienced diarrhea and about 25% reported having nausea. Loose stool was the predominant GI symptom that appeared more frequently among survivors versus controls—numerically almost twice as common.[107]

In terms of the mechanism of diarrhea due to COVID-19, it is believed that because the virus attaches to and enters cells through angiotensin-converting enzyme 2 (ACE2), which has significantly higher expression in the Small Intestine than the lung, and the gastrointestinal tract may play a key role in the infectivity of COVID-19.[108] Some researchers say that SARS-CoV uses the angiotensin-converting enzyme 2 (ACE2) and the serine protease TMPRSS2 for S protein priming. ACE2 and TMPRSS2 are not only expressed in the lung, but also in the small intestinal epithelia. ACE2 is expressed furthermore in the upper oesophagus, liver, and colon.[109]

Current treatment in modern medicine is supportive. It has been noticed that early extensive use of antibacterial and antiviral drugs could also lead to diarrhea in patients. Thus, treatment options for COVID-19 patients should be promptly adjusted.[110]

---

[107]John Gever. GI disruption lasts for months in many COVID survivors-persistently loose stools were most common after-effect. *MedPage Today*. 24 May 2021. https://www.medpagetoday.com/meetingcoverage/ddw/92766.

[108]Arno R. Bourgonje, *et al*. Angiotensin-converting enzyme 2 (ACE2), SARS-CoV-2 and the pathophysiology of coronavirus disease 2019 (COVID-19). *The Journal of Pathology*. 2020, 251(3): 228–248. https://doi.org/10.1002/path.5471.

[109]Ferdinando D'Amico, *et al*. Diarrhea during COVID-19 infection: Pathogenesis, epidemiology, prevention, and management. *Clin Gastroenterol Hepatol*. 2020, 18(8): 1663–1672. doi: 10.1016/j.cgh.2020.04.001.

[110]Qing Ye, *et al*. The mechanism and treatment of gastrointestinal symptoms in patients with COVID-19. *Am J Physiol — Gastrointest Liver Physiol*. 2020, 319: G245–G252. doi: 10.1152/ajpgi.00148.2020.

11.16.1 TCM understanding of Long COVID-associated diarrhea

In TCM's view, diarrhea is mainly caused by the disturbed transportation and transformation of the spleen, resulting in a mixture of water and food and the formation of damp-phlegm in the large intestine. It is related to the disorder in the stomach, heart, San Jiao, liver and kidney. The remaining external pathogenic factors, accumulation of damp-phlegm in the spleen, disharmony between the liver and spleen, and deficiency of qi and yang, etc, are the common factors in TCM for diarrhea related to Long COVID.

11.16.1.1 *Incomplete elimination of external pathogenic factors*

Although COVID-19 is mainly caused by the invasion of cold-damp or damp-heat with a pestilent toxin to the lung and heart, some other internal zang-fu organs can also be affected, such as the spleen, stomach and large intestine. When these pathogenic factors are not eliminated completely or in time, they could cause stagnation and latent accumulation in these organs, resulting in dysfunction of transportation, the transformation of the spleen, and diarrhea occurs.

11.16.1.2 *Emotional disturbance*

Severe emotional disturbance, including stress, excessive anger, sadness, over worrying, and frustration during COVID-19 could impair the free flow of the qi in the liver, resulting in stagnation of liver-qi and spleen-qi. According to the Five Elements theory, the Wood (liver) controls the Earth (spleen). When there is severe stagnation of liver-qi, the liver could over control the spleen, leading to disturbance of the spleen in transportation and transformation, which in turn could cause diarrhea.

11.16.1.3 *Accumulation of damp-phlegm*

The stomach and spleen are in charge of the acceptation, transportation and transformation of water and food to produce qi and blood in the body. Intake of unhygienic food, overeating of fatty and greasy food, too much alcoholic drinks, overeating of raw materials, irregular intake of diet, as well as intake of high dosage of antiviral drugs or antibiotics prior to or during COVID-19 could cause dysfunction of stomach and spleen, resulting in the formation of damp-phlegm. A mixture of damp-phlegm in the large intestine could result in diarrhea.

Dysfunction of the spleen and stomach, on the other hand, will affect the formation of qi, leading to weakness of the large intestine in transportation and formation of stool, thus loose stool or diarrhea occurs.

11.16.1.4 *Deficiency of qi or yang*

Prolonged persistence of COVID-19 could cause over consumption of the qi and yang in the body, resulting in weakness of the qi or yang in different zang-fu organs in dealing with water metabolism. Therefore, the transportation, transformation and vaporization will be impaired, resulting in the formation of damp-phlegm in the body. A mixture of water, damp-phlegm and stool in the large intestine may result in diarrhea. For instance, when there is a deficiency of qi and yang of the spleen and stomach, there would be diarrhea, accompanied by cold hands and feet, aversion to cold, and abdominal swelling, etc.

The heart is a fire organ according to the Five Elements theory in TCM. Deficiency of qi and yang of the heart could cause the failure of the spleen and stomach to be warmed and stimulated. Thus, the transportation and transformation of the spleen and stomach will be impaired, and diarrhea occurs.

The kidney is an organ, which contains both yin and yang. kidney-yang could also warm the spleen in physiology. In case of deficiency of kidney-yang (qi), the spleen will not be properly warmed and supported, the physiological functions of the spleen will be impaired, and diarrhea happens.

Constitutional weakness prior to COVID-19, especially weakness in the spleen and kidney, could cause constitutional damp-phlegm accumulation in the spleen or constitutional qi or yang deficiency in the kidney, thus diarrhea occurs.

11.16.2 TCM treatment of Long COVID-associated diarrhea

Diarrhea is in fact a natural way for the body to get rid of possible toxins and some pathogenic factors. Remaining or suppressing toxins may lead to serious complications.

Besides TCM treatment, it is encouraged to inform the patients to pay some attention to having a balanced diet, such as trying to avoid overly sweet and greasy foods, drinking enough water to avoid dehydration, eating well-cooked food with good nutritional value, adding aromatic herbs to create a good smell, and choosing a variety of food. In this way, the color, smell, and appearance of food could stimulate the appetite and activate the spleen and stomach.

11.16.2.1 *Incomplete elimination of cold-damp*

Remaining diarrhea since COVID-19, abdominal cramp, pain and distension, nausea or vomiting, poor appetite, preference to warmth, alleviation of abdominal pain and cramp by warmth, absence of thirst, sensitivity to cold and humid weather, occasional myalgia and headache, heaviness of the body and four limbs, a thin, white, and slightly greasy tongue coating, and a slippery pulse.

Principal of Treatment:
Eliminate external damp, harmonize the spleen and stomach, and relieve diarrhea.

Herbal Treatment:
Huo Xiang Zheng Qi San-*Agastache Powder to Rectify the Qi.*

Huo Xiang *Herba Agastaches seu Pogostemi* 10 g
Hou Po *Cortex Magnoliae Officinalis* 10 g
Cang Zhu *Rhizoma Atractylodis* 10 g
Zi Su Ye *Folium Perillae Frutescentis* 10 g
Bai Zhu *Rhizoma Atractylodis Macrocephalae* 10 g
Fu Ling *Sclerotium Poriae Cocos* 15 g
Zhi Ke *Fructus Citri Aurantii* 10 g
Zhi Ban Xia *Rhizoma Pinelliae Ternatae* 10 g
Chen Pi *Pericarpium Citri Reticulatae* 5 g
Gan Jiang *Rhizoma Zingiberis Officinalis* 5 g
Zhi Gan Cao *Radix Glycyrrhizae Preparata* 3 g

Explanations:
- Huo Xiang and Zi Su Ye eliminate the remaining external pathogenic disturbance, resolve damp-phlegm, harmonize the middle Jiao and relieve diarrhea.
- Hou Po, Cang Zhu and Zhi Ke promote qi circulation in the middle Jiao, resolve damp and regulate the ascending and descending functions of the qi in the spleen and stomach to harmonize the transportation and transformation.
- Zhi Ban Xia, Chen Pi, Fu Ling and Zhi Gan Cao, the complete composition of Er Chen Tang, resolve damp, eliminate phlegm, and relieve diarrhea.
- Bai Zhu and Gan Jiang activate the spleen and stomach, eliminate cold and warm the middle Jiao to stop diarrhea.

Herbal Remedy:
Huo Xiang Zheng Qi Wan-*Agastache Pill to Rectify the Qi.*

Acupuncture Treatment:
- Waiguan SJ-5 + Zulinqi GB-41, Lieque LU-7, Hegu L.I.-4, Fengchi GB-20, Neiguan P-6, Sanyinjiao SP-6, Yinlingquan SP-9 and Tianshu ST-25.

- An even method is applied to SJ-5 + GB-41 and a reducing method is applied to the rest of the points.
- Moxibustion is advisable to be applied on LU-7, L.I.-4, SP-9 and ST-25.

Explanations:
- A combination of SJ-5 + GB-41 regulates the Yangwei and Dai channels and eliminates the remaining pathogenic factors in the body.
- L.I.-4, the yuan-source point of the large intestine channel, and LU-7, the luo-connecting point of the lung channel, dispel damp, regulate the large intestine functions, relieve the external symptoms, and stop diarrhea.
- GB-20 calms the shen, promotes qi circulation, eliminates the remaining pathogenic factors at the upper parts of the body and relieves headaches.
- SP-6, the crossing point of three yin channels of the foot, SP-9, the he-sea point of the spleen channel, and ST-25, the front-mu point of the large intestine, eliminate damp, resolve phlegm in the body and stop diarrhea.
- P-6 harmonizes the stomach, regulates and improves digestion.
- Moxibustion is used to strengthen the effect of these points to dispel wind-damp and relieve diarrhea.

11.16.2.2 *Accumulation of damp-phlegm in the spleen*

Diarrhea with loose stool or watery diarrhea, a possible mixture of stool with sticky phlegm, tiredness, heaviness of the general body, heaviness in the head or in the four limbs, stomach and abdomen, poor appetite, clammy hands, somnolence, obesity, sometimes aversion to cold, greasy coating on the tongue, and a slippery pulse.

Principle of Treatment:
Activate the spleen, promote the qi transformation, resolve damp-phlegm, and relieve diarrhea.

Herbal Treatment:
Cang Fu Dao Tan Tang-*Atractylodes, Poria Phlegm-Dissipating Decoction.*

Cang Zhu *Rhizoma Atractylodis* 10 g
Zhi Shi *Fructus Immaturus Citri Aurantii* 10 g
Fu Ling *Sclerotium Poriae Cocos* 15 g
Zhi Ban Xia *Rhizoma Pinelliae Ternatae* 10 g
Chen Pi *Pericarpium Citri Reticulatae* 5 g
Shan Yao *Radix Dioscoreae Oppositae* 10 g
Bai Zhu *Rhizoma Atractylodis Macrocephalae* 10 g
Zhi Ke *Fructus Citri Aurantii* 10 g
Mu Xiang *Radix Aucklandiae Lappae* 10 g
Bian Dou *Semen Dolichoris Lablab* 10 g
Yi Yi Ren *Semen Coicis Lachryma-Jobi* 10 g
Zhi Gan Cao *Radix Glycyrrhizae Preparata* 3 g

Explanations:
- Cang Zhu and Zhi Shi strongly eliminate damp-phlegm, promote qi circulation, and relieve diarrhea.
- Zhi Ban Xia, Chen Pi, Fu Ling and Zhi Gan Cao, the composition of Er Chen Tang, eliminate damp, resolve phlegm, harmonize the middle Jiao and relieve diarrhea.
- Bai Zhu, Shan Yao, Yi Yi Ren and Bian Dou activate the spleen, eliminate damp, and relieve diarrhea.
- Mu Xiang and Zhi Ke promote qi circulation in the middle Jiao and relieve diarrhea.

Herbal Remedy:
Shen Ling Bai Zhu Wan-*Ginseng, Poria and Atractylodis Macrocephalae Pill.*

Acupuncture Treatment:
- Taibai SP-3, Sanyinjiao SP-6, Yinlingquan SP-9, Zusanli ST-36, Fenglong ST-40, Zhongwan REN-12, Hegu L.I.-4, Taichong LIV-3, Zhangmen LIV-13, Pishu BL-20 and Weishu Bl-21.

- A tonifying method is applied to SP-3, SP-6, ST-36, LIV-13, BL-20 and BL-21. A reducing method is applied to the rest of the points.

Explanations:
- SP-3 and SP-6, the yuan-source point of the spleen channel and the crossing point of the three yin channels of the foot respectively, ST-36, the he-sea point of the stomach channel, LIV-13, the front-mu point of the spleen, BL-20 and BL-21, the back-shu point of the spleen and stomach respectively, activate the spleen and stomach, promote the physiological functions of these two organs, tonify qi, eliminate damp-phlegm and relieve the diarrhea.
- SP-9, the he-sea point of the spleen channel, ST-40 and REN-12, the luo-connecting point of the stomach channel and the front-mu point of the stomach respectively, eliminate damp-phlegm in spleen and stomach and stop the diarrhea.
- L.I.-4 and LIV-3, the yuan-source point of the large intestine channel and liver channel respectively, promote the qi circulation in the body and relieve the fullness and heaviness in the body.

11.16.2.3 *Disharmony between the liver and spleen*

Diarrhea since COVID-19 onset, aggravation of diarrhea when nervous and stressed, irritability, abdominal distension and pain before diarrhea, frequent discharge of flatus, nausea, belching, acid reflux which can be triggered or aggravated by stress, frustration, headache, insomnia, poor appetite, thin and white coating on the tongue, and a wiry pulse.

Principal of Treatment:
Smooth the liver, harmonize the spleen, regulate the qi circulation, and stop diarrhea.

Herbal Treatment:
Tong Xie Yao Fang-*Important Formula for Painful Diarrhea.*

Chai Hu *Radix Bupleuri* 6 g
Bai Zhu *Rhizoma Atractylodis Macrociphalae* 10 g
Bai Shao Yao *Radix Paeoniae Alba* 10 g
Chen Pi *Pericarpium Citri Reticulatae* 5 g
Fang Feng *Radix Ledebouriellae* 5 g
Xiang Fu *Rhizoma Cyperi* 10 g
Mu Xiang *Radix Aucklandiae Lappae* 10 g
Shan Yao *Radix Dioscoreae Oppositae* 10 g
Yan Hu Suo *Rhizoma Corydalis* 10 g
Zhi Gan Cao *Radix Glycyrrhizae Preparata* 3 g

Explanations:
- Chai Hu and Bai Shao Yao, entering the liver and its channel, smooth the liver and relieve stagnation of liver-qi. Bai Zhu and Shan Yao, entering the spleen, activate and strengthen the spleen, dry damp, and resolve phlegm to relieve diarrhea. These four herbs regulate the function of the liver and spleen and build up the new balance between these two organs.
- Invasion of the spleen by the liver could cause disturbance of the spleen in transportation and transformation, and stagnation of qi together with formation of damp-phlegm. Xiang Fu, Mu Xiang, Yan Hu Suo, Chen Pi and Fang Feng regulate the qi in the middle Jiao and liver, stop abdominal pain, dry damp-phlegm and relieve diarrhea.
- Zhi Gan Cao is used to harmonize the prescription.

Herbal Remedy:
Chai Hu Shu Gan Wan-*Bupleurum Pill to Spread the Liver,* plus
Shen Ling Bai Zhu Wan-*Ginseng, Poria and Atractylodis Macrocephalae Pill.*

Acupuncture Treatment:
- Neiguan P-6 + Gongsun SP-4, Hegu L.I.-4, Shenmen HE-7, Taichong LIV-3, Zhangmen LIV-13, Qimen LIV-14, Yanglingquan GB-34, Tianshu ST-25, Zusanli ST-36, Taibai SP-3, Sanyinjiao SP-6, Ganshu BL-18 and Pishu BL-20.

- An even method is applied on P-6 + SP-4, a reducing method is applied on L.I.-4, HE-7, LIV-3, LIV-14, GB-34, BL-18, and ST-25, and a tonifying method is applied on LIV-13, ST-36, SP-3, SP-6 and BL-20.

Explanations:
- A combination of P-6 + SP-4 regulates emotion, smooths the liver, and promotes digestion.
- L.I.-4 and LIV-3, the yuan-source point of the large intestine channel and liver channel respectively, LIV-14, the front-mu point of the liver, GB-34, the he-sea point of the gallbladder channel, and BL-18, the back-shu point of the liver, smooth the liver, promote the circulation of liver-qi and sedate the abdominal pain.
- HE-7, the yuan-source point of the heart channel, regulates emotion, calms the shen and improves sleep.
- ST-25, the front-mu point of the large intestine, restores the physiological functions of the large intestine and relieves diarrhea.
- ST-36, the he-sea point of the stomach channel, LIV-13, the front-mu point of the spleen, SP-3 and SP-6, the yuan-source point of the spleen channel and the crossing point of the three yin channels of the foot respectively, and BL-20, the back-shu point of the spleen, activate the spleen, eliminate damp, and relieve the diarrhea.

11.16.2.4 *Deficiency of spleen-qi*

Intermittent occurrence of diarrhea after COVID-19, aggravation of diarrhea when eating raw, cold, and greasy food, dull pain in the abdomen which may be relieved by warmth or by pressure and aggravated by cold or hunger and fatigue, lassitude, aversion to cold, fatigue, pale complexion, low voice, poor appetite, thin and white coating on the tongue, pale tongue with some tooth marks, and a deep, weak, and thready pulse.

Principal of Treatment:
Tonify qi, activate the spleen and relieve diarrhea.

Herbal Treatment:
Si Jun Zi Tang-*Four Gentlemen Decoction.*

Dang Shen *Radix Codonopsis Pilosulae* 10 g
Bai Zhu *Rhizoma Atractylodis Macrocephalae* 10 g
Fu Ling *Sclerotium Poriae Cocos* 15 g
Chen Pi *Pericarpium Citri Reticulatae* 5 g
Zhi Ban Xia *Rhizoma Pinelliae Praeparatae* 10 g
Mu Xiang *Radix Aucklandiae* 10 g
Sha Ren *Fructus Amomi* 3 g
Zhi Gan Cao *Radix Glycyrrhizae Praeparata* 3 g

Explanations:
- Dang Shen, Bai Zhu, Fu Ling and Zhi Gan Cao, the complete composition of Si Jun Zi Tang, tonifies spleen-qi, activates the spleen and stomach and relieves diarrhea.
- Zhi Ban Xia and Chen Pi harmonize stomach-qi, transform phlegm and relieve diarrhea.
- Mu Xiang and Sha Ren promote qi circulation in the middle Jiao and relieve the pain and distension in the abdomen.

Herbal Remedy:
Si Jun Zi Pian-*Four Gentlemen Tablets.*

Acupuncture Treatment:
- Zusanli ST-36, Taibai SP-3, Pishu BL-20, Weishu BL-21, Qihai REN-6, Tianshu ST-25, Sanyinjiao SP-6 and Yinlingquan SP-9.
- A tonifying method is applied on ST-36, SP-3, BL-20, BL-21, REN-6, and Sanyinjiao SP-6. A reducing method is applied on ST-25 and SP-9.
- Moxibustion is applied on ST-36 and REN-6.

Explanations:
- ST-36, the low he-sea point of the stomach and the he-sea point of the stomach channel, SP-3, the yuan-source point of the spleen

channel, SP-6, the crossing point of the three yin channels of the foot, BL-20, and BL-21, the back-shu point of spleen and stomach respectively, tonify qi, activate the spleen and stomach, eliminate damp, and relieve diarrhea.

- SP-9, the he-sea point of the spleen channel, and ST-25, the front-mu point of the large intestine, eliminate damp-phlegm, regulate the large intestine, and relieve diarrhea.
- REN-6 tonifies qi in the body and strengthens the body.
- Moxibustion warms the stomach and spleen and eliminates interior cold in the body.

11.16.2.5 *Deficiency of yang of the spleen and kidney*

Persistent diarrhea after COVID-19, often having diarrhea before dawn, undigested food particles in the stool, aversion to cold, lower back pain, low libido, frequent clear urination, extreme cold hands, feet and abdomen, extreme tiredness, poor appetite, immediate diarrhea after eating raw and cold food, a thin, white and wet tongue coating, and a deep, thready and slow pulse.

Principal of Treatment:
Warm the spleen, tonify the kidney-yang and relieve diarrhea.

Herbal Treatment:
Si Shen Wan-*Four Miracle Pill.*

Rou Dou Kou *Semen Myristicae Fragrantis* 5 g
Wu Zhu Yu *Fructus Evodiae Rutaecarpae* 10 g
Gan Jiang *Rhizoma Zingiberis Officinalis* 10 g
Wu Wei Zi *Fructus Schisandrae Chinensis* 10 g
Bu Gu Zhi *Fructus Psoraleae Corylifoliae* 10 g
Dang Shen *Radix Codonopsis Pilosulae* 10 g
Shan Yao *Radix Dioscoreae Oppositae* 10 g
Fu Ling *Sclerotium Poriae Cocos* 15 g
Bian Dou *Semen Dolichoris Lablab* 10 g

Explanations:

- Rou Dou Kou and Bu Gu Zhi warm and tonify kidney-yang and dispel cold in the body.
- Wu Zhu Yu and Gan Jiang warm the spleen and eliminate interior cold in the middle Jiao.
- Dang Shen, Shan Yao, Fu Ling and Bian Dou tonify and activate the spleen and stomach, eliminate damp, and relieve diarrhea.
- Wu Wei Zi stops diarrhea.

Herbal Remedy:
Si Shen Wan-*Four Miracle Pill.*

Acupuncture Treatment:

- Guanyuan REN-4, Qihai REN-6, Taixi KID-3, Yingu KID-10, Pishu BL-20, Shenshu BL-23, Tianshu ST-25, Zusanli ST-36, Taibai SP-3 and Yinlingquan SP-9.
- A tonifying method is applied on REN-4, REN-6, KID-3, KID-10, ST-36, SP-3, BL-20 and BL-23. A reducing method is applied on ST-25 and SP-9.
- Moxibustion is applied on REN-4, REN-6 and ST-36.

Explanations:

- KID-3 and KID-10, the yuan-source point and the he-sea point of the kidney channel respectively, and BL-23, the back-shu point of the kidney, tonify the kidney and promote the physiological functions of the kidney.
- REN-4 and REN-6 with moxa strongly tonify the kidney, reinforce kidney-qi and kidney-yang and eliminate interior cold in the body.
- ST-36 and SP-3, the he-sea point of the stomach channel and the yuan-source point of the spleen channel respectively, and BL-20, the back-shu point of the spleen, activate the spleen, tonify the spleen and stomach, eliminate damp-phlegm and relieve the diarrhea.
- ST-25 and SP-9, the front-mu point of the large intestine and the he-sea point of the spleen channel respectively, eliminate damp-phlegm and relieve the diarrhea.

- Moxibustion warms the body, tonifies yang of the spleen and kidney and eliminates interior cold.

11.16.2.6 *Deficiency of yang of the heart and spleen*

Diarrhea during COVID-19, palpitations, cold and painful sensation in the chest, aversion to cold, somnolence, cold hands and feet, loose stool or watery stools, abdominal pain and cold feeling, poor appetite, muscle weakness, a thin, white and wet tongue coating, and a thready, deep, and weak pulse.

Principle of Treatment:
Tonify qi, warm heart-yang, activate the spleen and relieve diarrhea.

Herbal Treatment:
Gui Zhi Gan Cao Tang-*Cinnamon and Glycyrrhizae Decoction,* plus Shen Ling Bai Zhu San-*Ginseng, Poria and Atractylodis Macrocephalae Powder.*

Gui Zhi *Ramulus Cinnamomi Cassiae* 10 g
Zhi Gan Cao *Radix Glycyrrhizae Praeparata* 5 g
Dang Shen *Radix Codonopsis Pilosulae* 10 g
Huang Qi *Radix Astragali Membranacei* 10 g
Bai Zhu *Rhizoma Atractylodis Macrocephalae* 10 g
Fu Ling *Sclerotium Poriae Cocos* 15 g
Shan Yao *Radix Dioscoreae Oppositae* 10 g
Gan Jiang *Rhizoma Zingiberis Officinalis* 10 g
Bian Dou *Semen Dolichoris Lablab* 10 g

Explanations:
- Gui Zhi and Zhi Gan Cao warm the heart, strengthen the heart, and eliminate interior cold.
- Dang Shen, Bai Zhu, Fu Ling and Bian Dou activate the spleen, tonify the spleen-qi and the general body, and relieve diarrhea.

- Gan Jiang warms the spleen and eliminates cold in the middle Jiao.
- Huang Qi and Shan Yao activate the spleen, tonify spleen-qi, and relieve diarrhea.

Herbal Remedy:
Li Zhong Wan-*Pill to Regulate the Middle.*

Acupuncture Treatment:
- Guanyuan REN-4, Qihai REN-6, Zusanli ST-36, Zhangmen LIV-13, Taibai SP-3, Sanyinjiao SP-6, Shenmen HE-7, Tianshu ST-25, Xinshu BL-15, Pishu BL-20, and Shenshu BL-23.
- A tonifying method is applied on REN-4, REN-6, ST-36, LIV-13, SP-3, SP-6, HE-7, BL-15, BL-20, and BL-23. An even method is applied on ST-25.
- Moxibustion is applied on REN-4, REN-6, and ST-36.

Explanations:
- REN-4 and REN-6 tonify the yuan-qi in the body, warm yang, eliminate interior cold and strengthen the body.
- ST-36, the he-sea point of the stomach channel, SP-3 and SP-6, the yuan-source point and the crossing point of three yin channels of the feet, LIV-13, the front-mu point of the spleen, and BL-20, the back-shu point of the spleen, tonify and activate the spleen and stomach, eliminate interior cold and relieve diarrhea.
- HE-7 and BL-15, the yuan-source point of the heart channel and the back-shu point of the heart respectively, tonify qi and yang of the heart and strengthen the heart.
- BL-23, the back-shu point of the kidney, warms the kidney, tonifies qi and yang of the kidney and eliminates interior cold.
- ST-25, the front-mu point of the large intestine, regulates the large intestine and relieves diarrhea.
- Moxibustion warms the qi and yang of the body and eliminates interior cold.

11.17 Psychological and Neuropsychiatric Disorders

Since the first case of novel coronavirus (SARS-CoV-2) disease (COVID-19) was officially diagnosed and reported in December 2019, the pandemic has led to the loss of many lives and a huge impact on the global economy. Under the extraordinary circumstance of the pandemic, all aspects of our life—social, economic, and cultural—have been affected. Apart from the physical effects of the virus—in which various organs and systems are attacked and damaged—the neurological system can also be affected regardless of the mental health of all age groups. Various psychological problems and associated symptoms arise, including anxiety, depression, loneliness, frustration, upset, fury, insomnia, headache, restlessness, and mild cognitive impairment. Many survivors of COVID-19 infection report the resulting stigma, leading to a huge negative impact on their psychological health. There may also be overwhelming worries about recession, unemployment, debt, and subsequent alcoholic abuse in adults. Children may suffer from nervousness, hyperactive behavior and lack of concentration which affects their studies during lockdown and home-schooling. Due to this psychological impact, COVID-19 survivors can face more challenges that the disease brings to their health. No matter mild or severe symptoms, during the ongoing or the recovery stage of the infection, these influences of the infection on people's mental state are of sufficient importance, that require immediate attention for preventative management and useful intervention. We are not the only ones sharing the concern over this ongoing issue. Mental Health UK has issued psychological first aid guidance from the very beginning of the outbreak.[111] In fact, even if all the intense symptoms of the infection subside, it is not the end of the story. The recovery phase of COVID-19 has proved to be a long journey for many people. In the recent SAGE UK government meeting regarding COVID-19 as of 7 May 2020, minutes of the meeting noted "the

---

[111] Mental Health UK. Managing your mental health during the coronavirus outbreak. https://mentalhealth-uk.org/help-and-information/covid-19-and-your-mental-health/.

existence of the long-term health sequelae, including fatigue, breathing difficulty, memory loss, post-intensive care syndrome, flashback and emotional distress".[112]

"People's lives will not be the same after the COVID-19". NHS officers recognized that the National Health Service is facing the challenge to help patients of post-COVID-19 struggle back to their ordinary life.

There are different approaches to deal with these psychological and neuropsychiatric problems. Besides conventional methods, TCM provides another option, and has a long history and profound wisdom in dealing with these conditions. Although individual contexts of Western and Chinese medicine over the disorders are totally different, their theories and interpretations could be used to bridge the gaps between these two systems to understand and treat post-COVID neuropsychiatric disorders (PCND).

While SARS-CoV-2 is still sweeping across the globe, our understanding of COVID-19 is developing day by day. As part of this, the symptoms of neuropsychiatric disorders are raising growing concerns of medical professionals, and yet, due to the complexity of the neuropsychiatric system, post-COVID-19 patients are left with very few options in terms of treatment. We have reason to be concerned that COVID-19 may lead to severe and long-lasting neuropsychiatric suffering for patients. Without proper management and treatment of these symptoms, patients face a difficult, painful, and prolonged recovery physically and mentally.

Previous influenza pandemics have been associated with long-lasting neuropsychiatric consequences.[113] A systematic review[114] of

---

[112] Stephen Matthews. Coronavirus patients can suffer from shortness of breath and fatigue for MONTHS after their battle with the disease, government scientists warn. *Mail Online*. 1 June 2020. https://www.dailymail.co.uk/news/article-8375747/Coronavirus-patients-suffer-shortness-breath-fatigue-MONTHS.html.

[113] Adrianna P. Kępińska, *et al.* Schizophrenia and influenza at the centenary of the 1918–1919 Spanish influenza pandemic: Mechanisms of psychosis risk. *Front. Psychiatry.* 2020, 11: 72. http://doi.org/10.3389/fpsyt.2020.00072.

[114] Jonathan P. Rogers, *et al.* Psychiatric and neuropsychiatric presentations associated with severe coronavirus infections: A systematic review and meta-analysis with

SARS and MERS infection shows that almost one in three hospitalized cases went on to develop post-traumatic stress disorder (PTSD), rates of depression and anxiety were at roughly 15% one year after the illness, and more than 15% of patients also complained of fatigue, mood swings and sleep disorders. Although based on SARS and MERS, this review suggests a clear prospect over the potential future of post-COVID psychiatric symptoms. The possible impact of COVID-19 on neuropsychiatric system may include several aspects below.

- Psychological effects

As a global emergent event, this pandemic obviously holds a wider social impact. The governmental rulings, including physical distancing measures and quarantine can adversely affect the infected and non-infected population.[115,116] Reactions of the population include widespread anxiety, social isolation, high levels of stress particularly amongst healthcare and other essential workers,[117] and concerns over unemployment and financial difficulties.[118] Those infected by the virus tend to suffer even more, with fears about the outcome of

---

comparison to the COVID-19 pandemic. *The Lancet Psychiatry.* 2020, 7(7): 611–627. doi: 10.1016/S2215-0366(20)30203-0.

[115]Joseph A Lewnard and Nathan C Lo. Scientific and ethical basis for social-distancing interventions against COVID-19. *The Lancet Infect Dis.* 2020, 20(6): 631–633. doi: 10.1016/S1473-3099(20)30190-0.

[116]Samantha K. Brooks, *et al.* The psychological impact of quarantine and how to reduce it: Rapid review of the evidence. *The Lancet.* 2020, 395(10227): 912–920. https://doi.org/10.1016/S0140-6736(20)30460-8.

[117]Neil Greenberg, *et al.* Managing mental health challenges faced by healthcare workers during COVID-19 pandemic. *BMJ.* 2020, 368. https://doi.org/10.1136/bmj.m1211.

[118]Covadonga Chaves, *et al.* The impact of economic recessions on depression and individual and social well-being: The case of Spain (2006–2013). *Soc Psychiatry Psychiatr Epidemiol.* 2018, 53(9): 977–986. doi: 10.1007/s00127-018-1558-2.

their illness,[119] stigma,[120] and amnesia or traumatic memories of severe illness.[121]

• Central nervous system damage

It is estimated that more than one-third of patients with COVID-19 develop neuropsychiatric symptoms, including headache, paresthesia, and disturbed consciousness. Severe neuropsychiatric symptoms seem to be associated with more severe disease.[122] Although there is not yet adequate evidence to prove what exactly COVID-19 does to the Central Nerve System (CNS), reports suggest that the virus can enter the nervous system and cause damage to the brain and relevant nerves. In a recent case series in France, out of 58 patients under ICU care, 84% developed neuropsychiatric symptoms, including agitation, confusion, and dysexecutive syndrome of various prevalence.[123] It is also reported that up to 88% of patients developed anosmia or ageusia, thought to be secondary to invasion of the olfactory bulb by the virus, suggesting brain involvement.[124] A case series from Wuhan demonstrated that at least 20% of patients who eventually died from

---

[119]Yu-Tao Xiang, *et al*. Timely mental health care for the 2019 novel coronavirus outbreak is urgently needed. *The Lancet Psychiatry*. 2020, 7(3): 228–229. doi: 10.1016/S2215-0366(20)30046-8.

[120]Judy Yuen-man Siu. The SARS-associated stigma of SARS victims in the post-SARS era of Hong Kong. *Qual Health Res*. 2008, 18(6): 729–738. doi: 10.1177/1049732308318372.

[121]Christina Jones, *et al*. Psychological morbidity following critical illness—The rationale for care after intensive care. *Clin Intensive Care*. 1998, 9(5): 199–205. https://doi.org/10.3109/tcic.9.5.199.205.

[122]Ling Mao, *et al*. Neurologic manifestations of hospitalized patients with coronavirus disease 2019 in Wuhan, China. *JAMA Neurol*. 2020: E1–E8. doi: 10.1001/jamaneurol.2020.1127.

[123]Julie Helms, *et al*. Neurologic features in severe SARS-CoV-2 infection. *N Engl J Med*. 2020, 382: 2268–2270. doi: 10.1056/NEJMc2008597.

[124]Jerome R. Lechien, *et al*. Olfactory and gustatory dysfunctions as a clinical presentation of mild-to-moderate forms of the coronavirus disease (COVID-19): a multicenter European study. *Eur Arch Otorhinolaryngol*. 2020, 17: 13. doi: 10.1007/s00405-020-05965-1.

COVID-19 had evidence of encephalopathy.[125] The direct or indirect damage caused by the virus to the brain and nervous system will not disappear immediately even after all the symptoms of infection subside. We believe the process of recovery and repair of the brain and nervous system determines partially the severity and duration of the neuropsychiatric symptoms.

- Inflammatory and antiviral defense effect

In addition to contributing to the progression of the immune response against viral infection, cytokines activate the hypothalamic-pituitary-adrenal (HPA) axis, resulting in the release of adrenal glucocorticoids. In all, although there is not enough evidence to support that inflammatory reaction of the immune system has a direct impact on the brain and neuropsychiatric system, the subsequent result with cytokine storm (happening with many severe cases), can have profound and severe influence on patients physically and mentally. In the end the suffering as a result from the infection is complex.

- Neuro-endocrine impact

The stress experienced by patients facing severe illness hugely impacts the progress of the disease and their mental health. When Long COVID associated stress responses are triggered, the activation of the neuroendocrine HPA stress axis and the renin-angiotensin-aldosterone system (RAAS—an aspect of the endocrine system involved in the regulation of blood pressure and fluid balance) plays an important part in somatic psychiatric disturbance.[126] Angiotensin-converting enzyme 2 (ACE2) has been shown to have an effect on stress responses and anxiety. In COVID-19 patients, expression of ACE2 has been noted not only in the respiratory tract, lung, ileum,

---

[125] Guang Chen, *et al.* Clinical and immunological features of severe and moderate coronavirus disease 2019. *J Clin Invest.* 2020, 130(5): 2620–2629. doi: 10.1172/JCI137244.

[126] Haibo Zhang, *et al.* Angiotensin-converting enzyme 2 (ACE2) as a SARS-CoV-2 receptor: Molecular mechanisms and potential therapeutic target. *Intensive Care Med.* 2020, 46: 586–590. doi: 10.1007/s00134-020-05985-9.

bladder, esophagus, heart, and kidney, but also in the hypothalamus, pituitary and adrenal glands.[127,128] It is worth mentioning that in SARS patients, after the lung, the adrenal and pituitary glands showed the highest concentration of virus particles,[129] making it clear that the hypothalamic-pituitary-adrenal (HPA) axis is targeted during coronavirus infection. In such cases a tailored treatment to rebalance the HPA axis will help reduce patients' stress and anxiety level.

11.17.1 TCM understanding of Long COVID-associated psychological and neuropsychiatric disorders

As the encounter of humans with COVID-19 outbreak develops, we are facing the challenge of conflict between the soaring demand for healing and the limited knowledge about the disease. The psychological and neuropsychiatric sufferings of patients in the recovery stage of the disease tends to become clear when survivors emerge from the acute stage. While there is still a lot of uncertainty about the exact mechanism of the symptoms in modern medicine, we have searched TCM literature to help outline a framework that acupuncture treatment can resolve post-COVID symptoms.

TCM holds that a human being is composed of three important interacting aspects: xing (形, physical body and internal organs), qi (气, vital energy) and shen (神, mind, spirit).

- The xing, which is the body, provides the core of life activities, supplying essential substances of qi, blood, body fluids and jing

---

[127] Xin Zou, *et al.* Single-cell RNA-seq data analysis on the receptor ACE2 expression reveals the potential risk of different human organs vulnerable to 2019-nCoV infection. *Front Med.* 2020, 14(2): 185–192. doi: 10.1007/s11684-020-0754-0.

[128] Qiufeng Lv, *et al.* Effects of taurine on ACE, ACE2 and HSP70 expression of hypothalamic-pituitary-adrenal axis in stress-induced hypertensive rats. *Adv Exp Med Biol.* 2017, 975(Pt 2): 871–886. doi: 10.1007/978-94-024-1079-2_69.

[129] Yanqing Ding, *et al.* Organ distribution of severe acute respiratory syndrome (SARS) associated coronavirus (SARS-CoV) in SARS patients: Implications for pathogenesis and virus transmission pathways. *J Pathol.* 2004, 203: 622–630. doi: 10.1002/path.1560.

(essence) to provide stable support to the function of qi and shen. Xing determines the reaction of shen as well as the repair of impaired qi and shen.

- Qi moves constantly through the body to connect the shen and xing and enable communication. The proper distribution, circulation and physiological functions of qi link up the zang-fu (internal organs), along with the various body structures, tissues and channels, and the expression of emotions and mental state.
- Shen determines our mental state, our response to emotional stimulus, and crucially influences all physiological activities by affecting the movement of qi, influencing sleep, thought and consciousness. Shen is also a manifestation of the xing with its foundation in the zang-fu organs, with which it communicates through qi.

SARS-CoV-2 infection is characterized by an aggressive pathogenesis and a rapidly progressing, multi-dimensional and toxic nature. It can rapidly collapse into multiple internal organs and systems, creating a mixture of complications involving multiple dysfunctions. Post-COVID-19 psychological and neuropsychiatric disorders feature a mixture of disorders affecting the xing, qi and shen from the beginning until the end of the disease, which can last long after recovery from the initial infections. In this sense we can conclude that attempting to treat these disorders without consideration of a full picture, including the zang-fu, qi and shen, is likely to bring about poor and limited effects.

11.17.1.1 *Disorders of xing*

As COVID-19 progresses, the invasion of wind, cold-damp with toxic heat into the channels adversely affects the zang-fu. It initially impairs the lung, spleen and San Jiao, but quickly penetrates further to damage the heart (pericardium), liver and kidney at the severe and critical stage. All these conditions could lead to neuropsychiatric manifestations.

The main function of the lung is to disperse and descend qi in respiration. Lung is one of the major organs attacked by SARS-CoV-2, resulting in failure of dispersing and descending of the qi. In addition, being the upper source of the water metabolism system in the body, as well as a prime minister, assisting the emperor (the heart), the lung is to assist the heart's function on blood circulation. Meanwhile, the lung is responsible for promoting the qi circulation in the body. Being a Metal Element, it controls the liver Wood. When the lung loses its function to disperse the qi and to regulate the liver, it could cause stagnation of qi in the liver and in the general body. Therefore, if impaired, lung can contribute to sadness and tearfulness, chest tightness and breath-related anxiety and restlessness, along with signs of impeded qi and blood stagnation. In some cases, it can be related to anger and frustration due to the failure of Metal lung's proper control over the Wood liver.

The spleen is in charge of transportation and transformation of food and fluid, providing the production of qi and blood. According to the Five Elements theory, the spleen is associated with the Earth Element, the mother of metal lung. When the spleen fails in transportation and transformation, the resulting accumulation of phlegm and damp may end up in the lung. Moreover, due to the close relationship between the spleen, liver and kidney, dysfunction of the spleen can eventually lead to featuring mental and emotional symptoms, such as lassitude-related depression, loss of interest in life and mental fatigue, repetitive patterns of negative emotions such as frequent recalling of traumatic memories. Impaired concentration and attention may occur too.

The San Jiao is the passageway for yuan (original) qi and water. It also belongs to Shaoyang and is associated with the gallbladder and liver. The emotional symptoms of Shaoyang patterns are irritability and anger, bitter taste in the mouth, restlessness, anxiety, insomnia with difficulty falling asleep or repetitive waking at the same time through night, nightmares, depression with a stiff and heavy body, and waking in morning with symptoms better after exercise. As stated in *Su Wen* (Simple Questions) Chapter 8, "The gallbladder is responsible for what is exact and just; determination and decision stem from it". The gallbladder is thus not only involved in making right decisions, but also provides courage and initiative, and works with the liver to process appropriate responses toward changes in external circumstances. The gallbladder also helps an individual observe and live by guiding principles. The pandemic lockdown in many countries, in which the free movement and social contact of people was reduced for an unexpectedly long period, could in turn trigger an emotional response from the gallbladder, including frustration and lack of courage for life and future. Symptoms such as the lack of assertiveness and judgment, hesitation, timidity, poor self-image and fear,[130] can present as a result of the gallbladder failing its role as the pivot within the Shaoyang function, especially when the exterior pathology is yet not resolved.

At any stage, whether early or during the critical stages, the heart can be involved. The heart is regarded as the emperor in TCM, ruling the physiological functions of all the zang-fu organs, especially as it oversees blood circulation and regulating of the blood vessels. Impairment of the heart can cause blood stasis in various organs, tissues, and channels, leading to pain. As the heart is associated with the fire phase, when it is affected by heat/fire along with yin depletion, it causes hyperactivity of fire throughout the body, including heat in blood. Symptoms of heart disharmony are over-excitement, heart-racing associated anxiety, restlessness and panic attacks, insomnia with difficulty falling asleep, and in severe cases, delirium. On the other hand, the depletion of heart-qi/yang due to the impact of lingering cold-damp can evolve into Shaoyin disharmony, characterized by extreme tiredness, aversion to cold, water retention, low spirit, somnolence, and pressured speech. The heart governs the mind/shen, including all mental/emotional activities, therefore the functions of the brain and neuropsychiatric system overlap with

---

[130]John Stan. A "curious organ"—The gallbladder. *Eastern Currents*. 1 May 2017. https://www.easterncurrents.ca/for-practitioners/practitioners%27-news/eastern-currents-news/2017/05/01/a-curious-organ---the-gallbladder.

this function. In order to restore the balance of the mental state in cases of post-COVID-19 disease, it is often necessary to focus on replenishing heart yin, qi and yang, and promote blood circulation.

The liver is responsible for the smooth movement of qi, the storage and regulation of blood and hormone systems in the whole body. Moreover, the liver manages the smooth expression of emotions via its qi-regulating function. Liver impairment can lead to mental and emotional disorders. On the other hand, intense or prolonged emotional imbalances can cause impairment of the liver. Plus, the liver-wood is the mother of heart-fire and the organ responsible to assist the functions of the spleen. In terms of mental and emotional symptoms, liver dysfunction is characterized by anger, frustration, aggression, resentment, irritability, anxiety, and panic attacks and is also associated with hormonal disturbance and irregularity. From this context we can see clearly that in TCM, the liver is closely associated with the autonomous nervous and neuropsychiatric system. Working on liver's balance will benefit the quicker and better re-stabilization of psychological and neuropsychiatric disorders.

The kidney can be severely depleted by COVID-19, especially during the severe and critical stages of the disease. The kidney is considered as a water organ, located at the lower Jiao and connected with the lung and spleen (the upper and middle sources of water). These three organs govern water metabolism and respiration. The heart and kidney are closely connected via channels and collaterals. Because of this, when both organs are dominated by too much retained water, it could force cold water up the heart, resulting in somnolence, fear, loss of stamina, and loss of memory. When there is pronounced heat in heart, it will burn out the kidney-yin. In return, kidney-yin deficiency will lead to the flare-up of deficient heat and affect the heart-mind, causing emotional instability and sleeping disorders. Moreover, the liver and kidney share the same origin, mutually supporting and affecting each other. When the kidney is impaired, the liver can also be affected, causing bad temper, red eyes and face, headaches and rise of blood pressure. PTSD is one of typical symptoms implying the relevant pathology. Looking into western context, the kidney's function in TCM also includes the function of adrenal glands. In this sense we may bravely conclude that the heart–liver–kidney relation in TCM could be a mirror equivalence of the HPA axis. The COVID-19 mechanism on ACE2 receptors not only has physical, but also neuropsychiatric significance in the TCM interpretation.

11.17.1.2 *Disorder of qi*

Upward, downward, outward and inward are the four directions of qi movement in the body. If qi cannot travel smoothly in these directions, it could be life threatening for the patient. The different movements of qi require proper coordination between the internal organs and channels to maintain a harmonious balance. The emotional state easily affects the movement of qi, while qi stagnation in different zang-fu organs affects the smooth expression of emotion. Moreover, the qi should be sufficient and not in excess. Disorder of qi in movement or in quantity could cause sickness physically and mentally.

The disorder initiated by external diseases is a key factor in disturbing the channel system including the wei, qi, ying and blood. This can affect the xing, resulting in damage and disturbance of zang-fu organs, and disrupt the shen, affecting the brain and neuropsychiatric system. With qi working actively as the connector and conductor between the xing and shen, these disorders can happen separately or simultaneously.

The beginning of qi impairment from COVID-19 infection manifests in the blockage and disturbance of the three yang channels (according to differentiation using the six-channel system), or the wei and qi levels by differentiation of the four-level system. In other words, the exterior level. At this stage, mental and emotional symptoms depend on the different natures of the exterior pathogenic factors and are usually mild to moderate. Wind is associated with mild symptoms of alternating or sudden patterns of emotional changes, like stress. Cold and damp contribute to low spirit and lassitude, depression, or in severe cases, delirium. Heat and fire lead to irritability, restlessness, anxiety, and sleeping difficulties. Of course, the stronger and deeper the pathogenic factors, the more severe the symptoms become. As the disease develops, the qi impairment involves more depletion of qi and other body substances like blood, body fluid, yin and yang and inevitably, the depletion of the xing. It is worth noting that qi impairment can present throughout the whole process, even at the recovery stage of the infection. Because of the rapid progression of COVID-19, the qi disorders of the three yang channels, or wei and qi levels, may coexist with xing impairment. Ignoring the importance of resolving the qi impairment on the exterior may impede the efficiency of TCM treatment. In Western context, the qi impairment state represents the process of the disease when the immune system is most active to fight against the virus. Infective and inflammatory changes and relevant immune activity may persevere for a long time even after the early symptoms disappear. In addition, since the qi and blood are closely related, blockage of qi could cause blood stasis, which provides explanation to why many COVID-19 patients develop thrombosis and CVA. Formation of blood clotting is one of the main pathologies in severe cases of COVID-19. Treatments to promote the qi and blood circulation simultaneously should be considered during the peak of the disease and will also be beneficial at the recovery stage by encouraging the restoration of damages that were done to the internal organs and systems, especially to the brain and neuropsychiatric system.

11.17.1.3 *Disorder of shen*

TCM views the mind and spirit, shen, as an integral part of our health and well-being and cultivation of the spirit is considered essential for health maintenance.

During the pandemic, both infected and non-infected populations are put under a lot of emotional stress, which brought about both psychological and physical impacts. Emotional activity in TCM is classified into joy, anger, grief, melancholy, worry, fear, and fright, widely known as the seven emotions, which can directly affect the zang-fu organs, and disturb the circulation of qi and blood. According to the *Yellow Emperor's Classic of Internal Medicine-Simple*

Questions, anger injures the liver, joy injures the heart, grief and melancholy injures the lung, worry injures the spleen, and fear and fright injure the kidney. It is also stated that anger causes the qi to rise, joy causes it to move slowly, grief drastically consumes it, fear causes it to decline, fright causes it to be deranged, and worry causes it to stagnate. This clearly explains that intense emotions certainly have negative mechanisms on the movement of qi.

TCM also holds that the seven emotions are the expressive reactions of the zang-fu organs toward different stimuli, environment, and pathology. An imbalanced zang-fu organ often dominates the body by its own featuring emotion. To restore a healthy mental and emotional balance, we need to achieve a healthy internal organ system as well as balanced qi circulation. It is this interactive relation between the qi of the emotions and internal organs that forms the foundation for resolution of neuropsychiatric disorders. Therefore, we set out the framework for how shen disorders follow the five-organ sequence below.

The heart is the governor of all the emotions in the body, connecting the physiology of the brain. With the heart overseeing all the mental activities, all emotions go through the monitoring of the heart. Palpitations, insomnia, restlessness, forgetfulness, poor concentration, lack of enthusiasm and vitality, mental depression, and despair are symptoms indicating that the heart is not functioning well. Other emotions such as anger, frustration, anxiety, fear, sadness, and insecurity, are also the erratic patterns indicating the shaking of housing for shen.

The lung is also related to certain emotions, i.e., grief and sadness. Pathological changes of the lung due to COVID-19 can impair its function causing emotional changes. And at same time, overwhelming and lingering grief and sadness can affect the physiological functions of the lung. Social distancing, home isolation, loss of family members, poor or insufficient treatment, lack of adequate and prompt viral test, and uncertainty of future and expectation, etc. are all the possible emotional elements that cause severe disappointment with grief and sadness. This may eventually lead to pressure in the chest, hyperventilation, bad mood, and emotional turmoil.

Spleen impairment due to COVID-19 can manifest in patterns of worrying and brooding, including dwelling, repetitive recalling of traumatic memories, lack of concentration and attention, etc. Research shows that the spleen is now understood to be integral to the sensitization that happens after prolonged stress in mice, leading to anxiety and other cognitive problems down the road.[131]

By ensuring the smooth movement of qi and blood, the liver helps with the proper expression of all emotions. Under the circumstance of the pandemic, people all over the world have been confronted with immense stress and frustration. In particular, frontline healthcare workers have reported despair and frustration. In fact, one quarter to one third of them may suffer from PTSD for a long time.[132] This is a strong demonstration on how the emotional elements affect the liver. The impairment of liver then determines the mental sufferings in a longer term. There is a vicious circle, where stress, frustration and devastation impede liver's qi, which then generates the stagnant heat in liver. Hyperactivity of liver-yang then follows, leading to headache, dizziness, depression, anger, feeling upset, frustration, nervousness, agitation, restlessness, and sleeping disorders over the longer term. In practice, soothing the liver-qi and strengthening liver blood and yin can help to resolve many mental sufferings.

The kidney is closely associated with post traumatic sufferings, manifesting fears, fright, or terror. Meanwhile, fear arises from anxiety over a short or long term. The feeling of insecurity and uncertainty, weak willpower and isolation, lack of power in dealing with an intense change in life or unstable living conditions, can also contribute to the pathology of the kidney. On the other hand, we now

---

[131]Ohio State University. Role of spleen in prolonged anxiety after stress. *Science Daily*. 13 November 2016. https://www.sciencedaily.com/releases/2016/11/161113154748.htm.

[132]Joanne Lusher. COVID-19: Psychological support for healthcare workers during and after the pandemic. *Nursing Management*. 12 May 2020. https://rcni.com/nursing-management/opinion/comment/covid-19-psychological-support-healthcare-workers-during-and-after-pandemic-160991.

know that by strengthening the kidney, the body will be able to tackle and overcome these symptoms much quicker and better.

To summarize, an imbalanced shen can be a factor in COVID-19 disease by disturbing the movement of qi which in turn impairs the xing. However, a healthy and strong internal zang-fu system is the core to maintain a balanced shen. The COVID-19 pandemic certainly brought in a huge challenge on the psychological and neuropsychiatric system, but TCM can be used to identify how the mental/emotional conditions are linked with specific internal organs. TCM's success at treating the relevant psychological and neuropsychiatric symptoms is not achieved only by targeting at the mental symptoms but looking more into balance of the zang-fu balancing and qi regulation.

11.17.2 TCM treatment of Long COVID-associated psychological and neuropsychiatric disorders

11.17.2.1 *The strategy of herbal treatment*

The survivors during Long COVID may suffer from various psychological and neuropsychiatric disorders, such as depression, anxiety, panic, restlessness, aggression, agitation, insomnia and post-traumatic stress disorder (PTSD), etc. This results in not only disturbed thinking, mood swings, the inability to cope with daily tasks, impaired work performance, feelings of worthlessness, delusions, and difficulty relating to others and the society, but also insomnia, fatigue, weakness, lack of appetite, or even a compromised immune system and aggravation of some underlying medical conditions. Psychological and neuropsychiatric disorders, no matter mild or serious, temporary or permanent, are medical conditions that take on many forms and may affect people to varying degrees. In terms of the management of psychological and neuropsychiatric disorders, TCM believes that mental and physical states are not seen as separate entities as they are in Western medicine. Individuals, their specific symptoms and manifestations, their medical histories, and underlying conditions, are all important considerations to improve overall well-being.

From the perspective of TCM, there is often remainder of some external pathogenic factors, such as the accumulation of excessive heat, accumulation of damp-phlegm, disturbance to the zang-fu organs, and deficiency of qi, blood, yin, and yang during Long COVID. TCM treatment aims to eliminate pathogenic excess, tonify the deficiency and restore the balance in zang-fu organs and yin and yang to treat the mental and psychological symptoms. Harmonization between the xing, qi, and shen is always maintained dynamically.

11.17.2.1.1 *Remaining external pathogenic factors*

Difficulty in controlling emotions, persistence of slight dry cough after COVID-19, cough with expectoration of some diluted whitish phlegm, absence of thirst, slight aversion to cold, myalgia, headache, tight pulse, and a thin and whitish tongue coating.

Principle of Treatment:
Dispel wind, eliminate cold-damp, restore the lung-qi, and improve emotions.

Herbal Treatment:
Xing Su San-*Apricot Kernel and Perilla Leaf Powder*, plus
Qiang Huo Sheng Shi Tang-*Notopterygium Decoction to Overcome Damp.*

Jing Jie *Herba seu Flos Schizonepetae Tenuifoliae* 5 g
Fang Feng *Radix Ledebouriellae Divaricatae* 5 g
Xing Ren *Semen Pruni Armeniacae* 10 g
Zi Su Zi *Fructus Perillae Frutescentis* 10 g
Zhi Ban Xia *Rhizoma Pinelliae Ternatae Preparata* 10 g
Chen Pi *Pericarpium Citri Reticulatae* 5 g
Fu Ling *Sclerotium Poriae Cocos* 12 g
Zhi Ke *Fructus Citri Aurantii* 10 g
Qiang Huo *Rhizoma et Radix Notopterygii* 10 g

Gao Ben *Rhizoma et Radix Ligustici* 10 g
Bai Zhi *Radix Angelicae Dahuricae* 10 g
Bai He *Bulbus Lilii* 10 g
He Huan Pi *Cortex Albizziae Julibrissin* 10 g
Yuan Zhi *Radix Polygalae Tenuifoliae* 10 g

Explanations:
- Jing Jie and Fang Feng are applied in combination with Qiang Huo and Gao Ben to dispel the remaining pathogens and relieve external symptoms, such as myalgia, headache, and slight aversion to cold.
- Xing Ren, Zi Su Zi, Zhi Ban Xia, Fu Ling, and Chen Pi are applied to eliminate phlegm and relieve cough.
- Bai Zhi relieves headache and muscle pain.
- Zhi Ke promotes qi circulation in the body and benefits emotions.
- Bai He, He Huan Pi, and Yuan Zhi regulate emotions, calm shen, and improve sleep.

Herbal Remedy:
Zhi Sou San-*Stop Coughing Powder (Granulates)*, plus
An Shen Ding Zhi Wan-*Calm the Shen and Settle the Emotions Pill.*

11.17.2.1.2 *Accumulation of damp-phlegm*

Worrying too much, sadness, fear, diminished appetite, nausea, vomiting, lassitude, swollen epigastric region and abdomen, loose stool, heaviness of body and four limbs, white and greasy tongue coating, and a slippery and wiry pulse.

Principle of Treatment:
Eliminate damp, resolve phlegm, activate the spleen, and improve emotion.

Herbal Treatment:
Ping Wei San-*Calm the Stomach Powder*, plus

Xiang Sha Liu Jun Zi Tang-*Six Gentlemen Decoction with Aucklandia and Amomum.*

Hou Po *Cortex Magnoliae Officinalis* 10 g
Cang Zhu *Rhizoma Atractylodis* 10 g
Chen Pi *Pericarpium Citri Reticulatae* 5 g
Xiang Fu *Rhizoma Cyperi Rotundi* 10 g
Sha Ren *Fructus Amomi* 3 g
Zhi Ban Xia *Rhizoma Pinelliae Ternatae Preparata* 10 g
Dang Shen *Radix Codonopsis Pilosulae* 10 g
Fu Ling *Sclerotium Poriae Cocos* 12 g
Bai Zhu *Rhizoma Atractylodis Macrocephalae* 10 g
He Huan Pi *Cortex Albizziae Julibrissin* 10 g
Yuan Zhi *Radix Polygalae Tenuifoliae* 10 g
Shi Chang Pu *Rhizoma Acori Graminei* 10 g
Shen Qu *Massa Medica Fermentata* 15 g
Jiao Gu Ya *Fructus Oryzae Sativae Germinantus (grill)* 15 g
Zhi Gan Cao *Radix Glycyrrhizae Preparata* 3 g

In case of cold-damp, add Gui Zhi *Ramulus Cinnamomi Cassiae* 10 g and Gan Jiang *Rhizoma Zingiberis Officinalis* 6 g.

In the case of damp-heat, add Huang Lian *Rhizoma Coptidis* 5 g and Zhi Zi *Fructus Gardeniae Jasminoidis* 10 g .

Explanations:
- Hou Po, Cang Zhu, Chen Pi, and Zhi Gan Cao, the complete composition of Ping Wei San, eliminate damp, resolve phlegm, activate the spleen, and improve appetite.
- Dang Shen, Bai Zhu, Fu Ling, Zhi Gan Cao, Zhi Ban Xia, Chen Pi, Xiang Fu, and Sha Ren, the complete composition of Xiang Sha Liu Jun Zi Tang, activate the spleen and stomach, eliminate damp, resolve phlegm, and promote the qi circulation in the spleen and stomach.
- He Huan Pi, Yuan Zhi, and Shi Chang Pu eliminate damp-phlegm, regulate qi circulation and harmonize emotions.
- Shen Qu and Jiao Gu Ya promote digestion and improve appetite.

- Gui Zhi and Gan Jiang warm the spleen and stomach and eliminate cold in the body.
- Huang Lian and Zhi Zi clear heat and eliminate damp in the middle Jiao.

Herbal Remedy:
Xiang Sha Liu Jun Wan-*Six Gentlemen Pill with Aucklandia and Amomum*, plus
An Shen Ding Zhi Wan-*Calm the Shen and Settle the Emotions Pill.*

11.17.2.1.3 *Stagnation of liver-qi*

Depression, unhappiness, mood swings, headache, insomnia, fullness in the chest and epigastric region, belching, acid regurgitation, aggravation of above situations when being nervous, irregular menstruation in women, irritable, thin white coating on the tongue, and a wiry pulse.

Principle of Treatment:
Smooth the liver, promote qi circulation and improve emotions.

Herbal Treatment:
Xiao Yao San-*Rambling Powder.*

Chai Hu *Radix Bupleuri* 10 g
Bai Shao Yao *Radix Paeoniae Lactiflorae* 15 g
Zhi Ke *Fructus Citri Aurantii* 10 g
Dang Gui *Radix Angelicae Sinensis* 10 g
Xiang Fu *Rhizoma Cyperi Rotundi* 10 g
Chen Pi *Pericarpium Citri Reticulatae* 5 g
Sha Ren *Fructus Amomi* 3 g
Bai Zhu *Rhizoma Atractylodis Macrocephalae* 10 g
Shen Qu *Massa Medica Fermentata* 15 g
Jiao Gu Ya *Fructus Oryzae Sativae Germinantus (grill)* 15 g
Fu Shen *Sclerotium Poriae Cocos Paradicis* 12 g

Yuan Zhi *Radix Polygalae Tenuifoliae* 10 g
He Huan Pi *Cortex Albizziae Julibrissin* 10 g

Explanations:
- Chai Hu and Bai Shao Yao smooth the liver and relieve qi stagnation in the liver.
- Zhi Ke, Xiang Fu, Chen Pi, and Sha Ren promote the qi circulation in the middle Jiao and improve the appetite.
- Dang Gui nourishes the liver-blood and benefits the liver.
- Bai Zhu activates the spleen and stomach and improves appetite.
- Shen Qu and Jiao Gu Ya promote digestion and improve appetite.
- Fu Shen, Yuan Zhi, and He Huan Pi smooth emotions, regulate the shen, and improve sleep.

Herbal Remedy:
Xiao Yao Wan-*Rambling Pill*, plus
An Shen Ding Zhi Wan-*Calm the Shen and Settle the Emotions Pill.*

11.17.2.1.4 *Disturbance of heart and gallbladder by damp-heat*

Restlessness, insomnia, difficulty in falling asleep, dream disturbed sleep, mood swings, bitter taste in the mouth, headache, palpitations, fullness of the chest, epigastric discomfort, nausea, poor appetite, thin, yellowish, and greasy tongue coating, and a slippery and rapid pulse.

Principle of Treatment:
Eliminate damp, clear heat, harmonize the gallbladder, and calm the shen.

Herbal Treatment:
Huang Lian Wen Dan Tang-*Warm Gallbladder Decoction with Coptis.*

Huang Lian *Rhizoma Coptidis* 5 g
Zhi Ban Xia *Rhizoma Pinelliae Ternatae Preparata* 10 g
Fu Ling *Sclerotium Poriae Cocos* 12 g
Fu Shen *Sclerotium Poriae Cocos Paradicis* 12 g
Chen Pi *Pericarpium Citri Reticulatae* 5 g
Zhi Shi *Fructus Immaturus Citri Aurantii* 10 g
Zhu Ru *Caulis Bambusae in Taeniis* 10 g
Hou Po *Cortex Magnoliae Officinalis* 10 g
Gua Lou *Fructus Trichosanthis* 10 g
Yuan Zhi *Radix Polygalae Tenuifoliae* 10 g
He Huan Pi *Cortex Albizziae Julibrissin* 10 g
Zhi Gan Cao *Radix Glycyrrhizae Preparata* 3 g

Explanations:
- Zhi Ban Xia, Fu Ling, Chen Pi, and Zhi Gan Cao, the complete compositions of Er Chen Tang, eliminate damp and regulate digestion.
- Zhi Shi, Ru Zhu, Hou Po, and Gua Lou eliminate damp, promote the qi circulation, and benefit the gallbladder.
- Huang Lian clears heat and calms the shen to relieve the restlessness.
- Fu Shen, Yuan Zhi, and He Huan Pi regulate the emotions and calm the shen.

Herbal Remedy:
Wen Dan Tang Ke Li-*Warm Gallbladder Granule.*

11.17.2.1.5 *Deficiency of qi and blood*

Mood swings, anxiety, sadness, excessive worrying, headache with light and empty feeling in the head, tiredness, exhaustion, shortness of breath, forgetfulness, poor appetite, loose stool, lower back pain, aversion to cold, spontaneous sweating, prone to the common cold,

cold peripheral limbs, thin with whitish coating on the tongue, pale tongue, and a weak and thready pulse.

Principle of Treatment:
Tonify qi and blood, benefit jing, strengthen the body and improve emotions.

Herbal Treatment:
Shi Quan Da Bu Tang-*All Inclusive Great Tonifying Decoction.*

Zhi Dang Shen *Radix Codonopsis Pilosulae Praeparata* 10 g
Zhi Huang Qi *Radix Astragali Membranacei Praeparata* 10 g
Shan Yao *Radix Dioscoreae Oppositae* 10 g
Bai Zhu *Rhizoma Atractylodis Macrocephalae* 10 g
Shu Di Huang *Radix Rhemanniae Glutinosae Praeparata* 12 g
Dang Gui *Radix Angelicae Sinensis* 10 g
Wu Wei Zi *Fructus Schisandrae Chinensis* 10 g
Fu Ling *Sclerotium Poriae Cocos* 12 g
Gan Jiang *Rhizoma Zingiberis Officinalis* 5 g
Rou Gui *Cortex Cinnamomi Cassiae* 3 g
He Huan Pi *Cortex Albizziae Julibrissin* 10 g
Duan Long Gu *Os Draconis (calcin)*15 g
Zhi Gan Cao *Radix Glycyrrhizae Preparata* 3 g

Explanations:
• Zhi Dang Shen, Bai Zhu, Fu Ling, and Zhi Gan Cao activate the spleen and tonify the qi in the body.
• Zhi Huang Qi, Shan Yao, and Wu Wei Zi tonify qi, benefit the lung and relieve spontaneous sweating.
• Shu Di Huang and Dang Gui tonify the kidney and benefit jing.
• Gan Jiang and Rou Gui warm the body and dispel the interior cold.
• He Huan Pi and Long Gu calm shen and improve sleep.

Herbal Remedy:
Gui Pi Wan-*Restore the Spleen Pill.*

11.17.2.1.6 *Deficiency of yin*

Slight dry cough or cough with scanty phlegm, thirst, dryness of the throat, night sweating, hotness of the palms and soles, blurred vision, lower back pain, tiredness, dry stools, red tongue, scanty or peeled tongue coating, and a deep, thready, and rapid pulse.

Principle of Treatment:
Nourish yin, promote the production of body fluid, and improve emotion.

Herbal Treatment:
Tian Wang Bu Xin Dan-*Emperor of Heaven's Special Pill to Tonify the Heart.*

Sheng Di Huang *Radix Rehmanniae Glutinosae Recens* 10 g
Tian Men Dong *Tuber Asparagi Cochinchinensis* 10 g
Mai Men Dong *Tuber Ophiopogonis Japonici* 10 g
Xuan Shen *Radix Scrophulariae Ningpoensis* 10 g
Dan Shen *Radix Salviae Miltiorrhizae* 10 g
Bai Shao Yao *Radix Paeoniae Lactiflorae* 10 g
Dang Gui *Radix Angelicae Sinensis* 10 g
Wu Wei Zi *Fructus Schisandrae Chinensis* 10 g
Fu Shen *Sclerotium Poriae Cocos Paradicis* 10 g
Yuan Zhi *Radix Polygalae Tenuifoliae* 10 g
Suan Zao Ren *Semen Zizyphi Spinosae* 10 g
Bai Zi Ren *Semen Biotae Orientalis* 10 g
Zhi Mu *Radix Anemarrhenae Asphodeloidis* 10 g

Explanations:
- Sheng Di Huang, Tian Men Dong, Mai Men Dong, and Wu Wei Zi nourish the yin of the body and clear the deficient heat.
- Xuan Shen and Bai Shao Yao clear deficient heat and smooth the liver.
- Zhi Mu clears deficient heat and relieves night sweating.
- Dang Gui tonifies blood and benefits the yin in the body.

- Dan Shen, Fu Shen, Yuan Zhi, Suan Zao Ren, and Bai Zi Ren clear the heat in the heart, smooth the emotions and improve sleep.

Herbal Remedy:
Tian Wang Bu Xin Dan-*Emperor of Heaven's Special Pill to Tonify the Heart.*

11.17.2.2 *The strategy of acupuncture treatment*

Acupuncture presents a great potential for the treatment of the psychological and neuropsychiatric disorders of post-COVID-19. It is however worth noting that if no attention is paid to treat the root of the illness, acupuncture treatment may not be effective. The appropriate analysis based on syndrome differentiations and root causes, along with dedicated management to stabilize the emotional imbalance are key to successful treatment of the psychological and neuropsychiatric disorders of post-COVID-19. We recommend applying a three-step procedure in treatment: xing adjustment, qi regulation and shen balance.

11.17.2.2.1 *Adjustment of xing*

- **Selection of point for regulation of internal organ**
Although the lung is the organ most obviously involved during COVID-19, it is not the only one attacked. Multiple organs impairments are often found at the various stages, including the spleen, stomach, large intestine, San Jiao, and even the heart, liver and kidney. Therefore, corresponding methods and treatments should be put in place to regulate these organs. The recommendation is noted below.

- **Special category points**
Yuan-source points, he-sea points, Front-mu points, and Back-shu points for relevant affected organs should be directly selected in order to sufficiently support them in time. These points, in general, are seldom applied in the early stage of usual exterior-oriented

illness. However, during COVID-19, it is different since the disease progresses dramatically and life may be in danger within days.

- **Eight extraordinary confluence points**

We also are keen on the eight extraordinary confluence points, especially Neiguan P-6 + Gongsun SP-4 combination, Lieque LU-7+ Zhaohai KID-6 combination, Shenmai BL-62 + Houxi SI-3 and Waiguan SJ-5 + Zulinqi GB-41 combination. These points have multi-dimensional actions on both primary 12 meridians and extraordinary vessels.

- **Selection of point for tonification of zheng-qi**

The COVID-19 pandemic is an unusual disease which does not necessarily start with a constitution of zheng-qi deficiency for the EPFs to fall into. With prevalent destructive power exceeding the body's resistance capacity, it damages, impedes, and depletes the whole system. At the same time, the pre-existing condition of the patient's zheng-qi is extremely important in deciding the progression of COVID-19 as well as the recovery of post-COVID-19. We shall bear in mind that while external pathogenic factors are still present and blocking the way, one should be cautious of tonifying zheng-qi with herbal treatment. Thus, acupuncture to support zheng-qi is always helpful. For post stage COVID-19, supporting treatment for qi and blood may be applied along with methods to eliminate the external pathogens. A good overall restoration of qi and blood in the zang-fu organs will greatly benefit the balance of xing, qi and shen. The most used points to restore the zheng-qi are Qihai Ren-6, Guanyuan Ren-4, Zusanli ST-36, Taixi KID-3, and Sanyinjiao SP-6.

11.17.2.2.2 *Regulation of qi*

- **Selection of points for further eliminating pathogenic factors**

It is generally accepted that COVID-19 is initially caused by invasion of wind, cold and damp mixed with toxic heat. Based on a patient's constitution, lifestyle habits, diet and emotional circumstances, these pathogens can lead to various kinds of pathologies. Treatment to eliminate these pathological factors should be based on stage, including initial stage (minor symptoms under medical observation), clinical treatment stage (confirmed cases of mild and moderate severity), severe and critical condition stage, and convalescence stage.[133]

In terms of acupuncture treatment for post-COVID-19, with the three yang channels being the main lodging place for the pathogenic factors, the Shaoyang (gallbladder and San Jiao) channel is of particular importance, as it is associated with the half-yang half-yin stage that characterizes the lingering aspect of the illness. The Shaoyang channel is also closely related to emotion regulation through the connection between the gallbladder and San Jiao with the liver and pericardium respectively.

- **Selection of point for improving qi and blood circulation**

Due to blockage by external invasion of cold-damp with toxins (or formation of damp-phlegm or heat as a secondary pathology), the disturbance to the circulation of qi and blood can be pronounced and may worsen as the disease evolves further. Promotion of qi and blood circulation can play a very active part in helping with the repair of damage to body organs that COVID-19 causes and building a better connection between the shen and xing. In terms of acupuncture treatment, combinations such as Hegu L.I.-4 + Taichong LIV-3 combination, Yanglingquan GB-34 + Sanyinjiao SP-6 combination, or Geshu BL-17 + Taiyuan LU-9, are commonly used in the treatment of COVID-19 to treat stagnation of qi and blood.

11.17.2.2.3 *Stabilization of shen*

Generally speaking, acupuncture is well known to be effective in stabilizing the mental states. But in the case of COVID-19, acupuncture takes effect not only via the tranquil effect but also help speed up the repair and recovery of the brain and nerve impairment. Disturbance or damages of CNS due to COVID-19 generate many psychiatric symptoms. By giving stimulation directly on local regions

---

[133] Peilin Sun and Wen Sheng Zhou. Acupuncture in the treatment of COVID-19: An exploratory study. *J Chinese Med.* 2020, (123): 14–20.

or remote points of meridians, acupuncture can promote the response of certain cerebral and nerve regions, speed up the local oxygen supply, as well as promote blood circulation.

• Scalp acupuncture

Scalp acupuncture is one of the modern micro-system acupuncture techniques which combine Chinese acupuncture needling methods with western medical knowledge on neuroanatomy, physiology, pathology, and neurology, to allocate the mirror areas on the scalp to the corresponding zones on the cerebral cortex. During the treatment, needles are inserted into the specific stimulating areas on the scalp to achieve the desired therapeutic effects, which is mainly for brain-related conditions, including neurological and psychological conditions.[134]

The treatment principle should be focused on the major damaged areas of the CNS. Scalp acupuncture would be a special technique for the following types of brain-related diseases or symptoms:

- Agitation, confusion, memory loss: Spirit-emotion area, foot-motor sensory area.
- Hyposmia and hypogeusia: Head area (or nose-throat-mouth-tongue area), sensory area lower 2/5.
- Frequent urination: Foot-motor sensory area.

• Selection of Ben Shen points

During the development of acupuncture theory and practice, TCM has established a group of special points for the treatment of mental and emotional disorders that are associated with the zang organs. It could be observed that there are various clinical mental and emotional symptoms of post-COVID-19, involving different zang organs at different stages. Besides emphasizing on the heart in housing the shen, acupuncture also pays attention to the role of the other zang organs and the specific points in association with mind and spirits, including:

---

[134]Jason Jishun Hao and Linda Lingzhi Hao. *Chinese Scalp Acupuncture.* Blue Poppy Press. Boulder, USA. 2011.

○ Shentang BL-44 (Spirit Hall)

This point is responsible for shen, Fire phase, and heart and pericardium organs. It could be used to treat restlessness, nervousness, too much negative concern, hysteria, and agitation, etc.

○ Yishe BL-49 (Thought Home)

This point is responsible for *yi* (Thought), Earth phase, and spleen organ. It could be used to treat nostalgia, excessive worrying about future life, health and financial security, muse, and obsession, etc.

○ Pohu BL-42 (Soul Door)

This point is responsible for *po* (Instinct), Metal phase, and lung organ. It could be used to treat severe sadness over getting sick, someone dying, unemployment, excessive grief and sorrow, and self-pity.

○ Hunmen BL-47 (Courage Gate)

This point is responsible for *hun* (Courage), Wood phase, and liver organ. It could be used to treat depression, irritation, frustration, guilt, grudge, aggression, accusation, self-disapproval, anger, hostility, lack of motivation, bitterness, boredom, and apathy, etc.

○ Zhishi BL-52 (Will Chamber)

This point is responsible for *zhi* (Will), Water phase, and kidney organ. It could be used to treat superior fear, lack of willpower, terror, inferiority, distrust, suspicion, panic, and paranoia, etc.

- **Selection of Ben Shen points**

The idea of a combination of Ghost points comes from ancient analogy that the evil epidemic EPFs are taken as secret and sneaky "ghosts" into human, based on the phenomenon that COVID-19 occurs extremely suddenly and unexpectedly, and that its pathologies and clinical manifestations present drastic change which often leads to urgent treatment within a very short period. In addition, the Ghost points have always been applied as a systematic approach to treat mental diseases as a TCM tradition, especially for severe and complicated cases.

There are 13 Ghost points in total although it is not necessary to apply all these points. We suggest from our clinical experience, three or four Ghost points in the actual practice for post-COVID-19 treatment. Since there is no conscious or coma problem, Shuigou DU-26 (Ghost palace) is often omitted. We recommend using Shaoshang LU-11 (Ghost faith), Yinbai SP-1 (Ghost fortress), and Daling P-7 (Ghost heart).

Although the above techniques and points are traditional methods to deal with post-COVID-19 neuropsychiatric disorders, better effects can only be achieved in combination with different strategies to solve the causative factors with a wider holistic view.

The above three step procedure is to aim at the three aspects of disorders around the pathology of COVID-19 infection. We advise you to follow the three steps in selecting the acupoints for treatment. However, it is not strictly necessary to use all the points in all categories in every treatment. Flexibility based upon differential diagnosis prior to the treatment and patient's response toward the previous treatments shall always be followed as part of the core philosophy of TCM practice.

11.18 Excessive Sweating

Over a year from the onset of the pandemic, the medical world and scientific community are learning more about the long-term complications and effects of COVID-19.

Although the major presentations of Long COVID are fatigue, shortness of breath, muscle pain, joint pain, and cough, excessive sweating can also be a chief symptom related to Long COVID. On 16 July 2021, *National Post* offered information on the symptoms of Long COVID, pointing out that from brain fog to night sweats, Long COVID has more than 200 symptoms.[135]

Everyone may have experienced having wet hands or feet, wet patches from under the arms, and a glistened forehead during hot or

---

[135]Emma Sandri. Brain fog to night sweats: Long COVID has more than 200 symptoms, study finds. *National Post.* 16 July 2021. https://nationalpost.com/news/from-brain-fog-to-night-sweats-long-covid-has-over-200-symptoms-study-finds.

stressful situations, such as physical exercise, high temperatures and wearing overly thick clothes. This form of sweating is a normal and temporary body reaction to an extreme situation to regulate body temperature. However, profuse sweating after slight exertion, or waking up flushed and covered in perspiration are considered as excessive sweating, which is no longer a physical reaction, but a medical condition. Excessive sweating can affect the entire body but usually occurs in the palms, soles, armpits, or groin area since there are a lot of sweat glands.

Excessive sweating of Long COVID, including spontaneous sweating and night sweating, is defined as sweating beyond the physiological need of the body. It is not caused by a rise in temperature or physical activity, and it has no underlying medical cause. This is a common disorder affecting some patients, who have recovered from acute COVID-19 infection.

Spontaneous sweating refers to the condition in which the patients sweat more than they might expect based on the surrounding temperature, the activity level or stress level.

Spontaneous sweating is often associated with fatigue, pale complexion, shortness of breath, poor appetite, aversion to cold, cold hands and feet, etc.

Night sweating during Long COVID is different from spontaneous sweating, which occurs only during the night while sleeping and stops after waking up and is a repeated episode of extreme perspiration that may drench the night clothes or sheets. This includes occasionally waking up after having perspired excessively, particularly if the bedroom is unusually hot or due to wearing too many bedclothes. These episodes are usually not labelled as night sweating. In general, night sweating is often associated with tiredness, hot flush, hotness of palms and soles, restlessness, insomnia, thirst, dry mouth, and stool.

In modern medicine, excessive sweating could be caused by infections, hypoglycemia, hormone disorders, neurologic conditions, menopause, and cancers. When it is associated with fever, weight loss, localized pain, and cough, etc., a further medical investigation should be carried out and certain procedures should be taken to exclude the above diseases.

Excessive sweating not only disrupts daily activities, it can also cause social anxiety and embarrassment. It can also bring about extreme loss of strength and the depletion of minerals and body fluids. Besides, the psychological and emotional impact of excessive sweating due to Long COVID, there can be the creation of social, and psychological problems, leading to a negative influence on the sufferer's quality of life.

11.18.1 TCM understanding of Long COVID-associated excessive sweating

In TCM, sweating is considered an essential substance of the body. Abnormal sweating is classified as the Han Zheng (sweating syndrome). Physiologically, TCM holds that sweating is the body fluid of the heart, and "sweating is that yang works on yin". Pathologically, any excessive or deficient status of yin and yang, disharmony of ying qi (nutrient qi) and wei qi (defensive qi), or accumulation of damp-heat will cause a sweating syndrome.

TCM subdivides sweating syndrome into the following types according to its forms of reaction:

- Zi Han (spontaneous sweating): Continuous sweating, which gets worse after any activity or work.
- Dao Han (night sweating): Sweating that occurs during sleep and stops after waking up.
- Zhan Han (shivering sweating): Sweating with alternate fever and chills, or an aversion to cold.
- Huang Han (yellow sweating): Sweat that looks yellow in color.
- Tuo Han (exhaustive perspiration): Involuntary profuse sweating or greasy sweating with cold limbs and weak breath.

Sweating in TCM can also be divided into different types according to the place of perspiration, such as hand sweating, head sweating, chest sweating, back sweating, and genital sweating, etc. Normally, sweat is colorless and odorless. However, certain food and drugs can cause sweat to have an abnormal color and smell. Besides, changes can also be due to internal disharmonies disturbing the sweating process. For instance, accumulation of internal heat or damp-heat could cause sweating with an offensive smell.

11.18.1.1 *Disturbance of ying and wei systems*

Ying qi and wei qi are associated with skin, muscle, blood, and blood vessels.

The main physiological functions of ying and wei are to warm the skin, moisten the muscle and benefit the blood vessels so as to protect the body from being invaded by pathogenic factors. COVID-19 is mainly caused by the invasion of external pathogenic factors with a pestilent toxin to the body, especially the lung and heart. The lung is connected to the skin and the heart is connected to the blood and blood vessels. Invasion of pathogenic factors during COVID-19 could cause disharmony between the ying and wei systems, leading to failure of the skin and muscles to be properly warmed and the opening of the skin pores to be regulated, thus sweating occurs. During Long COVID, if there are remaining external pathogenic factors, this pathogenic condition may influence the harmonization of the ying and wei systems, resulting in the occurrence of sweating. In this case, the proper treatment to relieve sweating should be focusing on further elimination of external pathogenic factors and harmonization of ying and wei systems.

11.18.1.2 *Deficiency of qi and yin*

When the qi in the body is sufficient, it could protect the body and maintain a consolidation of the skin pores. Prolonged persistence of COVID-19, especially in old and weak patients, the lack of post-COVID-19 care for daily life and diet, and overstrain, etc., could cause consumption of qi, leading to deficiency of qi or even yang, resulting in failure of the qi to maintain a consolidation of the skin, and sweating happens.

Physiologically, yin and yang remain in a balance. However, prolonged sickness of COVID-19 could cause consumption of yin in the body too, leading to the formation of deficient fire. When this deficient fire stirs the blood and body fluid, it may cause fast movement of these materials and escape of body fluid from the body, thus sweating appears.

11.18.1.3 *Accumulation of excessive heat*

Constitutional yang excess, accumulation of heat in the body, having remaining external heat in the body after COVID-19, or dysfunction of the San Jiao in yuan-qi distribution, emotional upset, and disorder in diet, etc., during the recovery of COVID-19, could cause the formation of excessive heat and overactive of yang in the body, which may lead to an imbalance of yin and yang, and sweating occurs.

11.18.1.4 *Formation of damp-heat*

Obesity, lack of care in daily diet (such as overconsumption of alcohol, fatty and sweet food, etc.), before or during COVID-19, could cause the formation of damp-phlegm in the body. When it remains in the body for a long time, it could cause the formation of damp-heat, resulting in the disorder of body fluid in distribution, thus sweating happens.

11.18.2 TCM treatment of Long COVID-associated excessive sweating

11.18.2.1 *Disharmony between ying and wei*

Spontaneous sweating after COVID-19, sensitivity to wind and cold, occasional soreness of the muscles, blocked nose, occasional sneezing, slight running nose with clear discharge, catching a cold easily, white and thin tongue coating, and a slow and soft pulse.

Principle of Treatment:
Harmonize the ying qi and wei qi, regulate the lung and relieve sweating.

Herbal Treatment:
Gui Zhi Jia Long Gu Mu Li Tang-*Cinnamon Twig Decoction, plus Dragon Bone and Oyster Shell.*

Gui Zhi *Ramulus Cinnamomi Cassiae* 10 g
Bai Shao Yao *Radix Paeoniae Lactiflorae* 10 g
Fang Feng *Radix Ledebouriellae Divaricatae* 5 g
Wu Wei Zi *Fructus Schisandrae Chinensis* 10 g
Fu Xiao Mai *Semen Tritici Aestivi Levis* 10 g
Duan Long Gu *Os Draconis (calcin)* 15 g
Duan Mu Li *Concha Ostreae* 15 g
Da Zao *Fructus Zizyphi Jujubae* 5 g
Sheng Jiang *Rhizoma Zingiberis Officinalis Recens 5 g*
Zhi Gan Cao *Radix Glycyrrhizae Preparata* 3 g

Explanations:
- Gui Zhi and Bao Shao Yao are used in combination to harmonize the ying qi and wei qi and regulate the skin and blood vessels.
- Fang Feng opens the skin pores to eliminate the remaining pathogenic factors.
- Wu Wei Zi regulates the ying qi, benefits the yin and arrests sweating.
- Fu Xiao Mai, Duan Long Gu, and Duan Mu Li arrest sweating.
- Da Zao, Sheng Jiang and Zhi Gan Cao assist Gui Zhi and Bai Shao Yao to harmonize the ying qi and wei qi.

Herbal Remedy:
Gui Zhi Jia Long Gu Mu Li Wan-*Cinnamon Twig, plus Dragon Bone and Oyster Shell Pill.*

Acupuncture Treatment:

- Lieque LU-7 + Zhaohai KID-6, Hegu L.I.-4, Waiguan SJ-5, Taiyuan LU-9, Shenmen HE-7, Feishu BL-13, Xinshu BL-15, Zusanli ST-36 and Sanyinjiao SP-6.
- An even method is applied on LU-7 + KID-6, LU-9, BL-13, BL-15, ST-36, and SP-6. A reducing method is applied to L.I.-4 and SJ-5.

Explanations:

- The combination of LU-7 + KID-6, one group of the Eight confluence points, regulates and harmonizes ying qi and wei qi and relieves sweating.
  - L.I.-4, the yuan-source point of the large intestine channel, and Waiguan SJ-5, the luo-connecting point of the San Jiao, regulate the skin pores and eliminate the remaining pathogenic factors.
  - LU-9, the yuan-source point of the lung channel, and BL-13, the back-shu point of the lung, tonify the lung-qi and benefit the physiological functions of the lung to relieve sweating. ST-36 and SP-6, the he-sea point of the stomach channel and the crossing point of three yin channels of foot, tonify qi and blood and benefit the wei qi. HE-7 and BL-15, the yuan-source point of the heart channel and the back-shu point of the heart respectively, strengthen the heart and blood vessels and benefit the ying qi. When these points are used in combination, they could regulate and harmonize the ying qi and wei qi to relieve sweating.

11.18.2.2 *Deficiency of qi*

Spontaneous sweating after COVID-19, fatigue, slight shortness of breath, expectoration of slight white and diluted phlegm which gets worse after any activities, aversion to cold, pale complexion, low voice, lower back pain, poor appetite, aversion to wind and cold, pale tongue with thin and white coating, and a thready, slow, and weak pulse.

Principle of Treatment:
Tonify the qi, regulate the lung, strengthen the spleen and kidney, and relieve sweating.

Herbal Treatment:
Bu Fei Tang-*Tonify the Lungs Decoction,* plus
Yu Ping Feng San-*Jade Windscreen Powder.*

Zhi Huang Qi *Radix Astragali Membranacei Praeparata* 10 g
Fang Feng *Radix Ledebouriellae Divaricatae* 10 g
Jiao Bai Zhu *Rhizoma Atractylodis Macrocephalae (grill)* 10 g
Zhi Dang Shen *Radix Codonopsis Pilosulae Praeparata* 10 g
Shu Di Huang *Radix Rhemanniae Glutinosae Praeparata* 12 g
Wu Wei Zi *Fructus Schisandrae Chinensis* 10 g
Zi Wan *Radix Asteris Tatarici* 10 g
Fu Ling *Sclerotium Poriae Cocos* 12 g
Ma Huang Gen *Radix Ephedrae* 10 g
Fu Xiao Mai *Semen Tritici Aestivi Levis* 10 g
Zhi Gan Cao *Radix Glycyrrhizae Preparata* 3 g

Explanations:
- Zhi Huang Qi, Fang Feng and Jiao Bai Zhu, the complete composition of Yu Ping Feng San, consolidate the skin, tonify the wei qi and improve the resistance to wind and cold.
- Zhi Dang Shen, Bai Zhu, Fu Ling, and Zhi Gan Cao, the complete composition from Si Jun Zi Tang, activate the spleen and tonify the qi in the body.
- Wu Wei Zi and Zi Wan tonify the qi in the lung and benefit the lung.
- Shu Di Huang tonifies the kidney and benefits the lung.
- Ma Huang Gen and Fu Xiao Mai arrest sweating.

Herbal Remedy:
Yu Ping Feng Wan-*Jade Windscreen Pill.*

Acupuncture Treatment:
- Zhongfu LU-1, Lieque LU-7, Chize LU-5, Taiyuan LU-9, Shenmen HE-7, Feishu BL-13, Zusanli ST-36, Sanyinjiao SP-6, Taixi KID-3, Qihai REN-6 and Shenshu BL-23.
- An even method is applied on LU-7 and LU-5, and a tonifying method is applied on the rest of the points. Moxibustion could be applied on ST-36, KID-3 and REN-6.

Explanations:
- LU-1, the front-mu point of the lung, LU-7 and LU-5, the luo-connecting point and the he-sea point of the lung channel respectively, and LU-9, the yuan-source point of the lung channel, and BL-13, the back-shu point of the lung, tonify the qi of the lung, consolidate the skin and restore the physiological functions.
- ST-36, SP-6, REN-6, KID-3 and BL-23 tonify the qi of the spleen and kidney and support the lung-qi.
- HE-7, the yuan-source point of the heart channel, tonifies the heart, regulates the shen and relieves sweating.
- Moxibustion warms the qi and dispels cold in the body.

11.18.2.3 *Deficiency of qi and yin*

Spontaneous and night sweating after COVID-19, tiredness, pale complexion, aversion to cold and warmth, shortness of breath, restlessness, insomnia, nervousness, thirst, dry eyes, throat and stool, a hot sensation in the chest, palms and soles, loose stool, poor appetite, pale tongue, thin and white tongue coating, and a deep, thready, and weak pulse.

Principle of Treatment:
Tonify the qi and yin of the lung and kidney and relieve sweating.

Herbal Treatment:
Bu Fei Tang-*Tonify the Lungs Decoction*, plus
Sheng Mai San-*Generate the Pulse Powder*.

Ren Shen *Radix Ginseng* 10 g
Mai Men Dong *Tuber Ophiopogonis Japonici* 10 g
Wu Wei Zi *Fructus Schisandrae Chinensis* 10 g
Chuan Bei Mu *Bulbus Fritillariae Cirrhosae* 10 g
Jiao Bai Zhu *Rhizoma Atractylodis Macrocephalae (grill)* 10 g
Sheng Di Huang *Radix Rehmanniae Glutinosae Recens* 10 g
Shu Di Huang *Radix Rhemanniae Glutinosae Praeparata* 12 g
Zi Wan *Radix Asteris Tatarici* 10 g
Fu Ling *Sclerotium Poriae Cocos* 12 g
Ma Huang Gen *Radix Ephedrae* 10 g
Fu Xiao Mai *Semen Tritici Aestivi Levis* 10 g
Zhi Gan Cao *Radix Glycyrrhizae Preparata* 3 g

Explanations:
- Ren Shen, Mai Men Dong and Wu Wei Zi, the complete composition of Sheng Mai San, tonify qi and nourish yin of the body.
- Chuan Bei Mu and Zi Wan nourish the yin and benefit the lung. They could also relieve shortness of breath.
- Sheng Di Huang clears deficient heat in the body.
- Ren Shen, Jiao Bai Zhu, Fu Ling, and Zhi Gan Cao, the complete composition of Si Jun Zi Tang, activate the spleen and tonify the qi in the body.
- Shu Di Huang tonifies the kidney and benefits the lung.
- Ma Huang Gen and Fu Xiao Mai arrest sweating.

Herbal Remedy:
Sheng Mai San or Wan-*Generate the Pulse Powder or Pill*.

Acupuncture Treatment:
- Lieque LU-7, Chize LU-5, Taiyuan LU-9, Shenmen HE-7, Feishu BL-13, Zusanli ST-36, Sanyinjiao SP-6, Taixi KID-3, Zhaohai KID-6, Guanyuan REN-4, Qihai REN-6 and Shenshu BL-23.

- An even method is applied on LU-7 and LU-5, and a tonifying method is applied on the rest of the points.

Explanations:
- LU-7 and LU-5, the luo-connecting point and the he-sea point of the lung channel respectively, and LU-9, the yuan-source point of the lung channel, and BL-13, the back-shu point of the lung, tonify qi and yin of the lung, consolidate the skin and restore the physiological functions.
- ST-36, SP-6, REN-4, REN-6, Taixi KID-3, KID-6 and BL-23 tonify the qi of the spleen, benefit the qi and yin of the kidney and support the lung-qi.
- HE-7, the yuan-source point of the heart channel, tonifies the heart, regulates the shen and relieves sweating.

11.18.2.4 *Deficiency of yin with hyperactivity of deficient fire*

Night sweating after COVID-19, hot flush on the face, feverish feeling, restlessness, insomnia, nervousness, thirst, dry eyes, throat and stool, a hot sensation in the chest, palms and soles, irregular menstruation for women, tiredness, red tongue, scanty and peeled tongue coating, and a deep, thready, and rapid pulse.

Principle of Treatment:
Tonify the yin of the lung, liver and kidney, reduce the deficient fire and relieve sweating.

Herbal Treatment:
Dang Gui Liu Huang Tang-*Decoction of Chinese Angelica and Six Yellow Ingredients.*

Huang Lian *Rhizoma Coptidis* 5 g
Huang Qin *Radix Scutellariae Baicalensis* 10 g
Huang Bai *Cortex Phellodendri* 10 g
Dang Gui *Radix Angelicae Sinensis* 10 g

Zhi Huang Qi *Radix Astragali Membranacei Praeparata* 10 g
Sheng Di Huang *Radix Rehmanniae Glutinosae Recens* 12 g
Shu Di Huang *Radix Rhemanniae Glutinosae Praeparata* 12 g
Zhi Mu *Radix Anemarrhenae Asphodeloidis* 10 g
Ma Huang Gen *Radix Ephedrae* 10 g
Duan Mu Li *Concha Ostreae* 15 g

Explanations:
- The first seven herbs form the compositions of Dang Gui Liu Huang Tang, which is applied to nourish the yin and clear deficient heat. It is the treatment to solve the root cause of night sweating.
- Zhi Mu clears deficient heat and relieves the hotness of palms and soles.
- Ma Huang Gen and Duan Mu Li arrest night sweating.

Herbal Remedy:
Dang Gui Liu Huang Wan-*Pill of Chinese Angelica and Six Yellow Ingredients.*

Acupuncture Treatment:
- Lieque LU-7 + Zhaohai KID-6, Chize LU-5, Taiyuan LU-9, Shenmen HE-7, Yinxi HE-6, Laogong P-8, Feishu BL-13, Xinshu BL-15, Sanyinjiao SP-6, Taixi KID-3, Yingu KID-10, Qihai REN-6, and Shenshu BL-23.
- An even method is applied on LU-7 + KID-6, and a tonifying method is applied on the rest of the points.

Explanations:
- LU-7 + KID-6, one of the point combinations from eight confluence points nourishes the yin of the body.
- LU-5, the he-sea point of the lung channel, LU-9, the yuan-source point of the lung channel, and BL-13, the back-shu point of the lung, tonify the yin of the lung, consolidate the skin and restore the physiological functions.
- SP-6, REN-6, KID-3, KID-10 and BL-23 tonify the yin of the kidney and clear deficient heat.

- HE-7 and HE-6, the yuan-source point and the xi-cleft point of the heart channel respectively, P-8, the ying-spring point of the pericardium channel, and BL-15, the back-shu point of the heart, tonify the heart-yin, reduce deficient fire, regulate the shen and relieve sweating.

11.18.2.5 *Accumulation of internal heat*

Profuse sweating after COVID-19, sweating with an offensive smell, thirsty, preference to cold drinks, restlessness, flushed complexion, a hot sensation in the body, constipation, red tongue, yellow and slight dry tongue coating, and a forceful and rapid pulse.

Principle of Treatment:
Clear the internal heat, promote defecation, and relieve sweating.

Herbal Treatment:
Da Huang Huang Qin Xie Xin Tang-*Rhubarb and Scute Decoction to Drain the Epigastrium.*

Huang Qin *Radix Scutellariae Baicalensis* 10 g
Huang Lian *Rhizoma Coptidis* 5 g
Da Huang *Radix et Rhizoma Rhei* 10 g
Zhi Mu *Radix Anemarrhenae Asphodeloidis* 10 g
Sheng Di Huang *Radix Rehmanniae Glutinosae Recens* 12 g
Long Dan Cao *Radix Gentianae Longdancao* 10 g
Sang Ye *Folium Mori Albae* 10 g
Sang Bai Pi *Cortex Mori Albae Radicis* 10 g
Ma Huang Gen *Radix Ephedrae* 10 g
Duan Long Gu *Os Draconis (calcin)* 15 g

Explanations:
- Huang Qin, Huang Lian and Da Huang, the complete composition of Da Huang Huang Qin Xie Xin Tang, promote defecation, clear excessive heat, and reduce fever.
- Zhi Mu and Sheng Di Huang clear heat and remove toxins.

- Long Dan Cao and Sang Ye clear heat in the liver.
- Sang Bai Pi clears heat in the lung.
- Ma Huang Gen and Duan Long Gu arrest sweating.

Herbal Remedy:
Fang Feng Tong Sheng Pian-*Saposhnikovia Pill that Sagely Unblocks*.

Acupuncture Treatment:
- Neiguan P-6 + Gongsun SP-4, Hegu L.I.-4, Quchi L.I.-11, Chize LU-5, Shenmen HE-7, Laogong P-8, Tianshu ST-25, Feishu BL-13, Xinshu BL-15, Sanyinjiao SP-6, Xingjian LIV-2 and Neiting ST-44.
- An even method is applied on P-6 + SP-4, and a reducing method is applied on the rest of the points.

Explanations:
- P-6 + SP-4, one of the point combinations from eight confluence points, regulates the internal organs and clears heat in the body.
- L.I.-4 and L.I.-11, the yuan-source point and the he-sea point of the large intestine channel respectively, ST-25, the front-mu point of the large intestine, ST-44, the ying-spring point of the stomach channel, clear excessive heat and promote defecation.
- LU-5, the he-sea point of the lung channel, and BL-13, the back-shu point of the lung, clear heat in the lung and restore the physiological functions.
- HE-7, the yuan-source point of the heart channel, and P-8, the ying-spring point of the pericardium channel, and BL-15, the back-shu point of the heart, clear heat in the heart and calm the shen to arrest sweating.
- SP-6, the crossing point of three yin channels of the foot, tonifies yin. LIV-2, the ying-spring point of the liver channel, clears heat in the liver.

11.18.2.6 *Accumulation of damp-heat*

Slight sweating after COVID-19 (which is sticky in nature and offensive in smell), thirsty with no desire to drink, slight cough, lassitude, heaviness of the body and head, nausea, poor appetite, loose stools or defecation with a burning sensation in the anus, difficulty in urinating, red tongue, yellow and slight greasy tongue coating, and a slippery and rapid pulse.

Principle of Treatment:
Eliminate damp, clear the heat, regulate the liver and gallbladder, and relieve sweating.

Herbal Treatment:
Hao Qin Qing Dan Tang-*Sweet Wormwood and Scutellaria Decoction to Clear the Gallbladder,* plus
Lian Po Yin-*Coptis and Magnolia Bark Drink.*

Huang Lian *Rhizoma Coptidis* 5 g
Qing Hao *Herba Artemisiae Annuae* 10 g
Huang Qin *Radix Scutellariae Baicalensis* 10 g
Zhi Zi *Fructus Gardeniae Jasminoidis* 10 g
Zhu Ru *Caulis Bambusae in Taeniis* 10 g
Lu Gen *Rhizoma Phragmitis Communis* 10 g
Hou Po *Cortex Magnoliae Officinalis* 10 g
Zhi Ban Xia *Rhizoma Pinelliae Ternatae Preparata* 10 g
Fu Ling *Sclerotium Poriae Cocos* 10 g
Chen Pi *Pericarpium Citri Reticulatae* 5 g

Explanations:
- Qing Hao and Zhi Zi clear damp-heat in the liver and gallbladder.
- Huang Qin clears damp-heat in the upper Jiao and relieves cough.
- Huang Lian, Zhu Ru and Hou Po resolve damp in the middle Jiao, clear heat and descend the stomach-qi.
- Zhi Ban Xia, Fu Ling and Chen Pi eliminate damp-phlegm in the body and relieve cough and nausea.
- Lu Gen clears heat and relieves thirst.

Herbal Remedy:
Hao Qin Qing Dan Tang (Wan)-*Sweet Wormwood and Scutellaria Decoction to Clear the Gallbladder Pill.*

Acupuncture Treatment:
- Neiguan P-6 + Gongsun SP-4, Hegu L.I.-4, Quchi L.I.-11, Yangchi SJ-4, Shenmen HE-7, Zhongwan REN-12, Tianshu ST-25, Fenglong ST-40, Sanyinjiao SP-6, Yinlingquan SP-9, Yanglingquan GB-34, Qiuxu GB-40, and Xingjian LIV-2.

  - An even method is applied on P-6 + SP-4, and a reducing method is applied on the rest of the points.

Explanations:
- The combination of P-6 + SP-4 regulates the internal organs and clears damp-heat in the body.
- L.I.-4 and L.I.-11, the yuan-source point and the he-sea point of the large intestine channel respectively, and ST-25, the front-mu point of the large intestine, clear excessive heat and promote defecation.
- ST-40, the luo-connecting point of the stomach channel, SP-6 and SP-9, the crossing point of the three yin channels of the foot and the he-sea point of the spleen channel respectively, active the spleen and stomach and eliminate damp-heat.
- SJ-4, the yuan-source point of the San Jiao, and REN-12, the gathering point of the fu organs, eliminate damp-heat in the body.
- GB-34 and GB-40, the he-sea point and the yuan-source point of the gallbladder channel respectively, together with LIV-2, the ying-spring point of the liver channel, eliminate damp-heat in the liver and gallbladder.
- HE-7, the yuan-source point of the heart channel, clears heat, calms the shen, and relieves sweating.

11.19 Sleep Disorders

Sleep is a natural state of rest to maintain good health. On one hand, a good night's sleep is essential and vital for individuals of all ages to maintain a healthy condition for the physical body, cognitive reaction, emotional processing, and overall quality of life. On the other hand, physical and mental health could greatly influence the quality of sleep. There are two important issues to be considered for a good sleep: sleep quality and sleep quantity. Sleep quality is usually defined by falling asleep easily and quickly, sleeping straight through the night, waking up no more than once per night and falling asleep again without difficulty, resulting in the person feeling rested, restored, and energized upon waking up in the morning. Sleep quantity often refers to sleeping seven to eight hours per night for adults. According to TCM, sleeping about seven hours per night is a natural cycle. Sleeping for longer or shorter than seven hours a night is not healthy. Unfortunately, it is not always easy for many people to achieve good sleep, especially during the COVID-19 pandemic.

A systematic review showed national rates of insomnia symptoms rise from 20% to 45% during the COVID-19 pandemic.[136] A Chinese study of nearly 57,000 responders to an online survey reported emergent sleep and mental health symptoms from pandemic restrictions: 29.2% for insomnia, 27.9% for depression, 31.6% for anxiety, and 24.4% for acute stress.[137]

Sleep problems appear to be common during the ongoing COVID-19 pandemic. Moreover, sleep problems were found to be associated with higher levels of psychological distress.[138] In one study, a total of 1,733 out of 2,469 discharged patients with COVID-

---

[136] Jude Mary Cénat, *et al.* Prevalence of symptoms of depression, anxiety, insomnia, posttraumatic stress disorder, and psychological distress among populations affected by the COVID-19 pandemic: A systematic review and meta-analysis. *Psychiatr Res.* 2021, 295: 113599. doi: 10.1016/j.psychres.2020.113599.

[137] Le Shi, *et al.* Prevalence of and risk factors associated with mental health symptoms among the general population in China during the coronavirus disease 2019 pandemic. *JAMA Netw Open.* 2020, 3(7): e2014053. doi: 10.1001/jamanetworkopen.2020.14053.

[138] Zainab Alimoradia, *et al.* Sleep problems during COVID-19 pandemic and its' association to psychological distress: A systematic review and meta-analysis. *EClinicalMedicine.* 2021, 36: 100916. https://doi.org/10.1016/j.eclinm.2021.100916.

19 were enrolled after 736 were excluded. Patients had a median age of 57.0 (IQR 47.0–65.0) years and 897(52%) were men. A follow-up study was done from 16 June to 3 September, 2020, and the median follow-up time after symptom onset was 186.0(175.0–199.0) days. Fatigue or muscle weakness (63%, 1038 of 1655) and sleep difficulties (26%, 437 of 1655) were the most common symptoms. Anxiety or depression was reported among 23%(367 of 1617) of patients. At six months after symptom onset, fatigue or muscle weakness and sleep difficulties were the main symptoms of patients who had recovered from COVID-19. Risk of anxiety or depression was an important psychological complication and impaired pulmonary diffusion capacities were higher in patients with more severe illness.[139]

The outbreak of COVID-19 not only caused great public concern, but also brought about huge psychological distress, especially for medical staff. They worried a lot about their health and the health of their families, being afraid of virus contagion and their overall safety. Wang *et al.* reported higher prevalence of sleep problem among medical staff compared to non-medical staff comprising of students, community workers, and volunteers (66.1% vs. 47.8, $p < 0.01$) and frontline healthcare providers compared to non-frontline medical workers (68.1 vs. 64.5, $p = 0.14$).[140] This conclusion is supported by one study. 168 cross-sectional, four case-control, and five longitudinal design papers comprising 345,270 participants from 39 countries were identified. The corrected pool estimated that prevalence of sleep problems was 31% among healthcare professionals, 18% among the general population, and 57% among COVID-19 patients (all p-values < 0.05). Sleep problems were associated with depression among healthcare professionals, the general population, and COVID-19 patients, with Fisher's Z scores of –0.28,

---

[139]Chaolin Huang, *et al. op. cit.*

[140]Wei Wang, *et al.* Sleep disturbance and psychological profiles of medical staff and non-medical staff during the early outbreak of COVID-19 in Hubei Province, China. *Front Psychiatry.* 2020, 11: 733. 2020. https://doi.org/10.3389/fpsyt.2020.00733.

−0.30, and −0.36, respectively. Sleep problems were positively (and moderately) associated with anxiety among healthcare professionals, the general population, and COVID-19 patients, with Fisher's, z scores of 0.55, 0.48, and 0.49, respectively.[141]

Some research attempted to find out the causative factors behind insomnia. One study suggested that insomnia could be related to lower education, where 36.1% of medical staff suffered from insomnia among the 1,563 participants. The insomnia group had more psychological problems related to the COVID-19 outbreak. It was found that low educational level was one risk factor for insomnia. Other factors include being in an isolated environment, worrying about being infected by COVID-19, lack of psychological support from the news or social media regarding the COVID-19 outbreak, and extreme uncertainty regarding effective disease control of the COVID-19 outbreak. The above were all risk factors for insomnia, while being a medical staff was a protective factor. This research mentioned that the risk of insomnia among medical staff with an education level of high school or below was 2.69 times higher than that of those with a doctoral degree.[142] This result was consistent with another insomnia survey of the general population in China that found that a low education level was associated with a high possibility of insomnia.[143] However, one research, conducted during the SARS epidemic, found that sleep quality was not affected by the education level.[144]

---

[141]Zainab Alimoradi, *et al. op. cit.*

[142]Chenxi Zhang, *et al.* Survey of insomnia and related social psychological factors among medical staff involved in the 2019 novel coronavirus disease outbreak. *Front Psychiatry.* 2020, 11: 306. doi: 10.3389/fpsyt.2020.00306.

[143]Yu-Tao Xiang, *et al.* The prevalence of insomnia, its sociodemographic and clinical correlates, and treatment in rural and urban regions of Beijing, China: A general population–based survey. *Sleep.* 2008, 31(12): 1655–1662. doi: 10.1093/sleep/31.12.1655.

[144]Ruey Chen, *et al.* Effects of a SARS prevention programme in Taiwan on nursing staff's anxiety, depression and sleep quality: A longitudinal survey. *Int J Nurs Stud.* 2006, 43(2): 215–225. doi: 10.1016/j.ijnurstu.2005.03.006.

There could be some difference between these factors contributing to insomnia and psychological problems for different populations. For instance, the most important risk factors for insomnia and mental health problems during the COVID-19 pandemic for healthcare workers include a sudden onset of a globally contagious virus. The deadly nature of the viral illness exerts a great pressure on healthcare workers as they must deal with the illness, suffer from the high risk of death, and adapt to irregular work schedules and frequent shifts apart from worrying for themselves and their families. However, non-medical healthcare workers may also have some risk factors for insomnia and mental health problems, such as having an underlying illness, being at risk of contact with COVID-19 infected patients, being a woman living alone or living in rural areas, the uncertainty of future life and financial stability, being afraid of losing family members or friends, etc. Several policies implemented to reduce the spread of COVID-19, such as home isolation, quarantine, curfews, and lockdown could exert some negative influence on people.

Medications may be considered for patients with severe depression or anxiety disorders. Multicomponent interventions include obtaining a comprehensive history, a sleep diary highlighting potential behavioral changes, addressing dysfunctional beliefs, and use of stimulus control, sleep restriction and various relaxation methods based on patient and therapist preferences.[145]

11.19.1 TCM understanding of Long COVID-associated sleep disorders

Sleep disorders in TCM include the following manifestations:

- difficulty in falling asleep
- waking up easily
- superficial sleeping
- dream-disturbed sleeping

---

[145] Philip M. Becker. Overview of sleep management during COVID-19. *Sleep Med.* 2021, 91: 211–218. doi: 10.1016/j.sleep.2021.04.024.

- movement or walking in sleep
- speaking while sleeping
- snoring or apnea
- restlessness leg
- nycturia
- somnolence
- alternative insomnia, etc.

In TCM, the heart is the location where the shen resides, determining the overall vitality of an individual. Besides sleep, the physiological conditions are often observed through thinking, speaking, responses, complexion, and the eyes. To fulfill its physiological functions ultimately, the heart needs to maintain a harmonious relationship with different zang-fu organs. Any disorder in other organs could result in dysfunction of the heart, leading to the occurrence of sleep disorders. During COVID-19 and Long COVID, there are usually dysfunctions of some zang-fu organs, which finally influence the heart. Again, waking at certain hours, such as between 1:00–3:00 am, between 3:00–5:00 am, or between 5 till 7:00 am, all indicate different pathologies and involvement of different organs. For instance, waking between 1:00–3:00 am is typically an indication of a disorder in the liver and could relate to unresolved stress and anger. Waking between 3:00–5:00 am is typically a disorder due to an imbalance in the Metal Element and could relate to unresolved grief or a sense of loss. Waking between 5:00–7:00 am is typically an indication due to an imbalance in the Metal Element and large intestine.

11.19.1.1 *Incomplete elimination of external pathogenic factors*

Invasion of cold-damp or damp-heat with a pestilent toxin to the body during COVID-19 could cause dysfunction of lung, liver, spleen, stomach, San Jiao, and kidney, resulting in disorder in qi and blood circulation, and the heart could eventually be disturbed. When these pathogenic factors are not eliminated completely or in time, they could cause stagnation and latent accumulation in the body, resulting in disturbance and obstruction of the channels and collaterals, qi and blood circulation in the internal zang-fu organs, and sleep disorders happen.

11.19.1.2 *Emotional disturbance*

The liver plays an important role in emotional activities. It regulates qi circulation and stores blood. Overstress, resentment, and frustration during COVID-19 may cause retardation of liver-qi circulation, and stagnation of liver-qi occurs. It could happen to both medical and non-medical persons. Once stagnation of liver-qi occurs, it may influence the physiological functions in other organs. Since the liver is a Wood organ in TCM, which is considered the son of heart. Stagnation of liver-qi could result in dysfunction of the heart, sleep disorders happen.

Qi belongs to the yang energy, which should be in a state of constant movement. In case of prolonged liver-qi stagnation, it may cause the gradual formation of liver-fire. Fire is characterized by uprising and burning. When there is the formation of liver-fire, which rises, it could cause hyperactivity of Fire of the liver and heart, sleep disorders appear, resulting in restlessness, insomnia, palpitations, redness of face and eyes, swelling of eyes, nervousness, irritability, bitter taste in the mouth, red tongue, thin and yellow tongue coating, and a rapid and wiry pulse.

Since qi circulation promotes blood circulation, and qi stagnation results in blood stagnation, stagnation of liver-qi could also cause stagnation of blood in the body. The heart dominates the vessels and promotes blood circulation. Stagnation of blood in the body may cause dysfunction of the heart, and sleep disorders occur.

11.19.1.3 *Accumulation of damp-heat*

Incomplete elimination of damp-heat, various underlying illnesses prior to COVID-19, improper diet during Long COVID (such as alcohol addiction and overeating of fatty and greasy food), could cause accumulation of damp-heat in the body, resulting in disturbance to the heart, and sleep disorders follow.

11.19.1.4 *Deficiency of qi, blood, yin, and yang*

Prolonged persistent or severe COVID-19 symptoms could cause consumption of qi, blood, yin and yang. Besides, the accumulation of damp to the spleen could result in dysfunction of the spleen and stomach. The spleen and stomach are the acquired source for qi and blood production, thus dysfunction of the spleen and stomach during COVID-19 or Long COVID would cause deficiency of qi and blood, leading to failure of the heart to be nourished and supported, and sleep disorders occur.

Improper diets or too little eating during COVID-19 may cause weakness of spleen in transportation and transformation, qi and blood production would be impaired, and deficiency of qi and blood forms.

Deficiency of yin and yang in the body could also eventually cause disturbance to the physiological functions of the heart, sleep disorders happen.

11.19.2 TCM treatment of Long COVID-associated sleep disorders

Sleep is part of the natural rhythm, reflecting the conditions of qi, blood, yin and yang, zang-fu organs, as well pathogenic disturbance. Good sleep could never be obtained only by applying some acupuncture points or herbs to calm the shen. Also, sleep disorders never appear as an individual complaint. Thus, sleep disorders are always managed by means of syndrome differentiation by analyzing the etiologies and pathologies.

11.19.2.1 *Disturbed head by external damp*

Insomnia, feeling sick, slight headache with heavy sensation, sensitivity to weather changes, slight general body pain with heavy sensation, fatigue, thin, white, and greasy tongue coating, and a slippery and superficial pulse.

Principle of Treatment:
Dispel wind, eliminate damp, harmonize the collaterals, and improve sleep.

Herbal Treatment:
Qiang Huo Sheng Shi Tang-*Notopterygium Decoction to Overcome Damp.*

Qiang Huo *Rhizoma seu Radix Notopterygii* 10 g
Du Huo *Radix angelicae Pubescentis* 10 g
Gao Ben *Rhizoma Radix Ligustici* 10 g
Fu Ling *Sclerotium Poriae Cocos* 15 g
Chuan Xiong *Rhizoma Ligustici Chuanxiong* 10 g
Fang Feng *Radix Ledebouriellae* 6 g
Ji Xue Teng *Caulis Milletiae Reticulatae* 10 g
Ye Jiao Teng *Caulis Polygoni Multiflori* 10 g
He Huan Pi *Cortex Albizziae Julibrissin* 10 g
Zhi Gan Cao *Radix Glycyrrhizae Preparata* 3 g

Explanations:
- Qiang Huo, Du Huo and Fang Feng dispel wind, eliminate cold-damp, and relieve remaining external pathogenic factors.
- Chuan Xiong and Gao Ben expel wind, promote qi and blood circulation and relieve headaches.
- Fu Ling dries damp, eliminates phlegm, harmonizes the middle Jiao and improves sleep.
- Ji Xue Teng, Ye Jiao Teng, and He Huan Pi harmonize the collaterals, calm the shen and improve sleep.
- Zhi Gan Cao coordinates the effects of the other herbs in the recipe.

Herbal Remedy:
Qiang Huo Sheng Shi Pian-*Notopterygium Pill to Overcome Damp.*

Acupuncture Treatment:
- Hegu L.I.-4, Lieque LU-7, Waiguan SJ-5, Fengchi GB-20, Sanyinjiao SP-6, Yinlingquan SP-9, Yanglingquan GB-34, Fenglong ST-40, Taichong LIV-3, Neiguan P-6, Shaohai HE-3, Shenmen HE-7 and Extra Sishencong.
- A reducing method is applied on all the points.

Explanations:
- L.I.-4 and LIV-3, the yuan-source point of the large intestine channel and liver channel respectively, and GB-20, the crossing point of the foot Shaoyang and Yangwei channels, regulate qi circulation and relieve pain in the body.
- LU-7 and SJ-5, the luo-connecting point of the lung channel and San Jiao channel respectively, eliminate external pathogenic factors, relieve external symptoms and pain.
- SP-6, the crossing point of three yin channels of the foot, SP-9 and GB-34, the he-sea point of the spleen channel and gallbladder channel respectively, and ST-40, the luo-connecting point of the stomach channel, eliminate damp, promote qi and blood circulation, and activate the spleen and stomach.
- P-6, HE-3, HE-7 and Extra Sishencong regulate the emotions and improve sleep.

11.19.2.2 *Stagnation of qi in the liver and heart*

Sleep disorders, palpitations, occasional pressure in the chest, headache with pressure and tension, always feeling under stress, unstable emotional state, depression, painful neck, distension and pain in the hypochondriac region, insomnia, irregular menstruation in women, poor appetite or overeating, a thin and white tongue coating, and a wiry pulse.

Principle of Treatment:
Smooth the liver, promote qi circulation, calm the shen and improve sleep.

Herbal Treatment:
Xiao Yao San-*Rambling Powder.*

Chai Hu *Radix Bupleare* 10 g
Dang Gui *Radix Angelicae Sinensis* 10 g
Bai Shao Yao *Radix Paeoniae Lactiflorae* 10 g
Zhi Ke *Fructus Citri Aurantii* 10 g
Bai Zhu *Rhizoma Areactylodis Macrocephalae* 10 g
Fu Ling *Sclerotium Poriae Cocos* 15 g
Chuan Xiong *Rhizoma Ligustici Chuan Xiong* 10 g
Huang Qin *Radix Scutellariae Baicalensis* 10 g
Bo He *Herba Menthae Haplocalycis* 3 g
Ye Jiao Teng *Caulis Polygoni Multiflori* 10 g
He Huan Pi *Cortex Albizziae Julibrissin* 10 g
Fu Shen *Sclerotium Poriae Cocos Paradicis* 10 g
Zhi Gan Cao *Radix Glycyrrhizae Preparata* 3 g

Explanations:
- Chai Hu and Bai Shao Yao smooth the liver, promote the qi circulation in the liver and relieve the qi stagnation in the liver.
- Zhi Ke promotes the qi circulation in the body and relieves depression.
- Dang Gui and Chuan Xiong regulate the blood circulation in the liver, harmonize and smooth the liver, and relieve pain in the body.
- In most cases, the spleen and stomach will be invaded when there is stagnation of liver-qi. Bai Zhu and Fu Ling strengthen the spleen and stomach and improve the appetite.
- Huang Qin and Bo He clear internal heat resulting from the stagnation of liver-qi, and prevent further formation of liver-fire.
- Ye Jiao Teng, He Huan Pi and Fu Shen calm the shen and improve sleep.
- Zhi Gan Cao harmonizes the actions of the other herbs.

Herbal Remedy:
Xiao Yao Wan-*Rambling Pill.*

Acupuncture Treatment:
- Waiguan SJ-5 + Zulinqi GB-41, Hegu L.I.-4, Shuaigu GB-8, Fengchi GB-20, Jianjing GB-21, Taichong LIV-3, Qimen LIV-14, Neiguan P-6, Sanyinjiao SP-6, Shaohai HE-3, Shenmen HE-7 and Extra Sishencong.
- An even method is applied on SJ-5 + GB-41, and a reducing method is applied on the rest points.

Explanations:
- SJ-5 + GB-41 is a combination to harmonize Shaoyang channels, benefit the gallbladder and smooth the emotions.
- L.I.-4 and LIV-3, the yuan-source point of the large intestine channel and the liver channel respectively, and LIV-14, the front-mu point of the liver, smooth the liver, regulate the qi circulation in the body and relieve liver-qi stagnation. Meanwhile, they could relieve depression.
- P-6, the luo-connecting point of the pericardium channel, regulates qi circulation and calms the shen.
- HE-3, HE-7 and Extra Sishencong calm the shen, improve sleep and regulate the emotion.
- SP-6, the crossing point of the three yin channels of the foot, promotes the smooth qi and blood circulation in the liver.
- GB-8, GB-20 and GB-21 regulate the collateral of the gallbladder channel, smooth the emotions, relieve the neck tension, and promote qi circulation.

11.19.2.3 *Hyperactivity of fire of the liver and heart*

Sleep disorders, restlessness, palpitations, dream-disturbed sleep, redness of eyes, irritability, bitter taste in the mouth, body pain, irregular menstruation in women, deep yellow urine, constipation, red tongue, and a rapid and wiry pulse.

Principle of Treatment:
Reduce liver-fire, clear heat in the heart, calm the shen and improve sleep.

Herbal Treatment:

Long Dan Xie Gan Tang-*Gentiana Longdancao Decoction to Drain the Liver,* plus
Dao Chi San-*Guide Out the Red Powder.*

Long Dan Cao *Radix Gentianae Anomalae* 10 g
Huang Qin *Radix Scutellariae Baicalensis* 10 g
Zhi Zi *Fructus Gardenniae* 10 g
Ze Xie *Rhizoma Alismatis* 12 g
Chuan Xiong *Rhizoma Lagustici Chuanxiong* 10 g
Xia Ku Cao *Spica Prunellae* 10 g
Dang Gui *Radix Angelicae Sinensis* 10 g
Sheng Di Huang *Radix Rehmanniae Glutinosae Recens* 12 g
Huang Lian *Rhizoma Coptidis* 5 g
Dan Zhu Ye *Herba Lophatheri Gracilis* 10 g
Mu Tong *Caulis Akebiae Trifoliatae* 5 g
He Huan Pi *Cortex Albizziae Julibrissin* 10 g
Fu Shen *Sclerotium Poriae Cocos Paradicis* 10 g
Zhi Gan Cao *Radix Glycyrrhizae Preparata* 3 g

In case of hyperactivity of liver-yang, add Gou Teng *Ramulus cum Uncis Uncariae* 10 g and Tian Ma *Rhizoma Gastrodiae Elatae* 10 g.

Explanations:
- Long Dan Cao, Huang Qin, Xia Ku Cao and Zhi Zi clear heat in the liver, reduce liver-fire and calm the liver.
- Dang Gui and Chuan Xiong promote liver-qi circulation, smooth the liver, regulate blood circulation of blood, and relieve body pain.
- Huang Lian clears heat, reduces heart-fire in the heart and improves sleep.
- Sheng Di, Dan Zhu Ye, Mu Tong, Ze Xie and Zhi Gan Cao clear heat, promote urination and induce fire out of the body through urination.
- Gou Teng and Tian Ma calm the liver and suppress liver-yang.

Herbal Remedy:
Long Dan Xie Gan Wan-*Gentiana Longdancao Pill to Drain the Liver.*

Acupuncture Treatment:
- Waiguan SJ-5 + Zulinqi GB-41, Neiguan P-6 + Gongsun SP-4, Hegu L.I.-4, Shaohai HE-3, Shaofu HE-8, Fengchi GB-20, Jianjing GB-21, Xiaxi GB-43, Baihui DU-20, Xingjian LIV-2, Qimen LIV-14, Sanyinjiao SP-6 and Extra Anmian.
- An even method is applied on SJ-5 + GB-41, P-6 + SP-4, and a reducing method is applied on the rest of the points.

Explanations:
- A combination of SJ-5 + GB-41 harmonizes the Shaoyang channels, benefits the gallbladder, and clears heat in the liver.
- A combination of P-6 + SP-4 promotes the qi circulation and harmonizes the emotion.
- L.I.-4 and LIV-14, the yuan-source point of the large intestine channel and the front-mu point of the liver, smooth the liver, regulate the qi circulation in the body and relieve liver-qi stagnation.
- LIV-2 and GB-43, the ying-spring point of the liver channel and gallbladder channel respectively, and DU-20, clear heat, reduce liver-fire and relieve headache.
- HE-3 and HE-8, the he-sea point and the ying-spring point of the heart channel respectively, clear heat in the heart, calm the shen and improve sleep.
- GB-20 and GB-21 regulate the collateral of the gallbladder channel, smooth the emotions, and relieve the neck tension.
- SP-6, the crossing point of the three yin channels of the foot, and extra Anmian promote the smooth qi and blood circulation in the liver and in the heart and improve sleep.

11.19.2.4 *Stagnation of blood*

Sleep disorders, prolonged persistence of stabbing body pain or headache with fixed location, aggravation of the pain at night, before or during menstruation, dark and purplish menstruation with clots, purplish tongue or purplish spots on the tongue, and a thready or unsmooth pulse.

Principle of Treatment:
Promote circulation of blood, eliminate blood stasis, and improve sleep.

Herbal Treatment:
Tao Hong Si Wu Tang-*Four Substance Decoction with Safflower and Peach Pit.*

Tao Ren *Semen Pruni Persicae* 10 g
Hong Hua *Flos Carhami* 10 g
Dang Gui *Radix angelicae Sinensis* 10 g
Chuan Xiong *Rhizoma LiGustici Chuanxiong* 10 g
Chi Shao Yao *Radix Paeoniae Rubra* 10 g
Dan Shen *Radix Salviae Miltiorrhizae* 10 g
Pu Huang *Pollen Typhae* 10 g
Xiang Fu *Rhizoma Cyperi* 10 g
Zhi Qiao *Fructus Aurantii* 10 g
He Huan Pi *Cortex Albizziae Julibrissin* 10 g
Fu Shen *Sclerotium Poriae Cocos Paradicis* 10 g
Long Gu *Os Draconis* 20 g

Explanations:
- Tao Ren, Hong Hua and Pu Huang promote blood circulation, eliminate blood stasis and relieve body pain.
- Dang Gui, Chuan Xiong, Chi Shao Yao and Dan Shen promote blood circulation, smooth the blood vessels and the collaterals, and relieve body pain and painful menstruation.
- Since qi circulation promotes blood circulation, some herbs to promote qi circulation are prescribed here as well, such as Xiang Fu and Zhi Qiao.
- He Huan Pi, Fu Shen and Long Gu calm the shen and improve sleep.

Herbal Remedy:
Tao Hong Si Wu Tang Pian-Four Substance Tablets with Safflower and Peach Pit.

Acupuncture Treatment:
- Neiguan P-6 + Gongsun SP-4, Hegu L.I.-4, Taiyuan LU-9, Shaohai HE-3, Shenmen HE-7, Geshu BL-17, Sanyinjiao SP-6, Taichong LIV-3, Qimen LIV-14, Xinshu BL-15, and Ganshu BL-18.
- An even method is applied on P-6 + SP-4, and a reducing method is applied to the rest points.

Explanations:
- Qi circulation guides blood circulation. A combination of P-6 + SP-4 is used to promote qi circulation, smooth the emotions, and relieve body pain. Meanwhile, L.I.-4 and LIV-3, the yuan-source point of the large intestine channel and the liver channel respectively, and LIV-14, the front-mu point of the liver, regulate qi circulation to lead to blood circulation and relieve the body pain.
- SP-6, the crossing point of three yin channels of the foot, and BL-17, the influential point of blood, promote blood circulation, eliminate blood stasis, and relieve body pain.
- HE-3 and HE-7, the he-sea point and the yuan-source point of the heart channel respectively, and LU-9, the influential point of the vessel in the body, calm the shen, regulate emotions, promote blood circulation, and relieve body pain.
- BL-15 and BL-18, the back-shu point of the heart and liver respectively, regulate the heart and liver, smooth the emotions, calm the shen and improve sleep.

11.19.2.5 *Disturbance of damp-heat to the gallbladder and heart*

Sleep disorders, restlessness, palpitations, dream-disturbed sleep, bitter taste in the mouth, nausea, red tongue, yellow and greasy tongue coating, and a rapid and wiry pulse.

Principle of Treatment:
Clear heat, eliminate damp, calm the shen and improve sleep.

Herbal Treatment:
Huang Lian Wen Dan Tang-*Warm Gallbladder Decoction with Coptis.*

Huang Lian *Rhizoma Coptidis* 5 g
Zhi Ban Xia *Rhizoma Pinelliae Ternatae* 10 g
Chen Pi *Pericarpium Citri Reticulatae* 5 g
Fu Ling *Sclerotium Poriae Cocos* 15 g
Zhi Shi *Fructus Immaturus Citri Aurantii* 10 g
Zhu Ru *Caulis Bambusae in Taeniis* 10 g
Sheng Di Huang *Radix Rehmanniae Glutinosae Recens* 12 g
Zhi Zi *Fructus Gardenniae* 10 g
He Huan Pi *Cortex Albizziae Julibrissin* 10 g
Fu Shen *Sclerotium Poriae Cocos Paradicis* 10 g
Zhi Gan Cao *Radix Glycyrrhizae Preparata* 3 g

Explanations:
- Huang Lian eliminates damp-heat in the gallbladder and heart, clears the heart-fire and improves sleep.
- Zhi Ban Xia, Chen Pi, Fu Ling and Zhi Gan Cao eliminate damp, resolve phlegm in the body, harmonize the middle Jiao and relieve nausea.
- Zhi Shi and Zhu Ru harmonize the gallbladder and eliminate damp-heat in the body.
- Sheng Di Huang and Zhi Zi clear heat in the heart and eliminate the disturbance to the heart and gallbladder.
- He Huan Pi and Fu Shen calm the shen and improve sleep.

Herbal Remedy:
Huang Lian Wen Dan Pian-*Warm Gallbladder Pill.*

Acupuncture Treatment:

- Waiguan SJ-5 + Zulinqi GB-41, Hegu L.I.-4, Xingjian LIV-2, Qimen LIV-14, Shaohai HE-3, Shaofu HE-8, Fengchi GB-20, Xiaxi GB-43, Sanyinjiao SP-6, Zhongwan REN-12 and Extra Anmian.
- An even method is applied on SJ-5 + GB-41, and a reducing method is applied on the rest of the points.

Explanations:

- A combination of SJ-5 + GB-41 harmonizes the Shaoyang channels, benefits the gallbladder, and clears heat in the liver.
- L.I.-4 and LIV-14, the yuan-source point of the large intestine channel and the front-mu point of the liver, smooth the liver, regulate the qi circulation in the body and relieve liver-qi stagnation.
- LIV-2 and GB-43, the ying-spring point of the liver channel and gallbladder channel respectively, clear heat, reduce fire and relieve the disturbance to the gallbladder.
- LIV-14, the front-mu point of the liver, smooths the liver, promotes qi circulation, and improves emotion.
- HE-3 and HE-8, the he-sea point and the ying-spring point of the heart channel respectively, clear heat in the heart, calm the shen and improve sleep.
- GB-20 regulates the collateral of the gallbladder channel, smooths the emotions, and relieves the neck tension.
- Sanyinjiao SP-6, the crossing point of the three yin channels of the foot, and REN-12, the gathering point of fu organs, eliminate damp-heat in the body, resolve damp and improve sleep.

11.19.2.6 *Deficiency of qi of lung and heart*

Sleep disorders (especially waking easily), aggravation of insomnia after physical exertion, fatigue, general weakness, pale complexion, aversion to cold, cold hands, shortness of breath, spontaneous sweating, loose stools, poor appetite, low voice, thin and white tongue coating, pale tongue with tooth marks, and a slow and deep pulse.

Principle of Treatment:
Activate the spleen and stomach, tonify qi and improve sleep.

Herbal Treatment:
Bai Zi Yang Xin Wan-*Nourish the Heart Pill with Biotae.*

Bai Zi Ren *Semen Biotae Orientalis* 10 g
Dang Shen *Radix Codonopsis Pilosulae* 10 g
Huang Qi *Radix Astragali Membranacea* 10 g
Dang Gui *Radix Angelicae Sinensis* 10 g
Zhi Ban Xia *Rhizoma Pinelliae Ternatae* 10 g
Yuan Zhi *Radix Polygalae Tenuifoliae* 10 g
Suan Zao Ren *Semen Zizyphi Spinosae* 10 g
Ye Jiao Teng *Caulis Polygoni Multiflori* 10 g
Chuan Xiong *Radix Ligustici Wallichii* 10 g
Fu Ling *Clerotium Poriae Cocos* 15 g
Zhi Gan Cao *Radix Glycyrrhizae Praeparata* 3 g

Explanations:
- Dang Shen and Huang Qi tonify the qi of the body and relieve fatigue and general weakness.
- Fu Ling and Zhi Gan Cao activate the spleen and tonify the qi. Meanwhile, Fu Ling could improve sleep.
- Dang Gui and Chuan Xiong tonify blood and benefit the heart.
- Zhi Ban Xia benefits the middle Jiao and improves digestion.
- Bai Zi Ren, Suan Zao Ren, Ye Jiao Teng and Yuan Zhi benefit the heart, improve sleep, and relieve sleep disorders.

Herbal Remedy:
Bai Zi Yang Xin Wan-*Nourish the Heart Pill with Biotae.*

Acupuncture Treatment:
- Zusanli ST-36, Taibai SP-3, Sanyinjiao SP-6, Qihai REN-6, Pishu BL-20, Weishu BL-21, Shaohai HE-3, Shenmen HE-7 and Xinshu BL-15.
- A tonifying method is applied to these points. Moxibustion should be applied on ST-36 and REN-6.

Explanations:
- ST-36, the he-sea point of the stomach channel, SP-3, the yuan-source point of the spleen channel, BL-20 and BL-21, the back-shu point of the spleen and stomach respectively, activate the spleen and stomach, tonify qi and relieve fatigue and general weakness.
- REN-6 and SP-6, the crossing point of the three yin channels of the foot, tonify qi and blood at the same time and strengthen the body to relieve general fatigue and weakness.
- HE-3 and HE-7, the he-sea point, yuan-source point of the heart channel respectively, and BL-15, the back-shu point of the heart, tonify qi of the heart, calm the shen and improve sleep.
- Moxibustion promotes the yuan-source qi, benefits the body, and relieves the weakness and cold in the body.

11.19.2.7 *Deficiency of heart-blood*

Easily waking during the night, light sleeping, tiredness, dizziness, palpitation, poor memory, pale complexion, scanty menstruation in women, hair loss, dry skin or stools, pale tongue, thin and white tongue coating, and a thready and weak pulse.

Principle of Treatment:
Nourish blood, benefit the heart, calm the shen and improve sleep.

Herbal Treatment:
Gui Pi Tang-*Restore the Spleen Decoction.*

Dang Shen *Radix Codonopsis Pilosulae* 10 g
Fu Ling *Sclerotium Poriae Cocos* 15 g
Huang Qi *Radix Astragali Membranacea* 10 g
Dang Gui *Radix Angelicae Sinensis* 10 g
Shu Di Huang *Radix Rhemanniae Glutinosae Praeparata* 12 g
Huang Jing *Rhizoma Polygonati* 10 g
Yuan Zhi *Radix Polygalae Tenuifoliae* 10 g
Suan Zao Ren *Semen Zizyphi Spinosae* 10 g
Ye Jiao Teng *Caulis Polygoni Multiflori* 10 g

Bai Zi Ren *Semen Biotae Orientalis* 10 g
Mu Xiang *Radix Aucklandiae Lappae* 10 g
Zhi Gan Cao *Radix Glycyrrhizae Praeparata* 3 g

Explanations:
* Dang Shen, Huang Qi, Fu Ling and Zhi Gan Cao tonify the qi of the body and relieve fatigue and general weakness. Meanwhile, Fu Ling could improve sleep.
* Dang Gui, Shu Di Huang and Huang Jing tonify blood and benefit the heart.
* Mu Xiang promotes qi circulation and benefits the middle Jiao to improve digestion.
* Yuan Zhi, Suan Zao Ren, Ye Jiao Teng and Bai Zi Ren benefit the heart, improve sleep, and relieve sleep disorders.

Herbal Remedy:
Gui Pi Wan-*Restore the Spleen Pill.*

Acupuncture Treatment:
* Zusanli ST-36, Sanyinjiao SP-6, Guanyuan REN-4, Qihai REN-6, Taixi KID-3, Shenshu BL-23, Shaohai HE-3, Shenmen HE-7, Neiguan P-6, Xinshu BL-15, Extra Sishencong and Extra Anmian.
* An even method is used on Extra Sishencong and Extra Anmian. A tonifying method is applied to the rest of the points.

Explanations:
* ST-36, the he-sea point of the stomach channel, and SP-6, the crossing point of the three yin channels of the foot, activate the spleen and stomach, tonify qi and blood and relieve general weakness and fatigue.
* KID-3 and BL-23, the yuan-source point of the kidney channel and the back-shu point of the kidney respectively, tonify kidney-jing and benefit blood.
* REN-6 and REN-4 tonify qi and blood at the same time and relieve general weakness and fatigue.

- HE-3 and HE-7, the he-sea point and the yuan-source point of the heart channel respectively, P-6, the luo-connecting point, and BL-15, the back-shu point of the heart, tonify heart-blood, benefit the heart, calm the shen and improve sleep.
- Extra Sishencong and extra Anmian calm the shen and improve sleep.
- REN-6, and SP-6, the crossing point of the three yin channels of the foot, tonify qi and blood at the same time and strengthen the body to relieve general fatigue and weakness.
- Moxibustion promotes the yuan-source qi, benefits the body, and relieves the weakness and cold in the body.

11.19.2.8 *Deficiency of heart-yin with hyperactivity of deficient fire*

Sleep disorders (difficulty in falling asleep), restlessness, nervousness, irritability, palpitations, thirst, dry throat and stool, tiredness, dizziness, night sweating, dry skin or hair, red tongue, thin and scanty tongue coating, and a thready, weak, and rapid pulse.

Principle of Treatment:
Nourish yin, clear deficient heat, benefit the heart, calm the shen and improve sleep.

Herbal Treatment:
Tian Wang Bu Xin Dan-*Emperor of Heaven's Special Pill to Tonify the Heart.*

Mai Men Dong *Tuber Ophiopogonis Japonici* 10 g
Bai Shao *Radix Paeoniae Alba* 10 g
Tian Men Dong *Tuber Asparagi Cochinchinensis* 10 g
Sheng Di Huang *Radix Rehmanniae Glutinosae Recens* 12 g
Xuan Shen *Radix Scrophulariae Ningpoensis* 10 g
Wu Wei Zi *Fructus Schisandrae Chinensis* 10 g
Gui Ban *Plastrum Testudinis* 15 g

Yu Zhu *Rhizoma Polygonati Odorati* 10 g
Dan Shen *Radix Salviae Miltiorrhizae* 10 g
Dang Shen *Radix Codonopsis Pilosulae* 10 g
Fu Shen *Sclerotium Poriae Cocos Paradicis* 15 g
Duan Long Gu *Os Draconis (calcine)* 15 g
Bai Zi Ren *Semen Biotae Orientalis* 10 g
He Huan Pi *Cortex Albizziae Julibrissin* 10 g
Zhi Gan Cao *Radix Glycyrrhizae Preparata* 3 g

Explanations:
- Mai Men Dong, Tian Men Dong, Yu Zhu, Gui Ban and Wu Wei Zi nourish yin, promote the production of body fluid, and benefit the body.
- Bai Shao smooths the liver, nourishes liver-yin, and relieves spasms in the body.
- Sheng Di Huang and Xuan Shen clear deficient heat and relieve restlessness.
- Dan Shen clears heat in the heart and calms the shen.
- Dang Shen tonifies qi of the spleen to promote the production of qi and yin in the body.
- Fu Shen, Duan Long Gu, Bai Zi Ren, and He Huan Pi calm the shen and improve sleep.
- Zhi Gan Cao harmonizes the herbs in the prescription.

Herbal Remedy:
Tian Wang Bu Xin Dan-*Emperor of Heaven's Special Pill to Tonify the Heart.*

Acupuncture Treatment:
- Zusanli ST-36, Sanyinjiao SP-6, Taichong LIV-3, Ququan LIV-8, Taixi KID-3, Fuliu KID-7, Yingu KID-10, Shenmen HE-7, Xinshu BL-15, Ganshu BL-18, Shenshu BL-23, extra Sishencong and extra Anmian.
- An even method is applied on LIV-3, extra Sishencong and extra Anmian. A tonifying method is applied on these points.

Explanations:

- ST-36, the he-sea point of the stomach channel, activates the spleen and stomach, tonifies qi and blood and relieves general weakness and fatigue.
- SP-6, the crossing point of three yin channels of the foot, KID-3, the yuan-source point of the kidney channel, BL-23, the back-shu point of the kidney, LIV-8 and KID-10, the he-sea point of the liver channel and kidney channel respectively, and KID-7 tonify blood, yin and kidney-jing at the same time, relieve the general fatigue and weakness so as to improve sleep.
- LIV-3 and BL-18, the yuan-source point of the liver channel and the back-shu point of the liver respectively, smooth the liver, promote the qi circulation, and relieve tension in the body so as to improve sleep.
- HE-7 and BL-15, the yuan-source point of the heart channel and the back-shu point of the heart respectively, nourish yin of the heart, calm the shen, and improve sleep.
- Extra Sishencong and extra Anmian improve sleep and relieve insomnia.

11.20 Hearing Loss or Tinnitus

Besides various respiratory symptoms that arise during the coronavirus pandemic, hearing loss or tinnitus could also be one annoying and unbearable Long COVID related symptom. Severe tinnitus, i.e., a loud ringing or buzzing sound in the ears, could even cause a patient to commit suicide.

Long COVID associated hearing loss and tinnitus refers to the signs and symptoms that develop during or after an infection consistent with COVID-19, are not yet resolved 12 weeks after the start of acute COVID-19 and are not explained by an alternative diagnosis.

Hearing loss has elements of both conductive hearing loss and sensorineural hearing loss. Long COVID associated hearing loss could be both, especially the latter, where the inner ear can't process sound that should be sent to the brain. Hearing loss associated with COVID-19 has been reported across a wide age range and severity, ranging from mild to severe. There are several case reports of sudden loss of hearing in one ear, often accompanied by tinnitus. Tinnitus is a common condition, affecting around 17% of all adults. Most people with tinnitus also have hearing loss, suggesting a close link between the two.[146] In most studies of audio-vestibular dysfunction & COVID-19, tinnitus is not well-defined but has been described as a non-pulsatile white noise or specific to certain frequencies, intermittent or continuous. In addition to hearing loss, millions of people are expected to suffer from tinnitus after diagnosis of COVID-19.[147]

When the COVID-19 pandemic emerged, there was considerable literature focused on its prevalence and the various symptoms associated with the virus. However, the discussion on the relationship between COVID-19 and hearing or tinnitus had not been highlighted. In fact, awareness of hearing or tinnitus is very important since a prompt course of steroid treatment could be given to reverse this disabling condition. In April 2020, a first reported case of sensorineural hearing loss following COVID-19 infection in the UK was confirmed.[148] One study confirmed that there are multiple reports of hearing loss (e.g., sudden unilateral) and tinnitus in adults with a wide range of COVID-19 symptom severity. A pooled estimate of prevalence, based primarily on retrospective recall of symptoms, is

---

[146] Kevin Munro. COVID associated with hearing loss, tinnitus and vertigo–new study confirms link. *The Conversation.* 22 March, 2021. https://theconversation.com/covid-associated-with-hearing-loss-tinnitus-and-vertigo-new-study-confirms-link-157522.

[147] Sugata Bhattacharjee. Opinion: Millions of people have hearing loss after COVID-19. *NDTV.* 1 June 2021. https://www.ndtv.com/opinion/opinion-millions-of-people-have-hearing-loss-after-covid-19-2453615.

[148] First reported UK case of sudden permanent hearing loss linked to COVID-19. *BMJ Case Reports.* 13 October 2020. doi: 10.1136/bcr-2020-238419. https://www.bmj.com/company/newsroom/first-reported-uk-case-of-sudden-permanent-hearing-loss-linked-to-covid-19/.

7.6%(CI: 2.5-15.1) and 14.8%(CI: 6.3-26.1) for hearing loss and tinnitus respectively.[149]

Hearing threshold refers to the lowest level that sound can be heard 50% of the time. Using electro audiometry, the average hearing threshold for frequencies of 0.25–4 kHz was determined.

Based on the threshold, hearing acuity was classified into three tiers:

- Grade 1: 26–40 dB mild deafness
- Grade 2: 41–70 dB moderate deafness
- Grade 3: ≥71 dB severe deafness

The degree of ringing was graded on a six-tier scale:

- Level 1: Extremely slight ringing, faintly detectable.
- Level 2: Slight ringing, definitely detectable. Only occurs in a quiet environment. No impact on daily life and work.
- Level 3: Moderate ringing, detectable in a normal environment. No observable impact on daily life and work.
- Level 4: Ringing detectable in any environment. Sleep and concentration are affected. Slight impact on work.
- Level 5: Loud and noisy ringing. Sleep and work are severely affected. Signs of slight anxiety, irritability, depression, or other psychological issues.
- Level 6: Extremely loud ringing. Constantly affected by ringing. Inability to sleep and work. Major signs of anxiety, irritability, depression, or other psychological issues.[150]

It was proposed that several pathophysiological processes regarding hearing hoss and tinnitus (such as a direct impairment of inner ear structures or a virus-mediated immune response) are caused by

---

149 Ibrahim Almufarrij and Kevin Munro. *op. cit.*

150 HealthCMi. Acupuncture and herbs quiet tinnitus. 18 February 2018. https://www.nccaom.org/wp-content/uploads/pdf/Acupuncture%20and%20Herbs%20Quiet%20Tinnitus.pdf.

COVID-19. Blood vessels, lymphatics and nerves—and in some cases the meninges (as proposed by Degen *et al.* 8)—have been proposed as entry routes for the virus[151]; direct damage to the cochlear hair cell with a reduced amplitude of transient otoacoustic emissions (TEOAEs) in infected adults and even in newborn patients exposed to SARS-CoV-2 intrauterinely[152,153]; a potential inflammatory involvement of inner ear vessels or of the stria vascularis with eventual vasculitis or endothelitis[154]; brain microhaemorrhages,[155] or relatively high risk from some medications used to treat the coronavirus, e.g., quinine, cholorquine and hydroxychloroquine,[156] etc. Moreover, emotional factors, anxiety, and poor sleep quality experienced during COVID-19 can play a relevant role in developing or enhancing tinnitus, which appears to be more bothersome for those under quarantine.[157] Of course, previous history of noise exposure, head trauma, autoimmune diseases, exposure to ototoxic drugs, Ménière disease, anatomical alterations of the ear and other predisposing factors should be always ruled out before postulating a link to SARS-CoV-2.

---

[151] Chantal Degen, *et al.* Acute profound sensorineural hearing loss after COVID-19 pneumonia. *Mayo Clin Proc.* 2020, 95(8): 1801–1803. doi: 10.1016/j.mayocp.2020.05.034.

[152] Turgut Celik, *et al.* Evaluation of cochlear functions in infants exposed to SARS-CoV-2 intrauterine. *Am J Otolaryngol.* 2021, 42(4): 102982. doi: 10.1016/j.amjoto.2021.102982.

[153] Mohamed Wael Mohamed Mustafa. Audiological profile of asymptomatic COVID-19 PCR-positive cases. *Am J Otolaryngol.* 2020, 41(3): 102483. doi: 10.1016/j.amjoto.2020.102483.

[154] Toshiaki Iba, *et al.* The coagulopathy, endotheliopathy, and vasculitis of COVID-19. *Inflammation Research.* 2020, 69(12): 1181–1189. doi: 10.1007/s00011-020-01401-6.

[155] Alireza Radmanesh, *et al.* COVID-19–associated diffuse leukoencephalopathy and microhemorrhages. *Radiology.* 2020, 297(1): E223. https://doi.org/10.1148/radiol.2020202040.

[156] Joy Victory. COVID-19 and hearing loss: What we know. *Healthy Hearing.* 30 August 2021. https://www.healthyhearing.com/report/53127-Coronavirus-hearing-loss-tinnitus-covid.

[157] Eldré W. Beukes, *et al.* Changes in tinnitus experiences during the COVID-19 Pandemic. *Front Public Health.* 2020, 8: 592878. https://doi.org/10.3389/fpubh.2020.592878.

In addition, Magnetic Resonance Imaging (MRI) is required to exclude retro-cochlear pathology.[158]

A prompt course of steroid treatment is one of the recommended therapies for acute hearing loss or tinnitus. However, if Long COVID associated hearing loss or tinnitus already passed 12 weeks after onset of the infection, steroid treatment may not be the best choice for this complaint. However, as the knowledge and understanding of Long COVID associated with hearing loss and tinnitus continues to grow, a large comprehensive research effort with high-quality studies on this topic could reveal more treatment options.

11.20.1 TCM understanding of Long COVID associated hearing loss or tinnitus

The chapter "On the Brain" in the book *Ling Shu* (Miraculous Pivot) points out that "if the brain marrow is insufficient, vertigo and tinnitus will occur".

The chapter of "Jue Qi" in the same book says: "depletion of essence gives rise to deafness". The chapter "Jin Gui Zhen Yan Lun" of *Su Wen* (Plain Questions) says "The heart opens into the ear". Later, the book of *Sheng Ji Zong Lu* (General Collection for Holy Relief) modified it into "The heart has its orifice in the ear", which expresses the close ties between the heart and the ear. From the above, we can see that ancient TCM had some good understanding of the relationship between the ear and different zang-fu organs.

All six Yang channels go through the head area to benefit the brain and clear orifices. The gallbladder channel, small Intestine channels, San Jiao channel, and stomach channel, as well as all

---

[158]Virginia Fancello, *et al.* SARS-CoV-2 (COVID-19) and audio-vestibular disorders. *Int J Immunopathol Pharmacol.* 2021, 35: 20587384211027373. doi: 10.1177/20587384211027373.

Yangqiao mai and Yangwei mai pass through or run in front of the ear to maintain the physiological functions of the ear.

Besides, these channels have their mutual connections with different zang-fu organs, such as the liver and gallbladder, the heart and small intestine, and the Pericardium and San Jiao. Moreover, the Du channel and the liver channel also have their connection or distribution on the head. The kidney is the important organ to produce marrow and the Brain is the sea of marrow. The spleen transforms the essence of food into qi and blood, which nourishes the brain and the orifices. lung disperses qi to all the parts of the body, including the head and ear. The heart dominates blood circulation, blood vessels, and is in charge of mental activity. Moreover, blood is the basic energetic source for the physiological activity of the brain. Disorders in any one of these channels or internal organs during Long COVID will influence the qi and blood circulation in the head, leading to hearing loss or tinnitus.

11.20.1.1 *Damage to the collaterals by external pathogenic factors*

COVID-19 is mainly caused by the invasion of cold-damp or damp-heat with a pestilent toxin to the body, especially to the lung and heart. When the physiological functions are damaged by these pathogenic factors, the lung is not able to disperse the qi to the ear, or the heart is not able to regulate the vessel in the ear, and hearing loss or tinnitus happens.

Besides, invasion of these pathogenic factors could also damage some local channels or collaterals around the ear, leading to the occurrence of hearing loss or tinnitus.

11.20.1.2 *Emotional disturbance*

The liver plays an important role in emotional activities. It regulates qi circulation and stores blood. Overstressing, resentment, and frustration during COVID-19 may cause retardation of liver-qi circulation, and stagnation of liver-qi occurs. If there is stagnation of liver-qi, it may influence the physiological functions in the head, leading to stagnation of qi and blood in the clear orifices. Stagnation of liver-qi could also cause qi stagnation in differential collaterals, especially the gallbladder channel, where hearing loss or tinnitus occurs.

Qi belongs to yang in the body. In case of prolonged persistence of liver-qi stagnation, especially in those with underlying sickness, it may cause the formation of liver-fire. Moreover, improper diet during COVID-19 may accelerate this process of fire formation. When there is the formation of liver-fire in the body, it may rise to the head, disturbing qi and blood circulation, burning the channels around the ear. Moreover, prolonged persistence of flaring of liver-fire may cause hyperactivity of liver-yang. Whenever there is an accumulation of damp in the body, the uprising of liver-qi, fire or yang could stir damp, causing disturbance of the clear orifice by damp. All these situations could lead to the formation of hearing loss or tinnitus.

11.20.1.3 *Blockage of the ear by damp-phlegm*

COVID-19 is mainly caused by the invasion of cold-damp or damp-heat with a pestilent toxin to the body. When these pathogenic factors are not eliminated completely or in time, they could cause stagnation and latent accumulation in the spleen, resulting in further disturbance to the ascending and descending functions of the spleen and stomach, and there could be the formation of damp-phlegm internally.

Constitutional weakness, lack of life care during COVID-19, overconsumption of alcoholic drinking, and eating too much fatty and greasy food, could result in dysfunction of the spleen and stomach in transportation and transformation, thus formation of damp-phlegm occurs.

Accumulation of damp-phlegm in the body would cause the failure of the clear qi and yang to rise and turbid qi to descend, causing hearing loss or tinnitus.

11.20.1.4 *Deficiency of qi and blood*

Overconsumption of qi and blood, lack of dietary care or improper treatment during COVID-19 could cause deficiency of qi and blood, leading to failure of the head to be nourished, resulting in hearing loss or tinnitus.

11.20.2 TCM treatment of Long COVID associated hearing loss or tinnitus

11.20.2.1 *Damage to the collaterals by external pathogenic factors*

After the onset of COVID-19, most of the other pulmonary symptoms are under control. However, there is persistent hearing loss or tinnitus, possible headache or slight muscle pain, aversion to wind occasionally, a thin and white tongue coating, and a wiry pulse.

Principle of Treatment:
Dispel wind, eliminate damp, harmonize the collaterals, and relieve tinnitus.

Herbal Treatment:
Shu Jing Huo Xue Tang-*Relax the Channels and Invigorate the Blood Decoction.*

Qiang Huo *Rhizoma seu Radix Notopterygii* 10 g
Gao Ben *Rhizoma Radix Ligustici* 10 g
Fang Feng *Radix Ledebouriellae* 6 g
Bai Zhi *Radix Angelicae Dahuricae* 10 g
Wei Ling Xian *Radix Clematidis* 10 g
Hong Hua *Flos Carhami* 10 g
Dang Gui *Radix angelicae Sinensis* 10 g
Chuan Xiong *Rhizoma Ligustici Chuanxiong* 10 g
Chi Shao Yao *Radix Paeoniae Rubra* 10 g
Yuan Zhi *Radix Polygalae Tenuifoliae* 10 g

Shi Chang Pu *Rhizoma Acori Graminei* 10 g
Zhi Gan Cao *Radix Glycyrrhizae Preparata* 3 g

Explanations:
- Qiang Huo, Fang Feng and Bai Zhi dispel the remaining external wind, eliminate cold-damp from the upper parts of the body and relieve remaining external pathogenic factors.
- Gao Ben and Wei Ling Xian harmonize the collaterals and eliminate cold-damp.
- Hong Hua, Dang Gui, Chuan Xiong and Chi Shao Yao promote qi and blood circulation, eliminating blood stasis in the collaterals.
- Shi Chang Pu and Yuan Zhi eliminate damp, benefit the ear, and improve hearing.
- Zhi Gan Cao coordinates the effects of the other herbs in the prescription.

Herbal Remedy:
Shu Jing Huo Xue Tang Ke Li-*Relax the Channels and Invigorate the Blood Granulate.*

Acupuncture Treatment:
- Waiguan SJ-5 + Zulinqi GB-41, Hegu L.I.-4, Lieque LU-7, Shuaigu GB-8, Fengchi GB-20, Shenting DU-24, Tinghui GB-2, Sizhukong SJ-23, Tinggong SI-19, and Sanyinjiao SP-6.
- An even method is applied on SJ-5 + GB-41, and a reducing method is applied on the rest of the points.

Explanations:
- A combination of SJ-5 + GB-41 harmonize Shaoyang collaterals, dispel external pathogenic factors, benefit the ears, and improve hearing.
- L.I.-4, the yuan-source point of the large intestine channel, and LU-7, the luo-connecting point of the lung channel, promote the qi circulation in the head, eliminate damp in the upper Jiao and relieve external pathogenic factors.

- GB-8, a local point around the ear, and GB-20, the crossing point of the foot Shaoyang and Yangwei channels, dispel wind, harmonize the collaterals, and relieve tension around the neck and head.
- GB-2, SJ-23 and SI-19, all the local points around the ear which are connected with different channels, promote the qi and blood circulation, harmonize the collaterals, improve hearing and relieve tinnitus.
- DU-24 benefits the shen, opens the clear orifice and improves hearing and tinnitus.
- SP-6, the crossing point of the three yin channels of the foot, promotes blood circulation and relieves stagnation of blood in the collaterals.

11.20.2.2 *Stagnation of liver-qi*

Persistence of hearing loss or tinnitus after the onset of COVID-19 with occasional aggravation especially when nervous or stressed, spasm and tension sensation on the scalp or in the head, emotional instability, depression, painful neck, distension and pain in the hypochondriac region, insomnia, irregular menstruation in women, poor appetite or overeating, thin and white tongue coating, and a wiry pulse.

Principle of Treatment:
Smooth the liver, promote qi circulation, calm the shen and improve hearing.

Herbal Treatment:
Xiao Yao San-*Rambling Powder.*

Chai Hu *Radix Bupleare* 10 g
Dang Gui *Radix Angelicae Sinensis* 10 g
Bai Shao Yao *Radix Paeoniae Lactiflorae* 10 g
Chuan Xiong *Rhizoma Ligustici Chuan Xiong* 10 g
Bai Zhu *Rhiizoma Areactylodis Macrocephalae* 10 g
Fu Ling *Sclerotium Poriae Cocos* 15 g
Huang Qin *Radix Scutellariae Baicalensis* 10 g

Bo He *Herba Menthae Haplocalycis* 3 g
Bai Ji Li *Fructus Tribulli Terrestris* 10 g
Yuan Zhi *Radix Polygalae Tenuifoliae* 10 g
Ju Hua *Flos Chrysanthemi Morifolii* 10 g
Zhi Gan Cao *Radix Glycyrrhizae Preparata* 3 g

Explanations:
- Chai Hu and Bai Shao Yao smooth the liver, promote liver-qi circulation, and relieve the spasm in the liver and at the neck.
- Dang Gui and Chuan Xiong nourish blood in the liver, harmonize and smooth the liver and relieve tension and spasm in the scalp, head, and hypochondriac region. Meanwhile, they promote blood circulation and relieve blood stasis in the ear.
- Bai Zhu and Fu Ling strengthen the spleen and stomach and improve the appetite.
- Huang Qin, Ju Hua, and Bo He clear internal heat resulting from the stagnation of liver-qi and prevent further formation of liver-fire.
- Bai Ji Li and Yuan Zhi benefit the clear orifice and improve hearing loss and tinnitus.
- Zhi Gan Cao harmonizes the other herbs in the prescription.

Herbal Remedy:
Xiao Yao Wan-*Rambling Pill.*

Acupuncture Treatment:
- Waiguan SJ-5 + Zulinqi GB-41, Neiguan P-6 + Gongsun SP-4, Hegu L.I.-4, Shuaigu GB-8, Tinghui GB-2, Yifeng SJ-17, Sizhukong SJ-23, Tinggong SI-19, Fengchi GB-20, Jianjing GB-21, Taichong LIV-3, Qimen LIV-14 and Sanyinjiao SP-6.
- An even method is applied on SJ-5 + GB-41, P-6 + SP-4, and a reducing method is applied on the rest of the points.

Explanations:
- A combination of SJ-5 + GB-41 harmonizes Shaoyang channels, benefits the gallbladder, and relieves hearing loss and tinnitus.

- A combination of P-6 + SP-4 regulates emotions, harmonizes qi circulation in the body and benefits the liver and heart.
- L.I.-4 and LIV-3, the yuan-source point of the large intestine channel and the liver channel respectively, and LIV-14, the front-mu point of the liver, smooth the liver, regulate the qi circulation in the body and relieve liver-qi stagnation.
- GB-20 and GB-21 regulate the channel and collateral of the gallbladder, smooth emotions, benefit the head and relieve the neck tension.
- GB-2, GB-8, SJ-17, SJ-23, SI-19, all the local points around the ear, promote qi circulation, harmonize the collaterals, and improve hearing loss and tinnitus.
- SP-6, the crossing point of the three yin channels of the foot, promotes the smooth qi and blood circulation in the liver and in the head.

11.20.2.3 *Flaring-up of liver-fire*

Persistence of hearing loss or tinnitus after the onset of COVID-19 with occasional aggravation, occasional headache or pain in the ear or a burning sensation in the ear, redness of eyes, irritability, bitter taste in the mouth, restlessness, insomnia, irregular menstruation in women, poor appetite, deep yellow urine, constipation, red tongue, and a rapid and wiry pulse.

Principle of Treatment:
Reduce liver-fire, clear heat, calm the shen and improve hearing loss and tinnitus.

Herbal Treatment:
Long Dan Xie Gan Tang-*Gentiana Longdancao Decoction to Drain the Liver.*

Long Dan Cao *Radix Gentianae Anomalae* 10 g
Huang Qin *Radix Scutellariae Baicalensis* 10 g
Zhi Zi *Fructus Gardenniae* 10 g

Ze Xie *Rhizoma Alismatis* 12 g
Chuan Xiong *Rhizoma Lagustici Chuanxiong* 10 g
Xia Ku Cao *Spica Prunellae* 10 g
Che Qian Zi *Semen Plantaginis* 10 g
Dang Gui *Radix Angelicae Sinensis* 10 g
Sheng Di Huang *Radix Rehmanniae Glutinosae* 12 g
Chai Hu *Radix Bupleuri* 10 g
Bai Ji Li *Fructus Tribulli Terrestris* 10 g
Ju Hua *Flos Chrysanthemi Morifolii* 10 g
Zhi Gan Cao *Radix Glycyrrhizae Preparata* 3 g

In case of hyperactivity of liver-yang, add Gou Teng *Ramulus cum Uncis Uncariae* 10 g and Tian Ma *Rhizoma Gastrodiae Elatae* 10 g.

Explanations:
- Long Dan Cao, Huang Qin, Xia Ku Cao and Zhi Zi clear heat in the liver, reduce liver-fire and relieve burning sensation in the ear.
- Dang Gui, Chuan Xiong and Chai Hu promote liver-qi circulation and smooth the liver.
- Ze Xie and Che Qian Zi promote urination and induce fire out of the body through urination.
- Sheng Di clears heat in the liver and nourishes the yin of the liver and kidney.
- Bai Ji Li and Ju Hua smooth the liver and relieve dizziness.
- Zhi Gan Cao harmonizes the actions of the other herbs.
- Gou Teng and Tian Ma calm the liver and suppress liver-wind.

Herbal Remedy:
Long Dan Xie Gan Wan-*Gentiana Longdancao Pill to Drain the Liver.*

Acupuncture Treatment:
- Waiguan SJ-5 + Zulinqi GB-41, Hegu L.I.-4, Shaohai HE-3, Shaofu HE-8, Shuaigu GB-8, Tinghui GB-2, Yifeng SJ-17, Sizhukong SJ-23, Tinggong SI-19, Fengchi GB-20, Jianjing GB-21, Xiaxi GB-43, Xingjian LIV-2, Qimen LIV-14, and Sanyinjiao SP-6.

- An even method is applied on SJ-5 + GB-41, and a reducing method is applied on the rest of the points.

Explanations:
- A combination of SJ-5 + GB-41 harmonizes the Shaoyang channels, benefits the gallbladder, and improves hearing and tinnitus.
- L.I.-4 and LIV-14, the yuan-source point of the large intestine channel and the front-mu point of the liver, smooth the liver, regulate the qi circulation in the body and relieve liver-qi stagnation.
- LIV-2 and GB-43, the ying-spring point of the liver channel and gallbladder channel respectively, clear heat, reduce liver-fire and sedate tinnitus.
- HE-3 and HE-8, the he-sea point and the ying-spring point of the heart channel respectively, clear heat in the heart, calm the shen and smooth the liver as well.
- GB-20 and GB-21 regulate the collateral of the gallbladder channel, smooth the emotions, relieve the neck tension, promote qi circulation in the head and improve hearing and tinnitus.
- GB-8, GB-2, SJ-17, SJ-23, and SI-19, all the local points around the ear, harmonize the collaterals around the ear and improve hearing and tinnitus.
- SP-6, the crossing point of the three yin channels of the foot, promotes the smooth qi and blood circulation in the liver and in the head.

11.20.2.4 *Blockage of the clear-yang by damp-phlegm*

Persistence of hearing loss or tinnitus after the onset of COVID-19, dizziness, a heavy sensation in the head, the fullness of the chest and epigastric region, nausea, occasional vomiting, poor appetite, lassitude, white and greasy tongue coating, and a slippery or wiry and slippery pulse.

Principle of Treatment:
Activate the spleen, eliminate damp, resolve phlegm, harmonize the collaterals, and improve hearing loss and tinnitus.

Herbal Treatment:
Ban Xia Bai Zhu Tian Ma Tang-*Pinellia, Atractylodes Macrocephala and Gastrodia Decoction.*

Ban Xia *Rhizoma Pinelliae* 10 g
Bai Zhu *Rhizoma Atractylodis Macrocephalae* 10 g
Tian Ma *Rhizoma Gastrodiae* 10 g
Cang Zhu *Rhizoma Atractylodis* 10 g
Hou Po *Cortex Magnoliae Officinalis* 10 g
Fu Ling *Sclerotium Poriae Cocos* 15 g
Chen Pi *Pericarpium Citri Reticulatae* 5 g
Bai Ji Li *Fructus Tribulli Terrestris* 10 g
Shi Chang Pu *Rhizoma Acori Graminei* 10 g
Yuan Zhi *Radix Polygalae Tenuifoliae* 10 g
Di Long *Lumbricus* 10 g
Zhi Gan Cao *Radix Glycyrrhizae Preparata* 3 g

Explanations:
- Ban Xia and Chen Pi dry damp, resolve phlegm in the body and relieve nausea.
- Fu Ling and Bai Zhu activate the spleen, promote the physiological functions of the spleen, and eliminate damp in the body.
- Cang Zhu and Hou Po eliminate damp-phlegm in the body and relieve nausea.
- Tian Ma, Bai Ji Li, Shi Chang Pu, Yuan Zhi and Di Long calm the liver, eliminate damp, improve hearing, and relieve tinnitus.
- Zhi Gan Cao harmonizes the functions of other herbs in the prescription.

Herbal Remedy:
Ban Xia Bai Zhu Tian Ma Pian-*Pinellia, Atractylodes Macrocephala and Gastrodia Tablet.*

Acupuncture Treatment:
- Waiguan SJ-5 + Zulinqi GB-41, Neiguan P-6 + Gongsun SP-4, Hegu L.I.-4, Shuaigu GB-8, Tinghui GB-2, Yifeng SJ-17, Sizhukong

SJ-23, Tinggong SI-19, Touwei ST-8, Zhongwan REN-12, Fenglong ST-40, Sanyinjiao SP-6 and Yinlingquan SP-9.
- An even method is applied on SJ-5 + GB-41, and a reducing method is applied on the rest of the points.

Explanations:
- SJ-5 + GB-41 promote the circulation of qi circulation Shaoyang channels, harmonize the collaterals and improve hearing and tinnitus.
- P-6 + SP-4 regulate emotions, promote digestion, and eliminate damp-phlegm.
- L.I.-4, the yuan-source point of the large intestine channel, promotes qi circulation in the body.
- REN-12, the front-mu point of the stomach and the influential point for the fu organs, SP-6, the crossing point of three yin channels of the foot, SP-9, the he-sea point of the spleen channel, and ST-40, the luo-connecting point of the stomach channel, activate the spleen, eliminate damp-phlegm, and improve digestion.
- GB-8, GB-2, SJ-17, SJ-23, SI-19, ST-8, all the local points from the ear, promote qi circulation, harmonize the collaterals, and improve hearing and tinnitus.

11.20.2.5 *Deficiency of qi and blood*

Persistence of hearing loss or tinnitus after the onset of COVID-19, empty sensation in the head, aggravation of hearing capacity or tinnitus after physical exertion, fatigue, general weakness, pale complexion, aversion to cold, cold hands, shortness of breath, spontaneous sweating, dry eyes and skin, insomnia, poor appetite, low voice, thin and white tongue coating, pale tongue with tooth marks, and a slow and deep pulse.

Principle of Treatment:
Tonify qi, reinforce blood, benefit kidney-jing, and improve hearing and tinnitus.

Herbal Treatment:
Shi Quan Da Bu Tang-*All-Inclusive Great Tonifying Decoction.*

Dang Shen *Radix Codonopsis Pilosulae* 10 g
Bai Zhu *Rhizoma Atractylodis Macrocephalae* 10 g
Fu Ling *Sclerotium Poriae Cocos* 15 g
Huang Qi *Radix Astragali Membranacea* 10 g
Shu Di Huang *Radix Rehmanniae Praeparatae* 15 g
Dang Gui *Radix Angelicae Sinensis* 10 g
Bai Shao *Radix Paeoniae Alba* 10 g
Chuan Xiong *Rhizoma Ligustici Chuanxiong* 10 g
Huang Jing *Rhizoma Polygonati* 10 g
He Shou Wu *Radix Polygoni Multiflori* 10 g
Tian Ma *Rhizoma Gastrodiae Elatae* 10 g
Bai Ji Li *Fructus Tribulli Terrestris* 10 g
Zhi Gan Cao *Radix Glycyrrhizae Preparata* 3 g

Explanations:
- Dang Shen, Bai Zhu, Fu Ling and Zhi Gan Cao, forming a prescription as Si Jun Zi Tang, together with Huang Qi, activate the spleen and stomach, tonify qi of the general body, dispel internal cold and relieve tiredness.
- Shu Di Huang, Dang Gui, Bai Shao, Chuan Xiong, Huang Jing and He Shou Wu tonify blood and benefit kidney-jing.
- Tian Ma and Bai Ji Li benefit the head and improve hearing and tinnitus.

Herbal Remedy:
Shi Quan Da Bu Wan-*All-Inclusive Great Tonifying Pill.*

Acupuncture Treatment:
- Zusanli ST-36, Taibai SP-3, Sanyinjiao SP-6, Qihai REN-6, Pishu BL-20, Weishu BL-21, Baihui DU-20, Shenting DU-24, Shuaigu GB-8, Tinghui GB-2, Yifeng SJ-17, Sizhukong SJ-23, Tinggong SI-19, and Touwei ST-8.

- An even method is applied on GB-8, GB-2, SJ-17, SJ-23, SI-19 and ST-8. A tonifying method is applied to the rest points. Moxibustion should be applied on REN-6 and ST-36.

Explanations:
- ST-36, the he-sea point of the stomach channel, and SP-3, the yuan-source point of the spleen channel, BL-20 and BL-21, the back-shu point of the spleen and stomach respectively, activate the spleen and stomach, tonify qi and blood.
- REN-6, and SP-6, the crossing point of the three yin channels of the foot, tonify qi and blood at the same time and strengthen the body to relieve general fatigue and weakness.
- DU-20 and DU-24 lift-up qi and blood to the headache to benefit the head and improve hearing loss and tinnitus.
- GB-8, GB-2, SJ-17, SJ-23, SI-19 and ST-8, the local points around the ear, harmonize the collaterals, benefit hearing, and improve tinnitus.
- Moxibustion promotes the yang-qi movement, benefits the body, and relieves the weakness and cold in the body.

11.21 Brain Fog

In addition to various common Long COVID symptoms, such as fatigue, myalgia, headache, cough, and shortness of breath, some patients could also suffer from difficulty in thinking clearly or difficulty in concentration or memory, a condition known as brain fog. Brain fog, a kind of cognitive dysfunction, is caused by direct effects from COVID-19 on the brain. It is a condition to describe how individuals feel when their thinking is sluggish, fuzzy, and not sharp. In fact, it is neither a medical or scientific term, nor a diagnosis, but in fact a symptom, a personal and subjective feeling.

Of course, brain fog is not "something in the mind" of the patients but a real biological phenomenon.

Neurological and psychiatric sequelae of COVID-19 have been reported, but more data are needed to adequately assess the effects of COVID-19 on brain health. In order to provide robust estimates of incidence rates and relative risks of neurological and psychiatric diagnoses in patients in the six months following a COVID-19 diagnosis, one research was carried out. Among 236,379 patients diagnosed with COVID-19, the estimated incidence of a neurological or psychiatric diagnosis in the following six months was 33.62%(95% CI 33.17–34.07), with 12.84%(12.36–13.33) receiving their first diagnosis. The researchers also found that COVID-19 patients were more likely to experience these issues as compared to patients in the sample pool who are diagnosed with other respiratory infections like the flu.[159]

One research analyzed data in a cross-sectional study from April 2020 through May 2021 from a cohort of patients with COVID-19. These patients had serum antibody positivity and no history of dementia. A relatively high frequency of cognitive impairment several months after patients contracted COVID-19. Impairments in executive functioning, processing speed, category fluency, memory encoding, and recall were predominant among hospitalized patients. The relative sparing of memory recognition in the context of impaired encoding and recall suggests an executive pattern.[160]

Another study investigated the frequency of brain fog in a large cohort of patients with documented coronavirus disease-2019 (COVID-19) who survived the illness at least three months after their discharge from the hospital. The research also scrutinized the potential risk factors associated with the development of brain fog. In total, 2696 patients had the inclusion criteria, and 1680(62.3%) people reported Long COVID syndrome (LCS). LCS-associated brain fog was reported by 194(7.2%) patients. It was reported that chronic Long COVID "brain fog" has significant associations with gender (female),

---

[159]Maxime Taquet, *et al.* May 2021. *op. cit.*

[160]Jacqueline H. Becker, *et al.* Assessment of cognitive function in patients after COVID-19 infection. *JAMA Netw Open.* 2021, 4(10): e2130645. doi: 10.1001/jamanetworkopen.2021.30645.

respiratory symptoms at the onset, and the severity of the illness (ICU admission).[161]

With brain fog, the patients feel a sensation similar to "a foggy haze in their head" that makes it harder to access their thoughts or plans. Their thoughts and emotions may feel numb and different, and daily physical activities and duties require more effort. As such, their mental and physical states feel less sharp and flexible as usual. Some additional symptoms of patients with brain fog include:

- forgetting a simple and usual task they must complete
- having trouble organizing thoughts or activities
- difficulty in paying attention
- disorientation
- taking much longer than usual to complete tasks
- feeling frequently distracted
- feeling tired when studying and reading
- decline in the quality of life and productivity
- feeling confused
- feeling mentally fatigued
- being easily distracted

It's not yet clear why COVID-19 survivors are so likely to experience neurological symptoms, but the medical community is still researching potential causes of brain fog after COVID-19. Researchers have identified several possible causes, including[162]:

- lack of oxygen caused by lung damage
- inflammation affecting brain cells
- an autoimmune disorder that is causing the immune system to attack healthy cells in the body

---

[161] Ali A. Asadi-Pooya, *et al.* Long COVID syndrome-associated brain fog. *Journal of Medical Virology.* 2021, 94(3): 979–984.. https://doi.org/10.1002/jmv.27404.
[162] Hackensack Meridian *Health.* Can COVID-19 cause brain fog? 11 August 2021. https://www.hackensackmeridianhealth.org/HealthU/2021/08/11/can-covid-19-cause-brain-fog/.

- lack of blood flow caused by swelling of the small blood vessels in the brain
- Invasion of infectious cells into the brain

Meanwhile, adverse effects of some psychological and social factors, such as depression, anxiety, worry, uncertainty, insomnia, etc., could also play a role in brain fog.

For some patients, Long COVID brain fog goes away in about three months, but for others, it can last much longer. It is still unclear how long it could exactly last.

A treatment plan for Long COVID brain fog may employ various strategies. Besides, some life care, such as sleeping well, avoiding alcohol and drugs, eating a balanced meal, participating in some physical exercises, etc., are often recommended. However, there is no concrete and effective medication yet available. However, since brain fog is a symptom rather than a medical diagnosis, there is no specific treatment for it. Sometimes, brain fog is associated with depression and anxiety, etc., therefore medication, including anti-anxiety medication, antidepressants, or stimulants for ADHD, can be the treatment options.

11.21.1 TCM understanding of Long COVID-associated brain fog

The causes of brain fog during Long COVID are mostly due to blockage of the clear-yang by damp-phlegm, stagnation of liver-qi, deficiency of qi, blood and kidney-jing.

The organs chiefly involved are the liver, spleen and kidney. Disturbance to the clear-yang or shen is the chief pathological result.

11.21.1.1 *Blockage of clear-yang by damp-phlegm*

COVID-19 is mainly caused by the invasion of cold-damp or damp-heat with a pestilent toxin to the body, especially the lung, heart and spleen. If these pathogenic factors are not eliminated completely or in time, they could cause stagnation and latent accumulation in the spleen, resulting in further disturbance to the ascending and descending functions of the spleen and stomach, and there could be the formation of damp-phlegm internally.

Some preexisting sickness, such as obesity, slow digestion, or lack of life care during COVID-19 (such as alcoholic drinking and overconsumption of fatty and greasy food), could result in dysfunction of the spleen and stomach in transportation and transformation, and formation of damp-phlegm occurs.

When damp-phlegm in the body moves with qi and blood to the head, the clear-yang could be blocked, leading to failure of the turbid qi to move downward, and brain fog occurs.

11.21.1.2 Emotional disturbance

The liver plays an important role in emotional activities. It regulates qi circulation and stores blood. Overstress, resentment, and frustration during COVID-19 may cause retardation of liver-qi circulation, resulting in stagnation of liver-qi. When there is stagnation of qi and blood in the head, brain fog happens.

Due to the close physiological relationship between the liver and heart, stagnation of liver-qi could cause disturbance to the heart, bringing about the dysfunction of the heart in housing the shen, and brain fog starts.

11.21.1.3 *Deficiency of qi, blood and kidney-jing*

Overconsumption of qi and blood, or lack of dietary care or even improper treatment during COVID-19, could cause deficiency of qi and blood, leading to failure of the clear-yang or the heart to be nourished, and brain fog appears.

Pre-existing kidney-jing deficiency during COVID-19 could deteriorate during COVID-19 due to overconsumption of qi and blood, thus the brain fails to be nourished, and the marrow becomes deficient, causing brain fog.

11.21.2 TCM treatment of Long COVID-associated brain fog

11.21.2.1 *Blockage of the clear-yang by damp-phlegm*

Brain fog, poor concentration, slight dizziness, a heavy sensation in the head, the fullness of the chest and epigastric region, nausea, poor appetite, lassitude, somnolence, white and greasy tongue coating, and a slippery or wiry and slippery pulse.

Principle of Treatment:
Activate the spleen, eliminate damp, resolve phlegm, harmonize the collaterals, and relieve brain fog.

Herbal Treatment:
Ban Xia Bai Zhu Tian Ma Tang-*Pinellia, Atractylodes Macrocephala and Gastrodia Decoction.*

Ban Xia *Rhizoma Pinelliae* 10 g
Bai Zhu *Rhizoma Atractylodis Macrocephalae* 10 g
Tian Ma *Rhizoma Gastrodiae* 10 g
Cang Zhu *Rhizoma Atractylodis* 10 g
Hou Po *Cortex Magnoliae Officinalis* 10 g
Ge Gen *Radix Puerariae* 10 g
Fu Ling *Sclerotium Poriae Cocos* 15 g
Chen Pi *Pericarpium Citri Reticulatae* 5 g
Bai Ji Li *Fructus Tribulli Terrestris* 10 g
Shi Chang Pu *Rhizoma Acori Graminei* 10 g
Yuan Zhi *Radix Polygalae Tenuifoliae* 10 g
Zhi Gan Cao *Radix Glycyrrhizae Preparata* 3 g

Explanations:
- Ban Xia and Chen Pi dry damp, resolve phlegm in the body and relieve nausea.
- Fu Ling and Bai Zhu activate the spleen and eliminate damp.
- Cang Zhu and Hou Po eliminate damp-phlegm in the body and relieve nausea.

- Tian Ma, Bai Ji Li, Shi Chang Pu and Yuan Zhi calm the liver, eliminate damp, and relieve brain fog.
- Ge Gen ascends the clear-qi, descends turbid qi and relieves brain fog.
- Zhi Gan Cao harmonizes the functions of other herbs in the prescription.

Herbal Remedy:

Ban Xia Bai Zhu Tian Ma Pian-*Pinellia, Atractylodes Macrocephala and Gastrodia Tablet.*

Acupuncture Treatment:

- Waiguan SJ-5 + Zulinqi GB-41, Neiguan P-6 + Gongsun SP-4, Hegu L.I.-4, Shuaigu GB-8, Fengchi GB-20, Touwei ST-8, Extra Taiyang, Extra Yintang, Extra Sishencong, Zhongwan REN-12, Taichong LIV-3, Fenglong ST-40, and Yinlingquan SP-9.
- An even method is applied on SJ-5 + GB-41, P-6 + SP-4, and a reducing method is applied on the rest of the points.

Explanations:

- A combination of SJ-5 + GB-41 could regulate the Shaoyang channels, harmonize the collaterals on the head, and relieve brain fog.
- A combination of P-6 + SP-4 harmonizes the Yinwei channel, regulates the zang organs, promotes digestion and eliminates damp-phlegm.
- GB-8, ST-8, Extra Taiyang, Extra Yintang and Extra Sishencong eliminate damp-phlegm, remove the disturbance of damp-phlegm to the brain, benefit the clear-yang and relieve brain fog.
- L.I.-4 and LIV-3, the yuan-source point of the large intestine channel and liver channel respectively, promote qi circulation, calm the liver, and relieve the blockage in the brain by damp-phlegm.
- GB-20 smooths the tension at the neck, promotes the qi circulation in the gallbladder channel and calms emotions.
- REN-12, the front-mu point of the stomach and the influential point for the fu organs.

- SP-9, the he-sea point of the spleen channel, and ST-40, the luo-connecting point of the stomach channel, activate the spleen, eliminate damp-phlegm, and improve digestion.

11.21.2.2 *Stagnation of liver-qi*

Brain fog, spasm, and tension sensation on the scalp or in the head, aggravation of brain fog under stress or emotional disturbance, depression, stiffness of the neck, distension and pain in the chest or hypochondriac region, insomnia, irregular menstruation in women, poor appetite or overeating, abdominal swelling, thin and white tongue coating, and a wiry pulse.

Principle of Treatment:
Smooth the liver, promote qi circulation, calm the shen and relieve brain fog.

Herbal Treatment:
Xiao Yao San-*Rambling Powder.*

Chai Hu *Radix Bupleare* 10 g
Dang Gui *Radix Angelicae Sinensis* 10 g
Bai Shao Yao *Radix Paeoniae Lactiflorae* 10 g
Bai Zhu *Rhiizoma Areactylodis Macrocephalae* 10 g
Fu Ling *Sclerotium Poriae Cocos* 15 g
Chuan Xiong *Rhizoma Ligustici Chuan Xiong* 10 g
Huang Qin *Radix Scutellariae Baicalensis* 10 g
Bo He *Herba Menthae Haplocalycis* 3 g
Bai Ji Li *Fructus Tribulli Terrestris* 10 g
Yuan Zhi *Radix Polygalae Tenuifoliae* 10 g
Zhi Gan Cao *Radix Glycyrrhizae Preparata* 3 g

Explanations:
- Chai Hu and Bai Shao Yao smooth the liver, regulate and promote liver-qi circulation and relieve qi stagnation in the liver.

- Dang Gui and Chuan Xiong nourish and benefit the blood in the liver, harmonize and smooth the liver and relieve tension and spasm in the scalp, head, and the hypochondriac region.
- Bai Zhu and Fu Ling strengthen the spleen and stomach and improve the appetite.
- Huang Qin and Bo He clear internal heat resulting from the stagnation of liver-qi and prevent further formation of liver-fire.
- Bai Ji Li and Yuan Zhi benefit the brain, regulate the shen and relieve brain fog.
- Zhi Gan Cao harmonizes the actions of the other herbs in the prescription.

Herbal Remedy:
Xiao Yao Wan-*Rambling Pill.*

Acupuncture Treatment:
- Waiguan SJ-5 + Zulingqi GB-41, Hegu L.I.4, Shuaigu GB-8, Toulinqi GB-15, Yanglingquan GB-34, Extra Yintang, Extra Taiyang, Extra Sishencong, Fengchi GB-20, Jianjing GB-21, Taichong LIV-3, Qimen LIV-14, Neiguan P-6, and Sanyinjiao SP-6.
- An even method is applied on SJ-5 + GB-41, and a reducing method is applied on the rest of the points.

Explanations:
- SJ-5 + GB-41 is a combination to harmonize Shaoyang channels, benefit the gallbladder and relieve brain fog.
- L.I.-4 and LIV-3, the yuan-source point of the large intestine channel and the liver channel respectively, and LIV-14, the front-mu point of the liver, smooth the liver, regulate the qi circulation in the body and relieve liver-qi stagnation.
- P-6, the luo-connecting point of the pericardium channel, regulates qi circulation, calms the shen and benefits the stomach.
- Extra Sishencong calms the shen, improves sleep and regulates emotion.

- SP-6, the crossing point of the three yin channels of the foot, promotes the smooth qi and blood circulation in the liver and in the head.
- GB-8, GB-15, GB-20, GB-21 and GB-34 regulate the collateral of the gallbladder channel, smooth the emotions, benefit the head, relieve the neck tension, and promote qi circulation in the head to relieve brain fog.
- Extra Yintang and Extra Taiyang, the local points, relieve dizziness.

11.21.2.3 *Deficiency of qi*

Brain fog after COVID-19, empty sensation in the head, aggravation of brain fog after physical exertion, fatigue, general weakness, pale complexion, aversion to cold, cold hands, shortness of breath, spontaneous sweating, loose stools, poor appetite, low voice, thin and white tongue coating, pale tongue with tooth marks, and a slow and deep pulse.

Principle of Treatment:
Tonify qi, activate the spleen and stomach and relieve brain fog.

Herbal Treatment:
Bu Zhong Yi Qi Tang-*Tonify the Middle and Augment the Qi Decoction.*

Dang Shen *Radix Codonopsis Pilosulae* 10 g
Bai Zhu *Rhizoma Atractylodis Macrocephalae* 10 g
Fu Ling *clerotium Poriae Cocos* 15 g
Huang Qi *Radix Astragali Membranacea* 10 g
Sheng Ma *Rhizoma Cimicifugae* 5 g
Chen Pi *Pericarpium Citri Reticulatae* 5 g
Gan Jiang *Rhizoma Zingiberis Officinalis* 5 g
Mu Xiang *Radix Aucklandiae* 10 g
Sha Ren *Fructus Amomi* 3 g

Bai Ji Li *Fructus Tribulli Terrestris* 10 g
Shi Chang Pu *Rhizoma Acori Graminei* 10 g
Zhi Gan Cao *Radix Glycyrrhizae Praeparata* 3 g

Explanations:
- Dang Shen, Bai Zhu, Fu Ling and Zhi Gan Cao, known as Si Jun Zi Tang, activate the spleen and stomach, tonify spleen-qi and relieve general fatigue and weakness.
- Huang Qi and Sheng Ma tonify spleen-qi and lift the qi to the head to benefit it.
- Chen Pi, Mu Xiang and Sha Ren harmonize stomach-qi and promote appetite.
- Bai Ji Li and Shi Chang Pu resolve damp in the head and relieve brain fog.
- Zhi Gan Cao harmonizes the herbs in the prescription.

Herbal Remedy:
Bu Zhong Yi Qi Wan-*Tonify the Middle and Augment the Qi Tablets.*

Acupuncture Treatment:
- Baihui DU-20, Zusanli ST-36, Taibai SP-3, Sanyinjiao SP-6, Qihai Ren-6, Pishu BL-20, Weishu BL-21, Shenting DU-24, Touwei ST-8 and Extra Yintang.
- A tonifying method is applied to these points. Moxibustion should be applied on REN-6 and ST-36.

Explanations:
- ST-36, the he-sea point of the stomach channel, and SP-3, the yuan-source point of the spleen channel, BL-20 and BL-21, the back-shu point of the spleen and stomach respectively, activate the spleen and stomach, tonify qi and promote digestion.
- REN-6, and SP-6, the crossing point of the three yin channels of the foot, tonify qi and blood at the same time and strengthen the body to relieve general fatigue and weakness.

- DU-20 lifts qi to the headache to benefit the head and relieves brain fog.
- DU-24, GB-8 and Extra Yintang benefit the brain and clear-yang and regulate collaterals and relieve brain fog.
- Moxibustion promotes the yang-qi movement, benefits the body, and relieves the weakness and cold in the body.

11.21.2.4 *Deficiency of blood*

Brain fog after COVID-19, a hollow sensation in the head, aggravation of brain fog after physical exertion and alleviation of it by rest, dry eyes, hair loss, palpitations, listlessness, dry skin and stools, insomnia, pale complexion, irregular menstruation in women, poor appetite, pale tongue, thin and white tongue coating, and a thready and weak pulse.

Principle of Treatment:
Tonify blood, benefit kidney-jing, relieve weakness and brain fog.

Herbal Treatment:
Si Wu Tang-*Four Substances Decoction.*

Shu Di Huang *Radix Rehmanniae Praeparatae* 15 g
Dang Gui *Radix Angelicae Sinensis* 10 g
Bai Shao *Radix Paeoniae Alba* 10 g
Chuan Xiong *Rhizoma Ligustici Chuanxiong* 10 g
Huang Jing *Rhizoma Polygonati* 10 g
He Shou Wu *Radix Polygoni Multiflori* 10 g
Tian Ma *Rhizoma Gastrodiae Elatae* 10 g
Bai Ji Li *Fructus Tribulli Terrestris* 10 g
Zhi Gan Cao *Radix Glycyrrhizae Preparata* 3 g

If there is lower back pain and tinnitus due to deficiency of kidney-jing, add Rou Cong Rong *Herba Cistanches Deserticolae* 10 g and Sang Ji Sheng *Ramulus Loranthi* 10 g.

Explanations:
- Shu Di Huang, Dang Gui, Bai Shao, Chuan Xiong, Huang Jing and He Shou Wu tonify and nourish the blood, benefit kidney-jing and relieve brain fog.
- Tian Ma and Bai Ji Li benefit the head and relieve brain fog.
- Zhi Gan Cao harmonizes the herbs in the prescription.
- Rou Cong Rong and Sang Ji Sheng tonify kidney-jing and strengthen the lower back and relieve the weakness of the knees.

Herbal Remedy:
Shi Quan Da Bu Wan-*All-Inclusive Great Tonifying Pill.*

Acupuncture Treatment:
- Zusanli ST-36, Sanyinjiao SP-6, Taichong LIV-3, Ququan LIV-8, Taixi KID-3, Yingu KID-10, Xuanzhong GB-39, Shenmen HE-7, Shuaigu GB-8, Baihui DU-20, Shenting DU-24, Extra Taiyang, Extra Yintang and Extra Sishencong.
- An even method is applied on LIV-3, and a tonifying method is applied to the rest of the points.

Explanations:
- ST-36, the he-sea point of the stomach channel, and SP-6, the crossing point of three yin channels of the foot, activate the spleen and stomach, tonify qi and blood and relieve brain fog.
- Since kidney-jing and blood share the same origin and benefit each other constantly, some points should be used to tonify kidney-jing to tonify blood. KID-3, the yuan-source point of the kidney channel, LIV-8 and KID-10, the he-sea point of the liver channel and kidney channel respectively, tonify blood and jing at the same time, relieve the general fatigue and weakness so as to relieve brain fog.
- GB-39, the influential point for marrow, benefits blood and relieves blood deficiency.
- DU-20 and DU-24, benefit the head and relieve brain fog.
- GB-8, Extra Taiyang, Extra Yintang and Extra Sishencong benefit the head, harmonize the collateral and relieve brain fog.

- LIV-3, the yuan-source point of the liver channel, and HE-7, the yuan-source point of the heart channel, promote qi and blood circulation, calm the shen, improve sleep and relieve brain fog.

11.22 Hair Loss

It is a natural process that everyone at any point of time could lose about 50–100 hairs every day. However, it becomes a pathological condition when hair loss is accelerated, there is heavy hair loss, or when hair growth declines, leading to obvious appearance of thinning hair or even balding. People who suffer from hair loss could also notice that their luscious locks are not what they used to be anymore.

There are several types of hair loss, and it could be caused by different factors, such as gender, age, genetics, malnutrition, improper diet, environmental changes and pollution. Also, some sicknesses, such as thyroid disorders, autoimmunity, and anaemia could also cause hair loss. However, hair loss due to COVID-19 is something else.

Whenever a person experiences severe infection, including COVID-19, hair fall is not an unusual after-effect, since the body has sustained an attack and fought off the virus, which often occurs a few weeks post recovery from COVID-19. During this process, the hair falls at a rate of more than 100–200 per day, although it could be distressing for the patient. The hair growth patterns will return to normal after a few months. However, an overwhelming number of people are reporting severe hair fall post COVID-19 infection.

Hair loss due to Long COVID is not the same as a skin condition, called seborrheic dermatitis, wherein there is an excess production of sebum on the scalp, typically accompanied by itching, pain, flaking dandruff, oily and peeling scalp.

One finding revealed that 63% of the patients experienced fatigue or muscle weakness, 26% suffered with sleeping problems, 23% had anxiety or depression, and 22% suffered from hair loss. It also found that 76% of patients reported at least one symptom six months after the first symptom onset, with the proportion higher in women. Patients who were severely ill from the virus were more likely to suffer from the likes of muscle weakness and depression.[163]

There's no clear evidence yet that the novel coronavirus itself directly causes hair loss, but it is generally accepted that the hair entered the telogen phase prematurely, causing existing hair to shed in order to pave way for new healthy hair to grow during COVID-19 infection. It is a temporary procedure. It is also believed that the physical and emotional stress that accompanies a case of COVID-19 can lead to a reversible hair loss, a condition called telogen effluvium. Stress can cause temporary hair shedding, and even if people never developed a fever or COVID-19, it is still beneficial to observe hair shedding in some patients. Emotional issues such as stress, anxiety, and restlessness during the pandemic, can also force more hairs than normal into the shedding phase. Stress-induced telogen effluvium is characterized by diffused hair loss within months of a significant systemic stressor because of premature follicular transition from the anagen (active growth phase) to the telogen (resting phase). The telogen phase lasts approximately three months, after which excessive hair loss ensues.[164] "When there's a shock to the system, the body goes into lockdown mode and only focuses on essential functions. Hair growth is not as essential as other functions, so you end up with hair shedding" explained a dermatologist at the Ohio State University Wexner Medical Centre.[165]

In terms of treatment, moderate hair fall can be controlled at home with the help of diet, exercise, emotional coaches, meditation, and having appropriate rest and sleep. However, both moderate and severe hair loss should be managed properly to rebalance the patient's physical and mental conditions.

---

[163] Chaolin Huang, *et al. op. cit.*

[164] Fahham Asghar, *et al.* Telogen effluvium: A review of the literature. *Cureus.* 2020, 12(5): e8320. doi: 10.7759/cureus.8320.

[165] Joni Sweet. COVID-19 survivors are losing their hair—here's why. *Healthline.* 22 August 2020. https://www.healthline.com/health-news/covid-19-survivors-are-losing-their-hair-heres-why#Stress-may-be-to-blame.

11.22.1 TCM understanding of Long COVID-associated hair loss

In TCM, the hair is considered as the excess of blood, which means that the hair conditions reflect blood situations, including its quantity, quality, and movement. Besides, hair conditions are also related to qi circulation and kidney-jing. In physiology, all the six yang channels are going through the head area to nourish the scalp. Du channel and liver channel also have their connection or distribution on the head. The spleen transforms the essence of food into qi and blood, which nourish the scalp and hair. The lung disperses qi to all the parts of the body, including the head and scalp. The heart dominates blood circulation and is in charge of mental activity. Disorders in any one of these channels or internal organs during Long COVID will influence the qi and blood circulation, including their quality and quantity, which can lead to hair loss.

11.22.1.1 *Emotional disturbance*

The liver plays an important role in emotional activities. It regulates qi circulation and stores blood. Overstress, resentment, anger, emotional trauma, and frustration during COVID-19 may cause retardation in liver-qi circulation, resulting in stagnation of liver-qi. When there is stagnation of qi and blood, the circulation in the channels and collaterals on the head and scalp will be blocked, or the qi and blood distribution and movement in the body will be disturbed, and hair loss appears.

Due to the close physiological relationship between the liver and heart, stagnation of liver-qi could cause disturbance to the heart, bringing about the dysfunction of the heart in housing the shen and regulation of the vessels, and hair loss forms.

11.22.1.2 *Blockage of the collaterals by damp-phlegm*

When the invasion of cold-damp or damp-heat with a pestilent toxin to the body during COVID-19 is not completely eliminated in time, they could cause severe damage or disturbance to the channels and collaterals on the head and scalp, resulting in retardation of qi and blood circulation, and hair loss occurs.

Besides, invasion of external damp to the spleen and stomach could cause disturbance to the ascending and descending functions, and formation of internal damp-phlegm happens. Meanwhile, a pre-existing sickness, such as obesity, slow digestion, or lack of life care during COVID-19 (such as alcoholic drinking and overconsumption of fatty and greasy food), could result in dysfunction of the spleen and stomach in transportation and transformation, and formation of damp-phlegm occurs.

When damp-phlegm in the body moves with qi and blood to the head, it could block the channels and collaterals on the scalp, leading to hair loss.

11.22.1.3 *Stagnation of blood*

Emotional disturbance, accumulation of damp-phlegm, and deficiency of qi and blood could cause blood movement to slow down, leading to the occurrence of blood stagnation. When that happens in the channels and collaterals on the head and scalp, hair loss starts.

11.22.1.4 *Deficiency of qi, blood and kidney-jing*

Overconsumption of qi and blood, lack of dietary care or improper treatment during COVID-19 could cause deficiency of qi and blood, leading to failure of the head and scalp to be nourished, and hair loss appears.

Pre-existing kidney-jing deficiency prior to COVID-19 could deteriorate during COVID-19 due to overconsumption of qi and blood, resulting in weakness of marrow with deficiency of blood, and hair loss occurs.

11.22.2 TCM treatment of Long COVID-associated hair loss

11.22.2.1 *Stagnation of liver-qi*

Hair loss after COVID-19 infection, spasm or tension feeling on the scalp or in the head, aggravation of hair loss when stressed, depression, anxiety, easily angered, stiffness of the neck, distension and pain in the chest or hypochondriac region, insomnia, irregular menstruation in women, poor appetite or overeating, abdominal swelling, thin and white tongue coating, and a wiry pulse.

Principle of Treatment:
Smooth the liver, promote qi circulation, calm the shen and improve hair loss.

Herbal Treatment:
Xiao Yao San-*Rambling Powder.*

Chai Hu *Radix Bupleare* 10 g
Dang Gui *Radix Angelicae Sinensis* 10 g
Bai Shao Yao *Radix Paeoniae Lactiflorae* 10 g
Chuan Xiong *Rhizoma Ligustici Chuan Xiong* 10 g
Zhi Ke *Fructus Citri Aurantii* 10 g
Bai Ji Li *Fructus Tribulli Terrestris* 10 g
Fang Feng *Radix Ledebouriellae Divaricatae* 10 g
Jie Geng *Radix Platycodi Grandiflori* 10 g
Yuan Zhi *Radix Polygalae Tenuifoliae* 10 g
Ce Bai Ye *Cacumen Biotae Orientalis* 10 g
Zhi Gan Cao *Radix Glycyrrhizae Preparata* 3 g

Explanations:
- Chai Hu, Bai Shao Yao and Zhi Ke smooth the liver, regulate and promote liver-qi circulation and relieve qi stagnation in the liver.
- Dang Gui and Chuan Xiong nourish and benefit the blood in the liver, harmonize and smooth the liver and relieve tension and spasm in the scalp, head, and the hypochondriac region.
- Bai Ji Li, Jie Geng and Fang Feng guide the effect of the prescription to the head and scalp and harmonize the collaterals on the scalp.
- Yuan Zhi benefits the brain, regulates the shen and relieves insomnia.
- Ce Bai Ye strengthens hair growth and prevents further hair loss.

11.22.2.2 *Blockage of the collaterals by damp-phlegm*

Hair loss after COVID-19 infection, poor concentration, slight dizziness, a heavy sensation in the head, the fullness of the chest and epigastric region, nausea, poor appetite, lassitude, somnolence, white and greasy coating on the tongue, and a slippery or wiry and slippery pulse.

Principle of Treatment:
Activate the spleen, eliminate damp, resolve phlegm, harmonize the collaterals, and improve hair loss.

Herbal Treatment:
Qiang Huo Sheng Shi Tang-*Notopterygium Decoction to Overcome Dampness.*

Qiang Huo *Rhizoma seu Radix Notopterygii* 10 g
Du Huo *Radix angelicae Pubescentis* 10 g
Gao Ben *Rhizoma Radix Ligustici* 10 g
Chuan Xiong *Rhizoma Ligustici Chuanxiong* 10 g
Fang Feng *Radix Ledebouriellae* 6 g
Jie Geng *Radix Platycodi Grandiflori* 10 g
Yuan Zhi *Radix Polygalae Tenuifoliae* 10 g
Ce Bai Ye *Cacumen Biotae Orientalis* 10 g
Zhi Gan Cao *Radix Glycyrrhizae Preparata* 3 g

Explanations:
- Qiang Huo, Du Huo, Fang Feng and Gao Ben dispel wind, eliminating the remaining damp in the channels and collaterals.
- Chuan Xiong expels wind, promotes qi and blood circulation, and relieves stagnation in the channels and collaterals.
- Jie Geng guides the effect of the prescription on the head and scalp and harmonizes the collaterals on the scalp.
- Yuan Zhi benefits the brain, regulates the shen and relieves insomnia.
- Ce Bai Ye strengthens hair growth and prevents further hair loss.

- Zhi Gan Cao coordinates the effects of the other herbs in the recipe.

Herbal Remedy:
Qiang Huo Sheng Shi Pian-*Notopterygium Pill to Overcome Dampness.*

Acupuncture Treatment:
- Waiguan SJ-5 + Zulinqi GB-41, Hegu L.I.-4, Lieque LU-7, Fengchi GB-20, Shuaigu GB-8, Toulinqi GB-15, Yanglingquan GB-34, Sanyinjiao SP-6, Yinlingquan SP-9 and Fenglong ST-40.
- An even method is applied on SJ-5 + GB-41, and a reducing method is applied to the rest of the points.

Explanations:
- A combination of SJ-5 + GB-41 harmonizes Shaoyang channels, benefits the gallbladder, and relieves tension at the neck and lateral aspects of the head.
- L.I.-4, the yuan-source point of the large intestine channel, and LU-7, the luo-connecting point of the lung channel, promote the qi circulation, dispel external damp in the channels and collaterals on the head and scalp.
- GB-8, GB-15, GB-20, and GB-34 regulate the collateral of the gallbladder channel, smooth the emotions, benefit the head, relieve the neck tension, and promote qi circulation in the head to relieve hair loss.
- SP-6 and SP-9, the crossing point of three yin channels of the foot, and the he-sea point of the spleen channel respectively, and ST-40, the luo-connecting of the stomach channel, promote, activate the spleen and stomach and eliminate damp in the body.

11.22.2.3 *Stagnation of blood*

Hair loss after COVID-19 infection, possible stabbing headache at a fixed location, aggravation of headache at night, numbness on the scalp, insomnia, history of cerebral diseases, insomnia, thin and white tongue coating, purplish tongue or purplish spots on the tongue, and a thready or unsmooth pulse.

Principle of Treatment:
Promote circulation of blood, eliminate blood stasis, and improve hair loss.

Herbal Treatment:
Tong Qiao Huo Xue Tang-*Open the Portals and Quicken the Blood Decoction.*

Tao Ren *Semen Pruni Persicae* 10 g
Hong Hua *Flos Carhami* 10 g
Dang Gui *Radix angelicae Sinensis* 10 g
Chuan Xiong *Rhizoma LiGustici Chuanxiong* 10 g
Chi Shao Yao *Radix Paeoniae Rubra* 10 g
Dan Shen *Radix Salviae Miltiorrhizae* 10 g
Xiang Fu *Rhizoma Cyperi* 10 g
Zhi Qiao *Fructus Aurantii* 10 g
Pu Huang *Pollen Typhae* 10 g
Xian He Cao *Herba Agrimoniae Pilosae* 10 g
Zhi Gan Cao *Radix Glycyrrhizae Preparata* 3 g

Explanations:
- Tao Ren, Hong Hua, Pu Huang, Xian He Cao and Dan Shen promote blood circulation and eliminate blood stasis. Meanwhile, Dan Shen cools the heat in the blood due to stagnation of blood.
- Dang Gui, Chuan Xiong, Chi Shao Yao promote blood circulation, regulate blood and benefit blood. In this way, blood is not damaged by using some blood circulation herbs.
- Since qi circulation promotes blood circulation, some herbs to promote qi circulation are prescribed here as well, such as Xiang Fu and Zhi Qiao are used to promote qi circulation to lead blood circulation.
- Zhi Gan Cao harmonizes the effects of the prescription.

Herbal Remedy:
Huo Xue Tong Mai Pian-*Quicken the Blood and Smooth the Vessels Tablets.*

Acupuncture Treatment:
- Lieque LU-7 + Zhaohai KID-6, Shenmai BL-62 + Houxi SI-3, Hegu L.I.-4, Shenting DU-24, Shuaigu GB-8, Fengchi GB-20, Taiyuan LU-9, Shaohai HE-3, Shenmen HE-7, Geshu BL-17, Sanyinjiao SP-6 and Taichong LIV-3.
- An even method is applied to LU-7 + KID-6, and a reducing method is applied to the rest of the points.

Explanations
- A combination of LU-7 + KID-6 regulates qi and blood circulation and eliminates blood stasis in the body.
- A combination of BL-62 + SI-3 promotes circulation in the Yangqiao mai and relieves blood stasis in the head and scalp.
- Qi is the guide for blood. L.I.-4 and LIV-3, the yuan-source point of the large intestine channel and the liver channel respectively, regulate qi circulation for blood circulation and eliminate blood stasis.
- SP-6, the crossing point of three yin channels of the foot, and BL-17, the influential point of blood, promote blood circulation and eliminate blood stasis in the body and on the scalp.
- HE-3, HE-7 and LU-9, the influential point of the vessel in the body, calm the shen, regulate emotions, promote blood circulation, and improve sleep.
- GB-8, DU-24 and GB-20, the local points on the head, promote qi and blood circulation in the head and speed up hair growth.

11.22.2.4 *Deficiency of qi*

Hair loss after COVID-19 infection, light sensation in the head, aggravation of hair loss after physical exertion, fatigue, general weakness, pale complexion, aversion to cold, cold hands, shortness of breath, spontaneous sweating, loose stools, poor appetite, diarrhea, lower back pain, weakness of knees, low voice, thin and white tongue coating, pale tongue with tooth marks, and a slow and deep pulse.

Principle of Treatment:
Tonify qi, activate the spleen and stomach, benefit the kidney, and improve hair loss.

Herbal Treatment:
Da Bu Yuan Jian-*Great Tonify the Primal Decoction.*

Ren Shen *Radix Ginseng* 10 g
Shu Di Huang *Radix Rhemanniae Glutinosae Praeparata* 15 g
Shan Yao *Radix Dioscoreae Oppositae* 12 g
Du Zhong *Cortex Eucommiae Ulmoidis* 10 g
Shan Zhu Yu *Fructus Corni Officinalis* 10 g
Gou Qi Zi *Fructus Lycii* 10 g
Huang Jing *Rhizoma Polygonati* 10 g
Suo Yang *Herba Cynomorii Songarici* 10 g
Gou Ji *Rhizoma Cibotii Barometz* 10 g
Wu Wei Zi *Fructus Schisandrae Chinensis* 10 g
Bai Zhu *Rhizoma Atractylodis Macrocephalae* 10 g
Zhi Gan Cao *Radix Glycyrrhizae Praeparata* 3 g

Explanations:
- Ren Shen greatly tonifies yuan-source qi, improves lung-qi and spleen-qi and relieves general fatigue and weakness.
- Bai Zhu tonifies spleen-qi and activates the spleen.
- Shu Di Huang, Shan Zhu Yu, Shan Yao, Du Zhong, Gou Ji, Suo Yang and Gou Qi Zi tonify kidney-qi, benefit kidney-jing and relieve fatigue and lower back pain.
- Huang Jing and Wu Wei Zi tonify lung-qi and benefit the lung.
- Zhi Gan Cao harmonizes the effects of the other herbs in the prescription.

Herbal Remedy:
Da Bu Yuan Jian Ke Li-*Great Tonify the Primal Granulates.*

Acupuncture Treatment:
- Baihui DU-20, Zusanli ST-36, Taibai SP-3, Sanyinjiao SP-6, Qihai REN-6, Guanyuan REN-4, Pishu BL-20, Weishu BL-21, Shenshu BL-23, Shenting DU-24, Touwei ST-8 and Shuaigu GB-8.
- A tonifying method is applied to these points. Moxibustion should be applied on REN-6 and ST-36.

Explanations:
- ST-36, the he-sea point of the stomach channel, SP-3, the yuan-source point of the spleen channel, BL-20 and BL-21, the back-shu point of the spleen and stomach respectively, activate the spleen and stomach, tonify qi and relieve general fatigue and weakness.
- REN-4, REN-6, SP-6 and BL-23 tonify qi and blood at the same time and strengthen the body to relieve general fatigue and weakness.
- DU-20 lifts qi to the headache to benefit the head and scalp.
- DU-24, ST-8 and GB-8, all the local points, harmonize the collaterals and benefit the scalp to improve hair loss.

11.22.2.5 *Deficiency of blood*

Hair loss after COVID-19 infection, a hollow sensation in the head, aggravation of hair loss after physical exertion and alleviation of it by rest, dry eyes, palpitations, listlessness, dry skin and stools, insomnia, pale complexion, lower back pain, weakness of knees, scanty or delayed menstruation in women, poor appetite, pale tongue, thin and white tongue coating, and a thready and weak pulse.

Principle of Treatment:
Tonify blood, benefit kidney-jing, relieve weakness and improve hair loss.

Herbal Treatment:
Si Wu Tang-*Four Substances Decoction.*

Shu Di Huang Radix Rehmanniae Praeparatae 15 g
Dang Gui *Radix Angelicae Sinensis* 10 g
Bai Shao *Radix Paeoniae Alba* 10 g
Chuan Xiong *Rhizoma Ligustici Chuanxiong* 10 g
Huang Jing *Rhizoma Polygonati* 10 g
He Shou Wu *Radix Polygoni Multiflori* 10 g
Tian Ma *Rhizoma Gastrodiae Elatae* 10 g
Bai Ji Li *Fructus Tribulli Terrestris* 10 g
Zhi Gan Cao *Radix Glycyrrhizae Preparata* 3 g

If there is lower back pain and tinnitus due to deficiency of kidney-jing, add Rou Cong Rong *Herba Cistanches Deserticolae* 10 g and Sang Ji Sheng *Ramulus Loranthi* 10 g.

Explanations:
- Shu Di Huang, Dang Gui, Bai Shao, Chuan Xiong, Huang Jing and He Shou Wu tonify and nourish the blood, benefit kidney-jing and improve hair loss.
- Tian Ma and Bai Ji Li benefit the head and improve hair loss.
- Zhi Gan Cao harmonizes the herbs in the prescription.
- Rou Cong Rong and Sang Ji Sheng tonify kidney-jing, strengthen the lower back and relieve the weakness of the knees.

Herbal Remedy:
Shi Quan Da Bu Wan-*All-Inclusive Great Tonifying Pill.*

Acupuncture Treatment:
- Zusanli ST-36, Sanyinjiao SP-6, Taichong LIV-3, Ququan LIV-8, Taixi KID-3, Yingu KID-10, Xuanzhong GB-39, Shenmen HE-7, Shuaigu GB-8, Baihui DU-20, Shenting DU-24, Touwei ST-8, extra Yintang and extra Sishencong.

- An even method is applied on LIV-3, and a tonifying method is applied to the rest of the points.

Explanations:
- ST-36, the he-sea point of the stomach channel, and SP-6, the crossing point of three yin channels of the foot, activate the spleen and stomach, tonify qi and blood and improve hair loss.
- Since kidney-jing and blood share the same origin and benefit each other constantly, some points should be used to tonify kidney-jing to tonify blood. KID-3, the yuan-source point of the kidney channel, LIV-8 and KID-10, the he-sea point of the liver channel and kidney channel respectively, tonify blood and jing at the same time, relieve the general fatigue and weakness so as to improve hair loss.
- GB-39, the influential point of the marrow, benefits blood and relieves blood deficiency.
- DU-20 lifts blood and kidney-jing to the head, nourishes the scalp and improves hair loss.
- DU-24, GB-8, ST-8, Extra Yintang and Extra Sishencong benefit the head, harmonize the collateral and improve hair loss.
- LIV-3, the yuan-source point of the liver channel, and HE-7, the yuan-source point of the heart channel, promote qi and blood circulation, calm the shen, and improve sleep and hair loss.

12

Long COVID Case Study

12.1 Case 1

Male, 23 years old, a university student.
Chief complaints: Long COVID-associated breathlessness and fatigue.
First consultation: 20 October 2021.

In March 2020, his younger sister contracted COVID-19 virus at her middle school and infected him and his father at the same time. At that time, it was not possible to get confirmation through a PCR test due to the insufficiency of tests. He suffered from fever, headache, shortness of breath, loss of smell and taste, and fatigue. He was mainly taking some antipyretics to treat his fever symptomatically at home. All the symptoms remained till mid-May. In the end, his shortness of breath became so severe that he was taken into a hospital and a PCR test showed that he was still positive with the COVID-19 infection. He stayed in the hospital for ten days. From the onset of his first symptoms until hospital discharge , he lost 10 kg and felt extremely tired. From March onwards, he took antipyretics for almost three months. In the last one and a half years, he struggled with breathlessness, a spasm feeling in the diaphragm, fatigue, and myalgia. Meanwhile, he also suffered from a burning sensation in the stomach with acid regurgitation mostly due to too much intake of antipyretics. He also had insomnia (causing him to wake up seven times a night because of body pain), poor appetite, feverish feeling over the whole body, poor concentration, a lot of hair loss, and no morning erection since sickness. During the process, he gained 3 kg, had a red tongue with a thin and white coating, and a thready, deep, and wiry pulse.

TCM Diagnosis:
Long COVID due to deficiency of qi and yin of the lung and kidney.

Principle of Treatment:
Tonify qi, nourish yin, restore the lung and kidney, and regulate respiration.

Herbal Treatment:
Sheng Mai San-*Generate the Pulse Powder,* plus
Bu Fei Tang-*Tonify the Lungs Decoction.*

Dang Shen *Radix Codonopsis Pilosulae* 10 g
Mai Men Dong *Tuber Ophiopogonis Japonici* 10 g
Wu Wei Zi *Fructus Schisandrae Chinensis* 10 g
Zhi Huang Qi *Radix Astragali Membranacei Praeparata* 10 g
Bai Zhu *Rhizoma Atractylodis Macrocephalae* 10 g
Huang Jing *Rhizoma Polygonati* 10 g
Shan Yao *Radix Dioscoreae Oppositae* 10 g
Zi Wan *Radix Asteris Tatarici* 10 g
Sang Bai Pi *Cortex Mori Albae Radicis* 10 g
Shu Di Huang *Radix Rhemanniae Glutinosae Praeparata* 10 g
Xing Ren *Semen Armeniacae* 10 g
Gua Lou Pi *Pericarpium Trichosanthis* 10 g
Zhi Shi *Fructus Immaturus Citri Aurantii* 10 g
Yu Jin *Tuber Curcumae* 10 g
Chuan Bei Mu *Bulbus Fritillariae Cirrhosae* 10 g
The herbal treatment is in concentrated powder granules. Take three times a day, each time 2 g.

Explanations:
- Dang Shen, Zhi Huang Qi, Bai Zhu, and Huang Jing tonify the qi of the lung and spleen, improve the appetite and relieve fatigue.

- Shu Di Huang and Shan Yao tonify kidney-qi, benefit kidney-jing and relieve fatigue.
- Chuan Bei Mu and Mai Men Dong nourish the yin of the lung and benefit the lung.
- Wu Wei Zi and Zi Wan tonify lung-qi, nourish lung-yin and relieve shortness of breath.
- Xing Ren and Sang Bai Pi descend lung-qi and relieve shortness of breath.
- Zhi Shi, Gua Lou Pi and Yu Jin promote qi circulation in the chest and relieve spasm of the diaphragm.

Acupuncture Treatment:
- Neiguan P-6 + Gongsun SP-4, Tanzhong REN-17, Hegu L.I.-4, Chize LU-5, Guanyuan REN-4, Qihai REN-6, Zusanli ST-36, Sanyinjiao SP-6, Taixi KID-3, Taichong LIV-3, and Qimen LIV-14.
- An even method is applied on P-6 + SP-4, a reducing method is applied on L.I.-4, LIV-3, and LIV-14, and a tonifying method is applied on the rest of the points.
- Acupuncture treatment is given twice a week for the first two weeks, followed by once a week.

Explanations:
- A combination of P-6 + SP-4 regulates the respiration, relaxes the chest, harmonizes the stomach, and relieves shortness of breath.
- REN-17, the influential point of qi in the body, relaxes the chest, regulates the diaphragm, and relieves shortness of breath.
- L.I.-4, the yuan-source point of the large intestine, LIV-3 and LIV-14, the yuan-source point and the front-mu point of the liver respectively, promote qi circulation and relieve the spasm at the diaphragm.
- ST-36, the he-sea point of the stomach channel, SP-6, the crossing point of three yin channels of the foot tonify qi and yin of the lung and the qi of the spleen so as to relieve fatigue.
- LU-5, the he-sea point of the lung, tonifies qi and yin of the lung and relieves shortness of breath.

- KID-3, the yuan-source point of the kidney channel, tonifies qi and yin of the kidney and relieves fatigue.
- REN-4 and REN-6 greatly tonify the qi and yin of the body and relieve fatigue.

Two weeks later, his breathlessness improved, and his fatigue is also much better. In addition, his sleep quality changed, he reported almost no more waking at night, and his physical and mental conditions are much stronger. However, his appetite is still smaller than before. All his complaints, which have lasted for more than one and a half years, were alleviated in a short period of time. He is able to participate in some fitness activities again, and he could drive a car to the clinic. Meanwhile, on the last visit on 17 November 2021, he mentioned that his morning erection regained (not that strong but almost normal), and he has gained 1 kg. He is happy with his recovery now.

12.2 Case 2

Female, 37 years old, a physiotherapist and acupuncturist.
Chief complaints: Long COVID-associated diarrhea and fatigue.
First consultation: 8 September 2021.

The patient experienced diarrhea since January 2021. After the contraction of the viral infection, she developed headache, fatigue, and slight myalgia. Her general complaints were kept under control quickly, but her diarrhea remained the same, usually a few times a day with watery diarrhea. She had a poor appetite, felt extremely tired, had cold hands and feet, occasionally showed a purplish color on the fingers, had a weak feeling in the heart. On top of that, she had an aversion to cold, preference to warmth, lost some weight (current body weight is 48 kg), emaciation, superficial sleep, a pale tongue with tooth marks, thin and white tongue coating, and a thready, deep, and slow pulse.

When she was 11 years old, she suffered from Hodgkin's lymphoma and received chemotherapy and radiation, which damaged her heart and thyroid. She is always feeling tired. In December 2015, she entered the hospital emergency ward at a university hospital due to heart failure and received a heart transplant. She has been suffering from tiredness since the onset of Hodgkin's lymphoma, which did not improve even after her heart transplantation.

TCM Diagnosis:
Long COVID-associated diarrhea and fatigue due to deficiency of Yang of the heart and spleen.

Principle of Treatment:
Tonify yang of the heart and spleen, activate the spleen and relieve diarrhea and fatigue.

Herbal Remedies:
Shen Ling Bai Zhu San-*Ginseng, Poria and Atractylodis Macrocephalae Pill.*
Take three times a day, six pills each time after meals with warm water.

Explanations:
- Normally an herbal formula, Fu Zi Li Zhong Wan-*Prepared Aconite Pill* to regulate the middle, should be given. However, it was not available at the clinic. Besides, she is too weak, and would not be able to tolerate a big and complicated herbal decoction or concentrated powder granules. Thus, herbal remedy Shen Ling Bai Zhu Wan was used as a substitute.
- In TCM it is held that the heart is a fire organ, which is the mother organ of the spleen-earth. Constitutional damage to the heart-yang could lead to the failure of the spleen to be warmed and supported, resulting in weakness of the spleen in transportation and transformation. Although she has received a heart transplant successfully, her heart-yang did not recover completely as it should be, and an underlying pathogenic factor thus remains.

- During the COVID-19 infection, the external pathogenic factor, mainly cold-damp and pestilent toxins, which is a routine pathogenic factor, invaded the spleen, causing diarrhea together with headache and myalgia. Although her external symptoms are under control, the damage to the spleen is unsolved. That is the reason why diarrhea still exists eight months after the COVID-19 infection. Deficiency of yang of the heart and spleen could explain why she has fatigue, weakness, emaciation, and superficial sleep.
- This herbal remedy could activate the spleen, tonify spleen-qi, improve fatigue, eliminate damp in the spleen and relieve diarrhea. Meanwhile, acupuncture is also given to support the treatment. Besides, dietary advice was given to her, such as avoiding cold and raw food, no sweet and greasy food, and drinking one glass of red wine every day, etc.

Acupuncture Treatment:
- Neiguan P-6 + Gongsun SP-4, Lieque LU-7 + Zhaohai KID-6, Zhongwan REN-12, Shaohai HE-3, Shenmen HE-7, Guanyuan REN-4, Qihai REN-6, Zusanli ST-36, Sanyinjiao SP-6, Yinlingquan SP-9, Taixi KID-3 and Taichong LIV-3.
- An even method is applied on P-6 + SP-4, and LU-7 + KID-6, a reducing method is applied on LIV-3, REN-12 and SP-9, and a tonifying method is applied on the rest of the points.
- Acupuncture treatment is given twice a week for the first three weeks, and then once a week.

Explanations:
- A combination of P-6 + SP-4 harmonizes the stomach and relieves diarrhea.
- A combination of LU-7 + KID-6 regulates the Ren and Yinqiao channels and harmonizes the shen.
- ST-36, the he-sea point of the stomach channel, and SP-6, the crossing point of three yin channels of the foot respectively, tonify qi of the spleen, activate the spleen, improve the appetite, and relieve tiredness and diarrhea.

- SP-9, the he-sea point of the spleen channel, eliminates damp and relieves diarrhea.
- HE-3 and HE-7, the he-sea point and the yuan-source point of the heart channel respectively, tonify heart-yang, eliminate interior cold and calm the shen.
- REN-4 and REN-6 greatly tonify the qi and yang of the heart and spleen and relieve fatigue.
- KID-3, the yuan-source point of the kidney channel, tonifies qi and yang of the kidney and relieves fatigue.
- Usually, some more points to warm the yang of the heart and spleen and a moxibustion should be applied to some points. However, as she is so weak and emaciated, the treatment should be given smoothly without too sudden and strong effects.
- One day later, when she came for the second acupuncture treatment, she mentioned that after a single treatment with acupuncture and taking herbal remedy for one day, she felt much stronger and better. Her diarrhea stopped but she still had an aversion to cold. In the following weeks, her diarrhea is mostly under control. If she works too much or feels too tired, her stools become loose. Thankfully, it mostly happens once per day. Her tiredness and aversion to cold also gradually improved in the following treatment.
- On 25 October 2021, she mentioned that she has been taking female hormone pills in the last three years to stimulate her menstruation in order to maintain a good density of her bones. However, her menstruation did not come in the last few months. Thus, Shi Quan Da Bu Wan-*All-Inclusive Great Tonifying Pill* was given, three times a day, six pills each time. Her diarrhea remained under control and her tiredness continuously improved.

12.3 Case 3

Female, 38 years old, a nurse.
Chief complaints: Long COVID-associated fatigue, palpitation and lack of smell and taste.
First consultation: 6 September 2021.

The patient is a nurse, working in a hospital ICU unit. During the pandemic period in May 2020, she contracted COVID-19 infection from her work, manifesting as fever (often around 38.5 degrees or slightly higher), dizziness, myalgia, pain at the scapular regions and lower leg, headache, and loss of smell and taste. Different PCR tests were negative, but she was quarantined immediately and received some symptomatic treatment. Two weeks later, she still felt the same and finally got another chance to take another PCR test, which showed a positive result. Her husband and two children did not show any symptoms of infection and no PCR tests were conducted on them. Three weeks after the onset of her first symptoms, she returned to work at the hospital. She was so tired that she was only able to work half the time. Even so, she constantly suffered from fatigue, palpitation, muscle pain especially in her left scapular region, and dizziness. Her serum glutamic pyruvic transaminase (SGPT) increased too after COVID-19 infection. Her palpitations got so severe that she went for some cardiological examinations, but nothing abnormal was found. Sometimes, her heartbeat could reach more than 160 beats/min, so she was prescribed bisoprolol fumarate 1.25 mg film-coated tablets, a beta blocker medication, once per day. Even with this medication, her palpitations were still not completely under control. She stayed at home on sick leave until October 2020.

A few days after returning to her work in October 2020, she felt sick again with almost the same symptoms as that in May 2020, such as some fever and myalgia, etc. On 20 October, she received a PCR test, which was negative. Her family members got sick at the same time. Her husband had fever, cough, headache, and loss of smell and taste. Her elder son (14 years old), only had some dizziness. Her younger son (11 years old), became very sick, manifesting fever, diarrhea, and cramps in the abdomen. Through PCR tests, it confirmed a positive result for her husband and her younger son, while her elder son had a negative result.

When she came for a consultation, it was one and a half years after the first clinical symptoms of infection. She still suffers from severe fatigue, chest pain, severe palpitations, stress from her job, depression, unhappiness, and anxiety, and she also mentioned continuous crying. One week before, she also suffered from tachycardia with arrhythmia, and her heartbeat was above 160 beats per minute. She also had a constant pain at her diaphragm, tingling on both legs, tension at her head and neck, cold hands, cramps in the abdomen, occasional nausea, poor appetite, lack of taste and smell, a purplish tongue with a thin, white, and greasy coating, and a wiry and slippery pulse.

TCM Diagnosis:
Long COVID-associated fatigue due to accumulation of cold-damp and stagnation of liver-qi.

Principle of Treatment:
Eliminate cold, resolve damp, promote qi circulation, regulate the shen and improve fatigue.

Herbal Treatment:
Cang Fu Dao Tan Tang-*Atractylodes-Poria Phlegm-Dissipating Decoction,* plus
Huo Xiang Zheng Qi San-*Agastache Powder to Rectify the Qi.*

Cang Zhu *Rhizoma Atractylodis* 10 g
Xiang Fu *Rhizoma Cyperi Rotundi* 10 g
Zhi Shi *Fructus Immaturus Citri Aurantii* 10 g
Hou Po *Cortex Magnoliae Officinalis* 10 g
Bai Zhu *Rhizoma Atractylodis Macrocephalae* 10 g
Fu Ling *Sclerotium Poriae Cocos Rubrae* 10 g
Chen Pi *Pericarpium Citri Reticulatae* 5 g
Sha Ren *Fructus Amomi* 3 g
Huo Xiang *Herba Agastaches seu Pogostemi* 10 g
Chuan Xiong *Radix Ligustici Wallichii* 10 g
Zhi Ke *Fructus Citri Aurantii* 10 g
Dan Shen *Radix Salviae Miltiorrhizae* 15 g
Hong Hua *Flos Carthami Tinctorii* 10 g

Bai Zhi *Radix Angelicae Dahuricae* 10 g
Yan Hu Suo *Rhizoma Corydalis* 10 g
The herbal treatment is in concentrated powder granulates. Take three times a day, each time 2 g after meals with warm water.

Explanations:
- Cang Zhu, Zhi Shi and Hou Po strongly eliminate cold-damp, promote qi circulation and relieve myalgia.
- Xiang Fu and Zhi Ke promote qi circulation and relieve pain in the chest and abdomen.
- Chuan Xiong, Yan Hu Suo and Bai Zhi promote qi circulation and relieve myalgia, chest pain and abdominal pain. Meanwhile, Bai Zhi could improve the sense of smell.
- All the above herbs can promote qi circulation, smooth the liver, and relieve depression and stress.
- Bai Zhu and Fu Ling activate the spleen and stomach and eliminate damp in the body.
- Huo Xiang, Chen Pi and Sha Ren regulate the middle Jiao, promote digestion, descend stomach-qi, relieve nausea, and improve the sense of taste.
- Dan Shen and Hong Hua calm the shen, promote blood circulation and relieve chest pain and abdominal pain.

Acupuncture Treatment:
- Neiguan P-6 + Gongsun SP-4, Lieque LU-7 + Zhaohai KID-6, Hegu L.I.-4, Yingxiang L.I.-20, Taichong LIV-3, Qimen LIV-14, Shaohai HE-3, Sanyinjiao SP-6, Yinlingquan SP-9, Zusanli ST-36, Taixi KID-3, Qihai REN-6, Tanzhong REN-17, Zhongwan REN-12, Fengchi GB-20 and Jianjing GB-21.
- An even method is applied on P-6 + SP-4, and LU-7 + KID-6, a reducing method is applied to L.I.-4, LIV-3, LIV-14, REN-12, REN-17, SP-6, SP-9, GB-20, GB-21 and HE-3, and a tonifying method is applied to ST-36, KID-3, and REN-6.
- Acupuncture treatment is given twice a week for the first three weeks, followed by once a week.

Explanations:
It seems that there are too many acupuncture points selected but they are all logical and necessary.

- A combination of P-6 + SP-4 regulates the emotion, promotes qi circulation, harmonizes the stomach, and improves taste.
- A combination of LU-7 + KID-6 regulates the heart and spleen and harmonizes the shen.
- L.I.-4, the yuan-source point of the large intestine channel, LIV-3 and LIV-14, the yuan-source point and the front-mu point of the liver channel and the liver respectively, and REN-17, the influential point of the qi in the body, smooth the liver, promote qi circulation, relieve stagnation of qi, improve chest pain and abdominal pain, and alleviate depression.
- GB-20 and GB-21 regulate qi circulation in the gallbladder and its channel and relieve the tension at the head and neck.
- HE-3, the he-sea point of the heart channel, regulates the shen, calms the heartbeat and improves sleep.
- REN-12, the front-mu point of the stomach and the influential point of the fu organs, and SP-9, the he-sea point of the spleen channel, activate the spleen and stomach, eliminate cold-damp, and relieve the pain in the body.
- ST-36, the he-sea point of the stomach channel, and SP-6, the crossing point of three yin channels of the foot tonify qi of the spleen, activate the spleen and improve the appetite.
- REN-6 and KI-3 tonify qi of the kidney and relieve prolonged weakness.
- L.I.-20, the local point around the nose, activates the opening of the nose and relieves the loss of smell.

After receiving TCM treatment for two weeks, her fatigue and myalgia greatly improved, and she felt relaxed during her work. Her abdominal cramps and nausea also improved. The happiest point was that the pain in her legs were much alleviated. Four weeks later, she reported that she sometimes felt some irritability from the stress working at the hospital due to increased COVID-19 patients in the ICU. At this point, she still did not accept the COVID-19 vaccination. Xiao Yao Wan-Rambling Powder was then given as extra support for her situation.

Two months after the first visit, her general situation of fatigue, chest pain, myalgia, and abdominal cramp, etc., were all much better. The same herbal powder granulates were prescribed again, but she should take them only twice a day, each time 1 g to consolidate the therapeutic results.

12.4 Case 4

Female, 54 years old, a university professor.
Chief complaints: Long COVID-associated disorder of taste.
First consultation: 11 October 2021.

The patient suffered from a lot of stress and food allergy in the last two years. She is allergic to red wine, peanuts, cauliflower, etc. She contracted COVID-19 in October 2021, and everything went well except that her smell and taste did not return completely. She could taste something, but it was mainly a metal taste. She had a burning sensation in the stomach and esophagus, alternative loose stools or constipation, constant presence of phlegm in the throat, insomnia, waking easily during the night, tension at the neck, headache, dizziness, hypertension, 150/90 mmHg, nervousness, irritability, and painful eyes with redness. All the above situations worsened when she gets very nervous or stressed, and she had pressure in the chest, red tongue with a thick, yellow, and greasy coating, and a wiry and slippery pulse.

TCM Diagnosis:
Long COVID-associated with disorder of taste due to impairment of the collaterals, hyperactivity of liver-fire, and disharmony between the liver and stomach.

Principle of Treatment:
Harmonize the collaterals, restore the taste, reduce liver-fire, and regulate the liver and stomach.

Herbal Remedy:
Long Dan Xie Gan Wan-*Gentiana Longdancao Pill to Drain the Liver.*

Explanations:
- Usually, the loss of smell and taste during COVID-19 could last a few months, but this lady has been suffering from a disorder of taste for more than a year. The taste she described in her mouth is a metal taste. In TCM, Metal is an element belonging to the lung, and a metal taste is often a disorder from the lung.
- COVID-19 is a disease in which the pathogenic factors mainly damage the lung. Although her chief physiological functions of the lung have been restored, some minor dysfunction remains unsolved. This dysfunction is the impairment of the collaterals in lung.
- There are different pathological situations that should be considered at same time, but the liver is the key organ to be cared for besides treating her for loss of smell and taste. Long Dan Xie Gan Wan is suitable for this complicated case since it could clear heat and reduce fire in the liver. When liver-fire is under control, most clinical symptoms will improve.
- In terms of loss of smell and taste due to the impairment of the collaterals in the lung, acupuncture treatment could be the best choice.

Acupuncture Treatment:
- Neiguan P-6 + Gongsun SP-4, Lieque LU-7 + Zhaohai KI-6, Hegu L.I.-4, Yingxiang L.I.-20, Juliao ST-3, Dicang ST-4, Xingjian LIV-2, Qimen LIV-14, Shaohai HE-3, Sanyinjiao SP-6, Yinlingquan SP-9, Zhongwan REN-12, Tanzhong REN-17, Fengchi GB-20, and Jianjing GB-21.

- An even method is applied on P-6 + SP-4, and LU-7 + KID-6. A reducing method is applied to all the rest of the points.
- Acupuncture treatment is given twice a week for the first two weeks, and then followed by once a week.

Explanations:
- A combination of P-6 + SP-4 promotes qi circulation, regulates the emotion, harmonizes the stomach, and improves the sense of taste.
- A combination of LU-7 + KID-6 regulates the Ren and Yinqiao channels, harmonize the shen and improve the sense of smell.
- L.I.-20, ST-3 and ST-4, the local points around the nose and mouth, harmonize the collaterals, activate the opening of the nose and improve the sense of taste.
- L.I.-4, the yuan-source point of the large intestine channel, LIV-14, the front-mu point of the liver channel, and REN-17, the influential point of the qi in the body, smooth the liver, promote qi circulation, and relieve stagnation of liver-qi.
- GB-20 and GB-21 regulate qi circulation in the gallbladder and its channel, relieve the tension at the head and neck and improve dizziness.
- HE-3, the he-sea point of the heart channel, regulates the shen, calms the heartbeat and improves sleep.
- REN-12, the front-mu point of the stomach and the influential point of the fu organs, SP-6 and SP-9, the crossing point of three yin channels of the foot, and the he-sea point of the spleen channel respectively, activate the spleen and stomach, promote digestion, and relieve a burning sensation in the stomach and esophagus.

When the liver is smoothed, liver-fire is reduced, and the middle Jiao is restored, the physiological functions of the spleen will be promoted, thus the sense of taste could also be regulated at the same time. It could be seen from this sense that if only some local points around the nose and mouth are selected without choosing the above general points for the liver and middle Jiao, the total effects of the treatment will be limited.

After TCM treatment for two weeks, her sense of taste started to return. Meanwhile, her emotions are also greatly under control. She could sleep better. But there is still constipation. Thus Tianshu ST-25 is added into the above acupuncture prescription. On 10 October 2021, she mentioned that she felt occasional dizziness, thus Shuaigu GB-8 is added. After treatment for another four weeks, most of the metal taste in her mouth disappeared and her liver-fire situations are also greatly under control.

12.5 Case 5

Female, 21 years old, a university student.
Chief complaints: Long COVID-associated loss of smell and taste.
First consultation: 14 June 2021.

The patient suffered from vulvodynia for one year, which makes it impossible for her to have sexual contact. The persistent, unexplained pain in the vulva started gradually. She went to the gynecologist but nothing abnormal was discovered. Therefore, she was prescribed painkiller creams to be applied locally to relieve the pain. Even with this cream, she could not have copulation. She usually has cystitis a few times a year, and it is not always possible to detect a bacterial infection. Her situation usually becomes worse when she is stressed, as she faces a lot of stress with her university studies. Meanwhile, she also has stress-related headaches, tension at the neck, irritability, stomach pain, nausea, lack of appetite, abdominal cramps and diarrhea. As the end of year examinations was approaching, her vulvodynia was getting worse and worse. Herbal remedy Long Dan Xie Gan Wan-*Gentiana Longdancao Pill to Drain the Liver* was offered in combination with an acupuncture treatment to smooth the liver, promote qi circulation on the liver and relieve the vulvodynia. After six visits, everything went relatively well till the end of July.

In the middle of August 2021, she contracted COVID-19 infection, which was confirmed by a PCR test. She mainly developed a lack of smell and taste three days after her slight fever (which lasted for a day) and moderate myalgia. Cough was not present. She was quarantined at home for ten days, and then went on holiday with her boyfriend. Upon coming back from holidays at the end of August, she still has a lack of smell and taste, so she went to have another PCR test, which showed positive again. On 8 September, she came back for a consultation about her loss of smell and taste. Her vulvodynia returned, causing her to feel a slight pain during urination and she also complained about urgent urination. It was observed that she had a thin and white tongue coating and a wiry pulse.

TCM Diagnosis:
Long COVID-associated loss of smell and taste impairment of the collaterals and stagnation of liver-qi.

Principle of Treatment:
Harmonize the collaterals, benefit the clear orifices, smooth the liver, and promote urination.

Acupuncture Treatment:
- Neiguan P-6 + Gongsun SP-4, Lieque LU-7 + Zhaohai KID-6, Hegu L.I.-4, Yingxiang L.I.-20, Juliao ST-3, Dicang ST-4, Zanzhu BL-2, Shenting DU-24, Ligou LIV-5, Jimai LIV-12, Sanyinjiao SP-6, Yinlingquan SP-9, Shuidao ST-28, Fenglong ST-40, and Qugu REN-2.
- An even method is applied on P-6 + SP-4, and LU-7 + KID-6. A reducing method is applied to all the rest of the points.
- Acupuncture treatment is given once a week.

Explanations:
- A combination of P-6 + SP-4 promotes qi circulation, regulates the emotion, smooths emotion, harmonizes the stomach, and improves the sense of taste.

- A combination of LU-7 + KID-6 regulates the lung, heart and spleen, harmonize the shen and improve the sense of smell.
- Besides, based on the effects from the above extra meridians to benefit the lung, spleen, and liver, this acupuncture could treat lack of smell and taste and vulvodynia as well as Lin syndrome at the same time.
- L.I.-20, ST-3, ST-4 and BL-2, the local points around the nose and mouth, activate the opening of the nose and relieve the loss of smell and taste. DU-24 benefits the shen, opens the orifices and improves smell and taste. When these five points are applied together, their therapeutic results to improve the sense of smell and taste are strengthened.
- L.I.-4, the yuan-source point of the large intestine channel, and SP-6, the crossing point of three yin channels of the foot, promote qi and blood circulation and relieve qi stagnation.
- LIV-5, the luo-connecting point of the liver channel, and LIV-12, a local point nearby the complaint of vulvodynia, smooth the liver, promote liver-qi circulation, and relieve vulvodynia.
- SP-9, ST-28, ST-40, and REN-2 promote urination and relieve pain when urinating.

After only one acupuncture treatment, the patient came back on 14 September. Her smell and taste have greatly improved, and she could smell and taste almost everything. However, her painful urination and vulvodynia only improved slightly. Upon the next visit on 22 September, her taste recovered completely except that she is extremely sensitive to cigarette smoking. On 29 September 2021, her smell and taste restored completely, and her vulvodynia and painful urination were also within control.

Note:

Although this case does not belong to Long COVID associated with loss of smell and taste because it is not consistent with the timeline of Long COVID, it is still interesting to show how fast and effective acupuncture could help patients with their complaints. There is no doubt to point that the earlier the patient receives TCM treatment, the better therapeutic results will be.

12.6 Case 6

Female, 30 years old, an artist and musician.
Chief complaints: Long COVID-associated breathlessness and digestion dysfunction.
First consultation: 17 September 2021.

The patient contracted a COVID-19 viral infection in March 2020 abroad. She was one of approximately 40 colleagues who were infected at the same time in her company. She had a low-grade fever for only two days, and her main complaints were headache, diarrhea, loss of smell and taste, and fatigue. She was sick for three months. Due to severe breathlessness, she went for a chest CT examination and cardiological check-up in a hospital in May 2020, but everything was normal. Since then, she has been suffering from superficial breathing, difficulty to breathe deeply, chest pain when taking a deep breath, stomach pain with swollen feeling, acid regurgitation, aggravation of stomach pain after eating, poor appetite, occasional abdominal pain, afraid of sudden death, and insomnia. She was also facing a lot of stress in her life and at her work in the last few years, the sense of insecurity and agitation, and neck tension and pain. When she feels relaxed, the above situation becomes less intensive. She is careful with her diet and does not eat too much sweet and greasy food. Her stool is relatively normal. Her menstruation is regular with no pain. Her tongue has a thin, white, and greasy coating, and she has a wiry and slippery pulse.

TCM Diagnosis:
Long COVID-associated breathlessness and digestion dysfunction due to accumulation of damp-phlegm and stagnation of liver-qi.

Principle of Treatment:
Eliminate damp, resolve phlegm, smooth the liver, and descend the qi of the lung and stomach.

Herbal Remedy:
Xiang Sha Yang Wei Wan-*Aucklandia, Amomum Nourish Stomach Pill*, plus
Xiao Yao Wan-*Rambling Pill.*
Take six pills from both remedies after meals, three times a day.

Explanations:
- Invasion of cold-damp with pestilent toxins could be the chief causative factor for her COVID-19 infection during the acute phase. This is because she did not have a very high fever and suffered from diarrhea and breathlessness at the same time. Although she survived from this infection, external pathogenic factors in her body are not eliminated completely, which blocked the lung and stomach.
- Accumulation of cold-damp in the lung is the main cause for her superficial breathing, difficulty in breathing deeply, and chest pain when taking a deep breath. On the other hand, accumulation of cold-damp in the stomach is the main cause for her stomach complaints, such as stomach pain with swollen feeling, acid regurgitation, aggravation of stomach pain after eating, and poor appetite. Nevertheless, she has stagnation of liver-qi due to a lot of stress in her life and at work in the last few years, leading to the occurrence of fear of sudden death, insomnia, sense of insecurity and agitation, and neck pain and pain, etc. Additionally, stagnation of liver-qi also could bring about qi stagnation in the lung and stomach, resulting in aggravation of the above situations when being nervous.
- Xiang Sha Yang Wei Wan is a very good herbal remedy for stomach pain and distention, poor appetite, and acid regurgitation due to the accumulation of cold-damp in the stomach. Although this remedy is not capable of resolving cold-damp in the lung, acupuncture treatment could focus on this issue.

- Xiao Yao San is an excellent remedy to smooth the liver and promote qi circulation in the body. Besides, it could relieve stomach pain and painful chest pain due to qi stagnation.

Acupuncture Treatment:
- Neiguan P-6 + Gongsun SP-4, Hegu L.I.-4, Taichong LIV-3, Qimen LIV-14, Fengchi GB-20, Yanglingquan GB-34, Shenting DU-24, Sanyinjiao SP-6, Yinlingquan SP-9, Tianshu ST-25, Zusanli ST-36, Fenglong ST-40, Zhongwan REN-12, and Tanzhong REN-17.
- An even method is applied to P-6 + SP-4, and a reducing method is applied to all the rest of the points.
- Acupuncture treatment is given twice weekly during the first two weeks and followed by once a week after.

Explanations:
- A combination of P-6 + SP-4 promotes qi circulation, regulates respiration, smooths emotions, harmonizes the stomach, and improves appetite.
- L.I.-4, the yuan-source point of the large intestine channel, LIV-3 and LIV-14, the yuan-source point and the front-mu point of the liver channel respectively, REN-17, the influential point of the qi in the body, promote qi circulation in the liver and relieve qi stagnation.
- GB-34, the he-sea point of the gallbladder channel, and GB-20 promote qi circulation and relieve tension in the body and at the neck.
- DU-24 calms the shen and improves sleep.
- SP-6 and SP-9, the crossing point of three yin channels of the foot and the he-sea point of the spleen channel respectively, REN-12, the influential point of the fu organs and the front-mu point of the stomach, ST-25, ST-36 and ST-40, the front-mu point of the large intestine, the he-sea point, and the luo-connecting point of the stomach channel respectively, activate the spleen and stomach, eliminate cold-damp, descend stomach-qi, promote digestion and relieve pain.

When she came for the second acupuncture treatment on 21 September 2021, she reported that her sleeping patterns and emotions were much better, but her stomach pain and abdominal pain remained the same, and her digestive system was still weak. After another two weeks worth of treatment, her appetite improved, and the abdominal pain also diminished.

On 18 November 2021, two months after the first visit, most of her complaints were under control, and her breathing became much easier. She felt almost no pain in the chest, stomach, and abdomen. The same herbs are given once more to consolidate the therapeutic results.

- Zhi Gan Cao harmonizes the actions of the other herbs in the prescription.

Herbal Remedy:
Xiao Yao Wan-*Rambling Pill.*

Acupuncture Treatment:
- Waiguan SJ-5 + Zulinqi GB-41, Neiguan P-6 + Gongsun SP-4, Hegu L.I.-4, Shuaigu GB-8, Toulinqi GB-15, Yanglingquan GB-34, Extra Yintang, Extra Sishencong, Fengchi GB-20, Jianjing GB-21, Taichong LIV-3, Qimen LIV-14, Shenmen HE-7 and Ganshu BL-18.
- An even method is applied on SJ-5 + GB-41, P-6 + SP-4, and a reducing method is applied to the rest of the points.

Explanations:
- A combination of SJ-5 + GB-41 harmonizes Shaoyang channels, benefits the gallbladder, and relieves tension at the neck and lateral aspects of the head.
- A combination of P-6 + SP-4 smooths the liver, regulates qi and blood circulation, and calms the shen.
- L.I.-4 and LIV-3, the yuan-source point of the large intestine channel and the liver channel respectively, LIV-14, the front-mu point of the liver, BL-18, the back-shu point of the liver, and GB-34, the he-sea point of the gallbladder channel, smooth the liver, regulate the qi circulation in the body, relieve liver-qi stagnation and improve emotions.
- HE-7, the yuan-source point of the heart channel, and extra Sishencong, promote qi circulation, calm the shen and emotions and improve sleep.
- GB-8, GB-15, GB-20 and GB-21 regulate the collateral of the gallbladder channel, smooth the emotions, benefit the head, relieve the neck tension, and promote qi circulation in the head to relieve hair loss.
- Extra Yintang and Extra Taiyang, the local points, improve qi and blood circulation in the scalp and relieve hair loss.